Zabriskie's

Obstetrics for Nurses

Zabriskie's

Obstetrics

TENTH EDITION

J. B. LIPPINCOTT COMPANY

Philadelphia · Montreal

CONVERSION TABLE FOR WEIGHTS OF NEWBORN

(Gram equivalents for pounds and ounces)

For example, to find weight in pounds and ounces of baby weighing 3315 grams, glance down columns to figure nearest 3315 = 3317. Refer to number at top of column for pounds and number to far left for ounces = 7 pounds, 5 ounces.

Pounds→ Ounces↓	3	4	5	6	7	8	9	10
0	1361	1814	2268	2722	3175	3629	4082	4536
1	1389	1843	2296	2750	3203	3657	4111	4564
2	1417	1871	2325	2778	3232	3685	4139	4593
3	1446	1899	2353	2807	3260	3714	4167	4621
4	1474	1928	2381	2835	3289	3742	4196	4649
5	1503	1956	2410	2863	3317	3770	4224	4678
6	1531	1984	2438	2892	3345	3799	4252	4706
7	1559	2013	2466	2920	3374	3827	4281	4734
8	1588	2041	2495	2948	3402	3856	4309	4763
9	1616	2070	2523	2977	3430	3884	4338	4791
10	1644	2098	2551	3005	3459	3912	4366	4819
11	1673	2126	2580	3033	3487	3941	4394	4848
12	1701	2155	2608	3062	3515	3969	4423	4876
13	1729	2183	2637	3090	3544	3997	4451	4904
14	1758	2211	2665	3118	3572	4026	4479	4933
15	1786	2240	2693	3147	3600	4054	4508	4961

OR, to convert grams into pounds and *decimals* of a pound, multiply weight in grams by .0022. Thus, 3317 × .0022 = 7.2974, i.e., 7.3 pounds, or 7 pounds, 5 ounces.

To convert pounds and ounces into grams, multiply the pounds by 453.6 and the ounces by 28.4 and add the two products. Thus, to convert 7 pounds, 5 ounces, 7 × 453.6 = 3175; 5 × 28.4 = 142; 3175 + 142 = 3317 grams.

for Nurses

ELISE FITZPATRICK, R.N., M.A.
Assistant Professor of Obstetric Nursing, Frances Payne Bolton School of Nursing, Western Reserve University; and

NICHOLSON J. EASTMAN, M.D.
Professor of Obstetrics, Johns Hopkins University, Obstetrician-in-Chief, Johns Hopkins Hospital

Dedication

The authors and the publishers of this volume record
with profound sorrow the death of Louise Zabriskie on
December 12, 1957. For 30 years Miss Zabriskie was
the guiding genius of this text; and, as a tribute to her
memory, this book is now called *Zabriskie's Obstetrics
for Nurses.*

Preface

It is the purpose of the authors in this new edition, as it has been in previous ones, (1) to set forth those principles of the science and the practice of obstetrics which must be grasped by every student nurse if she is to approach the manifold problems in the field with intelligence and understanding, (2) to describe complete maternity care, in abnormal as well as normal cases, as she will see it carried out by doctors and nurses throughout the country and (3) to incorporate particularly the current underlying philosophy as well as the basic practices of obstetric nursing and their rationale.

A noteworthy feature of this edition is the sequence in which the subject matter is presented. Normal pregnancy, normal labor, the normal puerperium and the normal newborn are reviewed first. Consideration of the complications which may develop in each of these periods is deferred until the student nurse has become acquainted with the over-all picture of normal childbearing. This sequence would seem to be logical for several reasons. In the first place, it is in accord with the concept that childbearing is a physiologic process—a normal, biologic phase of the life cycle. In the second place, if the full significance of certain disorders of pregnancy are to be grasped, an acquaintance with normal labor, the normal puerperium and the normal newborn is essential. Finally, this is the sequence which is followed by most teachers of obstetric nursing as

well as by all instructors in medical schools and by all textbooks for medical students.

Another feature of this edition is the extensive consideration given to nursing care. Basic principles and technics have been stressed rather than specific procedures, which vary from hospital to hospital. In addition to good physical care, which is fundamental to high quality nursing, mental health concepts have been incorporated whenever appropriate. In this connection the family-centered approach to maternity care is stressed. Health teaching in relation to the mother and her newborn infant is included as a part of total maternity care.

Every chapter of the book has been extensively revised, rewritten and reorganized. In this process all the newer developments have been included, and considerable outmoded material has been eliminated. Two new chapters have been introduced: Home Delivery and Obstetrics During Emergency. Many new illustrations, both photographs and original drawings, have been added. In some instances drawings which appeared in the 9th edition have had their value enhanced by additional art work.

In sum, the authors, the illustrators and the publishers have made a coordinated effort to present a modern textbook for student nurses which is clear, orderly and well illustrated.

ELISE FITZPATRICK, R.N.
NICHOLSON J. EASTMAN, M.D.

Acknowledgments

We acknowledge with sincere gratitude the help of many friends and colleagues in the revision of this text. We are indebted to Miss Sara E. Fetter, Public Health Nursing Consultant in Maternal and Child Health, Division of Public Health Nursing, Maryland State Department of Health; Dr. John Whitridge, Chief, Bureau of Preventive Medicine, Maryland State Department of Health; and Col. John Welch, M.D., Chief, Medical Services, Civil Defense, Maryland State Department of Health, for giving permission to publish the section, "Disaster Insurance for Mothers and Babies." Miss Fetter has also given generously of her time and wise counsel on the subject of home delivery.

We are also grateful to Dr. William A. Cull, Assistant Professor of Anesthesia, Western Reserve University School of Medicine, for his guidance and assistance in revising and rewriting the chapter on Analgesia and Anesthesia. This section not only presents current methods of providing pain relief during labor but also provides information that the nurse should have in order to render safe, effective nursing care to patients receiving analgesic and anesthetic medications.

In addition, the book and its authors owe much to those who contributed illustrative material. Mrs. Ranice Birch Davis, Assistant Professor and Director of the Department of Art as Applied to Medicine, the Johns Hopkins University School of Medicine, has contributed many superb medical illustrations to this edition. Moreover, Mrs. Davis gave the authors invaluable assistance in critically evaluating the drawings and the photographs in the book. Miss Helen Fisk, Chief, Division of Public Health Nursing, Maryland State Department of Health, has graciously allowed us to use the materials compiled by her agency. Mr. Howard Bartner, Clinical Illustrator, National Institutes of Health, has also contributed a number of excellent illustrations. Likewise, we are indebted to Mr. George LeMaster, Department of Photography, University Hospitals of Cleveland, and to Mr. Lindsey Burch, Department of Photography, the Johns Hopkins Hospital, for their outstanding photography.

To Dr. Eleanor P. Hunt, Assistant Chief, Program Analysis Branch, Division of Research, Children's Bureau, we are indebted for generous assistance in compiling data on vital statistics. We are grateful also to Dr. Robert A. Hingson, Professor of Anesthesia, Western Reserve University School of Medicine, for his editorial assistance in this edition. To Miss Jane E. Wynn, Assistant Professor of Public Health Nursing, Boston University School of Nursing, the authors are grateful for untiring assistance. To Mrs. Geraldine Mink, Librarian, School of Nursing, Western Reserve University, and to Mrs. Ella A. Richer, who typed the greater part of the new manuscript, we wish also to express our thanks.

Gratitude is due as well to various professional organizations, publishers, manufacturers and individuals who have contributed to this book. It is particularly fitting that we acknowledge the many new photographs in this edition given by the Gordon Armstrong Company in memory of the late Mr. Gordon

Armstrong whose unwavering interest in the welfare of newborn infants is known to many of us.

Finally, the authors take this opportunity to thank the J. B. Lippincott Company, particularly Mr. Barton H. Lippincott, Mr. Walter Kahoe and Mr. Stanley A. Gillet, for their interest, cooperation and help.

THE AUTHORS

Contents

UNIT TWO

NURSING IN PREGNANCY

ORIENTATION

UNIT THREE
NURSING DURING LABOR AND DELIVERY
ORIENTATION

UNIT FOUR
NORMAL PUERPERIUM
ORIENTATION

UNIT SEVEN

ABNORMALITIES OF OBSTETRICS

UNIT EIGHT

ABNORMALITIES OF THE FETUS AND THE NEWBORN

UNIT NINE
RELATED INFORMATION

UNIT ONE

Human Reproduction

ORIENTATION

What is obstetrics? What are its aims? How can nurses further these aims? In order that the student nurse may appreciate early the immeasurable importance of obstetrics to the women and the children of our country, as well as the contributions which she herself can make to this field, these fundamental questions are considered in the first chapter.

The subsequent chapters of this Unit survey the anatomy and the physiology of the female reproductive organs and the development of the unborn baby (the fetus). Since childbirth entails the passage of the infant through an unyielding bony canal, the pelvis, the anatomy of this structure is of the utmost importance in obstetrics. The physiologic mechanism by which conception takes place and a new human being develops is not only a fascinating story in itself but also one which has far-reaching practical implications in respect to the welfare of both mother and child.

The study of obstetrics includes not only the mechanics of anatomy and physiology but also, in its full meaning, the study of human development and relationships. All that a human being comes to be depends upon many factors present at the time of his birth: heritage, care before birth, care at birth, and his care and training in infancy and childhood.

The Unit concludes with a consideration of the various positions which the fetus in utero may occupy. A clear grasp of the material in this Unit, including as it does many basic definitions, is essential to any intelligent understanding of obstetrics. The illustrations should be studied in close correlation with the text, and every effort should be made to visualize the anatomic relationships and the physiologic phenomena described.

CHAPTER ONE

Orientation to Obstetric Nursing

OBSTETRICS DEFINED

Obstetrics is the art and the science of caring for the childbearing woman and her newborn baby. It deals essentially with 3 distinct periods: pregnancy (from the time of conception to the beginning of labor); labor (the series of processes by which the baby and the placenta are expelled from the mother's body into the outside world); and the puerperium (the period during which the organs of reproduction are restored to approximately their former size and condition).

The word "obstetrics" is derived from an old Latin verb *obsto,* which means to "stand by." Thus, in ancient Rome, a person who cared for women at childbirth was known as an "obstetrix," or a person who "stood by" the laboring mother. While the original employment of the term doubtless referred to the physical act of standing beside the woman, scholars point out that the word also means to "stand by" in the sense of "to protect"—as one ship stands by another in possible danger. Accordingly, it may be said that by the very derivation of the term, obstetrics involves standing by and protecting the childbearing woman throughout pregnancy, labor and the puerperium. The viewpoint that this branch of medicine has to do with protecting the expectant mother throughout her childbearing epoch is a most important one for the nurse to grasp early in the course, for obstetrics is largely concerned with preventing possible dangers and hence is truly a phase of preventive medicine.

AIMS OF OBSTETRICS

It is the ultimate aim of obstetrics that every pregnancy culminate in a healthy mother and a healthy infant. In attaining this goal it strives to reduce to a very minimum the number of women and infants who die or are left injured as the result of childbearing; to minimize the discomforts of pregnancy, labor and the puerperium; and at the same time so to safeguard the whole process that mother and child will conclude the experience in a healthy condition, both physically and mentally. If it is hoped to reduce the number of mothers and infants who die in the birth process, it first becomes desirable to know how many such deaths occur in this country annually and under what circumstances they occur.

3

Statistics

In this country these data are expressed officially by the National Office of Vital Statistics. Maternal deaths, stillbirths and infant deaths amounted to 183,401 in 1957. To understand the significance of the statistics quoted in the following discussion, the nurse should be familiar with the following terms, explained according to the definitions of the National Office of Vital Statistics.

Birth Rate. The number of births per 1,000 population

Marriage Rate. The number of marriages per 1,000 total population

Neonatal Death. One in which an infant dies within the first 4 weeks of life

Neonatal Death Rate. The number of neonatal deaths per 1,000 live births

Fetal Death or "Stillbirth." One in which the infant of 20 weeks or more gestational age dies in utero prior to birth

Perinatal Mortality. Definitions in current use vary somewhat. The sum of all deaths classified as neonatal deaths and fetal deaths of 20 or more weeks of gestation (stillbirths)

Infant Mortality Rate. The number of deaths before the first birthday per 1,000 live births

Maternal Mortality Rate. The number of maternal deaths per 10,000 live births

Birth Rate

The number of registered births each year clearly indicates the magnitude of obstetrics as a branch of medical practice. During the 1930's there was an average of 19 births per 1,000 population. There was a sharp rise during and immediately after World War II to a birth rate of 25.8 in 1947, but after this peak the birth rate for the total population declined slightly and has maintained itself at about 25.0. The birth rate for the nonwhite population has shown no such decrease but has continued to rise. According to the vital statistics of the U. S. for 1957, the number of live births registered was 4,254,784. There were 2,667,872 births in excess of deaths in that year; thus, the population of the U. S. increased nearly 12.9 per cent between 1950 and 1957 (Table 1).

One factor which influences the birth rate is the marriage rate. The estimated number of marriages for 1957 was 1,518,000, only slightly lower than in 1955; although in these 2 years there were fewer marriages than in 1953. It is of interest to note that the increase in couples now having a third or a fourth child is continuing.

The Birth Certificate

In 1915, the Federal Government began to collect data on registered births and organized birth registration. At first only 10 states and the District of Columbia were included in this method of

TABLE 1. LIVE BIRTHS AND POPULATION, UNITED STATES, 1940-1957*

| YEAR | LIVE BIRTHS, ADJUSTED FOR UNDER REGISTRATION | | | POPULATION OF CONTINENTAL U. S. |
	TOTAL	WHITE	NONWHITE	
1957	4,254,784	3,621,456	633,328	171,196,000
1954	4,078,055	3,474,811	603,244	162,409,000
1950	3,631,485	3,107,638	523,847	151,132,000
1945	2,858,449	2,470,502	387,947	139,928,000
1940	2,558,647	2,198,911	359,736	131,820,000

* Birth Statistics: Department of Health, Education and Welfare. Social Security Administration. Children's Bureau. Based on data from the National Office of Vital Statistics.

Total Population: Department of Commerce. Bureau of the Census. Current Population Survey P-25, No. 195, Feb. 18, 1959.

reporting births, but it gradually expanded so that by 1933 the entire country was included. The Dependencies were admitted to the area: the Virgin Islands in 1924, the Territory of Hawaii in 1929, Puerto Rico in 1943 and Alaska in 1950. At the present time, all 50 states and the District of Columbia demand that a birth certificate be filled out on every birth and that it be submitted promptly to the local registrar. After the birth has been registered, the local registrar sends a notification to the parents of the child. Also, a complete report is forwarded from the local registrar to the State authorities, and then to the National Office of Vital Statistics in Washington.

Complete and accurate registration of births is a legal responsibility (see Fig. 174). The birth certificate gives evidence of age, citizenship and family relationships and, as such, often is required for military service, passports and even in order to collect benefits on retirement. On the basis of birth certificates, information which is essential to those agencies concerned with human reproduction is compiled by the National Office of Vital Statistics. The brief reports of statistics presented in this chapter are only a fraction of the volume of such studies compiled by that office.

THE PROBLEM OF MATERNAL MORTALITY

During 1957, the number of women who died as a direct result of childbearing was 1,746 in the course of 4,254,784 live births, or a rate of 4.1 maternal deaths per 10,000 live births. The reduction in maternal mortality rates since 1915 has been dramatic, but more particularly since 1930—from a rate of 67.3 in white women in 1930 to 2.8 in 1957, and the corresponding rate in nonwhite women from 117.4 in 1930 to 11.8 in 1957 (Fig. 1).

However, if we hope to reduce the number of mothers who die in childbirth, first we must know why these women succumb. They die of 3 main causes: hemorrhage, puerperal infection and the toxemias of pregnancy—which are responsible for about 75 per cent of all maternal deaths (see Fig. 2). Subsequently, these 3 conditions will be discussed in detail, but it would seem important to stress here the fact

TABLE 2. REGISTERED LIVE BIRTHS BY ATTENDANT AND COLOR IN METROPOLITAN AND NONMETROPOLITAN COUNTIES, UNITED STATES, 1957

| AREA AND COLOR | TOTAL | ATTENDED BY PHYSICIAN | | ATTENDED BY MIDWIFE | ATTENDED BY OTHER OR NOT SPECIFIED ATTENDANT |
		IN HOSPITAL (PHYSICIAN'S ATTENDANCE ASSUMED)	NOT IN HOSPITAL		
All Counties:					
White	3,621,456	3,557,028	42,816	16,404	5,208
Nonwhite	633,328	513,408	32,298	84,526	3,096
Total	4,254,784	4,070,436	75,114	100,930	8,304
Metropolitan Counties:					
White	2,176,622	2,156,202	13,862	4,176	2,382
Nonwhite	378,920	359,888	10,060	7,994	978
Total	2,555,542	2,516,090	23,922	12,170	3,360
Nonmetropolitan Counties:					
White	1,444,834	1,400,826	28,954	12,228	2,826
Nonwhite	254,408	153,520	22,238	76,532	2,118
Total	1,699,242	1,554,346	51,192	88,760	4,944

Note: The category "Metropolitan Counties" includes all counties within the States that are in "Standard Metropolitan Areas" as defined by the Bureau of the Census in 1950, except in New England where the counties are those in the "Metropolitan State Economic Areas," also as defined by the Bureau of the Census in 1950. The category "Nonmetropolitan Counties" includes all other counties.

Source: Department of Health, Education, and Welfare. Social Security Administration. Children's Bureau. Based on data from the National Office of Vital Statistics.

that deaths from these causes are for the most part preventable.

Various improvements in obstetric care, together with newer drugs, have caused the death rate from puerperal infection and the toxemias of pregnancy to fall more dramatically than from hemorrhage. Consequently, hemorrhage has become the predominant cause of death in childbirth. According to the *official classification,* only the direct cause of death is considered, even though the predisposing cause may be an important factor. For example, in a case in which the mother has a massive hemorrhage and then (in her weakened condition) develops a puerperal infection which eventually causes her death, it is classified as death due to puerperal infection. Hemorrhage is often a predisposing factor, and in this manner its toll in maternal mortality probably exceeds all other causes combined.

Puerperal infection is a wound infec-

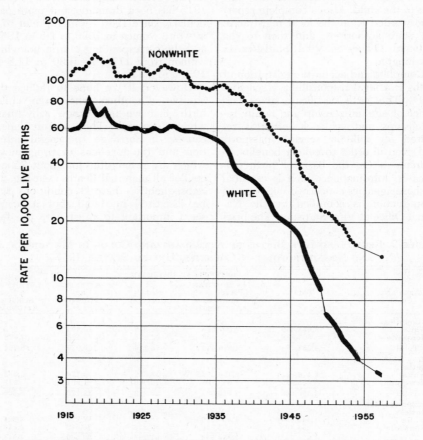

Fig. I. Maternal mortality rates by race; birth registration states 1915-1957. Deaths from delivery and complications of pregnancy, childbirth and puerperium per 10,000 live births in each specified group.

Note: Deaths for 1949-1957 classified according to the 6th revision of the International Lists of Diseases, Injuries and Causes of Death, WHO, Geneva.

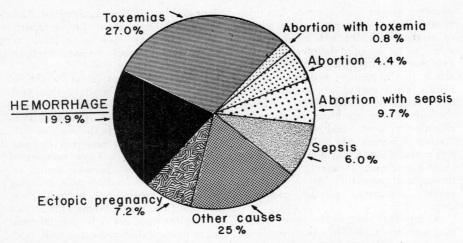

Fig. 2. Causes of maternal death; percentage distribution by cause, 1957. (Department of Health, Education, and Welfare. Social Security Administration. Children's Bureau. Based on data from the National Office of Vital Statistics)
Note: The official classifications of causes of death considers only the *direct* cause, even though the predisposing cause of the complication which finally brings about the maternal death may be in itself an important factor in the outcome.

tion of the birth canal after childbirth, which sometimes extends to cause phlebitis or peritonitis. The nurse can play an important role in helping to prevent such infections, not only in terms of flawless technic in performing nursing procedures, but also in protecting the mother from exposure to anyone with an infection.

The toxemias of pregnancy are certain disturbances peculiar to gravid women, characterized mainly by hypertension, edema, albuminuria and, in some severe cases, by convulsions and coma. Antepartal care plays an important role in prevention or early detection of symptoms, and with suitable treatment the disturbance often can be allayed.

In a study made by Mrs. Mary Breckinridge, R.N., director of the Frontier Nursing Service, a comparison was made between the number of American women who have died in childbirth during a 96-year period and the number of American men who have

died in battle during the same period (Mexican War, Civil War, Spanish-American War and World War I). Her calculations, which are most meticulous and conservative, show that the number of soldiers who died over this period was 858,430, while the number of mothers who died in childbirth was over 1,000,000. This illustrates clearly the tremendous progress made in preventive care when compared with recent statistics. Many factors are responsible for achieving the over-all reduction in maternal mortality in this country during the past 25 years. Most important perhaps is the development of widespread training and educational programs in obstetrics which have provided more and better qualified specialists, professional nurses and other personnel in maternity programs. Better hospital facilities, multiple safeguards provided in the modern maternity hospitals and advances in therapy have all played major roles.

The distinct change in attitudes of

doctors, nurses and parents has also contributed to this progressive saving of mothers. Childbirth is no longer an event to be awaited helplessly by the expectant mother with what fortitude she is able to muster; instead, it is the climax of a period of preparation—a true state of preparedness attained through the co-operation of the physician, the nurse and the expectant mother or parents. As indicated before, this preparation for childbirth, based on careful medical and nursing supervision throughout pregnancy, is called antepartal (sometimes termed prenatal) care.

Antepartal care is the most important advance which has been made in obstetrics during the present century, and it will be of interest to the nurse to know that this salutary contribution to the mother's welfare was initiated by the nursing profession. It had its beginning in 1901, when the Instructive Nursing Association in Boston began to pay antepartal visits to some of the expectant mothers who were to be delivered at the Boston Lying-In Hospital. This work gradually spread until, in 1906, all these women, prior to confinement, were paid at least one visit by a nurse from the association. By 1912, this association was making about three antepartal visits to each patient. In 1907, another pioneer effort in prenatal work was instituted when George H. F. Schrader gave the Association for Improving the Condition of the Poor, in New York City, funds to pay the salary of 2 nurses to do this work. In 1909, the Committee on Infant Social Service of the Women's Municipal League, of Boston, organized an experiment in antepartal work. The pregnant women were visited every 10 days— oftener if necssary. Blood pressure readings and urine tests were made at each visit. This important work was limited because of the effort to make it as nearly self-supporting as possible; therefore, only mothers under the care of physicians and hospitals were accepted. Thus began this movement for antepartal care which has done more than any other single agency to save mothers' lives in our time.

Another important factor in the reduction of maternal mortality has been the development of maternal hygiene programs in State Departments of Public Health, particularly the work of public health nurses in maternal hygiene. These nurses visit a large number of the mothers who otherwise would receive little or no medical care, bringing them much-needed aid in pregnancy, labor and the puerperium. This service fills a great need not only in rural areas but in metropolitan centers as well.

Still another factor responsible for the decline in maternal mortality is the trend toward hospitalization for childbirth—a trend that is gaining ground every year. In the early years of the century women rarely went to a hospital for such care. In 1935, 37 per cent of the live births occurred in hospitals, and in 1957, 95.6 per cent were hospitalized. This means that the percentage of hospital births has more than doubled during a 20-year period. In our larger cities, the vast majority of babies are born in hospitals.

THE PROBLEM OF INFANT MORTALITY

The 2 groups of cases of infant mortality which are of chief concern in obstetric practice are (1) those in which the fetus dies in the uterus prior to birth (so-called "stillbirth") and (2) those in which it dies within a short period of time after birth (neonatal death). The phrase *perinatal mortality* often is used to designate all deaths in these two categories.

In May, 1950, in an effort to end confusion arising from usage of a variety of terms such as stillbirth, abortion, miscarriage, etc., the World Health Or-

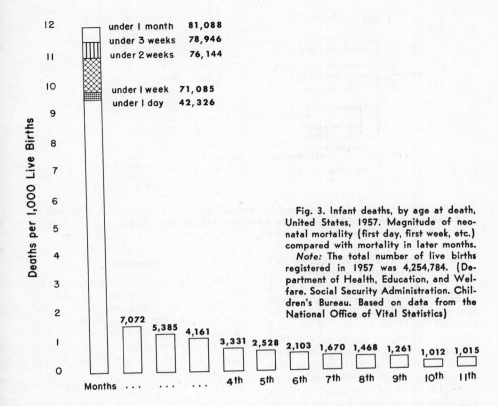

Fig. 3. Infant deaths, by age at death, United States, 1957. Magnitude of neonatal mortality (first day, first week, etc.) compared with mortality in later months. *Note:* The total number of live births registered in 1957 was 4,254,784. (Department of Health, Education, and Welfare. Social Security Administration. Children's Bureau. Based on data from the National Office of Vital Statistics)

ganization recommended the adoption of the following definition of fetal death:

Fetal death is a death prior to complete expulsion or extraction from its mother of a product of conception, irrespective of duration of pregnancy; the death is indicated by the fact that after such separation, the fetus does not breathe or show any other evidence of life such as beating of the heart, pulsation of the umbilical cord, or definite movement of voluntary muscles.*

It further defined it into 4 subgroups, according to gestation age in weeks.

* National Summaries: Fetal Deaths, U. S., 1954, National Office of Vital Statistics, vol. 44, no. 11, August 17, 1956.

In the United States in 1957, 69,561 stillbirths (according to the present classification) and a total of 112,094 infant deaths before the first birthday were reported. Approximately 37.8 per cent of the infant deaths occurred on the first day after birth and 72.3 per cent under 28 days of age. Despite the fact that this decline in infant mortality is indeed gratifying, it is not comparable with the fall in maternal mortality. The great toll taken in the first day of life is compared in Figure 3 with the number of deaths occurring in the rest of the year.

There are many causes responsible for the staggering infant mortality. The huge number of infant deaths is the result of several main causes: premature

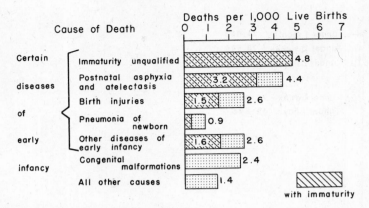

Fig. 4. Main causes of neonatal mortality, United States, 1957. (Department of Health, Education, and Welfare. Social Security Administration. Children's Bureau. Based on data from the National Office of Vital Statistics)

birth, asphyxia and atelectasis, congenital malformations and birth injury (see Fig. 4). During the first 4 weeks of life, prematurity is the most important cause of death. Brain injury, i.e., cerebral injury as a result of anoxia in utero or traumatic injury to the brain suffered in passing through the birth canal, is the second most common cause of neonatal death. Subsequently, these conditions will be discussed in detail. It suffices to say here that the first and most important of them, prematurity, is largely a nursing problem. Indeed, in all the wide range of nursing care there is no area which offers such a challenge to the nurse, or such lifesaving possibilities, as that of caring for the premature infant.

The welfare of approximately 4,000,-000 babies born annually in the United States is very much the concern of obstetrics and one of its main objectives. To reduce the huge loss of newborn lives, to protect the infant not only at birth but also in the prenatal period, and during his early days to lay a solid foundation for his health throughout life—this is the problem and the challenge.

Abortion

The huge number of infants lost by abortion, the spontaneous or artificial termination of pregnancy prior to the period of viability, is a matter of grave importance. The abortion rate in this country exceeds stillbirths and neonatal deaths in fetal wastage. About 10 per cent of all pregnancies terminate in spontaneous abortion due to such factors as: faulty germ plasm; unsatisfactory environmental conditions, hormonal and otherwise; many unknown etiologic causes; and an unknown number of criminal interruptions. The nurse should be aware of 3 considerations in this last category: (1) the immediate danger for the mother, (2) that the effects of such practices often impair the women's future childbearing career and (3) the legal implications for those involved.

THE SCOPE OF OBSTETRIC NURSING

Modern obstetrics has broadened its focus, and simultaneously the scope of obstetric nursing has expanded. Many factors have influenced the evolution of

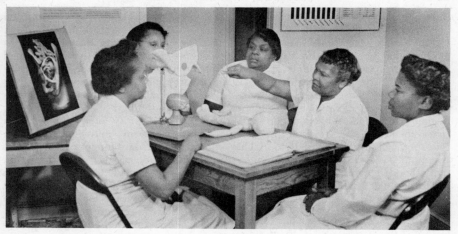

Fig. 5. The certified nurse-midwife, a member of the Public Health Nursing staff of Charles County Health Department, LaPlata, Maryland, conducting a class for nonprofessional midwives. (Maryland State Department of Health)

new definitions of the functions of nursing in the promotion of maternal and child health. Increased educational opportunities and experiences have afforded improved quantity and quality of trained personnel. Research as a whole, new discoveries in medicine, the expanding programs in various fields such as public health, the construction of facilities to permit more patient-centered care, and the function of health workers as a team to give comprehensive services to the expectant family have all contributed to and encouraged more continuity of nursing care for maternity patients. Federal legislation and the continuous efforts of such organizations as the American Association for Maternal and Infant Health, the Maternity Center Association, the Frontier Nursing Service and the Maternity Consultation Service, Inc., have played a most important role in providing better facilities and better prepared personnel.

In 1912, the Children's Bureau of the United States Department of Labor was created by an act of Congress for the purpose of promoting maternal and child health "among all classes of people." It was said to be a public health nurse who first conceived the idea of a Federal bureau of this kind and originally suggested the plan to President Theodore Roosevelt in 1905. The Children's Bureau has continually stressed the importance of public health nursing in maternal and child welfare. Between the years 1921 and 1929, public health nursing consultants were employed by the Bureau, and their services were offered to the states for maternal and infant hygiene. In rural areas public health nursing services throughout the United States were greatly extended, and 2,978 centers for prenatal and child health work were established.

The amount of public health nursing service available in this country has changed only slightly for the past few years. The latest census (Jan. 1, 1957) showed that 29,396 nurses were employed for public health work in the United States, in Hawaii, Alaska, Puerto Rico and the Virgin Islands. A relatively large proportion of these nurses render care which contributes to maternal and child health. In addition to the more traditional services to mothers and babies, health teaching in the preconceptional period is of major importance. The public health nurse is now teaching classes to many groups (such as high school students) on general hygiene, nutrition, sex education, attitudes toward family relationships and the responsibility of parenthood. The community is aware that preparation for parenthood is a related series of learning experiences which begin early in life; thus it is ready to receive this kind of guidance.

Public health and hospital nurses have combined forces in their efforts to approach realistically a plan for family-centered maternity care. For example, co-operative policies and procedures have been developed between public health agencies and hospitals for combined conferences and referral systems. This kind of interagency communication is a valuable adjunct in the care of patients.

The present trend in our population, with increasing numbers of the very young and the very old groups, has affected the demand for public health services. Pearl McIver has described 5 areas in the public health nursing program which reflect the developments in the whole field of public health.[*] The first of these she summarizes with the following statement:

There is an expansion in our service for expectant mothers, infants and pre-school and school children. Disease is still a problem, but the emphasis is on growth and development and the emotional needs of children and families.

At the present time, a relatively small percentage of all pregnancies and labors in the United States are without benefit of medical attention (see Table 2). While it is the ultimate goal to provide all these underprivileged women with

[*] The Yearbook of Modern Nursing, New York, Putnam, 1956.

complete medical, nursing and hospital care, years may elapse before that aim can be realized. For this reason it is recognized increasingly that the certified nurse-midwife has a place in maternity programs for certain areas and among certain population groups where medical care is limited.

To the majority of people in this country the term "midwife" means an untrained person, thought of as ignorant and superstitious. In recent years an effort has been made to train and license these midwives (Fig. 5). A teaching and supervisory program for this group is also in effect in several states.

"A certified nurse-midwife is a graduate registered nurse who has successfully completed a recognized course in midwifery, covering theory and practice. She has a sound knowledge of accepted public health practices and usually has had practical and theoretical experience in public health nursing or special hospital experience in obstetrics, including teaching and supervision.

"A certified nurse-midwife is qualified to manage the antepartal, intrapartal, and postpartal periods of such maternity patients who have been examined by a qualified physician with special experience in obstetrics and approved by him for nurse-midwife care. When any abnormality occurs during any one of the periods, the certified nurse-midwife requests medical direction. When such direction is not immediately available, or until such time as medical assistance arrives, the nurse-midwife, by virtue of her training and experience, handles the abnormal condition to the best of her ability, following standing orders."[†]

The important contribution which such highly trained nurse-midwives can make to the maternity program of a nation has been demonstrated in certain foreign countries, notably in Norway

[†] Maryland State Department of Health, Division of Public Health Nursing.

and Sweden. There some 85 per cent of the deliveries are attended by such trained personnel with excellent results. Of course, the training, the practice and the supervision of these midwives is regulated most carefully by law, and upon the development of the slightest abnormality in any patient, a physician is summoned at once.

The first use of the trained nurse-midwife in this country was made in 1925 when an organization was established in the mountains of eastern Kentucky to handle the maternity problem in the rural and isolated areas of that territory—the now famous Frontier Nursing Service (Figs. 6 and 7). The staff is composed not only of nurses but of certified midwives as well; a physician is available for consultation in complicated cases. This organization has demonstrated clearly that graduate nurses trained in midwifery can help to lower the maternal mortality rates in rural and isolated areas. Thus, in a series of 5,500 deliveries conducted by the Frontier Nursing Service, there occurred only four maternal deaths, and two of these were not related to the pregnancy. In the fall of 1939, the Frontier Nursing Service inaugurated the Frontier Graduate School of Midwifery in Hayden, Kentucky.

In 1931, the Maternity Center Association in New York established the first school of nurse-midwifery in the United

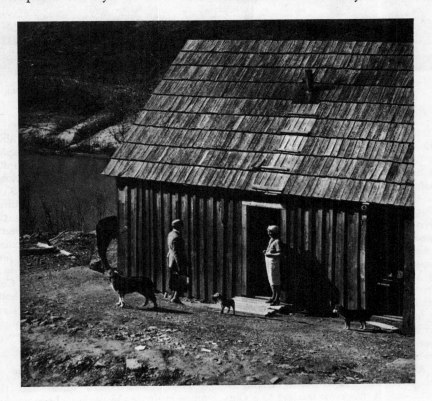

Fig. 6. Antepartal visit. Outside the cabin. (Frontier Nursing Service, Wendover, Ky. Photo by Marvin Breckinridge)

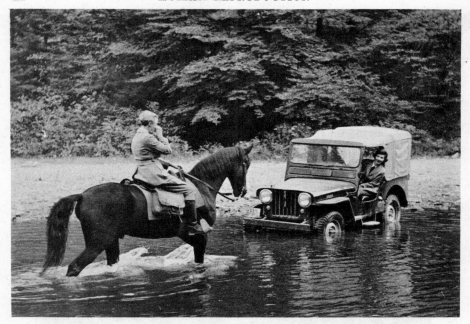

Fig. 7. By horse and by jeep. (Louisville Courier-Journal Photo—Thomas V. Miller, Jr.;
Frontier Nursing Service, Wendover, Ky.)

States for graduate nurses. The Loben-stine Midwifery Clinic was established to provide a field service for this school. It trained about 12 students a year in a 6-month course which provided obstet-ric theory and supervised practice by an obstetrician and by graduate nurse-mid-wives. In 1935, the Maternity Center Association and the Lobenstine Mid-wifery Clinic applied to the State of New York to consolidate under the name of Maternity Center Association. In its first 20 years, 231 nurse-midwives were graduated from this school.

In October, 1945, the Catholic Ma-ternity Institute School of Midwifery was established at Santa Fe, New Mex-ico (Fig. 8).

At the present time there are four schools in the United States offering 6- to 12-month programs leading to a Cer-tificate in Nurse-Midwifery: the Ma-ternity Center Association, School of Nurse-Midwifery in New York, in affili-ation with The Johns Hopkins Hospital in Baltimore and Kings County Hospital in Brooklyn; the Frontier Graduate School of Midwifery in Hayden, Ken-tucky; the Catholic Maternity Institute in Santa Fe, New Mexico; and the School of Nurse-Midwifery of the Puerto Rico Department of Health. There are, in addition, three graduate nursing pro-grams in obstetric nursing leading to a Master of Science Degree and a Cer-tificate in Nurse-Midwifery: Catholic University of America School of Nurs-ing, Columbia University Faculty of Medicine Department of Nursing and Yale University School of Nursing.

Obstetric Nursing in Wartime

The public health nurse and the nurse-midwife always have been needed in our maternity programs. Today this need has definitely multiplied, due to

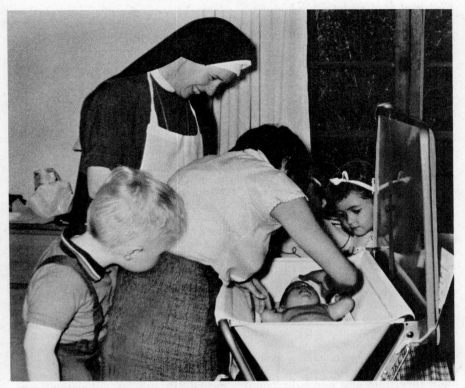

Fig. 8. Postpartal care and teaching in the home provided by the certified nurse-midwife. (Catholic Maternity Institute, Santa Fe, New Mexico)

the increase in birth rate, the lack of sufficient maternity hospital beds to meet the need and fewer doctors preferring rural to urban practice. According to the last available statistics (1957), about 184,348 mothers were delivered at home. For vast portions of our population the public health nurse and the trained nurse-midwife represent the only possible solution to the problem. This is a heavy responsibility, but the nursing profession must meet it.

During World War II another obstetric problem was created when millions of women workers took jobs in industrial plants. Since many women are still engaged in industry, the problem persists. In this connection a number of questions arise. Should pregnant women be allowed to work in factories? If so, for how long? What type of work should be forbidden them? How soon may they return to work after childbirth? These and many related questions will be brought to nurses engaged in industrial work, as well as to public health nurses (p. 155).

THE RELATIONSHIP OF OBSTETRICS TO OTHER FIELDS

Obstetrics is a many-sided subject, and its relationships to the other branches of medicine are numerous and close. Thus, the newborn baby and his problems link obstetrics intimately with pediatrics; and to be a good obstetric nurse, one must also be a good pediatric nurse. Moreover, obstetrics may be regarded as a surgical specialty, and a competent obstetric nurse must be thoroughly grounded in the principles of asepsis and in practical operating-room technic. Since a pregnant woman may contract the same diseases as the nonpregnant, the nurse will be confronted with various medical complications of pregnancy. Whenever a medical disease is present or develops in the course of pregnancy, the complication may be aggravated by the pregnancy, or the pregnancy itself may be endangered by the disease. Rheumatic heart disease, diabetes mellitus, tuberculosis and untreated syphilis are some of the diseases in which one or both of these adverse effects sometimes may be observed. In such situations the obstetric nurse must have an adequate knowledge of medical nursing, as well as obstetric nursing, to be able to administer intelligent, effective nursing care. Pregnancy, in many instances, creates an added economic problem, as well as concern about family responsibilities. Since these problems affect the family unit, the obstetric social worker is often the connecting link between the family and the doctor and the nurse (p. 145). Finally, obstetrics is related to psychiatry, since pregnancy sometimes disturbs the mental and emotional balance of the patient; and, in all cases, there is need for emphasis on a cheerful, wholesome mental attitude.

Obstetrics differs from some of the other subjects previously studied by the nurse in that it deals with the normal physiologic processes of the reproductive organs. Under ideal conditions, pregnancy is a constructive period. It has to do with the beginning of a new life. All attitudes and anticipations should point toward a normal outcome. For the patient, any difficulties associated with the experience have the compensation of the new baby to which she looks forward. For the nurse this is a wholly new phase of nursing. Past teachings have been based on the "curative" point of view, and the previous experience of the nurse has been based upon the observation of the symptoms of pain and discomfort, the acquisition of a knowledge of surgical technic and the art of making patients comfortable. In the earlier courses in her nursing education, the nurse has been given a general idea of the functions of the various systems of the human body, but in this course in obstetrics there is opportunity to pursue the study of the generative organs in detail in order to understand the changes during pregnancy, the climax during labor and delivery and the adjustments involved during the return to normal in the postpartal period and the months following. She must also have some understanding of the emotional reactions which accompany this whole maternity cycle.

In few fields is so much responsibility placed upon the nurse as in obstetrics. In few, also, are there so many opportunities for originality of thought and initiative. The fact that such monumental advances as our current antepartal care and the related work of the Children's Bureau had their genesis in the nursing profession is proof enough of what can be accomplished in this field by women of vision.

SUGGESTED READING

Adair, Fred L.: Maternity as the frontier of human welfare, The Mother 5:5, 1943.

Breckinridge, Mary: Wide Neighborhoods, New York, Harper, 1952.

Children's Bureau: Four Decades of Action for Children (Pub. No. 358), Washington, D. C., U. S. Dept. of Health, Education, and Welfare, Social Security Agency, 1956.

Deming, Dorothy: Public health nursing test, Pub. Health Nursing 43:271, 1951.

Eastman, N. J.: Maternity care looks to the future, Children 1:5, 1954.

Hospital Services in the United States, J.A.M.A. **146**:109, 1951.

Hospital Statistics, Hospitals **30**:10, 1956.

Jackson, Edith: New trends in maternity care, Am. J. Nursing **55**:584, 1955.

Kamperman, George: An evaluation of the newer obstetrics, Am. J. Obst. & Gynec. **60**:239, 1950.

Kirkwood, Samuel B.: Twenty years of maternal care, Children **2**:133, 1955.

Maternity Center Association: Twenty Years of Nurse-Midwifery, New York, Maternity Center Association, 1955.

Public Health Service: International Recommendations on Definitions of Live Births and Fetal Death (Pub. No. 39), Washington, D. C., Federal Security Agency, Public Health Service, National Office of Vital Statistics, 1950.

——: Special Reports on Maternal and Infant Statistics, Washington, D. C.,

U. S. Dept. of Health, Education, and Welfare, Public Health Service, National Office of Vital Statistics.

Reid, Duncan E., and Cohen, Mandel E.: Trends in obstetrics, J.A.M.A. **142**:615, 1950.

Schwartz, Doris: Nurse-midwives in the mountains, Am. J. Nursing **51**:102, 1951.

Stitt, Pauline: Who wants to know?, Children **2**:213, 1955.

Wishik, Samuel: Maternal Care Today —What is Needed for Tomorrow?, Transactions of the Fifth American Congress on Obstetrics and Gynecology, pp. 178ff, 1952.

World Health Organization: Manual of the International Statistical Classification of Diseases, Injuries and Causes of Death, 6th rev. of the Lists of Diseases, Injuries and Causes of Death, Geneva, World Health Organization, 1948.

CHAPTER TWO

Anatomy as a Basis for Obstetrics

PELVIS

The pelvis, so called from its resemblance to a basin (*pelvis*, a basin), is a bony ring interposed between the trunk and the thighs. The vertebral column, or backbone, passes into it from above, transmitting to it the weight of the upper part of the body, which the pelvis, in turn, transmits to the lower limbs. From an obstetric point of view, however, we have to consider it as the cavity which contains the generative organs, and particularly as the canal through which the baby must pass during birth.

Structure

The pelvis is made up of 4 united bones: the 2 hip bones (or innominate bones) situated laterally and in front, and the sacrum and the coccyx behind (Figs. 9-11). Anatomically, the hip bones are divided into 3 parts: the ilium, the ischium and the pubis. These bones become firmly joined into one by the time the growth of the body is completed, i.e., at about the age of 20 to 25, so that on examining them in the prepared pelvis no trace of the original edges or divisions of these 3 bones can be discovered. Each of these bones may be roughly described as follows.

The ilium, which is the largest portion of the bone, forms the upper and back part of the pelvis. Its upper flaring border forms the prominence of the hip or crest of the ilium (hip bone). The ischium is the lower part below the hip joint; from it projects the tuberosity of the ischium on which the body rests when in a sitting posture. The pubis is the front part of the hip bone; it extends from the hip joint to the joint in front between the 2 hip bones, the symphysis pubis, and then turns down toward the ischial tuberosity, thus forming with the bone of the opposite side the arch below the symphysis, the pubic or subpubic arch. This articulation closes anteriorly the cavity of the pelvis.

The sacrum and the coccyx form the lowest portions of the spinal column. The former is a triangular wedge-shaped bone, consisting of 5 vertebrae fused together; it serves as the back part of the pelvis. The coccyx consists of 4 very small vertebrae which form a tail end to the spine. The coccyx is usually movable at its attachment to the sacrum (the sacrococcygeal joint) and may become pressed back during labor to give more room for the passage of the fetal head.

18

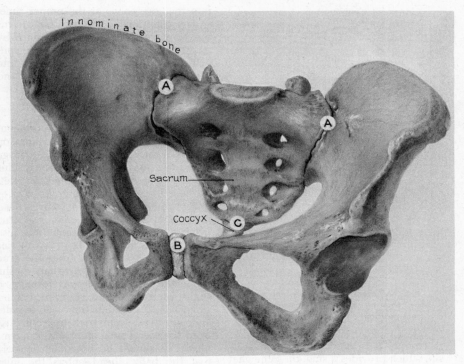

Fig. 9. Pelvis. (A) Sacro-iliac articulations (synchrondroses). (B) Symphysis pubis. (C) Sacrococcygeal articulation.

Of special importance is the marked projection which is formed by the junction of the last lumbar vertebra with the sacrum; this is known as the sacral promontory and is one of the most important landmarks in obstetric anatomy.

Articulation and Surfaces

The articulations (joints) of the pelvis, which possess obstetric importance, are 4 in number. Two are behind, between the sacrum and the ilia on either side, and are termed the sacro-iliac synchondroses (Fig. 9, A); one is in front, between the two pubic bones, and is called the symphysis pubis (Fig. 9, B); and the fourth, of little consequence, is between the sacrum and coccyx, the sacrococcygeal articulation (Fig. 9, C). All of these articular surfaces are lined with fibrocartilage, which becomes thickened and softened during pregnancy; likewise, the ligaments which bind the pelvic joints together become softened and, as a result, greater mobility of the pelvic bones develops. A certain definite, though very limited, motion in the joints is desirable for a normal labor; however, there is no change in the actual size of the pelvis. From a practical standpoint, one of the most important facts for the nurse to know about these joints is that the increased mobility which they develop in pregnancy produces a slight "wobbliness" in the pelvis and throws greater strain on the surrounding muscles and ligaments. This accounts, in large part, for the frequency of backache and legache in the latter months of pregnancy.

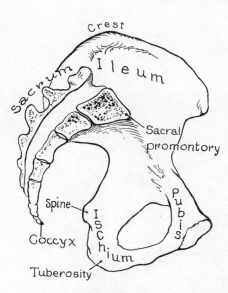

Fig. 10. Lateral view of left innominate bone showing its 3 constituent parts (erect position).

The pelvis is lined with muscular tissue which provides a smooth, somewhat cushioned surface over which the fetus has to pass during labor; these muscles also help to support the abdominal contents.

Divisions

Regarded as a whole, the pelvis may be described as a two-storied, bony basin that is divided by a natural line of division (the inlet or brim) into 2 parts. These parts are called the false pelvis (above) and the true pelvis (below) (Fig. 12).

The false pelvis, or upper flaring part, is much less concerned with the problems of labor than is the true pelvis, but it is considered in obstetrics because it offers certain landmarks for the practice of pelvimetry or pelvic measurements and because its shape and inclination aid in estimating the nature of the true pelvis. It also supports the uterus during late pregnancy and directs the fetus

into the true pelvis at the proper time.

The true pelvis, or lower part, forms the bony canal through which the baby must pass during parturition; for convenience in description it is divided into 3 parts: an inlet or brim, a cavity and an outlet.

Pelvic Inlet

Continuous with the sacral promontory and extending along the ilium on each side in circular fashion is a ridge called the linea terminalis (brim). This bounds an area or plane called the inlet, so named because it is the entryway or inlet through which the baby's head must pass in order to enter the true pelvis. The pelvic inlet, sometimes also referred to as the pelvic brim or superior strait, divides the false from the true pelvis. It is roughly heart-shaped, the promontory of the sacrum forming a slight projection into it from behind (Fig. 13); it is widest from side to side, and narrowest from back to front, i.e., from the sacral promontory to the symphysis. It should be noted particularly that the baby's head enters the inlet with its longest diameter (anteroposterior) in the transverse diameter of the pelvis. In other words, as shown in Figure 13, the greatest diameter of the head accommodates itself to the greatest diameter of the inlet. As the inlet is entirely surrounded by bone, the measurements of its diameters can be estimated accurately; and for the same reason, these measurements are very important, since variations from the normal (e.g., smaller in size or flattened) may cause grave difficulty at the time of labor.

Pelvic Outlet

When viewed from below, the pelvic outlet is a space bounded in front by the symphysis pubis and the pubic arch, at the sides by the ischial tuberosities, and behind by the coccyx and the greater sacrosciatic ligaments. It requires only a little imagination to see

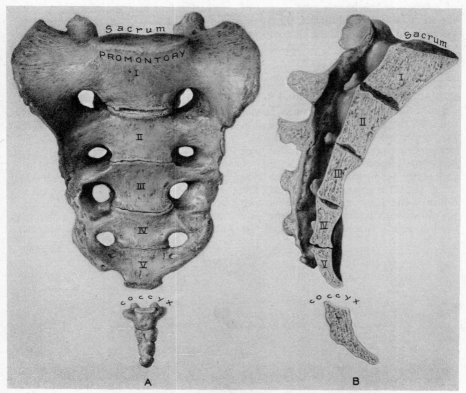

Fig. 11. Sacrum and coccyx. (A) Front view. (B) Median section; note how promontory of sacrum juts forward.

that the front half of the outlet resembles a triangle, the base of which is the distance between the ischial tuberosities, and the other two sides of which are represented by the pubic arch. From an obstetric point of view, this triangle is of great importance, since the baby's head must make use of this space to gain exit from the pelvis and the mother's body (Fig. 14). For this reason Nature has provided a wide pubic arch in females, whereas in males it is narrow (see Fig. 20). If the pubic arch in women were as narrow as it is in men, natural childbearing would be extremely difficult, since the baby's head, unable to squeeze itself into the narrow anterior triangle of the outlet, would be forced backward against the coccyx and the sacrum where its progress would be impeded.

As has been stated, the greatest diameter of the inlet is the transverse (from side to side), whereas the greatest diameter of the outlet is the anteroposterior (from front to back). Moreover, the baby's head, as it emerges from the pelvis, passes through the outlet in the anteroposterior position, again accommodating its greatest diameter to the greatest diameter of the passage. Since the baby's head enters the pelvis in the transverse position and emerges in the anteroposterior, it is obvious that the head must rotate some 90° as it passes through the pelvis. This process of rotation of the baby's head is one of the most important phases of the mechanism of labor and will be discussed in more detail later on pages 220-222.

Pelvic Cavity

The pelvic cavity is the space between the inlet above, the outlet below and the anterior, posterior and lateral walls of the pelvis. The pelvic canal is practically cylindric in shape in its upper portion and curved only in its lower half. It is important to note the axis of the cavity when viewed from the side (Fig. 15). It is apparent that during the delivery the head must descend along the downward prolongation of the axis until it nearly reaches the level of the

ischial spines and then begins to curve forward. The axis of the cavity determines the direction which the baby takes through the pelvis in the process of delivery. As might be expected, labor is made more complicated by this curvature in the pelvic canal because the baby has to accommodate itself to the curved path as well as to the variations in the size of the cavity at different levels.

Pelvic Variations

The pelvis presents great individual variations—no two pelves are exactly alike. Even those patients with normal measurements may present differences in contour and muscular development

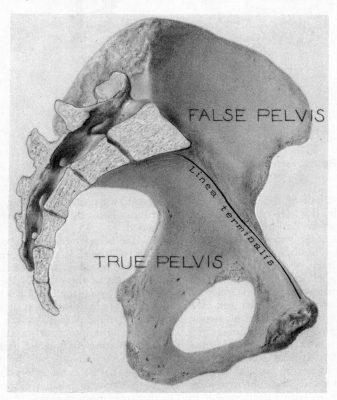

Fig. 12. False and true pelves, sagittal section.

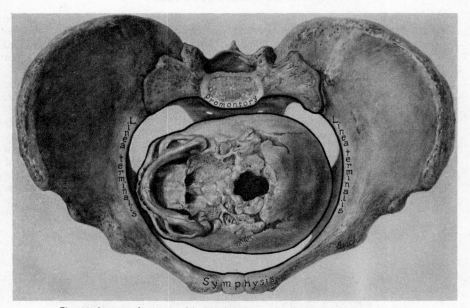

Fig. 13. Largest diameter of baby's head entering largest diameter of inlet. Therefore, it enters transversely.

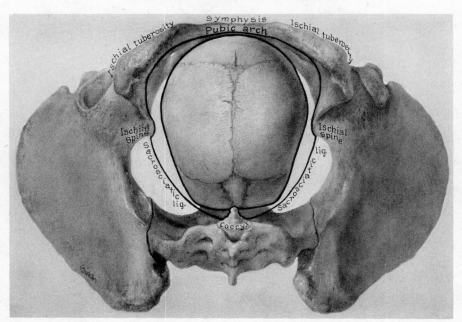

Fig. 14. Largest diameter of baby's head passing through largest diameter of outlet. Therefore, it passes through outlet anteroposteriorly.

which influence the actual size of the pelvis. These varying differences are due in part to heredity, disease, injury and development. Heredity may be responsible for passing on many racial and sexual differences. Such diseases as tuberculosis and rickets cause malformations. Accidents and injuries during childhood or at maturity result in deformities of the pelvis or other parts of the body which affect the pelvis. Adequate nutrition and well-formed habits related to posture and exercise have a very definite influence upon the development of the pelvis.

It must be remembered also that the pelvis does not mature until between the ages of 20 and 25 years, and until that time complete ossification has not taken place.

There are many so-called borderline cases of abnormal pelvic development. Such pregnant patients should be supervised closely. At periodic intervals the size of the fetus is estimated (by palpation of the abdomen), and definite arrangements are made for the type of delivery indicated.

There are several types of pelves. Even pelves whose measurements are

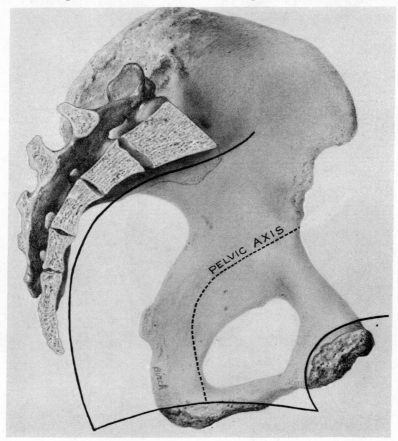

Fig. 15. Pelvic cavity. Heavy black line indicates location of soft parts, vagina, etc.

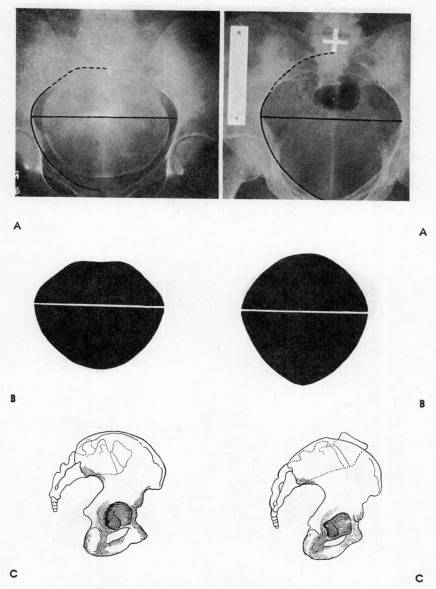

Fig. 16. (*Left*) Gynecoid (normal female) pelvis. Inlet is well rounded in hind- and fore-pelvis (A, B). Sacrosciatic notch is curved, moderate in width and depth (C).

Fig. 17. (*Right*) Anthropoid pelvis. Inlet is deep in hind- and fore-pelvis, increased in anteroposterior diameter (A, B). Sacrosciatic notch is broad, shallow (C).

(Roentgenograms from W. E. Caldwell, M.D., and H. C. Moloy, M.D., Sloane Hospital for Women, New York)

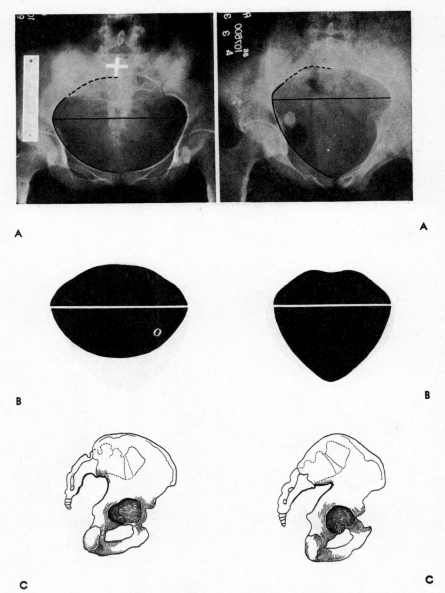

Fig. 18. (*Left*) Platypelloid pelvis. Inlet is a transverse oval, well-curved but decreased in anteroposterior diameter (A, B). Sacrosciatic notch is curved, small (C).

Fig. 19. (*Right*) Android pelvis. Inlet is wedged-shaped with shallow hind-pelvis and pointed fore-pelvis (A, B). Sacrosciatic notch is narrow, deep, pointed (C).

(Roentgenograms from W. E. Caldwell, M.D., and H. C. Moloy, M.D., Sloane Hospital for Women, New York)

FEMALE   MALE

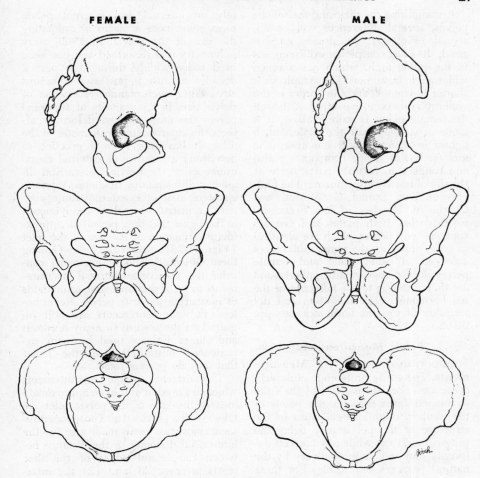

Fig. 20. Female pelvis contrasted with male in lateral, front and inlet views.

normal differ greatly in the shape of the inlet, in the proximity of the greatest transverse diameter of the inlet to the sacral promontory, in the size of the sacrosciatic notch, and in their general architecture. Dr. H. C. Moloy and the late Dr. W. E. Caldwell, of the Sloane Hospital for Women, New York City, have utilized these characteristics in establishing a classification of pelves which has been of great interest and value to obstetricians. The four main

types, according to this classification, are shown in Figures 16 to 19. The manner in which the baby passes through the birth canal and, consequently, the type of labor vary considerably in these pelvic types.

In addition, of course, there are many pelvic types which result from abnormal narrowing of one or the other diameters. These contracted pelves will be described in a subsequent chapter (see p. 440).

In comparing the male and the female pelves, several differences will be observed (Fig. 20). As already emphasized, the most conspicuous difference is in the pubic arch, which has a much wider angle in women. The symphysis is shorter in women, and the border of the arch probably is more everted. Although the female pelvis is more shallow, it is more capacious than the male, much lighter in structure and smoother. The male pelvis is deep, compact, conical and rougher in texture, particularly at the site of muscle attachments. The findings of Drs. Daniel G. Morton and Charles T. Hayden, of San Francisco, indicate that both males and females start life with pelves which are identical in type, and that the major differences observed in adult male and female pelves do not appear until puberty and are therefore due to the influence of the sex hormones. (For definition and description of the sex hormones, see pp. 60-62.)

Pelvic Measurements

Importance of Pelvic Measurements. The entire problem in childbirth centers on the safe passage of the fully developed fetus through the pelvis of the mother. Slight irregularities in the structure of the pelvis may delay the progress of labor, while any marked deformity may render the delivery by the natural passages impossible. For these reasons the pelvis of every pregnant woman should be measured accurately in the antepartal period to enable the physician to determine, before labor begins, whether or not there is anything in the condition of the mother's pelvis that may complicate the delivery. This examination is a part of the antepartal examination. In addition to a general physical examination, the pelvic measurements are made and compared with the dimensions of the normal pelvis.

Types of Pelvic Measurements. For many years the physician had to rely on internal and external pelvic measurements as a means of estimating the size of the pelvis. In 1900, x-ray pelvimetry was described and has been used more widely during the past 2 decades because it possesses numerous advantages over manual estimation of pelvic size. In the majority of abnormal pelves the most marked deformity affects the anteroposterior diameter of the inlet. It has long been a practice to determine a number of external measurements of the pelvis (intercristal diameter, interspinous diameter, intertrochanteric diameter, external conjugate) with an instrument called a pelvimeter, in the belief that they permit an approximate estimation of the size of the inlet (Figs. 21-26). Authorities today (among them Greenhill, Thoms, Eastman) consider the transverse external measurements to be of dubious value as methods of measuring the true pelvis. Nevertheless, these measurements are still required on the records in many hospitals and clinics and are used by many experienced obstetricians in the belief that they do possess some value.

The external pelvic measurements which are used to obtain an approximate idea of the size of the pelvic inlet are taken with a pelvimeter. Those measurements most commonly made are: (1) the intercristal diameter or the distance between the lateral edges of the iliac crests, average 28 cm.; (2) the interspinous diameter or the distance between the external aspects of the anterior superior iliac spines, average 25 cm.; (3) intertrochanteric diameter or the distance between the external aspects of the trochanters of the femurs, average 31 cm.; (4) the external conjugate (Baudelocque's diameter) or the distance between the anterior aspect of the symphysis pubis in front and the depression below the spine of the 5th lumbar vertebra behind, average 18 to 20 cm. In addition, some physicians measure the right and the left oblique

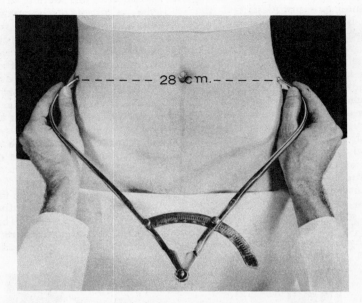

Fig. 21. Method of measuring intercristal diameter.

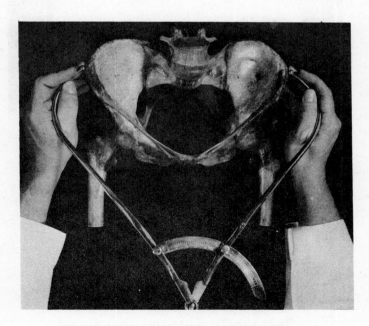

Fig. 22. Intercristal diameter measured on bony pelvis.

external diameters. For all the pelvic measurements just described, the patient lies on her side or on her back, according to the diameter to be measured, with the abdomen exposed.

The internal pelvic measurements are made to determine the actual diameters of the inlet. The chief internal measurement taken is the *diagonal conjugate* or the distance between the sacral promontory and the lower margin of the symphysis pubis. The patient should be placed on her back on the examining table with her knees drawn up and her feet supported by stirrups. Two fingers are introduced into the vagina, and, before measuring the diagonal conjugate, some evaluation of the pelvis is made by palpation: the height of the symphysis pubis and the shape of the

pubic arch, the motility of the coccyx, the inclination of the anterior wall of the sacrum and the side walls of the pelvis and the prominence of the ischial spines. In order to obtain the length of the diagonal conjugate, the 2 fingers passed into the vagina are pressed inward and upward as far as possible until the middle finger rests on the sacral promontory. The point on the back of the hand just under the symphysis is then marked by putting the index finger of the other hand on the exact point (Fig. 27), after which the fingers are withdrawn and measured. The distance from the tip of the middle finger to the point marked represents the *diagonal conjugate measurement*. This distance may be measured with a rigid measuring scale attached to the wall (Fig. 28)

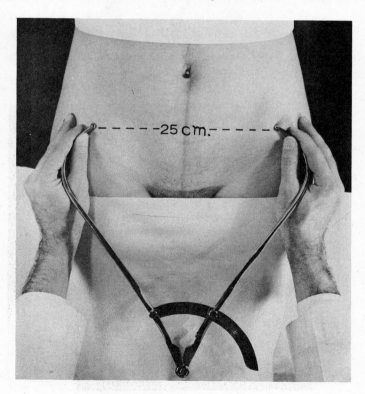

Fig. 23. Method of measuring interspinous diameter.

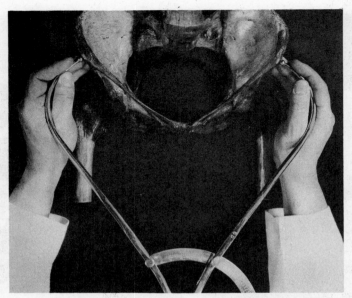

Fig. 24. Interspinous diameter measured on bony pelvis.

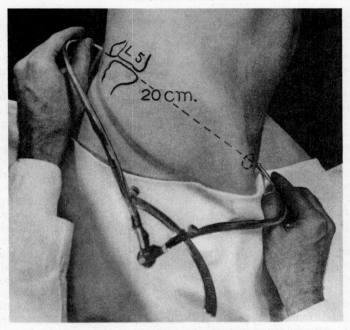

Fig. 25. Method of measuring external conjugate diameter
(Baudelocque's diameter).

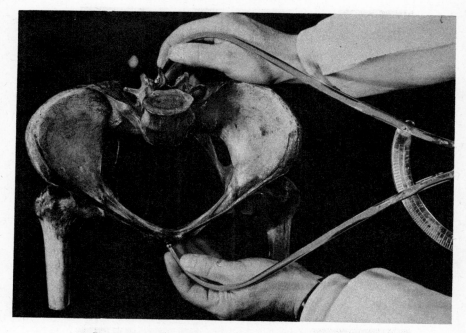

Fig. 26. External conjugate diameter measured on bony pelvis.

or with a pelvimeter (Fig. 29), but the former is preferred because there is less chance of error. If the measurement is greater than 11.5 cm. it is justifiable to assume that the pelvic inlet is of adequate size for childbirth. In common medical parlance this measurement is often referred to as the "C.D." (conjugata diagonalis).

An extremely important internal diameter is the *true conjugate* or, in Latin, the conjugata vera (C.V.), which is the distance between the posterior aspect of the symphysis pubis and the promontory of the sacrum. However, direct measurement of this diameter cannot be made except by means of a roentgenogram; consequently, it has to be estimated from the diagonal conjugate measurement. It is believed that if 1.5 cm. is deducted from the length of the diagonal conjugate the true conjugate is obtained. For instance, if the diagonal conjugate is 12.5 cm., the conjugata vera may be estimated as being about 11.0 cm. In this method the problem consists of estimating the length of one side of a triangle, the conjugata vera; the other two sides, the diagonal conjugate and the height of the symphysis pubis, are known. If the symphysis pubis is high and has a marked inclination, the physician takes this into consideration and may deduct 2 cm. The length of the true conjugate, or conjugata vera, is of utmost importance, since it is about the smallest diameter of the inlet through which the baby's head must pass. Indeed, the main purpose in measuring the diagonal conjugate is to give an estimate of the size of the conjugata vera.

Next to the diagonal conjugate measurement the most important clinical dimension of the pelvis is the transverse diameter of the outlet, the diameter

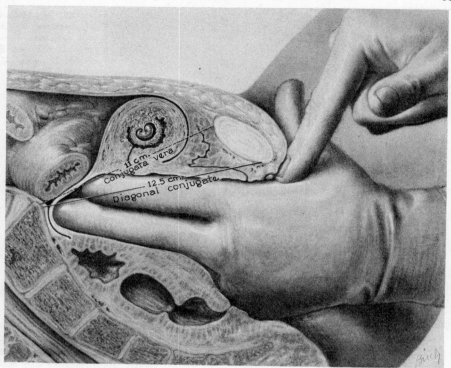

Fig. 27. Method of obtaining diagonal conjugate diameter.

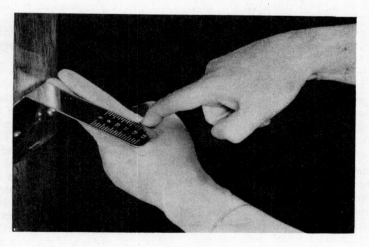

Fig. 28. Method of measuring diagonal conjugate diameter as obtained
in Figure 27, using wall bracket.

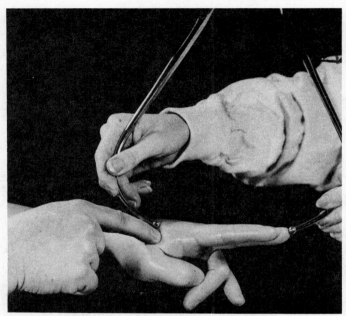

Fig. 29. Method of measuring diagonal conjugate diameter as obtained in Figure 27, using pelvimeter.

between the ischial tuberosities. This is sometimes called the *tuberischii diameter* (often abbreviated T.I.), or bi-ischial diameter, or intertuberous diameter (Figure 31). This measurement is taken with the patient in the lithotomy position, well down on the table and with the legs widely separated. The measurement is taken from the innermost and lowermost aspect of the ischial tuberosities, on a level with the lower border of the anus. The instruments usually employed are the Williams' pelvimeter (Figs. 32 and 33) or the Thoms' pelvimeter. A diameter in excess of 8 cm. is considered average.

X-ray Pelvimetry

As stated before, there is no manual procedure which permits measurement of the transverse diameter of the inlet. For these reasons both roentgenologists and obstetricians have striven to perfect an x-ray method which will not only yield precise measurements but also will give a clear picture of the entire inlet and of the general pelvic architecture.

A number of such methods are now available and are being used more and more frequently, particularly in cases in which pelvic abnormalities are suspected.

Possibly the most widely used method, and one of the simplest, is that of Dr. Herbert Thoms of New Haven, Conn., a pioneer worker in this field. For a complete study two roentgenograms are made as follows.

1. The patient is placed on the x-ray table in a semirecumbent position so that her pelvic inlet is horizontal and as nearly parallel as possible with the plate beneath her (Fig. 34). The exact plane in which the patient's inlet lies, both front and back, is now determined and recorded. After an exposure of the film has been made, the patient is removed from the table, and a lead plate or grid containing perforations, a centimeter apart, is placed in the plane previously occupied by the inlet of the patient. Another exposure is now made on the same film. When the latter is developed, the outline of the inlet is shown, as are also the dots produced by the perforations

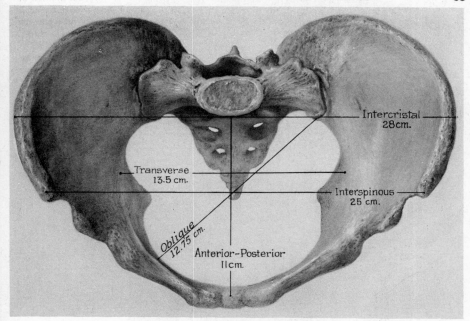

Fig. 30. Measurements of inlet.

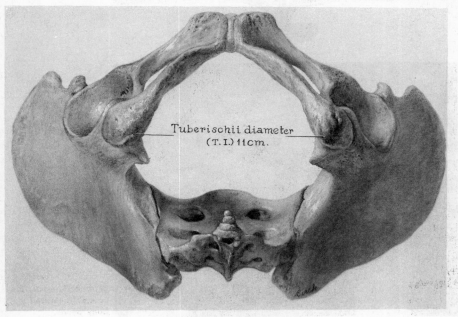

Fig. 31. Measurement of outlet.

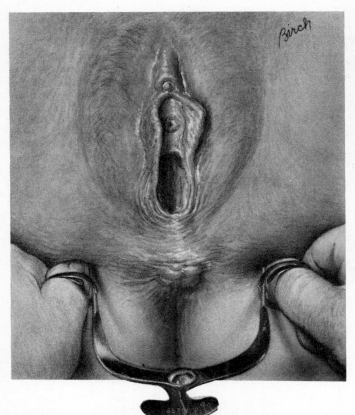

Fig. 32. Method of measuring tuberischii or intertuberous diameter of outlet, using the Williams pelvimeter. The measurement is made on a line with the lower border of the anus.

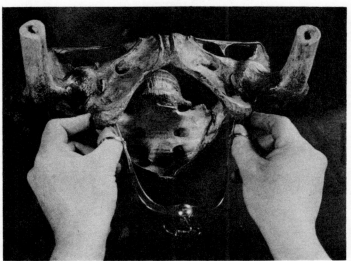

Fig. 33. Tuberischii or intertuberous diameter measured on bony pelvis.

Fig. 34. Pelvis inlet roentgenogram. The scale represents corrected centimeters for various levels of the pelvic canal. The top line is used for measuring the diameters of the inlet. The other levels are established on the lateral roentgenogram. Pelvic morphology is readily established by viewing both lateral and inlet views. (Herbert Thoms, M.D., Yale School of Medicine)

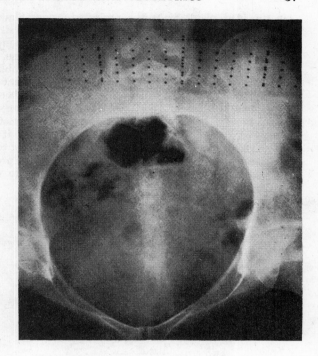

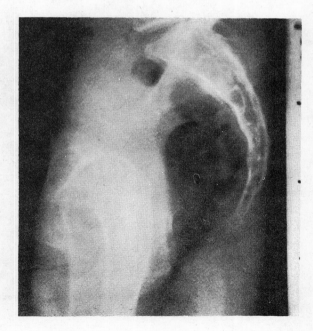

Fig. 35. Lateral roentgenogram. The scale represents corrected centimeters in the midplane of the body. By means of calipers the various diameters may be measured. The lateral morphologic aspects are readily visualized. (Herbert Thoms, M.D., Yale School of Medicine)

in the lead plate. Since the projected dots on the film represent centimeters in the plane of the inlet, the diameters of the inlet can be read off directly as centimeters.

2. A somewhat similar procedure is carried out with the patient standing and from the lateral view (Fig. 35). Here, however, an upright lead and iron rod, with a centimeter scale notched on its edge, is placed posterior to the patient and close to the gluteal fold. After an exposure has been made, the devel-

oped film will show a lateral view of the symphysis pubis, the sacral promontory, other bony landmarks and, in addition, of course, the notched centimeter scale for establishing the distance between important points. Diameters which may be measured are the obstetric conjugate, posterior sagittal at the inlet, midpelvis and outlet, and the anteroposterior diameter at the midpelvis and outlet.

Other technics entail the use of stereoscopic procedures which allow the physician to view the films with 3-dimen-

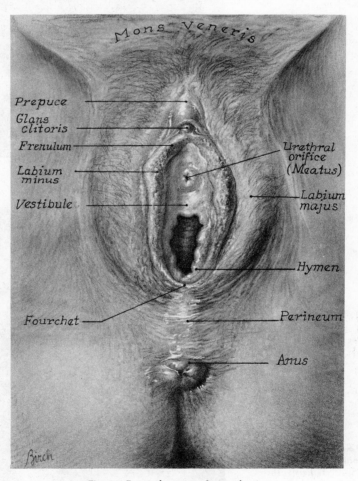

Fig. 36. External organs of reproduction.

sional vision and thus gain a clear image of all pelvic relationships.

When roentgenograms are made late in pregnancy by any of these methods, it is possible to secure also an impression of the size of the baby's head. When this is considered in relation to the pelvic picture, helpful information may be obtained in forecasting whether or not this particular pelvis is large enough to allow this particular baby to pass through.

Preventive Care Based on Pelvimetry. The importance of the knowledge gained through skillful performance of external and internal pelvimetry cannot be overestimated. Especially should it never be neglected in the case of a woman pregnant for the first time, nor in any case in which the patient has suffered previously from difficult or tedious labors.

FEMALE ORGANS OF REPRODUCTION

The female organs of reproduction are divided into two groups—the external and the internal (Figs. 36-41).

External Organs

The external female reproductive organs are called the *vulva* (L.-covering). This includes everything which is visible externally from the lower margin of the pubis to the perineum, namely, the mons veneris, the labia majora and minora, the clitoris, the vestibule, the hymen, the urethral opening and various glandular and vascular structures (Fig. 36). The term vulva often has been used to refer simply to the labia majora and minora.

The mons veneris is a firm, cushionlike formation over the symphysis pubis and is covered with crinkly hair.

The labia majora are 2 prominent longitudinal folds of adipose tissue covered with skin which extend downward and backward from the mons veneris and disappear in forming the ante-

rior border of the perineal body. These 2 thick folds of skin are covered with hair on their outer surfaces after the age of puberty but are smooth and moist on their inner surfaces. At the bottom they fade away into the perineum posteriorly, joining together to form a transverse fold, the posterior commissure, situated directly in front of the fourchet. This fatty tissue is supplied with an abundant plexus of veins which may rupture as the result of injury sustained during labor and give rise to an extravasation of blood or hematoma.

The labia minora are 2 thin folds of reddish tissue covered entirely with thin membrane and situated between the labia majora, with their outer surfaces in contact with the inner surfaces of the labia majora; the labia minora extend from the clitoris downward and backward on either side of the orifice of the vagina. In the upper extremity each labium minus separates into two branches which when united with those of the opposite side enclose the clitoris. The upper fold forms the prepuce and the lower the frenum of the clitoris. At the bottom the labia minora pass almost imperceptibly into the labia majora or blend together as a thin fold of skin forming the anterior edge of the perineum or perineal body. This thin edge is known as the fourchet.

The clitoris is a small, highly sensitive projection composed of erectile tissue, nerves and blood vessels and is covered with a thin epidermis. It is analogous to the penis in the male and is regarded as the chief seat of voluptuous sensation. The clitoris is so situated that it is partially hidden between the anterior ends of the labia minora.

The vestibule is the almond-shaped area which is enclosed by the labia minora and extends from the clitoris to the fourchet. It is perforated by 4 openings: the urethra, the vaginal opening, the ducts of the Bartholin's glands and the ducts of the Skene's glands. Bartho-

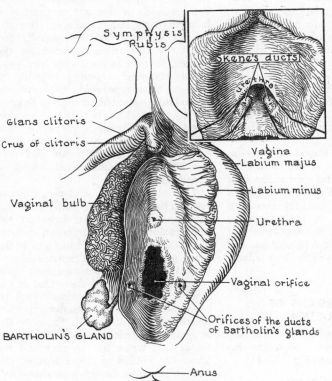

Symphysis Pubis

Skene's ducts

Urethra

Glans clitoris

Crus of clitoris

Vaginal bulb

Vagina
Labium majus

Labium minus

Urethra

Vaginal orifice

Orifices of the ducts of Bartholin's glands

BARTHOLIN'S GLAND

Anus

Fig. 37. The vestibule, showing the urethra, the vaginal orifice and Bartholin's glands. Insert shows the orifices of the ducts of Skene's glands which open just within the urethral meatus.

lin's glands are 2 small glands situated beneath the vestibule on either side of the vaginal opening. During sexual excitement varying amounts of mucoid material are secreted by these glands. In women infected with gonorrhea, these ducts sometimes harbor gonococci, which may cause the glands to suppurate, so that the entire labia become distended by pus. Skene's ducts open upon the vestibule on either side of the urethra (Fig. 37).

The hymen marks the division between the internal and the external organs. It is a thin fold of mucous membrane situated at the orifice of the vagina. It may be entirely absent or it may form a complete septum across the lower end of the vagina. In women who have had children the irregularity of torn edges remains. The hymen presents marked differences in shape and consistency. In the newborn child it projects beyond the surrounding parts. In adult virgins it is a membrane of varying thickness which closes the vaginal opening more or less completely and presents an aperture which varies in size from a pin point to one which will readily admit 1 or even 2 fingers. The opening is circular or crescentic in shape. In rare instances the hymen may be imperforate and cause retention of menstrual discharge if it occludes the vaginal orifice completely.

The perineum consists of muscles and fascia of the urogenital diaphragm, which lies across the pubic arch, and the pelvic diaphragm, which consists of the coccygeus and the levator ani muscles. The levator ani is the larger and consists of 3 portions: the iliococcygeus,

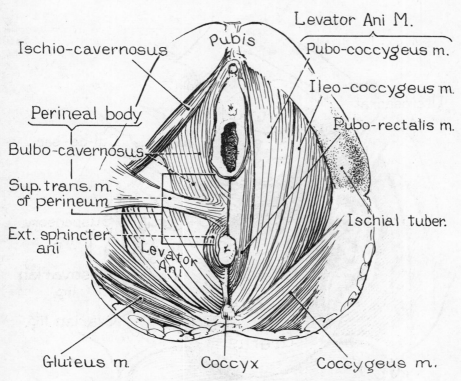

Fig. 38. Muscles of the pelvic floor (after Dickinson).

the pubococcygeus and puborectalis. These muscles form a slinglike support for the pelvic structure, and between them pass the urethra, the vagina and the rectum (Fig. 38). Between the anus and the vagina the levator ani is reinforced by a central tendon of the perineum to which 3 pairs of muscles converge: the bulbocavernosus, the superficial transverse muscles of the perineum and the external sphincter ani. These structures constitute the perineal body and form the main support of the perineal floor. They often are lacerated during delivery.

Internal Organs

The internal organs of reproduction are the vagina, the uterus, the fallopian tubes and the ovaries.

Ovaries. The ovaries are 2 small almond-shaped organs situated in the upper part of the pelvic cavity, one on either side of the uterus. Their chief functions are the development and the expulsion of ova and the provision of certain internal secretions (hormones). These organs correspond to the testes in the male. They lie embedded in the posterior fold of the broad ligament of the uterus (Fig. 39) and are supported by the suspensory, the ovarian and the mesovarian ligaments.

Each ovary contains in its substance at birth a large number of germ cells or ovules (primordial ova) (p. 55). This huge store of primordial follicles present at birth more than suffices the woman for life. It is usually believed that no more are formed and that this

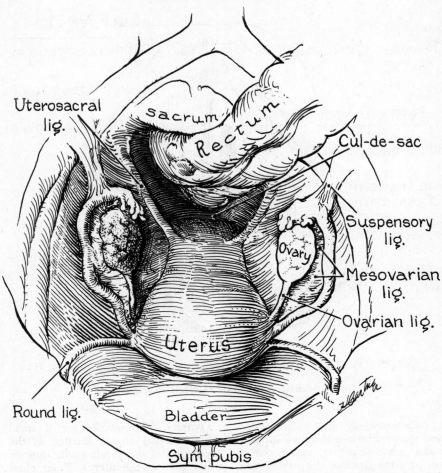

Fig. 39. Pelvic contents from above, showing the position of the pairs of ligaments and the relationship to the uterus, the tubes and the ovaries. (After Dickinson)

large initial store is gradually exhausted during the period of sexual maturity. Beginning at about the time of puberty, 1 (or possibly 2) of the follicles which contain the ovules enlarges each month, gradually approaches the surface of the ovary and bursts (Fig. 46). The ovum and the fluid content of the follicle are liberated on the exterior of the ovary into the abdominal cavity; then they are swept into the tube and so pass

into the uterus. The development and the maturation of the follicles (containing the ova) and the ova continue from puberty to menopause.

The arteries which supply the ovary are 4 or 5 branches that arise from the anastomosis of the ovarian artery with the ovarian branch of the uterine (see Fig. 42). The veins proceeding from the ovary become tributary to both the uterine and the ovarian plexus.

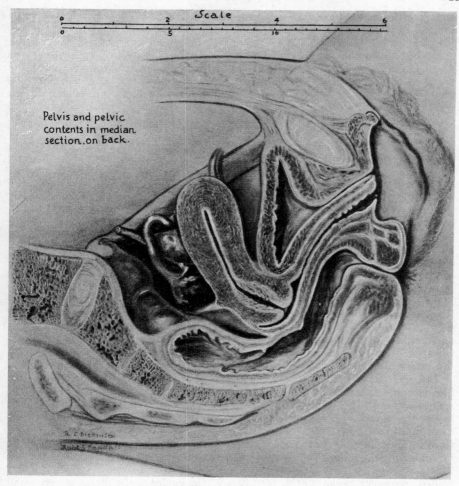

Fig. 40. Pelvic contents in median section with the subject on her back.
(Robert L. Dickinson, M.D., New York)

The nerves supplying the ovaries are derived from the craniosacral and the thoracolumbar sympathetic systems. The postganglionic and visceral afferent fibers form a plexus surrounding the ovarian artery, which in turn is formed by contributions from the renal and the aortic plexuses and corresponds to the spermatic plexus in the male.

Fallopian Tubes. The fallopian tubes (see Figs. 39 and 52) are 2 trumpet-shaped, thin, flexible, muscular tubes, about 4½ inches long and somewhat thinner than a lead pencil. They extend from the upper angles of the uterus, the cornua, in the upper margin of the broad ligament, toward the sides of the pelvis. They have 2 openings: one into the uterine cavity and the other into the abdominal cavity. The opening into the uterine cavity is minute and will admit only a fine bristle; the abdominal opening is somewhat larger and is surrounded by a large number of fine fringes, hence the term "fimbriated end." The fimbriated extremity lies in the neighborhood of the ovary, but it is not necessarily in direct contact with it. It is generally believed that the cilia upon the fimbriated end of the tube give rise to a current in the capillary layer of fluid lying between the various pelvic organs. The fallopian tubes convey the discharged ova by peristaltic action from the ovaries to the cavity of the uterus; by their tentaclelike processes the fimbriated ends of the tube draw the escaped ova into the tube. Thus, the function of the fallopian tube is to conduct the ovum along the canal by peristaltic action until it reaches the uterus.

The tubes are lined with mucous membrane containing ciliated epithelium. The muscular layer is made up of longitudinal and circular fibers which provide peristaltic action. The serous membrane covering the tubes is a continuation of the peritoneum, which lines the whole abdominal cavity.

The fallopian tubes receive their blood supply from the ovarian and the uterine arteries. The veins of the tubes follow the course of these arteries and empty into the uterine and the ovarian trunks. The nerves which supply the uterus supply the tubes (see Fig. 42).

Uterus. The uterus is a hollow thick-walled, muscular organ (Figs. 39, 40 and 41). It serves two important functions: (1) it is the organ of menstruation and (2) during pregnancy it receives the fertilized ovum and retains and nourishes it until it expels the products of conception at the time of labor.

The uterus varies in size and shape according to the age of the individual and whether or not she has borne children. The uterus of the adult nullipara weighs approximately 60 Gm. and measures 5.5 to 8 cm. in length. It resembles a flattened pear in appearance and has two divisions: the upper triangular portion, the corpus, and the lower constricted cylindric portion, the cervix, which projects into the vagina. The fallopian tubes extend from the cornu (L.-horn) of the uterus at the upper outer margin on either side. The upper rounded portion of the uterus between the points of insertion of the fallopian tubes is called the fundus (Fig. 41).

The nonpregnant uterus is situated in the pelvic cavity between the bladder and the rectum. Almost the entire posterior wall and the upper portion of the anterior wall is covered by peritoneum. The lower portion of the anterior wall is united to the bladder wall by a thick layer of connective tissue. The lower posterior wall of the uterus and the upper portion of the vagina are separated from the rectum by an area called Douglas' cul-de-sac. Due to its muscular composition, the uterus is capable of enlarging to the size of a pumpkin; at the termination of pregnancy it weighs about 2 pounds. It is made up of involuntary muscle fibers arranged in all directions, making expansion possible in every direction to accommodate the products of conception. Due to the nature of this arrangement of the muscle, the uterus is able to expel its contents at the termination of normal labor (Fig. 92). Arranged between these muscular layers are many blood vessels, lymphatics and nerves.

The cavity of the uterus is very small and somewhat triangular in shape, being widest at the fundus, between the very small openings into the canals of the fallopian tubes, and narrowest below at the opening into the cervix. The anterior and the posterior walls lie almost in contact, so that if a cross section of the uterus could be examined the cavity between them would appear as a mere slit. The uterus is lined with mucous membrane (endometrium) and is divided into 2 parts: the cavity of the body of the uterus and the cavity of the cervix.

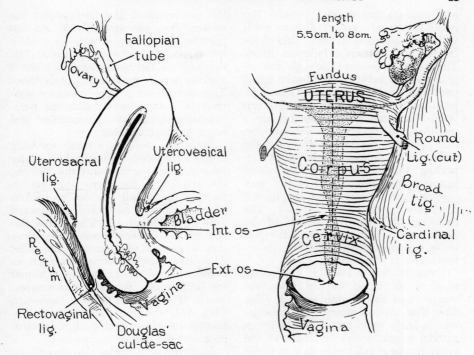

Fig. 41. Lateral and anterior views of the uterus. The ligaments which support the uterus in the pelvic cavity are the broad ligaments (2), the round ligaments (2), the uterosacral ligaments (2), the uterovesical ligament (1), and the rectovaginal ligament (1).

The cervix is less freely movable than is the body of the uterus. Its muscular wall is not so thick, and the mucous membrane lining its cavity (cervical endometrium) is different in that it is much folded and contains more glands, which produce mucus and are the chief source of the mucous secretion during pregnancy. The cervix has an upper opening called the internal os, leading from the cavity of the uterine body into the cervical canal, and a lower opening called the external os, opening into the vagina. The cervix is very small in the nonpregnant woman, barely admitting a probe, but at the time of labor it dilates to a size sufficient to permit the passage of the fetus (Fig. 131).

LIGAMENTS. The uterus is supported in two ways: by ligaments (Fig. 41)

and by the muscles of the pelvic floor (Fig. 38). The ligaments which support the uterus in the pelvic cavity are the broad ligaments (2), the round ligaments (2), the uterosacral (2), the uterovesical (1) and the rectovaginal (1). The broad ligaments are 2 wing-like structures which extend from the lateral margins of the uterus to the pelvic walls and serve to divide the pelvic cavity into an anterior and a posterior compartment. Each consists of folds of peritoneum which envelop the fallopian tubes, the ovaries and the round and the ovarian ligaments. Its lower portion, the cardinal ligament, is composed of dense connective tissue which is firmly united to the supravaginal portion of the cervix. The median margin is connected with the lateral margin of the uterus and encloses the uterine vessels. The round ligaments are 2 fibrous cords which are attached on either side of the fundus just below the fallopian tubes. They extend forward through the inguinal canal and terminate in the upper portion of the labia majora. These ligaments aid in holding the fundus forward. The uterosacral ligaments are 2 cordlike structures which extend from the posterior cervical portion of the uterus to the sacrum. These aid in supporting the cervix. The uterovesical ligament is merely a fold of the peritoneum which passes over the fundus and extends over the bladder. The rectovaginal ligament is a fold of the peritoneum which passes over the posterior surface of the uterus and is reflected on to the rectum.

UTERINE BLOOD SUPPLY. The uterus receives its blood supply from the ovarian and the uterine arteries (Fig. 42). The uterine artery, the principal source, is the main branch of the hypogastric, which enters the base of the broad ligament and makes its way to the side of the uterus. The ovarian artery is a branch of the aorta. It enters the broad ligament and on reaching the ovary breaks up into smaller branches which enter that organ, while its main stem makes its way to the upper margin of the uterus where it anastomoses with the ovarian branch of the uterine artery.

The uterovaginal plexus returns the blood from the uterus and the vagina. These veins form a plexus of exceedingly thin-walled vessels which are embedded in the layers of the uterine muscle. Emerging from this plexus, the trunks join the uterine vein, which is a double vein. These veins follow on either side of the uterine artery and eventually form one trunk which empties into the hypogastric vein, which makes its way into the internal iliac.

UTERINE NERVE SUPPLY. The uterus possesses an abundant nerve supply derived principally from the sympathetic nervous system but partly from the cerebrospinal and parasympathetic system. Both the sympathetic and the parasympathetic nerve supplies contain motor and a few sensory fibers. The functions of the nerve supply of the 2 systems are in great part antagonistic. The sympathetic causes muscular contraction and vasoconstriction; the parasympathetic inhibits contraction and leads to vasodilatation.

Since the uterus is a freely movable organ suspended in the pelvic cavity between the bladder and the rectum, the position of the uterus may be influenced by a full bladder or rectum which pushes it backward or forward (see Figs. 40 and 44). The uterus also changes its position when the patient stands, lies flat or turns on her side. Also, there are abnormalities such as anteflexion, where the fundus is tipped too far forward (Fig. 44); retroversion, where it is tipped too far backward (Fig. 44); and prolapse, due to the relaxation of the muscles of the pelvic floor and the uterine ligaments.

LYMPHATIC VESSELS. The lymphatic vessels drain into the lumbar lymph nodes.

Vagina. The vagina is a dilatable passage lined with mucous membrane situated between the bladder and the rectum. The vaginal opening occupies the lower portion of the vestibule and in the virgin appears almost completely closed by the hymen. The vagina is from 3 to 5 inches in length, and at the upper end is a blind vault, commonly called the fornix, into which the lower portion of the cervix projects. The fornices (plural of fornix) are divided into 4 parts for convenience of description. The lateral fornices are the spaces between the vaginal wall on either side and the cervix; the anterior fornix is between the anterior vaginal wall and the cervix; the posterior fornix is between the posterior vaginal wall and the cervix. The posterior fornix is considerably deeper than the anterior since the vagina is attached higher up on the

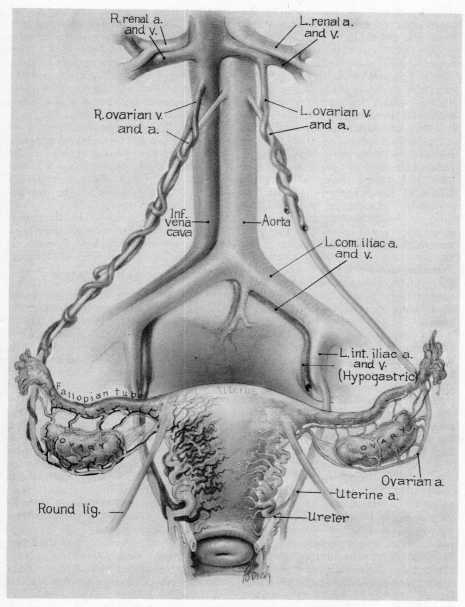

Fig. 42. Blood supply of the uterus and the adnexa.

posterior than the anterior wall of the cervix. The fornices are important because the physician is usually able to palpate the internal pelvic organs through their thin walls. The vagina serves 3 important functions: it represents the excretory duct of the uterus through which its secretion and the menstrual flow escape, it is the female organ of copulation and it forms part of the birth canal during labor. Its walls are arranged into thick folds, the columns of the vagina, and in women who have not borne children, numerous ridges or rugae extend outward and almost at right angles to the vaginal columns and give the surface a corrugated appearance. Normally, the anterior and the posterior walls of the vagina lie in contact, but they are capable of stretching to allow marked distention of the passage, as in the process of childbirth. The vagina is kept moist by a small amount of secretion from the uterus.

The vagina receives its abundant blood supply from branches of the uterine, the inferior vesical, the median hemorrhoidal and the internal pudic arteries. The passage is surrounded by a venous plexus; the vessels follow the course of the arteries and eventually empty into the hypogastric veins. The lymphatics empty into the inguinal, the hypogastric and the iliac glands.

Related Pelvic Organs

Bladder. The bladder is a thin, muscular sac which serves as a reservoir for the urine. It is situated in front of the uterus and behind the symphysis pubis. When empty or only moderately distended it remains entirely in the pelvis, but if it becomes greatly distended it rises into the abdomen. Urine is conducted into the bladder by the ureters, 2 small tubes which extend down from the basin of the kidneys over the brim of the pelvis and open into the bladder at about the level of the cervix. The bladder is emptied through the urethra, a short tube which terminates in the meatus (Fig. 36). Lying on either side of the urethra and almost parallel with it are 2 small glands, less than 1 inch long, known as Skene's glands. Their ducts empty into the urethra just above the meatus. Often in cases of gonorrhea, Skene's glands and ducts are involved (see Fig. 37).

Anus. The anus is the entrance to the rectal canal. The rectal canal is surrounded at the opening or anus by its sphincter muscle, which binds it to the coccyx behind and to the perineum in front. It is supported by the muscles passing into it (see Fig. 38).

The muscles involved are those that aid in supporting the pelvic floor. The rectum is considered here because of the proximity to the field of delivery.

MAMMARY GLANDS

Breasts. The breasts, or mammary glands, are 2 highly specialized cutaneous glands located on either side of the anterior wall of the chest between the third and the seventh rib (Fig. 43). Because they are abundantly supplied with nerves, formerly it was believed that direct nervous system connection existed between the uterus and the breasts. But the demonstration that lactation can be established after excluding the spinal nervous mechanism by severing all nerves supplying the breasts clearly indicated that some other factor must be involved in the explanation of mammary changes in pregnancy. It is evident that the stimulation to growth of the mammary gland is hormonal and not nervous in origin.

The internal mammary and the intercostal arteries supply the breast gland, and the mammary veins follow these arteries. Also, there are many cutaneous veins which become dilated during lactation. The lymphatics are abundant, especially toward the axilla. These breast glands are present in the male, but only in the rudimentary state, and are not connected by the sympathetic

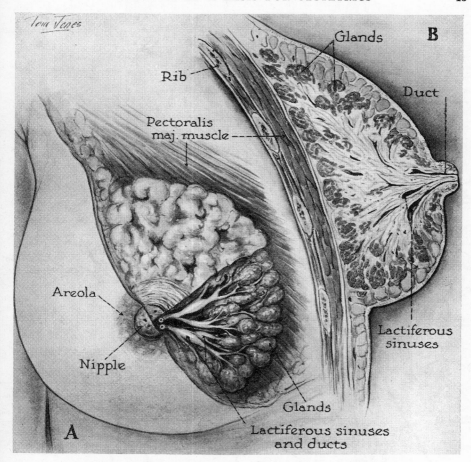

Fig. 43. (A) Mammary gland, showing the lactiferous ducts and sinuses. (B) Cross section of the breast.

system to the male generative organs.

INTERNAL STRUCTURE. The breasts of a woman who never has borne a child are, in general, conic or hemispheric in form, but they vary in size and shape at different ages and in different individuals. In women who have nursed one or more babies they tend to become pendulous. At the termination of lactation, certain exercises aid in restoring the tone of the breast tissue.

The breasts are made up of glandular tissue and fat. Each organ is divided into 15 or 20 lobes, which are separated from each other by fibrous and fatty walls. Each lobe is subdivided into many lobules, and these contain numerous acini which are lined with a single layer of cells enveloped in a capillary network. By the process of osmosis the products necessary for the milk are filtered from the blood, but the secretion of the milk really begins in the acini cells. As the ducts leading from the lobules to the lobes and from the lobes approach the nipple they are di-

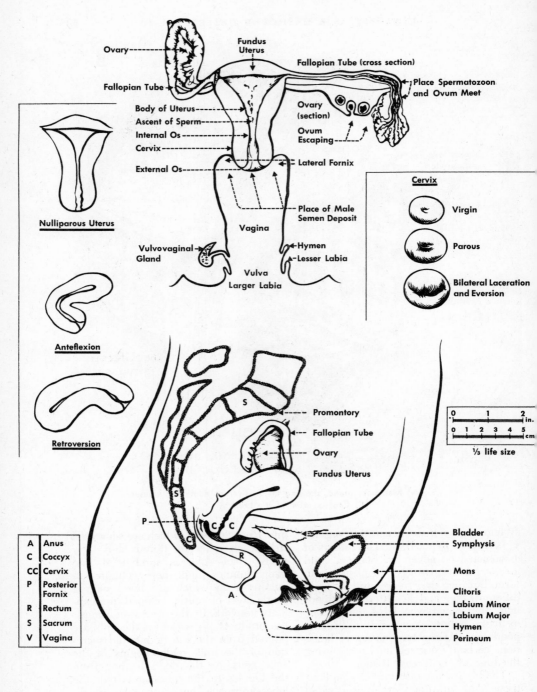

Nulliparous Uterus

Ovary

Fundus
Uterus

Fallopian Tube (cross section)

Fallopian Tube

Place Spermatozoon
and Ovum Meet

Body of Uterus
Ascent of Sperm
Internal Os
Cervix

Ovary
(section)

Ovum
Escaping

External Os

Lateral Fornix

Place of Male
Semen Deposit

Vagina

Vulvovaginal
Gland

Hymen
Lesser Labia

Vulva
Larger Labia

Cervix

Virgin

Parous

Bilateral Laceration
and Eversion

Anteflexion

Retroversion

Promontory

Fallopian Tube

Ovary

Fundus Uterus

| 0 | | 1 | | 2 | in. |
| 0 | 1 2 3 4 5 | | | | cm |

⅓ life size

Bladder
Symphysis

Mons

Clitoris
Labium Minor
Labium Major
Hymen
Perineum

A	Anus
C	Coccyx
CC	Cervix
P	Posterior Fornix
R	Rectum
S	Sacrum
V	Vagina

Fig. 44. Female anatomy. (Dickinson, Robert L.: Human Sex Anatomy,
Baltimore, Williams & Wilkins)

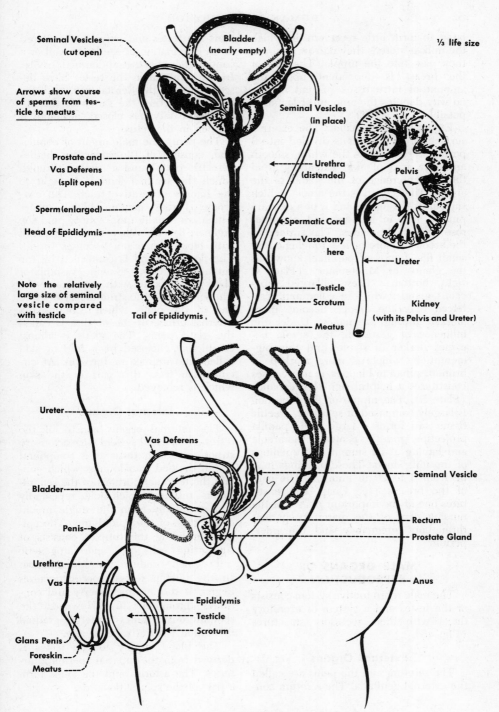

Seminal Vesicles
(cut open)

Bladder
(nearly empty)

⅓ life size

Arrows show course
of sperms from tes-
ticle to meatus

Seminal Vesicles
(in place)

Urethra
(distended)

Pelvis

Prostate and
Vas Deferens
(split open)

Sperm (enlarged)

Head of Epididymis

Spermatic Cord

Vasectomy
here

Ureter

Note the relatively
large size of seminal
vesicle compared
with testicle

Testicle

Scrotum

Tail of Epididymis

Kidney
(with its Pelvis and Ureter)

Meatus

Ureter

Vas Deferens

Seminal Vesicle

Bladder

Rectum

Penis

Prostate Gland

Urethra

Vas

Anus

Epididymis

Testicle

Scrotum

Glans Penis

Foreskin

Meatus

Fig. 45. Male anatomy. (Dickinson: Human Sex Anatomy, Williams & Wilkins)

lated to form little reservoirs in which the milk is stored; they narrow again as they pass into the nipple. The size of the breast is dependent upon the amount of fatty tissue present and in no way denotes the amount of lactation possible.

EXTERNAL STRUCTURE. The external surface of the breasts is divided into 3 portions. The first is the white, smooth and soft area of skin extending from the circumference of the gland to the areola. The second is the areola, which surrounds the nipple and is of a delicate pinkish hue in blondes and a darker rose color in brunettes. The surface of the areola is more or less roughened by small fine lumps of papillae, known as the glands of Montgomery (Plate 4, right, bottom). These enlarged sebaceous glands, white in color and scatterred over the areola, become more marked during pregnancy. Under the influence of gestation, the areola becomes darker in shade, and this pigmentation, which is more marked in brunettes than in blondes, in many cases constitutes a helpful sign of pregnancy (Plate 5). The nipple or third portion is largely composed of sensitive, erectile tissue and forms a large conic papilla projecting from the center of the areola and having at its summit the openings of the milk ducts. These openings may be from 3 to 20 in number. The care of the breasts (see Chap. 8) constitutes one of the important phases of the nursing care of the maternity patient throughout pregnancy and the puerperium.

MALE ORGANS OF REPRODUCTION

The male reproductive system consists of the testes and a system of excretory ducts with their accessory structures (Fig. 45).

External Organs

The scrotum and the penis are called the external genitalia. The scrotum contains the testes and may be considered as an evagination of the body wall or a continuation of the abdominal cavity. In the adult male the testes have descended into the scrotal sac, and the canal connecting the sac with the abdominal cavity has closed, although it is open in the fetus.

The penis, the male organ of copulation, consists of the cavernous bodies (erectile parts) and a urethra through which the seminal fluid is brought to the female generative tract. The cavernous bodies contain blood spaces which are usually quite empty, and the organ is flaccid. When these spaces fill with blood the organ becomes turgid. The flow of blood is controlled by the autonomic nervous system (vasodilator fibers) and varies with sexual activity. The enlarged conic structure at the free end of the penis which contains the external orifice of the urethra is called the glans penis. The glans is almost completely enclosed by a fold of skin called the prepuce or foreskin. At circumcision it is this part of the skin which is removed.

Internal Organs

The internal organs consist of the testes and a canal system with accessory structures. Each testis is a compound gland, divided into lobules which contain the terminal portions of the seminiferous tubules which join repeatedly and eventually form the single muchcoiled tube of the epididymis. The epithelium lining the tubules consists of supporting cells and spermatogenetic cells which produce the spermatozoa. In the human testes, spermatogenesis begins at the age of puberty and continues throughout life. However, the seminiferous tubules undergo gradual involution with advancing age.

The blood supply to the testes is derived from the internal spermatic arteries. The arteries and the veins form a part of the spermatic cords.

The lymphatic vessels accompany the blood vessels in the spermatic cord, and eventually the lymphatics empty into the lumbar lymph nodes.

The efferent nerves which supply the testes are derived from the thoracolumbar and sacral divisions of the autonomic system. They are distributed chiefly to the walls of the blood vessels. Afferent fibers convey impulses from these structures to the central nervous system.

The canal system consists of the epididymis (which is made up of numerous seminiferous tubules), the ductus deferens (which passes from the epididymis to the ejaculatory duct), the ejaculatory duct (formed by the union of the ductus deferens and the duct of the seminal vesicle) and the urethra, which is surrounded by the prostate gland and terminates in the penis.

The accessory structures consist of the seminal vesicles (sacculated structures located behind the bladder and in front of the rectum), the prostate gland (which surrounds the base of the urethra and the ejaculatory duct) and the bulbo-urethral glands or Cowper's glands (which lie at the base of the prostate and on either side of the membranous urethra).

SUGGESTED READING

Caldwell, W. E., and Moloy, H. C.: Anatomical variations in the female pelvis and their effect in labor with a suggested classification, Am. J. Obst. & Gynec. **26**:479, 1933.

Dippel, A. L.: The diagonal conjugate versus x-ray pelvimetry, Surg., Gynec. & Obst. **68**:642, 1939.

Greisheimer, Esther M.: Physiology and Anatomy, ed. 7, Philadelphia, Lippincott, 1955.

Mengert, W. F., and Eller, W. C.: Graphic portrayal of relative pelvic size, Am. J. Obst. & Gynec. **52**:1032, 1946.

Netter, Frank H.: Reproductive System, Summit, N. J., Ciba Pharmaceutical, 1954.

Thoms, H.: Outlet pelvimetry, Surg., Gynec. & Obst. **83**:399, 1946.

——: A discussion of pelvic variations and a report on the findings, Am. J. Obst. & Gynec. **52**:248, 1946.

CHAPTER THREE

Physiology in Relation to Obstetrics

Only a brief statement of the most elementary facts of physiology, the science dealing with the functions of the organs and tissues of the body, can be attempted here, but such a review is essential, in order that the nurse may better understand the special relation of physiology to the problems in obstetrics.

SEXUAL MATURITY

Evidences of sexual maturity in the female begin at the time of puberty with the establishment of the specific reproductive functions of ovulation and menstruation. At puberty certain well-defined changes take place; the establishment of the menses, the monthly bloody discharge from the uterus, is an indication that the internal organs have matured. Changes in the external organs, such as an increase in size and the appearance of axillary and pubic hair are other evidences of this period of development; the breasts at this time also become larger and more prominent. Along with these physical changes are emotional changes as well.

Puberty

Puberty usually occurs between the ages of 12 and 16, although heredity, race, climate and environment may influence its early or late appearance; for example, maturity tends to appear earlier in warm climates and later in cold regions. The reproductive period covers about 30 years, from the beginning of menstruation, at or about the age of 12, until its cessation during the menopause, at about the age of 45.

Ovulation and Menstruation

Ovulation. Each month, with considerable regularity, a blisterlike structure about half an inch in diameter develops on the surface of one or the other ovary. Inside this bubble, almost lost in the fluid about it, lies a tiny speck, scarcely visible to the naked eye; a thimble would hold 3 million of them. This little speck is the human ovum—a truly amazing structure. It possesses within its diminutive compass not only the potentialities of developing into a human being with all the complicated physical organization entailed, but also embodies the mental as well as the physical traits of the woman and her forbears: perhaps her own brown eyes or her father's tall stature, possibly her mother's love of music or her grandfather's genius at mathematics. These and a million other potentialities are all wrapped in this little speck, or ovum, so small that it is about one fourth the size of the period at the end of this sentence.

With the exact periodicity which characterizes so many of Nature's works, one blister on one ovary bursts at a definite time each month and discharges an ovum, a process known as *ovulation*. The precise day on which ovulation occurs is a matter of no small importance. For instance, since the ovum can be fertilized (or impregnated by the male germ cell) only within the 36-hour period after its escape from the ovary, this is the only time when a woman is really fertile. During the rest of the monthly cycle, theoretically at least, it is impossible for her to conceive. Evidence of various sorts indicates that ovulation usually occurs between the 10th and the 16th days of the menstrual cycle, counting from the day on which bleeding begins. Ordinarily, then, the most fertile time is a week to 10 days after the cessation of menstruation. While this is the rule, there are many exceptions, and ovulation may take place at any time between the 9th and the 18th days of the cycle. The fact that ovulation rarely occurs during the last 10 days of a 28-day cycle has given rise to the birth-control doctrine of the "safe period," or "rhythm," according to which it is impossible to conceive after the 18th day. Theoretically, this claim is altogether sound; practically, not a few women appear to have conceived during this period, so that it would seem that occasionally ovulation may take place later than theory would indicate.

Graafian Follicle. In delving further into this process of ovulation, we find that at birth each ovary contains a huge number of undeveloped ova, probably more than 100,000. These are rather large round cells with clear cytoplasm and a good-sized nucleus occupying the center. Each of these ova is surrounded by a layer of a few small, flattened or spindle-shaped cells. The whole structure—ovum and surrounding cells—is spoken of as a "follicle," while in its underdeveloped state at birth it is referred to as a "primordial follicle." It is the consensus that the manufacture of these primordial follicles ceases at birth or shortly after, and that the large number contained in the ovaries of the newborn represents a lifetime's supply. Nevertheless, the majority of these disappear before puberty so that there are then perhaps 30,000 or so left in each ovary. This disintegration of follicles continues throughout the reproductive period, with the result that usually none are found after the menopause.

Meanwhile, from birth to the menopause, a certain few of these primordial follicles show signs of development. The surrounding granular layer of cells begins to multiply rapidly until they are several layers deep, at the same time becoming cuboidal in shape. As this proliferation of cells continues, a very important fluid develops between them, the follicular fluid. After puberty this accumulates in such quantities that the multiplying follicle cells are pushed toward the margin, and the ovum itself is almost surrounded by fluid, being suspended from the periphery of the follicle by only a small neck or isthmus of cells. The structure is now known as the *graafian follicle*, after the famous Dutch physician who in 1672 first described it (Figs. 46 and 47). While increasing in size so enormously, the graafian follicle naturally pushes aside other follicles, forming each month, as has been said, a very noticeable, blisterlike projection on the surface of the ovary. At one point the follicular capsule becomes thin, and as the ovum reaches full maturity, it breaks free from the few cells attaching it to the periphery and floats in the follicular fluid. The thinned area of the capsule now ruptures, and the ovum is expelled into the peritoneal cavity.

Changes in the Corpus Luteum. After the discharge of the ovum, the ruptured follicle undergoes a change. It becomes filled with large cells containing a special yellow colored matter called lutein. The follicle is then known as the corpus luteum or yellow body. If pregnancy does not occur, the corpus luteum reaches full development in about 8 days, then retrogresses and is gradu-

Fig. 46. Ovary with
graafian follicle.

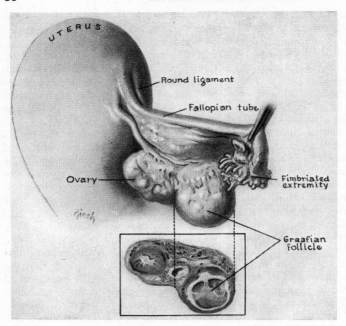

ally replaced by fibrous tissue, corpus albicans. If pregnancy does occur, the corpus luteum enlarges somewhat and persists throughout the period of gestation, reaching its maximum size about the 4th or 5th month and retrogressing slowly thereafter. The corpus luteum secretes an extremely important substance, *progesterone*, which will be considered in a later section of this chapter.

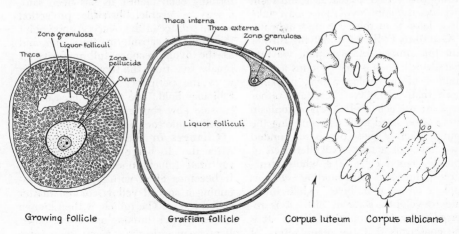

Fig. 47. Development of the graafian follicle.

BASAL TEMPERATURE RECORD

NAME _Jane Doe_ ADDRESS _10 Main St._ PHONE _24107_

FOR DR. _Wm. Smith_ ADDRESS _8 State St._ PHONE _25621_

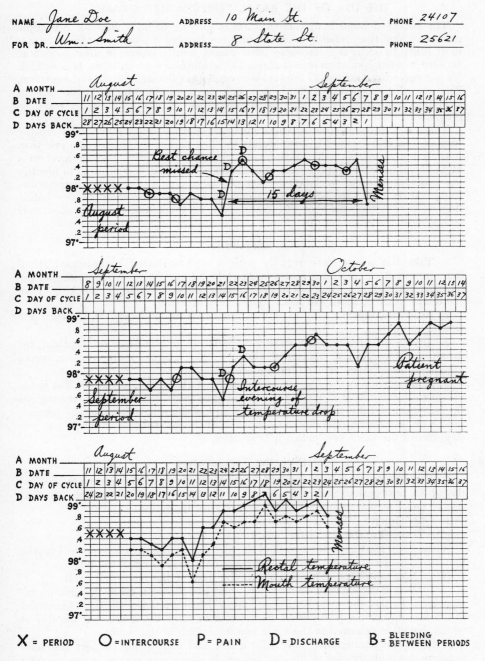

X = PERIOD   O = INTERCOURSE   P = PAIN   D = DISCHARGE   B = BLEEDING BETWEEN PERIODS

PUBLISHED UNDER THE AUSPICES OF THE MEDICAL COMMITTEE OF THE PLANNED PARENTHOOD FEDERATION OF AMERICA, INC.

Fig. 48. Directions for using this chart are given on the 2 following pages.

THE USE OF THE BASAL TEMPERATURE GRAPHS

The taking of basal body temperatures is proving to be a valuable procedure in determining the probable ovulation and in planning a pregnancy. Pregnancy is most likely to occur if intercourse takes places shortly before or after ovulation. In most women, ovulation occurs about 14 days before menstruation. It is difficult for patients whose menstrual interval is irregular to calculate the date of ovulation. The use of a temperature graph may help to determine the probable time of ovulation, and hence the time when intercourse is mostly likely to result in pregnancy.

There is a slight rhythm of variation in the normal temperature of a healthy woman. Her temperature is lower during the first part of the menstrual cycle than it is during the latter half. Furthermore, the transition from a lower level to a higher level occurs about the time of ovulation. Therefore, it is possible to identify the probable date of ovulation by keeping a record of the body temperature. Temperature may vary slightly from day to day from one tenth to one half a degree, so it is essential that the temperature be taken and recorded accurately according to the following directions:

Directions

1. Take the temperature rectally with a well-lubricated blunt-tipped rectal thermometer for *Five (5) Minutes by the Clock Immediately After* waking in the morning and *Before* getting out of bed, talking, eating, drinking or smoking. Take the temperature at about *the Same Time Every Morning*.

2. Read the thermometer to within one tenth of a degree and record the reading accurately.

3. Any known cause for temperature variation should be noted on the chart, for example, interrupted or shortened sleep, a cold, grippe, indigestion, a severe emotional disturbance or even indulgence in alcohol.

4. Some women can recognize ovulation by a characteristic pain in the lower abdomen. Others have slight vaginal bleeding or increased clear, slippery vaginal discharge around the time of ovulation. If any of these manifestations is present, note it on the chart on the day of occurrence. If the pain occurs on more than one day, record the exact hour when it is greatest.

Plotting the Temperature

1. The menstrual cycle is counted from the first day of one period to the first day of the next period. Start a new graph at the beginning of the period. The first day of menstruation is marked as the first day of the cycle.

2. (A) MONTH—Write the month on this line.

(B) DATE—Put the day of the month on this line.

Write down the day of the month of the first day of menstruation above 1 on the line for "day of cycle" and continue with the days to the end of the line.

(C) DAYS OF CYCLE—This line shows the days of the menstrual cycle.

(D) DAYS BACK—When the next menstrual period starts, fill in this line beginning with the day the period starts and from then on number the days backward to the first day of the past period. This serves to show the number of the day at which ovulation occurred in the cycle and the length of the cycle.

3. Chart the temperature daily with a dot, and with a line connect this temperature dot with the dot of the day before. If intercourse occurs in the morning

encircle the dot. If it takes place at night mark the circle on the line between that dot and the temperature dot of the next morning.

4. It is necessary to continue the graph for at least two menstrual cycles before the probable time of ovulation can be judged. Sexual abstinence for several days before ovulation allows time for the male to store up sperm and probably increase the chance of fertilization.

5. The temperature will fall and rise within a range of ½ to 1 degree. Watch for a drop in temperature about 15 days before the expected period. The last drop in the cycle (usually the largest) is the important one, and intercourse should take place that day or evening.

Mouth Temperature

Temperature may be taken by mouth immediately upon awakening, *Before Getting Out of Bed and Before Talking, Eating, Drinking or Smoking*. Mouth temperatures show the same variations as rectal. However, mouth temperatures are not usually as marked as the rectal.

MENSTRUAL CYCLE

Menstruation in Relation to Pregnancy

Menstruation is the periodic discharge of blood, mucus and epithelial cells from the uterus. If the individual is normal, it occurs throughout the reproductive period at fairly regular intervals of about 28 days, except during pregnancy and lactation when it is usually suppressed entirely. Accordingly, the span of years during which childbearing usually is possible—that is, from the age of about 12 to 45—corresponds to the period during which menstruation occurs. In general, moreover, a woman who menstruates is able to conceive, whereas one who does not is probably sterile. There is good reason for believing, therefore, that these two phenomena are closely interlinked, and, since no process of Nature is purposeless, that menstruation must play some vital and indispensable role in childbearing. What is this role?

If, day by day, we were privileged to watch the endometrium or lining membrane of the uterus, we should observe some remarkable alterations. Immediately following the termination of a menstrual period, this membrane is very thin, measuring perhaps a twen-tieth of an inch in depth. Each day thereafter it becomes a trifle thicker and harbors an increasing content of blood, while its glands become more and more active, secreting a rich nutritive substance which used to be called "uterine milk." About a week before the onset of the next expected period this process reaches its height; the endometrium is now of the thickness of heavy, downy velvet and has become soft and succulent with blood and glandular secretions. At this time the egg, if one has been fertilized, embeds itself into this luxuriant lining.

All these changes have only one purpose: to provide a suitable bed in which the fertilized ovum may rest, secure nourishment and grow. If an egg is not fertilized, these alterations are unnecessary; accordingly, through a mechanism which even today is obscure, the swollen endometrium disintegrates, and the encased blood and glandular secretions escape into the uterine cavity; passing through the cervix they flow out through the vagina, carrying the egg with them. In other words, menstruation represents the abrupt termination of a process designed to prepare board and lodging, as it were, for a fertilized ovum; it betokens the breakdown of a bed which was not needed because the "boarder" did not materialize; its purpose then is to clear away the old bed in order that a new and fresh one may be created the next month.

Hormonal Control of Menstruation

If, while watching the changes in the endometrium during the menstrual cycle, as described above, it were possible to inspect the ovaries from day to day, it would be noted that the uterine alterations are directly related to certain phenomena which take place in the ovary.

Immediately following menstruation, it will be recalled, the endometrium is very thin. During the subsequent week or so it proliferates markedly. The cells on the surface become taller, while the glands which dip into the endometrium become longer and wider. As the result of these changes the thickness of the endometrium increases 6-fold or 8-fold. During this phase of the menstrual cycle (from the 5th to the 14th day, approximately) a graafian follicle each month is approaching its greatest development and is manufacturing increasing amounts of follicular fluid. This fluid contains a most important substance, the estrogenic hormone—or, as it is sometimes called, "estrogen." A hormone, it will be remembered, is a specific organic substance which is produced by an endocrine or ductless gland and passes directly into the blood stream which transports it to other parts of the body where it performs a specific function. The word "hormone" comes from a Greek word which means "I bring about," and in the case of estrogen it brings about (among other things) the thickening of the endometrium described. Each month, then, after the cessation of menstruation, a developing graafian follicle manufactures this hormone, estrogen, as an ingredient of the follicular fluid; and estrogen acts on the endometrium to build it up. For this reason this phase of the menstrual cycle is often referred to as the follicular or estrogenic phase. However, it is more commonly referred to as the *proliferative phase*. The first four or five days of this phase are sometimes called the *resting* or *postmenstrual phase*.

Following rupture of the graafian follicle (ovulation), the cells which form the corpus luteum begin to secrete, in addition to estrogen, another important hormone, progesterone. This supplements the action of estrogen on the endometrium in such a way that the glands become very tortuous or corkscrew in appearance and are greatly dilated. This change is due to the fact that they are swollen with a secretion containing large amounts of glycogen and mucin. Meanwhile, the blood supply of the endometrium is increased, with the result that it becomes very vascular and succulent. Since these effects are directed at providing a bed for the fertilized ovum, it is easy to understand why the hormone which brings them about is called "progesterone," meaning "for gestation." It is also clear why this phase of the cycle (from the 14th to the 28th day, approximately) is sometimes called the *progestational phase*, and also why occasionally it is referred to as the *luteal phase*. More commonly, perhaps, it is called the *secretory*, or *premenstrual, phase*.

Unless the ovum is fertilized, the corpus luteum is short-lived, and its activity ceases after about 10 days (or around the 25th day of the cycle). Since corpus luteum cells secrete not only progesterone but also estrogen, cessation of corpus luteum activity means a withdrawl of both of these hormones which have been responsible for building up the endometrium. As a result, the endometrium degenerates. This is associated with rupture of countless small blood vessels in the endometrium with innumerable minute hemorrhages. Along with the blood, superficial fragments of the endometrium, together with mucin from the glands, are cast

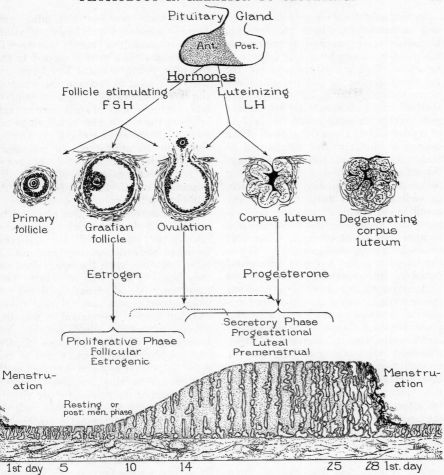

Fig. 49. Hormonal control of the normal menstrual cycle.

away, and all this constitutes the menstrual discharge (Fig. 49). Naturally, this phase of the cycle (the 1st to the 5th day, approximately) is called the *menstrual phase*.

The pituitary gland is of considerable importance in the function of the reproductive system. The *anterior lobe* of the pituitary, the "master clock," secretes, among other hormones, two hormones whose function is to produce these ovarian alterations at fairly regular monthly intervals during the repro-

ductive years. One is called the follicle-stimulating hormone (sometimes abbreviated as FSH), active from the 5th to the 15th day of the cycle, and the other is the luteinizing hormone (LH), active during the luteal phase. The posterior lobe of the pituitary produces internal secretions which are also important in obstetrics but have altogether different functions for the present discussion. A third hormone, gonadotropin, derived from the chorion, is discussed on page 125.

In addition to their role in controlling menstruation, these two ovarian hormones, estrogen and progesterone, have other far-reaching and important functions. Estrogen is responsible for the development of the secondary sex characteristics, that is, for all those distinctive sex manifestations which are not directly concerned with the process of reproduction. Thus, the growth of the breasts at puberty, the distribution of body fat, the appearance of pubic hair, the size of the larynx and its resulting influence on the quality of the voice, as well as mating instincts are all the result of estrogenic action. We may almost say, therefore, that a woman is a woman because of estrogen. Often this hormone is used therapeutically. When the nurse is called upon to administer estrogen intramuscularly, she should understand that it may be labeled on the ampule or other container by various trade names devised by the several pharmaceutical companies. Among these are: Theelin, Theelol, Amniotin, Oestrin, Follicular Hormone and Progynon B. During recent years a synthetic (artificially manufactured) form of estrogen, named stilbestrol, has been used widely. Its effects are essentially the same as estrogen.

Aside from its action on the endometrium, progesterone plays a most important role in preserving the life of the embryo during the first two or three months of pregnancy. It also has a relaxing action on the uterine muscle. For these two reasons, sometimes it is employed therapeutically in cases in which there is a tendency to abort (miscarry —see p. 404). In this connection, the nurse will usually encounter it under the trade name Proluton.

Clinical Aspects of Menstruation

From what has been said concerning the underlying mechanism of menstruation, it is clear that the monthly flow of blood is only one phase of a marvelous cyclic process which not only makes childbearing possible but also profoundly influences both body and mind. For this reason the time of the onset of menstruation is a critical period in the life of a young woman. The term menarche is used to indicate the onset of the first menstruation. The term puberty has a much broader connotation and refers to the whole transitional stage between childhood and maturity. During this time the appearance of secondary sex characteristics and the development of sex consciousness are other equally important manifestations. Not only do notable bodily changes occur, but a radical transformation takes place in the mental attitude of the girl. She matures rapidly in mind, and her interests broaden. Nevertheless, her emotions are often unstable, with the result that she may laugh or cry without reason. This transition period from girlhood to womanhood is sometimes a most trying one, but a good foundation in sex education from early childhood so that knowledge of the physical bodily changes and careful observance of the rules of general hygiene, together with tolerance, sympathy and understanding on the part of parents and those closely associated with the adolescent, will do much to secure a normal adjustment.

The average age of the onset of menstruation is between 13 and 14 years. It may be as early as the tenth year or as late as the seventeenth year and still be within normal limits. Although the interval of the menstrual cycle, counting from the beginning of one period to the onset of the next, averages 28 days, there are wide variations even in the same woman. Indeed, there is scarcely a woman who menstruates exactly every 28 or 30 days. This question has been the subject of several studies on normal young women, chiefly student nurses, who have conscientiously recorded the time and the nature of each period. These investigations show that the majority of women (almost 60%) experience variations of at least 5 days in the length of their menstrual cycles; differences in the same woman of even 10 days are not uncommon and may occur without explanation or apparent detriment to health. For reasons which even today are obscure, menstrual blood does not clot.

Normal menstruation should not be accompanied by pain, although quite often there is some general malaise, together with a feeling of weight and discomfort in the pelvis. Frequent, also, are such disturbances as a sense of fatigue, headache, backache, sensitivity in the breasts and unstable emotional reactions. If there is great irregularity or extremely profuse flow or marked pain, a pathologic condition may be present. Painful menstruation is known as *dysmenorrhea*. Absence of the menses is known as *amenorrhea*. The most common cause of amenorrhea is pregnancy, but sometimes it is brought about by emotional disturbances, such as fear, worry or fatigue, or disease (anemia, tuberculosis), and occasionally it may be the result of a decided change in climate.

The cessation of menstrual function usually occurs between the ages of 45 and 50. The period over which this alteration takes place is known as the *menopause,* or *climacteric,* but generally it is referred to by the laity as the *"change of life."* About one half of all women cease menstruating between these years, about one fourth stop before 45, and another quarter continue to menstruate until past 50.

INFERTILITY

Although the problem of infertility is considered in the field of gynecology, it is a factor which has complicated the childbearing of many women. Thus, the obstetric nurse needs to be aware of its implications.

Dr. Abraham Stone stated that the United States Census Bureau's records show that more than 15 per cent of all married women never bear any children, and most of this childlessness is involuntary. Within the last quarter of a century many very important scientific advances have been made in the field of human infertility. Two newer concepts are of particular significance. One is that impaired fertility is most often due not to a single cause but to a multiplicity of factors. Systemic, local, nutritional, glandular and emotional conditions affect both the husband and the wife; therefore, in each instance it is necessary to make a complete study of the history of the health situation and mode of life of the couple. The second concept is that the husband bears a far greater responsibility as a factor in sterile matings than had been recognized previously. Indeed, modern investigations indicate that about 40 per cent of cases of sterility are attributable to deficiencies on the part of the husband.

A few of the causes in women may be failure of ovulation, obstructions in the genital tract, especially in the cervix or the fallopian tubes, or disturbances in the development of the uterus and its lining which interfere with the implantation and the growth of the fertilized ovum. In the male the causes may be deficiency in the seminal fluid and particularly in the quantity and the quality of the spermatozoa, or obstructions in the seminal ducts which prevent the spermatozoa from passing through. Lack of sperm production may be caused by developmental anomalies, glandular disturbances, local injuries or infections and constitutional diseases.

Due to modern developments in the field of human infertility, about 30 per cent of the barren marriages can be rendered fertile. Today there is continued research in the physiologic and psychological aspects of reproduction, and physicians have available better technics and methods for the diagnosis and the treatment of infertility.

MENOPAUSE

In a general way, the earlier puberty

occurs, the later the menopause; conversely, the later puberty is experienced, the earlier the menopause. The menopause is usually a gradual process; the periods first become scanty, then one may be absent, and finally they cease altogether.

The cause of the menopause is cessation of ovarian activity. Having functioned for some 30 years, the ovary now shrivels up into a small, flat organ composed mostly of scar tissue. As a consequence, estrogen is no longer produced. This permanent and complete withdrawal of estrogen results in atrophy of the uterus, the fallopian tubes, the vagina and the vulva. The absence of the hormone sometimes also produces certain nervous symptoms, such as flushing of the face and the body, sensations of heat ("hot flashes") and cold, sweating, hyperexcitability and irritability. Estrogen, either as the pure hormone or as stilbestrol, finds its greatest therapeutic usefulness in these menopausal disorders. The better one's general health, the more surely one can look forward to an uneventful menopause.

SUGGESTED READING

Corner, G. W.: The Hormones in Human Reproduction, Princeton, 1942.

Guttmacher, A. F.: Life in the Making, New York, Viking, 1933.

——: Into This Universe, New York, Viking, 1937. (Published also under the title "The Story of Human Birth," Blue Ribbon Books, 1939.)

——: Babies by unknown fathers, Parents Magazine, Feb., 1949.

Kurzrock, Raphael: The menopause *in* Transactions of the Third American Congress on Obstetrics and Gynecology, p. 282, St. Louis, Mosby.

Tyler, Edward T.: Semen studies and fertility, J.A.M.A. **146**:307, 1951.

CHAPTER FOUR

Development and Physiology
of the Fetus

In all Nature's wide universe of miracles there is no process more wondrous, no mechanism more incredibly fantastic, than the one by which a tiny speck of tissue, the human egg, develops into a 7-pound baby. So miraculous did primitive peoples consider this phenomenon that they frequently ascribed it all to superhuman intervention and even overlooked the fact that sexual intercourse was a necessary precursor. Throughout unremembered ages our own primitive ancestors doubtless held similar beliefs, but now we know that pregnancy comes about in only one way: from the union of a female germ cell, the egg or ovum, with a male germ cell, the spermatozoon (Fig. 50). These two gametes, ovum and spermatozoon, become fused into one cell or zygote which contains the characteristics of both the female and the male from which these gametes originated.

MATURATION OF OVUM AND
SPERM CELLS

By the time the two sex cells or gametes, ovum and spermatozoon, in humans are matured or ready for union, a number of peculiar changes have occurred previously, as shown in Figure 51.

Typical cells of the testes and the ovary are shown at the top of the dia-

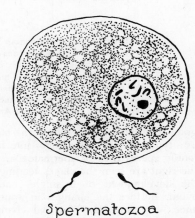

Fig. 50. Relative size of spermatozoa and ovum. (After Eastman)

65

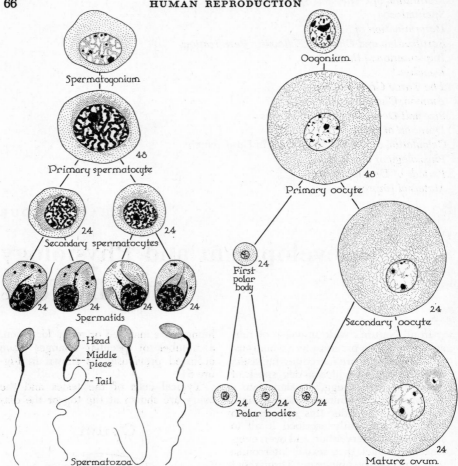

Fig. 51. Diagram of gametogenesis with maturation. The various stages of spermato-genesis are indicated on the left; one spermatogonium gives rise to 4 spermatozoa. On the right, the oogenesis of the ovum is indicated; from each oogonium, 1 mature ovum and 3 abortive cells are produced. In maturation, the chromosomes are reduced to one half the number characteristic for the general body cells of the species, as indicated; in man, the number in the body cells is 48, and that in the mature spermatozoon and ovum is 24. (Greisheimer, E. M.: Physiology and Anatomy, ed. 7, Philadelphia, Lippincott)

gram. On the left are shown the steps as a typical testes cell changes into four motile sperm cells or spermatozoa. On the right are seen the stages leading to the development of a single mature ovum. Besides the changes in appearance, very important internal changes have also taken place. The chromo-somes, normally 48* in all cell tissues of man, have been reduced in number in both kinds of sex cells—ovum and sper-matozoon. Each motile spermatozoon now has 24 chromosomes in its nucleus; the number at each stage in the forma-tion of the spermatozoon is indicated by small figures at the lower right at each

* This text presents the classic interpretation—48 chromosomes with their factors of 24 and 96. Recent research indicates the greater likelihood of 46 (44 regular plus "X" plus "Y") and the resultant factors of 23 and 92.

stage. The ovum, too, contains only 24 chromosomes, its chromosomes having been reduced not by division but by extrusion of chromosome material, called "polar bodies" because they were observed at one pole of the developing ovum. Their remnants are shown in the cells in the top row of Figure 55. They finally become lost and need not be considered here, as they play no active part in reproduction.

The maturation of the ovum takes place about the time of ovulation and is probably complete before the ovum is discharged from the graafian follicle. The spermatozoon is also fully matured before it is discharged.

The chromosomes differ in form and size, ranging from small spherical masses to long rods which are often bent to resemble the letters V and J.

Every human cell—whatever the tissue—has 48 chromosomes. The reduction to 24 in each gamete means that the fertilized ovum has 48 chromosomes, the number characteristic of all human cells. In every cell division from now on to adulthood and throughout the differentiation of all tissues, each will have 48 chromosomes. This is accomplished by an internal change in the cell before division, in which the 48 chromosomes split into halves, and each of the two new cells receives half of the 96 halves or 48 chromosomes. This splitting and halving is continued in all dividing cells until growth ceases.

It is only as a preparation for reproduction by the fertilization of an ovum by a spermatozoon that this number varies, as described above.

Within the chromosomes are contained the ultramicroscopic self-perpetuating bodies called genes, and each gene carries one or more special characteristics. To these genes are attributed such differences as color of hair and eyes, body build and facial characteristics. Each gamete, ovum and spermatozoon comes from a different person with a different ancestral history and different genes in its 24 chromosomes. Since a single gene may carry more than one character, there may be numerous variable results in the offspring of any two parents. The hereditary possibilities discarded or retained in the mature gametes is a matter of chance, but the nature of the combination of the germ plasm which occurs in each generation when two gametes fuse in fertilization is of great significance. If either parent brings defective germ plasm, the result may affect the zygote and the characteristics of the child which results.

Biologists have estimated that at the time of the reduction division some 17 million different combinations are possible due to the interchange of genes. Apparently there is sufficient stability produced during this intricate interchange process to ensure characteristics of the progenitors.

Ova

As described in Chapter 3, ova normally are discharged from the human ovary at the rate of 1 a month. The ovum at this time is a relatively large cell, measures about 0.2 millimeters (1/125 of an inch) and is just visible to the naked eye. The nucleus is small in comparison with the amount of cytoplasm and contains many strands or filaments of deeply staining material. These minute particles are called chromosomes and are the all-important links in the endless chain of heredity; they were discussed in more detail in a previous paragraph of this chapter. The large amount of cytoplasm surrounding the nucleus contains a small quantity of nutritive material in the form of yolk granules. The surface of the ovum is immediately surrounded by a thick membrane, the zona pellucida (translucent belt).

Transport Through the Fallopian Tube

After the ovum has been discharged

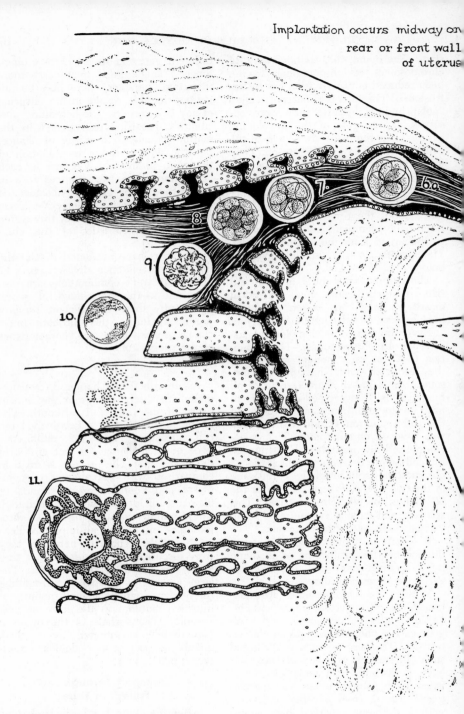

Implantation occurs midway on
rear or front wall
of uterus

Fig. 52. Travel of egg from ovary through implantation, with alterations en route: 3 days in tube, 4 days in uterus before implantation. (Robert L. Dickinson, M.D., New York, adapted from Sellheim, with suggestions from Streeter, Frank and Hartman)

1. Follicle bursts.
2. Ovum with adhering granulosa cells.
   First polar body.
   2nd. maturation spindle.
3. Sperm enters egg.
   2nd. maturation division
4. Male and Female pronuclei

5. Pronuclei fusing
   Fertilization accomplished
   5a. First cleavage division
6-7 Early cleavage
   8. Morula.
9-10. Early and later gastrula
   11 Fully implanted growing embryo. (Miller.)

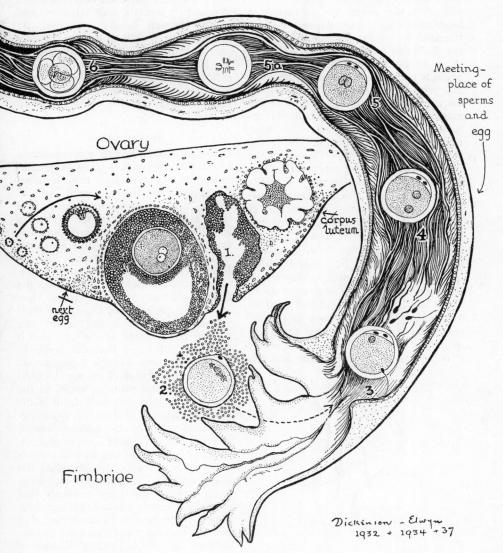

Meeting-place of sperms and egg

Ovary

corpus luteum

next egg

Fimbriae

Dickinson - Elwyn
1932 + 1934 + 37

from the ovary it faces a 10-day journey. Its goal is the cavity of the uterus, more than 3 inches away (Fig. 52). The only pathway of approach is the tortuous fallopian tube, whose lining is wrinkled unevenly by the folds of tubal epithelium, and whose passageway at the inner end is no larger than a bristle. Moreover, the ovum has no means of locomotion but must depend on extraneous forces for propulsion through the fallopian tube. Offhand it would seem to be impossible; actually, the ovum is not only able to make this journey with apparent ease but has been known to reach its destination after the most unbelievable meanderings. For instance, if one fallopian tube has been removed by an operation, the ovum may migrate to the opposite side of the uterus and enter the other tube. This whole "transportation system" is made possible, it seems, through two factors. In the first place, currents in the film of fluid which bathes the lining of the tube waft the ovum downward. If this lining were inspected with a microscope, there would be observed little hairlike projections, called cilia, which wave or beat in such a manner as to direct any overlying fluid (as well as any particle afloat thereon) in the direction of the uterine cavity. Once the ovum has been expelled from the ovary, it is drawn by these currents into the

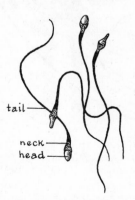

Fig. 53. Spermatozoa.

funnel-like opening of the tube and is then propelled down the tube by these same currents. The second factor responsible for the migration of the ovum down the tube is found in the peristaltic action of the tubal musculature. But the ovum is scarcely a third of the way down the tube when the supreme event happens: it meets a spermatozoon, and a new human being is created. As Margaret Shea Gilbert has so happily expressed it in her book, *Biography of the Unborn,* "Life begins for each of us at an unfelt, unknown, and unhonored instant when a minute wriggling sperm plunges headlong into a mature ovum or egg."

Spermatozoa

These minute, wriggling spermatozoa are in some respects even more remarkable than the ova which they fertilize. In appearance they resemble microscopic tadpoles, with oval heads and long, lashing tails about ten times the length of the head. The human spermatozoon consists of 3 parts: the head, the middle-piece (or neck) and the tail (Fig. 53). The nucleus, and consequently the chromatin material, is in the head; the tail serves for propulsion. They are much smaller than the ovum, their over-all length measuring about one quarter the diameter of the egg, and it has been estimated that the heads of 2 billion of them—enough to regenerate the entire population of the world—could be placed, with room to spare, in the hull of a grain of rice. As a result of the wriggling motion of the tails, spermatozoa swim with a quick vibratory motion and have been "timed" under the microscope at rates as fast as one seventh of an inch a minute. In ascending the uterus and the fallopian tube they must swim against the same currents that waft the ovum downward; nevertheless, they seem to be able to reach the outer part of the tube within an hour or two. Perhaps the most amazing feature of spermatozoa is their huge number. At each ejaculation, the climax of inter-

Fig. 54. The sex of the offspring is determined at the time of fertilization by the combination of the sex chromosome of the spermatozoon (either "X" or "Y") and that of the ovum ("X"). The ovum fertilized by a sperm cell containing the "X" chromosome produces a female (46 regular chromosomes + 2 "X" chromosomes). If it is fertilized by a spermatozoon containing the "Y" chromosome, the union produces a male (46 regular chromosomes + "X" + "Y").

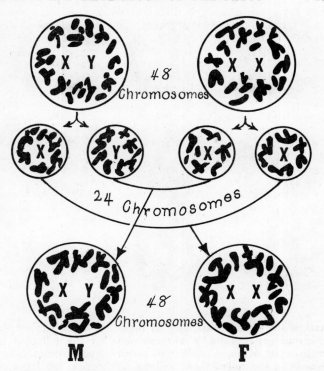

course in the male, about 300 million are discharged; if each of these could be united with an ovum, the babies which would thus be created would exceed the total number born in the United States during the past hundred years—all from a single ejaculation. So lavish is Nature in her effort to perpetuate the species! Although many million spermatozoa die in the vagina as the result of the acid secretion there myriads survive, penetrate the neck of the uterus and swarm upward to the uterine cavity and into the fallopian tube. There they lie in wait for the ovum (Fig. 52).

DETERMINATION OF SEX

In the human being, age, state of health and natural physical strength have nothing to do with the determination of sex of the offspring. The sex is determined at the time of fertilization by the spermatozoon—not by the ovum.

All spermatozoa and ova have 48 chromosomes originally. Each spermatozoon has 46 regular chromosomes and an "X" and a "Y" chromosome, whereas each ovum contains 46 regular chromosomes and two "X" sex chromosomes. When maturation occurs, each spermatozoon and ovum divides into 2 cells. Each of the 2 ovum cells contains 23 regular chromosomes and an "X" chromosome, but one half of the spermatozoon cells contain 23 regular chromosomes and an "X" chromosome and the other half of the spermatozoon (or sperm) cells contain 23 regular chromosomes and a "Y" chromosome. If a sperm cell containing 23 chromosomes and an "X" chromosome fertilizes an ovum, a female will result because in the union of the sperm and the ovum there will be 46 regular chromosomes and an "X" chromosome from the ovum and an "X" chromosome from the spermatozoon. If, on the other

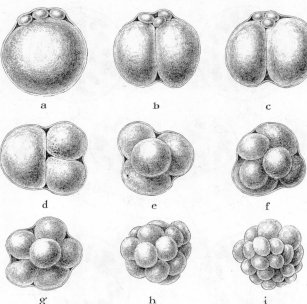

Fig. 55. Segmentation of the fertilized ovum. The ovum divides into two, each of the two into two, making four, and so on to form a solid mass of cells, called a *morula*. (Modified from Sobotta)

hand, a sperm cell containing 23 regular chromosomes and a "Y" chromosome fertilizes an ovum, a male will result because in the union there will be 46 regular chromosomes and an "X" chromosome from the ovum and a "Y" chromosome from the spermatozoon (Fig. 54). It is definitely a matter of chance, as far as is known today, whether a sperm with an "X" or a "Y" chromosome will fertilize an ovum. This is evidenced by the fact that almost universally about 94 female babies are born to every 100 male babies in single births. Although many attempts have been made to influence Nature's roulette wheel of sex, to the end that a child of a desired sex may be had, no success has been met. Nor can a physician predict with any degree of assurance, even late in pregnancy, whether the baby will be a girl or a boy.

FERTILIZATION AND CHANGES FOLLOWING FERTILIZATION

The process of union of ovum and spermatozoon is known as fertilization. It usually takes place in the outer third of the fallopian tube. As soon as the ovum comes near the army of spermatozoa, the latter, as though they were tiny bits of steel drawn by a powerful magnet, fly at the ovum. One penetrates, but only one. It appears that the entrance of one sperm into an egg causes a change in the surface of the egg which prevents entrance of other spermatozoa. The union of ovum and spermatozoon is followed at once by profound changes in the nuclei, which result in cell division and multiplication and the development of a new being. Seemingly electrified, all the particles which make up the ovum (now fused with the sperm) exhibit vigorous agitation, as though they were being rapidly churned about by some unseen force; this becomes more and more violent until it amounts to such an upheaval that the fertilized ovum divides into two cells. Before division the male and the female chromosomes and their genes are mingled and finally split, forming two sets of 48 chromosomes, one set of

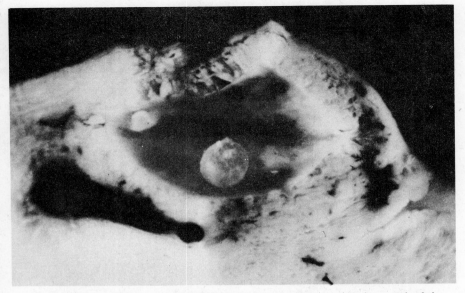

Fig. 56. The youngest human twin embryos yet seen are shown in this photograph of the gestation sac. The embryos are the small round objects, one on the floor, the other on the roof of the chorionic cavity which is the dark spot near the top of the picture. (Carnegie Institution of Washington, through Science Service, Inc.)

48 going to each of the 2 new cells. This process is repeated again and again, until masses containing 16, 32 and 64 cells are produced successively, and so on endlessly. These early cell divisions produce a solid ball of cells called the "morula," because they resemble a mulberry (Fig. 55). It is believed that the 16-cell stage is reached about 96 hours after ovulation. Meanwhile, this growing aggregation of cells is being carried down the fallopian tube in the direction of the uterine cavity.

The journey of the ovum down the fallopian tube is believed to require about 3 days, and then it spends a period of some 4 days in the uterine cavity before actual embedding takes place, a total interval of some 7 days between ovulation and implantation. Meanwhile, important changes are taking place in the internal structure of the fertilized ovum. The cells in the center of the mulberry mass secrete a fluid which pushes the remaining cells to the periphery of the sphere. At the same time it becomes apparent that this external envelope of cells is actually made up of two different layers, an inner and an outer. A specialized portion of the inner layer, after some 260 days, will develop into the long-awaited baby. The outer layer is a sort of foraging unit, called the "trophoblast" (trophectoderm), which means "feeding" layer; it is the principal function of these cells to secure food for the embryo (Figs. 56 and 57).

While the ovum is undergoing these changes, the lining of the uterus, it will be recalled, is making preparations for its reception. Considering that ovulation took place on the 14th day of the menstrual cycle and that the tubal journey and the uterine sojourn required 7 days, 21 days of the cycle will have passed before the ovum has developed its trophoblastic layer of cells. This is the

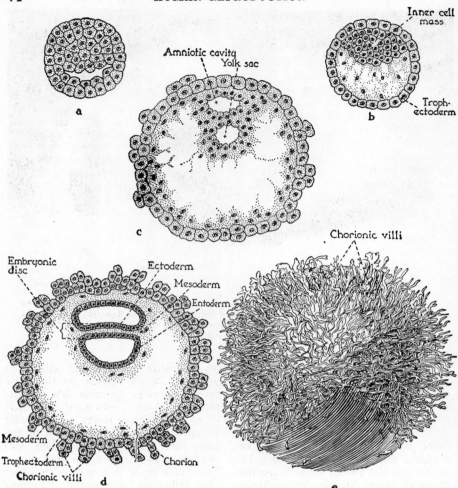

Fig. 57. Early stages of development. (a, b) The cells are separated into a peripheral layer and an inner cell mass; the peripheral layer is called the trophoblast or trophectoderm; the entire structure is called a blastodermic vesicle. (c) The formation of the amniotic cavity and yolk sac is indicated. The former is lined by ectoderm; the latter, by entoderm. (d) The location of the embryonic disk and the three germ layers are shown, together with the beginning of the chorionic villi. (e) The external appearance of the developing mass is shown; the chorionic villi are abundant. (Greisheimer: Physiology and Anatomy, Philadelphia, Lippincott)

period when the lining of the uterus has reached its greatest thickness and succulence. In other words, the timing has been precisely correct; the bed is prepared, and the ovum has so developed that it is now ready to embed itself.

IMPLANTATION OF THE OVUM

The embedding of the ovum is the work of the outer "foraging" layer of cells, the trophoblast, which possesses the peculiar property of being able to digest or liquefy the tissues with which it comes into contact. This process is carried out by means of enzymes. In this manner these cells not only burrow into the uterine lining and eat out a nest for the ovum but also digest the walls of the many small blood vessels that they encounter beneath the surface. The mother's blood stream is thus tapped, and presently the ovum finds itself deeply sunk in the lining epithelium of the uterus, with tiny pools of blood around it (Fig. 58). Sprouting out from the trophoblastic layer, quivering, fingerlike projections now develop and extend greedily into the blood-filled spaces. Another name for the trophoblast, and one more commonly employed as pregnancy progresses, is the chorion, and the fingerlike projections mentioned above become known as chorionic villi (Fig. 57). These chorionic villi contain blood vessels connected with the fetus and are extremely important because they are the sole means by which oxygen and nourishment are received from the mother. The entire ovum becomes covered with villi, which grow out radially and convert the chorion into a shaggy sac.

DECIDUA

The thickening of the uterine endometrium, which occurs during the premenstrual phase of menstruation, has been described already. If pregnancy ensues, this endometrium becomes even more thickened, the cells enlarge, and the structure becomes known as the decidua. It is simply a direct continuation in exaggerated form of the already modified premenstrual mucosa.

For purposes of description, the decidua has been divided into three portions. That part which lies directly under the embedded ovum is known as the decidua basalis, or serotina. That portion which is pushed out by the embedded and growing ovum is called the decidua capsularis or reflexa. The remainder of the decidua, or that portion which is not in immediate contact with the ovum, is known as the decidua parietalis or vera. As pregnancy advances, the decidua capsularis expands rapidly over the growing embryo and at about the fourth month lies in intimate contact with the decidua vera.

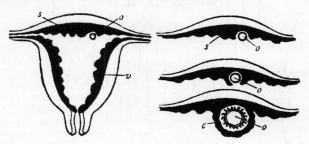

Fig. 58. Various stages in the process of implantation; the relation of the uterine mucosa to the embryonic vesicle during implantation is shown: (s) decidua basalis, (v) decidua vera, (c) decidua capsularis, and (o) the ovum or embryonic vesicle. (Greisheimer: Physiology and Anatomy, Philadelphia, Lippincott)

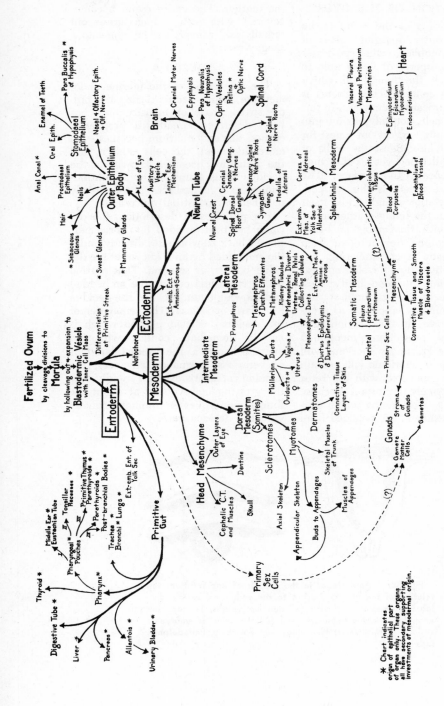

Fig. 59. Derivation of various parts of the body by progressive differentiation and divergent specialization. Note especially how the origin of all the organs can be traced back to the three primary germ layers. (Patten, B. M.: Human Embryology, New York, Blakiston)

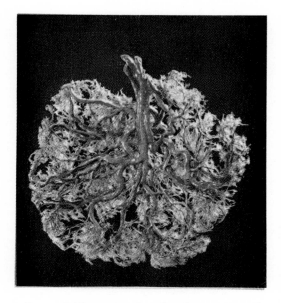

PLATE 1. Placenta stripped to the main vessels. Arteries are red; veins, blue. (Life Magazine. Picture taken by Rudolph Skarda Research Anatomist, University of California, San Francisco, Calif.)

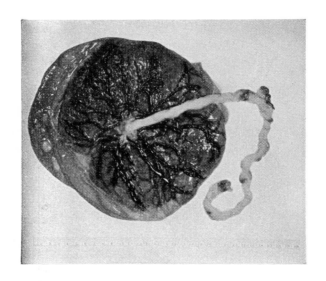

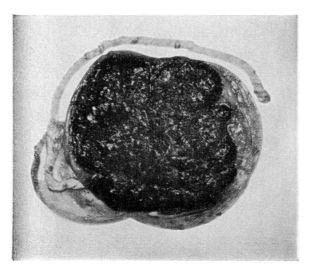

PLATE 2. (*Top*) Fetal surface of placenta.
(*Bottom*) Maternal surface of placenta.

THE THREE GERM LAYERS

With nutritional facilities provided, the cells which are destined to form the baby grow rapidly. At first they all look alike, but soon after embedding, groups of cells here and there assume distinctive characteristics and differentiate into 3 main groups: an outer covering layer, a middle layer and an internal layer. These are called, respectively, the ectoderm, the mesoderm and the entoderm.

From the *ectoderm* the following structures arise: epithelium of skin, hair, nails, sebaceous glands, sweat glands,

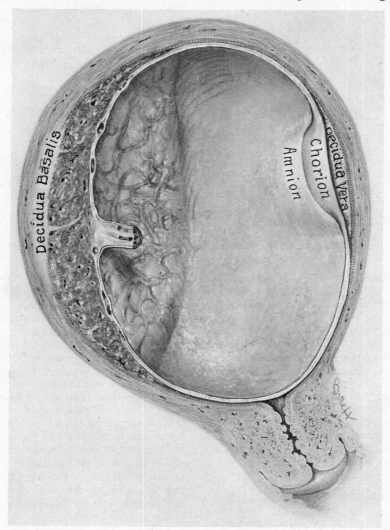

Fig. 60. Amniotic cavity, placenta and membranes (amnion and chorion).

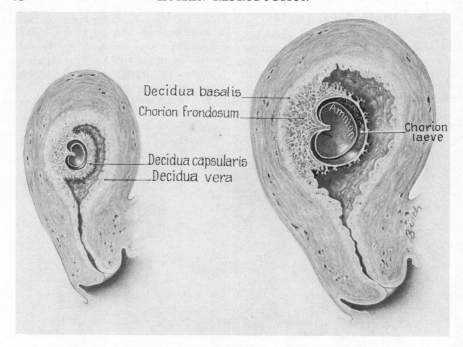

Fig. 61. Development of decidua basalis, capsularis and vera; chorion frondosum.

epithelium of the nasal and oral passages, salivary and mucous glands of the mouth and nose, enamel of the teeth, and the nervous system. From the *mesoderm* are derived: muscles, bone, cartilage, dentin of teeth, ligaments, tendons, areolar tissue, kidneys, ureters, ovaries, testes, heart, blood, lymph and blood vessels, and lining of pericardial, pleural and peritoneal cavities. From the *entoderm* arise: the epithelium of the digestive tract, of glands which pour their secretion into the tract, of the respiratory tract and of the bladder, the urethra, the thyroid and the thymus (Fig. 59).

AMNION, CHORION AND PLACENTA

Amnion. Even before these structures become evident, however, a fluid-filled space develops about the embryo,

a space which is lined with a smooth, slippery, glistening membrane, the amnion. The space is the amniotic cavity; being filled with fluid, often it is spoken of as the bag of waters; in this the fetus floats and moves (Fig. 60). At full term, this cavity normally contains from 500 to 1,000 cc. of liquor amnii, or the "waters." The amniotic fluid has a number of important functions: it keeps the fetus at an even temperature, cushions it against possible injury and provides a medium in which it can move easily; furthermore, it is known that the fetus drinks this fluid. At the end of the 4th month of pregnancy the bag of waters has enlarged to the size of a large orange and, with the fetus, occupies the entire interior of the uterus.

Chorion. As explained, the early ovum is covered on all sides by shaggy chorionic villi, but very shortly those villi which invade the decidua basalis enlarge and multiply rapidly. This portion of the trophoblast is known as the chorion frondosum (leafy chorion) (Fig. 61). Contrariwise, the chorionic villi covering the remainder of the fetal envelope degenerate and almost disappear, leaving only a slightly roughened membrane. This latter is called the chorion laeve (bald chorion). The chorion laeve lies outside of the amnion, of course, with which it is in contact on its inner surface, while its outer surface lies against the decidua vera. The fetus is thus surrounded by two membranes, the amnion and the chorion, and in ordinary clinical discussions these are usually referred to simply as "the membranes."

Placenta. By the third month another important structure has formed, the placenta. This is a fleshy, disklike organ; late in pregnancy it measures about 8 inches in diameter and 1 inch in thickness. It receives its name from a Latin word meaning cake, which this structure resembles somewhat in shape. The placenta is formed by the union of the chorionic villi and the decidua basalis. An analogous situation is seen when a tree or a plant sends down its roots into a bed of earth for nourishment; when the plant is removed a certain amount of the earthy bed clings to the interlocking roots. Similarly, a thin layer of the uterine bed clings to the branching projections of chorionic villi, and together they make up this organ which supplies food to the fetus, as the roots and the earth provide nourishment for a plant. At term the placenta weighs about 500 Gm., or 1 pound. Its fetal surface is smooth and glistening, being covered by amnion, and beneath this membrane may be seen a number of large blood vessels (Plates 1 and 2). The maternal surface is red and fleshlike in character and is divided into a number of segments, about an inch in diameter, called cotyledons.

The placenta and the fetus are connected by means of the *umbilical cord,* or funis, which is usually about 20 inches in length and about three quarters of an inch in diameter. The cord leaves the placenta near the center and enters the abdominal wall of the fetus at the umbilicus, a trifle below the middle of the median line in front. It contains 2 arteries and 1 large vein, which are twisted upon each other and are protected from pressure by a transparent, bluish-white, gelatinous substance called Wharton's jelly.

SIZE AND DEVELOPMENT OF THE FETUS

Size at Various Months

The physician, as well as the nurse, is sometimes called upon to estimate the intra-uterine age of a fetus which has been expelled prematurely.

Generally speaking, the length affords a more accurate criterion of the age of the fetus than its weight. Hasse's rule suggests that for clinical purposes the length of the embryo in centimeters may be approximated during the first 5 months by squaring the number of the month to which the pregnancy has advanced; in the second half of pregnancy, by multiplying the month by 5. Conversely, the approximate age of the fetus may be obtained by taking the square root of its length in centimeters during the first 5 months, and thereafter by dividing its length in centimeters by 5. For instance, a fetus 16 cm. long is about 4 months old; a 35-cm. fetus is about 7 months old.

Development Month by Month

Most women consider themselves one month pregnant at the time of the first missed menstrual period, 2 months pregnant at the second missed period, and so on. Since conception does not ordinarily take place until some 14 days after the onset of menstruation, it is obvious that an embryo does not attain the age of one month until about a fort-

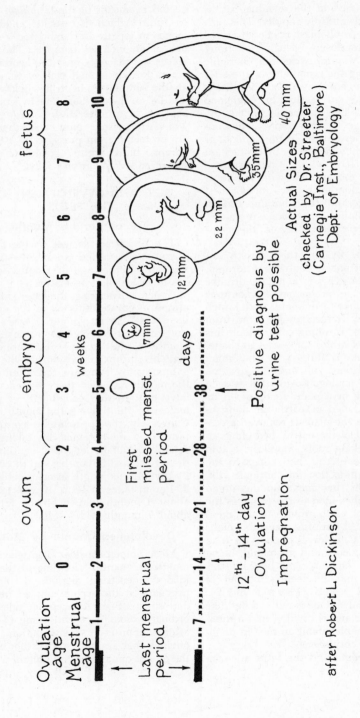

Fig. 62. Growth of ovum, embryo and fetus during the early weeks of pregnancy.

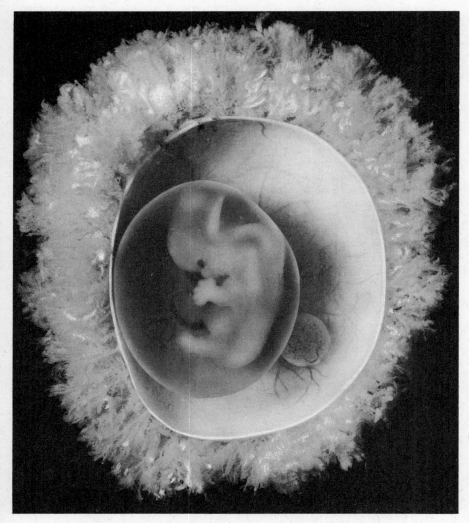

Fig. 63. Human embryo photographed by Chester F. Reather. This specimen represents about 40 days' development and is shown in the opened chorion. It is reproduced at a magnification of 1.7. (Carnegie Institution, Washington, D. C.)

night after the first missed period (assuming a 28-day cycle), and its "birthday" by months regularly falls two weeks or so after any numerically specified missed period. This should be remembered in reading the monthly development of the fetus. Thus, in speaking of the age of a pregnancy in "months," physicians refer to "lunar months," that is, periods of four weeks. Since a lunar month corresponds to the usual length of the menstrual cycle, they find it easier to "figure" in this way (Fig. 62).

Month by month the development of the fetus is something as follows:

End of First Lunar Month. The embryo is about one quarter of an inch long if measured in a straight line from head to tail—for it does have a tail at this early stage—and recognizable traces of all organs have become differentiated. The backbone is apparent but is so bent upon itself that the head almost touches the tip of the tail. At one end of the backbone the head is extremely prominent, representing almost one third of the entire embryo. (Throughout intra-uterine life the head is always very large in proportion to the body, a relationship which is still present, although to a lesser degree, at birth.) The rudiments of the eyes, the ears and the nose now make their appearance. The tube which will form the future heart has been formed, producing a large, rounded bulge on the body wall; even at this early age this structure is pulsating regularly and propelling blood through microscopic arteries. The rudiments of the future digestive tract are also discernible—a long, slender tube leading from the mouth to an expansion in the same tube which will become the stomach; connected with the latter the beginnings of the intestines may be seen. The incipient arms and legs are represented by small nubbins that resemble buds.

End of Second Lunar Month. The fetus, the term used to refer to the product of conception after the fifth week of gestation, now begins to assume human form (Fig. 63). Due to the development of the brain, the head becomes disproportionately large so that the nose, the mouth and the ears become relatively less prominent. It has an unmistakably human face and also arms and legs, with fingers, toes, elbows and

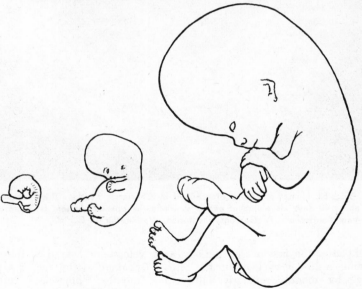

Fig. 64. Actual size of fetus at approximately one month, two months and three months, respectively. (Eastman: Expectant Motherhood, Boston, Little)

knees. During the past 4 weeks it has quadrupled in length and measures about 1 inch from head to buttocks; its weight is approximately one thirtieth of an ounce. The external genitalia become apparent, but it is difficult to distinguish between male and female. During the second month the human tail reaches its greatest development, but by the end of the month it is less prominent and then undergoes retrogression.

End of Third Lunar Month. The fetus now measures somewhat over 3 inches in length and weighs almost an ounce. The sex can now be distinguished because the external genitalia are beginning to show definite signs of sex. Centers of ossification have appeared in most bones; the fingers and the toes have become differentiated, and the fingernails and the toenails appear as fine membranes. Early in this month buds for all the temporary "baby" teeth are present, and sockets for these develop in the jawbone. Rudimentary kidneys have developed and secrete small amounts of urine into the bladder, which in all probability escape later into the amniotic fluid. Movements of the fetus are known to occur at this time, but they are too weak to be felt by the mother (Fig. 64).

End of Fourth Lunar Month. The fetus from head to toe is now 6½ inches long and about 4 ounces in weight. The sex as evidenced by the external genital organs is now quite obvious (Fig. 65).

End of Fifth Lunar Month. The length of the fetus now approximates 10 inches, while its weight is about 8 ounces. A fine downy growth of hair, *lanugo,* appears on the skin over the entire body. Usually, about this time the mother becomes conscious of slight fluttering movements in her abdomen which are due to movements of the fetus. Their first appearance is referred to as *quickening,* or the perception of life. At this period the physician often is able to hear the fetal heart for the first time. If a fetus is born now it may make a few efforts to breathe, but its

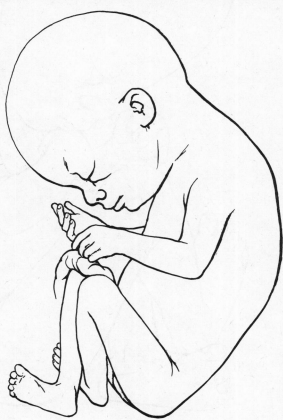

Fig. 65. Actual size of fetus at approximately 4 months.

lungs are insufficiently developed to cope with conditions outside the uterus and it invariably succumbs within a few hours at most (Fig. 66).

End of Sixth Lunar Month. The length of the fetus is 12 inches and its weight is 1½ pounds. It now resembles a miniature baby, with the exception of

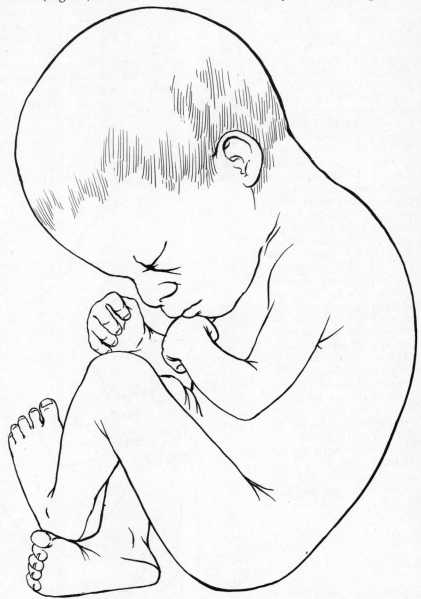

Fig. 66. Actual size of fetus at approximately 5 months.

the skin which is wrinkled and red with practically no fat beneath it. At this time, however, the skin begins to develop a protective covering called "vernix caseosa," which means "cheesy varnish." This fatty, cheesy substance adheres to the skin of the fetus and at term may be an eighth of an inch thick. Although a few cases are on record in which fetuses of this size have survived, the outlook must be regarded as practically hopeless.

End of Seventh Lunar Month. The fetus measures about 15 inches in length and weighs approximately 2½ pounds. If born at this time it has some chance of survival, perhaps one in ten. There is a widespread notion, quite incorrect, that infants born at the 7th month are more likely to survive than those born at the 8th month. This is another of those old superstitions which have descended through more than two thousand years from the time of the ancient Greek physicians. They believed that the fetus is born by means of its own effort, that is, it pushes with its legs against the upper part of the womb and wriggles out into the world. It was their opinion that the fetus first attempts to escape from the uterus at the 7th month and, if strong, it succeeds. If the attempt fails, it is repeated at the 8th month. However, if it now succeeds it is so exhausted as the result of the previous attempt that it is more likely to die than if it had been successful in the prior attempt a month earlier. We now know, of course, that the fetus is entirely passive, that it is expelled from the mother's body solely through the muscular action of the uterus, and that this old belief is wholly fallacious. The fetus born at the 8th month stands a much better chance of survival than one born at the 7th.

End of Eighth Lunar Month. The fetus measures about 16.5 inches and weighs some 4 pounds. Its skin is still red and wrinkled, and vernix caseosa and lanugo are still present. In appearance it resembles a little old man. With proper incubator and good nursing care, infants born at the end of the 8th month have better than even chances of survival, possibly as high as two chances out of three.

End of Ninth Lunar Month. For all practical purposes, the fetus is now a mature infant, measures some 19 inches and weighs around 6 pounds. Due to the deposition of subcutaneous fat, the body has become more rotund and the skin less wrinkled and red. As though to improve its appearance before making its debut into the world, the fetus devotes the last two months in the uterus to putting on weight and during this period gains ½ pound a week. Its chances of survival are now quite as good as though born at full term.

Middle of Tenth Lunar Month. Full term has now been reached, and the fetus weighs on an average about 7 pounds if a girl and 7½ if a boy; its length approximates 20 inches. Its skin is now white or pink and thickly coated with the cheesy vernix. The fine, downy hair which previously covered its body has largely disappeared. The fingernails are firm and protrude beyond the end of the fingers (Plate 3).

DURATION OF PREGNANCY

The length of pregnancy varies greatly; it may range, indeed, between such wide extremes as 240 days and 300 days and yet be entirely normal in every respect. The average duration, counting from the time of conception, is 9½ lunar months, that is, 38 weeks, or 266 days. Counting from the first day of the last menstrual period, its average length is 10 lunar months, or 40 weeks or 280 days. That these average figures mean very little, however, is shown by the following facts. Scarcely one pregnancy in 10 terminates exactly 280 days after the beginning of the last period. Less than one half terminate within 1 week of this 280th day. In 10 per cent of cases birth occurs a week or more before the theoretical end of pregnancy,

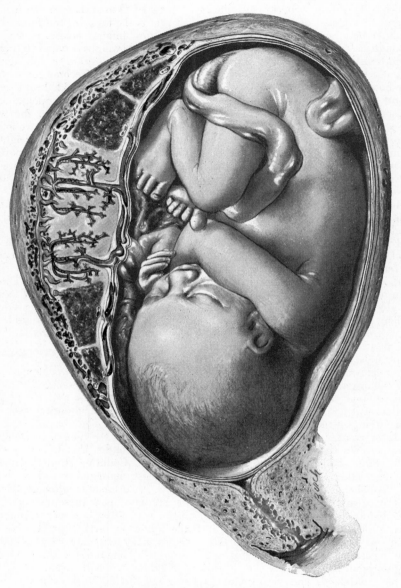

Plate 3. Full-term fetus in utero, with placental circulation shown in color.

and in another 10 per cent it takes place more than 2 weeks later than we would expect from the average figures cited above. Indeed, it would appear that some fetuses require a longer time, others a shorter time, in the uterus for full development.

CALCULATION OF THE EXPECTED DATE OF CONFINEMENT

In view of the wide variation in the length of pregnancy, it is obviously impossible to predict the expected day of confinement (often abbreviated EDC) with any degree of precision. The time-honored method, based on the above "average figures," is simple. Count back three calendar months from the first day of the last menstrual period and add seven days (Naegele's Rule). For instance, if the last menstrual period began on June 10, we would count back three months to March and, adding seven days, arrive at the date of March 17. An easier way to calculate this is to substitute numbers to designate the months. Then, this example becomes: 6/10 minus 3 months equals 3/10, plus 7 days equals 3/17. While it may be satisfying to the curiosity to have this date in mind, it must be understood that less than 5 per cent of all pregnant women go into labor on the estimated date of confinement, and in 35 per cent a deviation of from 1 to 5 days, before

or after this date, may be expected (Table 3).

Yet, whether pregnancy terminates a week before or 2 weeks later than the day calculated, the outlook for mother and baby is usually as good as though it had ended at "high noon" on the due date. Actually, women seldom go "over-term"; in most of these cases it is the system of calculation and not Nature which has erred. For example, ovulation and hence conception may have occurred some days later than calculated; this error would make the beginning and the end of pregnancy that many days later. If, superimposed on this circumstance, we were dealing with a baby which required a slightly longer stay in the uterus for complete development, it would be clear that the apparent delay was quite normal and for the best.

PHYSIOLOGY OF THE FETUS

Nutrition; Placental Transmission

During the period when the ovum lies unattached in the uterine cavity, its nutriment is provided by an endometrial secretion which is rich in glycogen and has been called "uterine milk." With the burrowing of the ovum into the endometrium, it lies in a lake of fluid representing the broken-down product of endometrial cells and obtains nourishment from this source (see Fig. 58).

Very early in pregnancy, certainly by

TABLE 3. DEVIATION FROM CALCULATED DATE OF CONFINEMENT, ACCORDING TO NAEGELE'S RULE, OF 4,656 BIRTHS OF MATURE INFANTS[*]

DEVIATION IN DAYS	EARLY DELIVERY	DELIVERY ON CALCULATED DATE	LATE DELIVERY
0		189 (4.1)	
1– 5	860 (18.5)		773 (16.6)
6–10	610 (13.1)		570 (12.2)
11–20	733 (15.7)		459 (9.9)
21–30	211 (4.5)		134 (2.9)
31 and over	75 (1.6)		42 (0.9)

The menstrual cycles of the mothers were 28±5 days. The infants were at least 47 cm. in length and 2,600 Gm. in weight (Burger and Korompai).

[*] Eastman, N. J.: Williams Obstetrics, ed. 11, p. 216, New York, Appleton, 1956.

the 3rd or the 4th week, the chorionic villi have blood vessels within them (connected with the fetal blood stream) and since these villi have already opened up the maternal blood vessels, nourishment is available from the maternal blood by the process of osmosis. In this connection it must be clearly understood that the maternal and the fetal bloods are never in contact and never intermingle. Indeed, even such substances as oxygen and glucose in the maternal blood must diffuse through several layers of tissue of the chorionic villi to reach the fetus. These layers are the cellular epithelium covering the villus, the loose connective tissue within it and finally the endothelium of the capillary blood vessel in the center of the villus. In this manner oxygen passes into the fetal circulation, while the fetal waste product, carbon dioxide, diffuses in the opposite direction. The placenta thus serves as the "lungs" of the baby in utero. Simple food substances, such as glucose, salt, calcium, phosphorus, iron, amino acids and fatty acids, all diffuse through the chorionic villus to the fetus by this process of osmosis.

It is particularly important to note that most drugs pass readily to the fetus and, if given to the mother very shortly before birth, may affect the behavior of the newborn baby (p. 226). In addition, it is interesting to observe that estrogen is transmitted to the fetus and produces certain effects in the newborn which may be very striking. In the first place, as the result of the action of this hormone, the breasts of both boy and girl babies may become markedly enlarged during the first few days of life and even secrete milk—the so-called "witch's milk" (See chap. 21, Breast engorgement). Secondly, estrogen causes the endometrium of the female fetus to hypertrophy, as it does that of an adult woman. After birth, when this hormone is suddenly withdrawn, the endometrium breaks down, and sometimes bleeding occurs. For this reason perhaps one girl baby in every 15 mani-

fests a little spotting on the diaper during the first week of life. This is entirely normal and clears up of itself within a few days.

Fetal Circulation

Since the placenta acts as the intermediary organ of transfer between the mother and fetus, the fetal circulation differs from that required for extra-uterine existence. To meet this situation the fetal circulation contains certain special vessels which may be regarded as "bypasses" or "detours" which shunt the blood around the lungs, with only a small amount going through them for nutritional purposes (Fig. 67).

The arterial (oxygenated) blood flows up the cord, through the umbilical vein and passes into the ascending vena cava, partly through the liver, but chiefly through the special fetal structure, the ductus venosus, which connects these 2 vessels. It is because of the fact that the liver receives a considerable supply of freshly vitalized blood direct from the umbilical vein that it is, proportionately, so large in a newborn baby.

From the ascending vena cava the current flows into the right auricle and directly on to the left auricle through a special fetal structure, the foramen ovale, thence into the left ventricle and out through the aorta. The blood which goes up the arms and the head returns through the descending vena cava to the right auricle again, but instead of passing through the foramen ovale, as before, the current is deflected downward into the right ventricle and out through the pulmonary arteries, partly to the lungs (for purposes of nutrition only), but mainly into the aorta, through the special fetal structure, the ductus arteriosus.

The blood in the aorta, with the exception of that which goes to the head and the upper extremities, which has been accounted for, passes downward to supply the trunk and the lower extremities. The greater part of this blood

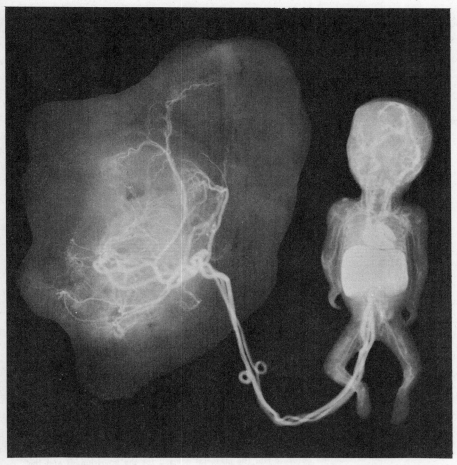

Fig. 67. Roentgenogram showing fetal and placental circulation at 11 weeks gestation, injected with Thorotrast (a contrast medium) by Charles H. Hendricks, M.D., and Frederick P. Zuspan, M.D. (Department of Obstetrics and Gynecology, Western Reserve University, Cleveland, Ohio)

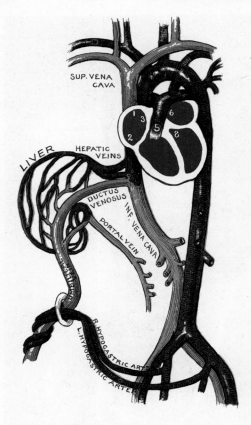

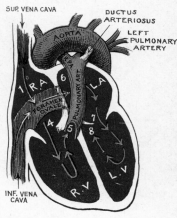

1 OPENING OF SUP. VENA CAVA
2 OPENING OF INF. VENA CAVA
3 FORAMEN OVALE
4 TRICUSPID VALVE TO R. VENTRICLE
5 PULMONARY VALVE
6 OPENING FROM PULMONARY VEINS
7 BICUSPID OR MITRAL VALVES
8 AORTIC VALVE

Fig. 68   Fig. 69

Fig. 68. Fetal Circulation Before Birth. The material needed for the nourishment and the development of the fetus is brought to it from the placenta by way of the umbilical vein. Since the lungs do not function in the exchange of gases, the placenta serves as the respiratory organ in supplying oxygen to the fetus and also serves as an excretory organ for waste products. After the blood is purified in the placenta it is sent with its nutritive material to the fetus by way of the umbilical vein, which vein divides into two branches after entering the abdominal wall. One of these branches joins directly to the portal vein which empties its blood into the liver, from which it is carried to the inferior vena cava by way of the hepatic veins. The other branch, the ductus venosus, joins directly the inferior vena cava, from which the blood is then carried to the right auricle of the heart. From the right auricle it goes through the foramen ovale to the left auricle and then to the left ventricle to the upper extremity by way of the aorta.

The blood returning from the upper extremity through the superior vena cava enters the right auricle, then the right ventricle, and then goes to the lungs by way of the pulmonary artery. Since the lungs do not function before birth only a small portion of this blood gains access to them. Most of the blood from the pulmonary artery is diverted through the ductus arteriosus to the aorta and is then carried to the trunk and lower extremities.

(Continued on facing page)

finds its way through the internal iliac, or hypogastric arteries, and so back through the cord to the placenta, where it is again oxygenated; but a small amount passes back into the ascending vena cava to mingle with fresh blood from the umbilical vein and again make the circuit of the entire body.

Circulation Change at Birth

The fetal circulation is so arranged that this passage of blood to the placenta through the umbilical arteries and back through the umbilical vein is possible up to the time of birth, but it ceases entirely the moment the baby breathes and so begins to take its oxygen directly from its own lungs. During intra-uterine life, the circulation of blood through the lungs is for the nourishment of the lungs and not for the purpose of securing oxygen (Figs. 68 and 69).

In order to understand, even in a general way, the course of the blood current and how it differs from the circulation after birth, it must be borne in mind that in infants after birth, as in the adult, the venous blood passes from the 2 venae cavae into the right auricle of the heart, thence to the right ventricle and through the pulmonary arteries to the lungs, whence it gives up its waste products and takes up a fresh supply of oxygen. After oxygenation the so-called arterial blood flows from the lungs, through the pulmonary veins to the left auricle, thence to the left ventricle and out through the aorta, to be distributed through the capillaries to all parts of the body and eventually collected, as venous blood, in the venae cavae and discharged again into the right auricle.

Circulation Path After Birth

As soon as the baby is born and breathes, the function of the lungs is established, and the placental circulation ceases (the baby no longer is dependent upon his mother's blood for oxygen but is a separate being and breathes to oxygenate his own blood). This change not only alters the character of the blood in many vessels but also makes many of these vessels of no use as such; the umbilical arteries within the baby's body become filled with clotted blood and ultimately are converted into fibrous cords, and the umbilical vein within the body becomes the round ligament of the liver, after occlusion of the vessel. After the umbilical cord is tied and separated, the large amount of blood returned to the heart from the lungs, which are now functioning, causes more or less equal pressure in both of the auricles—this pressure causes the foramen ovale to close. The foramen ovale remains closed and eventually disappears, and the ductus arteriosus and the ductus venosus finally shrivel up and are converted into fibrous cords or ligaments in the course of two or three months. The instantaneous closure of the foramen ovale changes the entire course of the blood current and converts the fetal circulation into the adult type.

The changes in the fetal circulation after birth may be tabulated as given on page 92.

Figure 69 *(Continued from facing page)*

Fig. 69. Fetal Circulation After Birth. Pulmonary circulation becomes established with birth. The umbilical cord circulation ceases. The arteries and the vein become obliterated immediately at the body junction. Shortly the hypogastric arteries, which are a continuance of the umbilical arteries after entrance into the body, become obliterated at their distal ends, followed by occlusion and obliteration of the umbilical vein and ductus venosus. The ductus arteriosus and the foramen ovale undergo a slower metamorphosis, finally occluding the circulation through the ductus arteriosus and closure of the foramen ovale. (Philips J. Carter, M.D., Louisiana State University, New Orleans)

CHANGES IN FETAL CIRCULATION AFTER BIRTH

Structure	Before Birth	After Birth
Umbilical vein	Brings arterial blood to liver and heart	Obliterated. Becomes the round ligament of liver
Umbilical arteries	Bring arteriovenous blood to the placenta	Obliterated. Become vesical ligaments on anterior abdominal wall
Ductus venosus	Shunts arterial blood into inferior vena cava	Obliterated. Becomes ligamentum venosum
Ductus arteriosus	Shunts arterial and some venous blood from the pulmonary artery to aorta	Obliterated. Becomes ligamentum arteriosum
Foramen ovale	Connects right and left auricles (atria)	Obliterated usually. At times open
Lungs	Contain no air and very little blood	Filled with air and well supplied with blood
Pulmonary arteries	Bring little blood to lungs	Bring much blood to lungs
Aorta	Receives blood from both ventricles	Receives blood only from left ventricle
Inferior vena cava	Brings venous blood from body and arterial blood from placenta	Brings venous blood only to right auricle

(Williams, J. F.: Anatomy and Physiology, ed. 7, Philadelphia, Saunders)

PERIODS OF DEVELOPMENT

Human life may be divided into periods. The successive periods, with the duration of each, are indicated below.

The period of the ovum extends from fertilization to implantation, about the close of the second week of prenatal life. (The term ovum is used in a strict sense to denote the female germ cell and also to indicate the developing zygote [fertilized ovum] previous to implantation.)

The period of the embryo extends from the 3rd to the 5th week of gestation, during which time the various organs are developed and a definite form is assumed.

The period of the fetus extends from after the 5th week to the time of birth.

The period of the newborn (neonatal) extends from birth to the close of the first month of postnatal life.

The period of infancy extends from the close of the first month to the close of the second year of life (Nelson's Textbook of Pediatrics, Saunders, 1959).

The period of childhood extends from the close of the 2nd year to about the 14th year in females and to about the 16th year in males. Puberty ends the period of childhood.

The period of adolescence extends from puberty to the last years of the second decade (late teens) in females and to the first years of the third decade (early twenties) in males.

The period of maturity extends from the end of the adolescent period to senility (old age).

Development goes on throughout life; during senility, retrogressive or degenerative changes occur.

MATERNAL IMPRESSIONS

One of the commonest superstitions relating to childbearing is the old belief that the mental condition of the mother may modify the development of the unborn infant or, as they used to say, "mark it." For instance, if a pregnant woman were frightened by some ugly beast, let us say, it used to be thought that when the baby was born it might be "marked" or distorted in the likeness of the animal. Very often the "marking" took the form of reddish blotches on the skin of the infant, which, in the mother's imagination, seemed to resemble the beast. Or, sometimes it was thought that the blotch resembled some article of food which the pregnant woman particularly craved.

This belief, like most obstetric superstitions, is of hoary antiquity; the Biblical story of Jacob and the "speckled and spotted" cattle and goats and the "brown" sheep reflects it, while dramatists and novelists from Shakespeare to Dickens have perpetuated the idea in stirring plots. The facts are these. There is no nervous connection between mother and fetus—in other words, no possible pathways along which any such impulses, pleasant or otherwise, could travel. The blood of the mother is likewise separate and distinct from that of the fetus. Furthermore, the anlagen for the various organs of the fetus are developed by the sixth week of pregnancy, that is, at a period when most women scarcely realize that they are pregnant; and, almost without exception, the causative mental shock or experience which is alleged to have brought about the "marking" occurred much later, long after the organ in question was in its final state of formation. Lastly, all modern experience refutes the belief. Obstetricians of vast experience, as well as maternity hospitals with thousands of deliveries annually, never have reported an authentic case.

How, then, is this age-old superstition to be explained? A number of factors probably contribute to it, chiefly coincidence. Approximately one baby in every 200 is born with some kind of blemish. In the event that such a blemish is present—let us say a reddish blotch on the buttocks of the baby—would it not be easy for an introspective mother, who had been told of this legend, to think finally of some object, some animal, or possibly some article of diet that she craved during pregnancy and, in her imagination, correlate it with the little red blotch?

SUGGESTED READING

Arey, L. B.: Developmental Anatomy, ed. 6, Philadelphia, Saunders, 1954.

Cook, Robert C., and Burks, Barbara S.: How Heredity Builds Our Lives, Washington, American Genetic Association.

Corner, G. W.: Ourselves Unborn; An Embryologist's Essay on Man, New Haven, Yale, 1944.

Davis, M. E., and Potter, Edith: Intrauterine respiration of the human fetus, J.A.M.A. **131**:1194, 1946.

Gilbert, M. S.: Biography of the Unborn, Baltimore, Williams & Wilkins, 1938.

Greisheimer, Esther M.: Physiology and Anatomy, ed. 7, Philadelphia, Lippincott, 1955.

Patten, Bradley M.: Human Embryology, ed. 2, New York, Blakiston Div. of McGraw-Hill, 1953.

Potter, Edith: Fundamentals of Human Reproduction, New York, McGraw-Hill, 1947.

Scheinfeld, Amram: You and Heredity, Philadelphia, Lippincott, 1950.

Snyder, Lawrence A.: The Principles of Heredity, Boston, Heath, 1946.

CHAPTER FIVE

Presentations and Positions

FETAL HABITUS

By habitus, or attitude, of the fetus is meant the relation of the fetal parts to one another. The most striking characteristic of the fetal habitus is flexion. The spinal column is bowed forward, the head is flexed with the chin against the sternum, and the arms are flexed and folded against the chest. The lower extremities are also flexed, the thighs on the abdomen and the calves of the lower legs against the posterior aspect of the thighs. In this state of flexion the fetus assumes a roughly ovoid shape, occupies the smallest possible space and conforms to the shape of the uterus. In this attitude it is about half as long as if it were completely stretched out. However, there are times when the fetus assumes many other positions.

FETAL HEAD

From an obstetric viewpoint, the head of the fetus is the most important part. If it can pass through the pelvic canal safely there is usually no difficulty in delivering the rest of the body, although occasionally the shoulders may cause trouble.

The cranium, or skull, is made up of 8 bones. Four of the bones—the sphenoid, the ethmoid and the 2 temporal bones—lie at the base of the cranium, are closely united and are of little ob-

stetric interest. On the other hand, the 4 bones forming the upper part of the cranium are of great importance; these are the frontal, the occipital and the 2 parietal bones. These bones are not knit closely together at the time of birth but are separated by membranous interspaces called *sutures*. The intersections of these sutures are known as *fontanels* (Fig. 70).

By means of this formation of the fetal skull the bones can overlap each other somewhat during labor and so diminish materially the size of the head during its passage through the pelvis. This process of overlapping is called "molding," and after a long labor with a large baby and a snug pelvis, the head is often so definitely molded that several days may elapse before it returns to its normal shape.

The most important sutures are: the sagittal, between the 2 parietal bones; the frontal, between the 2 frontal bones; the coronal, between the frontal and the parietal bones; and the lambdoid, between the posterior margins of the parietal bones and the upper margin of the occipital bone. The temporal sutures, which separate the parietal and temporal bones on either side, are unimportant in obstetrics because they are covered by fat parts and cannot be felt on the living baby.

The fontanels of importance are the

94

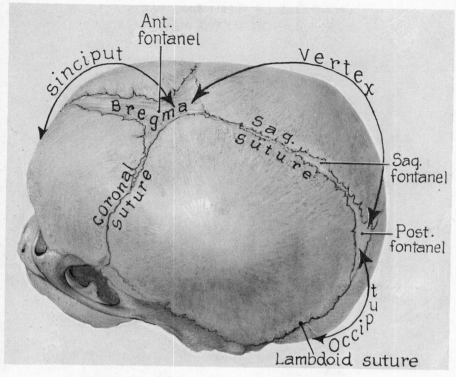

Fig. 70. Fetal skull, showing sutures and fontanels.

anterior and the posterior. The anterior fontanel, large and diamond-shaped, is at the intersection of the sagittal and the coronal sutures, while the small triangular posterior fontanel lies at the junction of the sagittal and the lambdoid suture. The sutures and the posterior fontanel ossify shortly after birth, but the anterior fontanel remains open until the child is over a year old, constituting the familiar "soft spot" just above the forehead of an infant. By feeling or identifying one or another of the sutures or fontanels, and considering its relative position in the pelvis, the physician is enabled to determine accurately the position of the head.

PRESENTATION

The term "presentation" or "presenting part" is used to designate that portion of the infant's body which lies nearest the internal os, or, in other words, that portion which is felt by the examining fingers of the physician when they are introduced into the cervix. When the presenting part is known, by abdominal palpation, it is possible to determine the relation between the long axis of the baby's body and that of the mother.

Head or *cephalic presentations* are the most common, being present in about 97 per cent of all cases at term. Cephalic presentations are divided into groups, according to the relation which the infant's head bears to its body. The most common is the *vertex presentation,* in which the head is sharply flexed so that the chin is in contact with the thorax, then the vertex is the presenting part. The *face presentation,* in which

POSITIONS OF PRESENTING PARTS
IN RELATION TO THE PELVIS

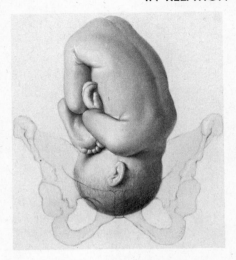

Fig. 71. Left-occipito-anterior (L.O.A.).

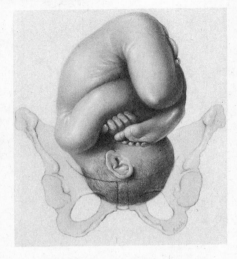

Fig. 73. Right-occipitotransverse (R.O.T.).

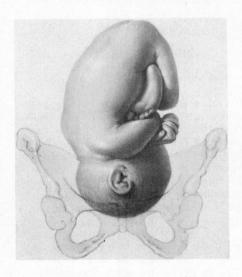

Fig. 72. Right-occipito-anterior (R.O.A.).

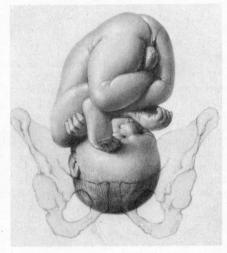

Fig. 74. Right-occipitoposterior (R.O.P.).

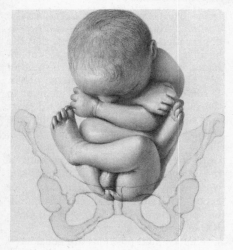

Fig. 75. Left-sacroposterior (L.S.P.).

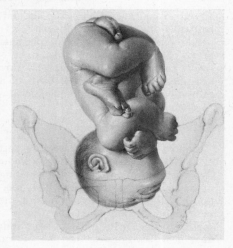

Fig. 76. Left-mento-anterior (L.M.A.).

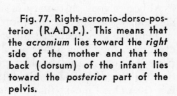

Fig. 77. Right-acromio-dorso-posterior (R.A.D.P.). This means that the *acromium* lies toward the *right* side of the mother and that the back (dorsum) of the infant lies toward the *posterior* part of the pelvis.

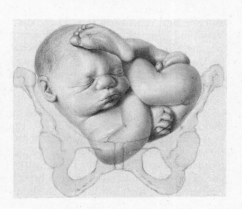

the neck is sharply extended so that the occiput and the back come in contact, is more rarely observed.

Next to the cephalic presentation, *the breech presentation* is the most common, being present, however, in only about 3 per cent of all cases. In breech presentations, the thighs may be flexed and the legs extended over the anterior surface of the body (*frank breech presentation*), or the thighs may be flexed on the abdomen and the legs on the thighs (*full breech presentation*), or one or both feet may be the lowest part (*foot or footling presentation*).

When the fetus lies crosswise in the uterus the shoulder is the presenting part—*shoulder presentation*. The common causes of a "transverse lie" are:

(1) abnormal relaxation of the abdominal walls due to great multiparity, (2) pelvic contraction, and (3) placenta previa. Shoulder presentations are relatively uncommon, and, with very rare exceptions, the spontaneous birth of a fully developed child is impossible in a "persistent transverse lie."

POSITIONS

Besides knowing the presenting part of the baby, it is important to know the exact position of this presenting part in relation to the pelvis. This relationship is determined by finding the position of certain points on the presenting surface with regard to the four imaginary divisions or regions of the pelvis. For this purpose the pelvis is considered to be divided into quadrants: left anterior, left posterior, right anterior and right posterior. These divisions aid the physician in indicating whether the presenting part is directed toward the right or the left side and toward the front or the back of the pelvis. Certain points on the presenting surface of the baby have been arbitrarily chosen as points of direction in determining the exact relation of the presenting part to the quadrants of the pelvis. In vertex presentations the occiput is the guiding point; in face presentations, the chin (mentum); in breech presentations, the sacrum; and in shoulder presentations, the scapula (acromion process).

Position, then, has to do with the relation of some arbitrarily chosen portion of the fetus to the right or the left side of the mother's pelvis. Thus, in a vertex presentation, the back of the head (occiput) may point to the front or to the back of the pelvis. The occiput rarely points directly forward or backward in the median line until the second stage of labor, but usually is directed to one side or the other.

The various positions are usually expressed by abbreviations, using the first letter of each word which describes the position: thus, left-occipito-anterior is abbreviated L.O.A. This means that the head is presenting with the occiput directed toward the left side of the mother and toward the front part of the pelvis. If the occiput were directed straight to the left with no deviation toward front or back of the pelvis, it would be termed left-occipitotransverse, or L.O.T. The occiput might also be directed toward the back or posterior quadrant of the pelvis, in which case the position would be left-occipito-posterior, or L.O.P. There are also three corresponding postions on the right side: R.O.A., R.O.T. and R.O.P.

The occipital positions are considered the most favorable for both mother and baby, and of these, the L.O.A. position is preferred. The same system of terminology is used for face, breech and shoulder presentations, as indicated in the following list of abbreviations (S, indicating breech; M, chin or face; and A, shoulder).

Although it is customary to speak of all "transverse lies" of the fetus simply as shoulder presentations, the examples of terminology sometimes used to express position in the shoulder presentation are listed. Left-acromio-dorso-anterior (L.A.D.A.) means that the acromion is to the mother's left and the back is anterior.

Positions—Vertex Presentation

L.O.A.—Left-occipito-anterior (Fig. 71)
L.O.T.—Left-occipitotransverse
L.O.P.—Left-occipitoposterior
R.O.A.—Right-occipito-anterior (Fig. 72)
R.O.T.—Right occipitotransverse (Fig. 73)
R.O.P.—Right-occipitoposterior (Fig. 74)

Positions—Breech Presentation

L.S.A.—Left-sacro-anterior
L.S.T.—Left-sacrotransverse
L.S.P.—Left sacroposterior (Fig. 75)
R.S.A.—Right-sacro-anterior
R.S.T.—Right-sacrotransverse
R.S.P.—Right-sacroposterior

Fig. 78. Fetal head, showing transverse diameters.

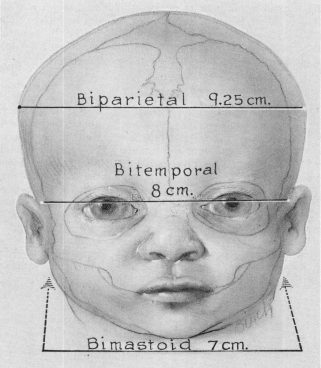

POSITIONS—FACE PRESENTATION

L.M.A.—Left-mento-anterior (Fig. 76)
L.M.T.—Left-mentotransverse
L.M.P.—Left-mentoposterior
R.M.A.—Right-mento-anterior
R.M.T.—Right-mentotransverse
R.M.P.—Right-mentoposterior

POSITIONS—SHOULDER PRESENTATION

L.A.D.A.—Left-acromio-dorso-anterior
L.A.D.P.—Left-acromio-dorso-posterior
R.A.D.A.—Right-acromio-dorso-anterior
R.A.D.P.—Right-acromio-dorso-posterior
(Fig. 77)

Figures 78 and 79 show the principal measurements of the fetal skull. The most important transverse diameter is the biparietal; it is the distance between the biparietal protuberances and represents the greatest width of the head. It measures, on an average, 9.25 cm. There are three important anteropos-

terior diameters: the suboccipitobregmatic, which extends from the undersurface of the occiput to the center of the anterior fontanel and measures about 9.5 cm.; the occipitofrontal, which extends from the root of the nose to the occipital prominence and measures about 12.0 cm.; and the occipitomental, which extends from the chin to the posterior fontanel and averages about 13.5 cm.

In considering these three anteroposterior diameters of the fetal skull, it is important to note that with the head in complete flexion and the chin resting on the thorax, the smallest of these, the suboccipitobregmatic, enters the pelvis, whereas if the head is extended or bent back (with no flexion whatsoever), the greatest anteroposterior diameter presents itself to the pelvic inlet. Herein lies the great importance of flexion; the more the head is flexed the smaller is the anteroposterior diameter which enters the pelvis. Figures 80 to 82 show this basic principle in diagrammatic form.

DIAGNOSIS OF FETAL POSITION

Diagnosis of fetal position is made in four ways: (1) abdominal palpation; (2) vaginal and rectal examination; (3) combined auscultation and examination; (4) in certain doubtful cases, the roentgenogram.

Inspection

Nurses should thus be able to determine whether a presentation is normal or otherwise, as work in rural, sparsely settled localities may often require of her knowledge not demanded in her hospital experience. Only under most unusual conditions would she be expected to ascertain this in any other way than by palpation.

Palpation

The nurse should familiarize herself thoroughly with this method. She will find it extremely helpful to palpate the abdomen before listening to the fetal heart tones. The region of the abdomen in which the fetal heart is heard most plainly varies according to the presentation and the extent to which the presenting part has descended. The location of the fetal heart sounds by itself does not give very important information as to the presentation and position of the child, but it sometimes reinforces the results obtained by palpation. In order to obtain satisfactory information by

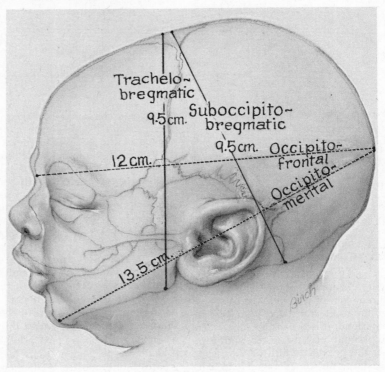

Fig. 79. Fetal head, showing anteroposterior diameters.

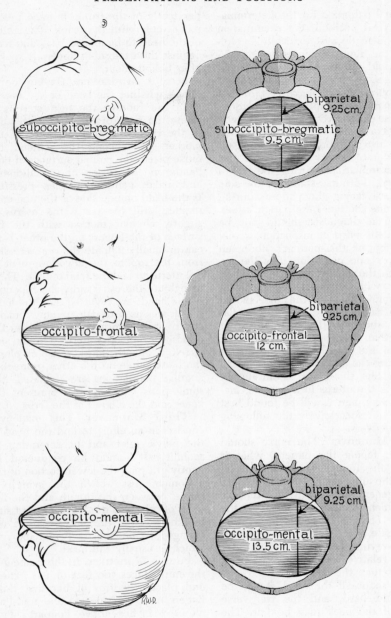

Fig. 80. (*Top*) Complete flexion allows smallest diameter of head to enter pelvis.
Fig. 81. (*Center*) Moderate extension causes larger diameter to enter pelvis.
Fig. 82. (*Bottom*) Marked extension forces largest diameter against pelvic brim, but it is too large to enter.

abdominal palpation for the determination of fetal position, the examination should be made systematically by following the four maneuvers suggested by Leopold, often called the *Leopold maneuvers*.

The nurse should make certain that the patient has emptied her bladder before the procedure is begun. This will not only contribute to the patient's comfort but also will aid the nurse to gain more accurate results in the latter part of the examination. During the first 3 maneuvers the nurse stands at the side of the bed facing the patient; during the last one she faces the patient's feet. Although a diagnosis should not be made on the basis of inspection, actual observation of the patient's abdomen should precede palpation. For the examination the patient should lie flat on her back, with her knees flexed, to relax the abdominal muscles; the nurse should lay both hands gently, and at first, flat upon the abdomen. If done in any other manner than this, or if her hands are not warm, the stimulation of her fingers will cause the abdominal muscles to contract. She should accustom herself to palpate the uterus in a definite, methodical way, and it will be found best to carry out successively the following four maneuvers.

First Maneuver. The nurse should ascertain, facing the patient, what is lying at the fundus of the uterus by feeling the upper abdomen with both hands; generally she will find there a mass, which is either the head or the buttocks (breech) of the fetus. She must decide which pole of the fetus this is by observing three points (Fig. 83):

1. Its relative consistency: the head is harder than the breech.

2. Its shape: if the head, it will be round and hard, and the transverse groove of the neck may be felt. The breech has no groove and usually feels more angular.

3. Mobility: the head will move inde-

pendently of the trunk, but the breech moves only with the trunk. The ability of the head to be moved back and forth against the examining fingers is spoken of as ballottement.

Second Maneuver. Having determined whether the head or the breech is in the fundus, the next step is to locate the back of the fetus in relation to the right and the left sides of the mother. Still facing the patient, the nurse places the palmar surfaces of both hands on either side of the abdomen and makes gentle but deep pressure. If the hand on one side of the abdomen remains still to steady the uterus, a slightly circular motion with the flat surface of the fingers on the other hand can gradually palpate the opposite side from the top to the lower segment of the uterus to feel the fetal outline. Then, to palpate the other side, the functions of the hands are reversed, i.e., the hand which was used to palpate now remains steady and the other hand palpates the opposite side of the uterus. On one side is felt a smooth, hard, resistant plane, the back, while on the other, numerous angular nodulations are palpated, the small parts; these latter represent the knees and the elbows of the fetus.

Third Maneuver. This maneuver consists in an effort to find the head at the pelvic inlet and to determine its mobility. It should be conducted by gently grasping the lower portion of the abdomen, just above the symphysis pubis, between the thumb and the fingers of one hand and then pressing together. If the presenting part is not engaged, a movable body will be felt, which is usually the head.

Fourth Maneuver. In this maneuver the nurse faces the feet of the patient and places the tips of her first three fingers on both sides of the mid-line, about 2 inches above Poupart's ligament. Pressure is now made downward and in the direction of the birth canal, the movable skin of the abdomen being

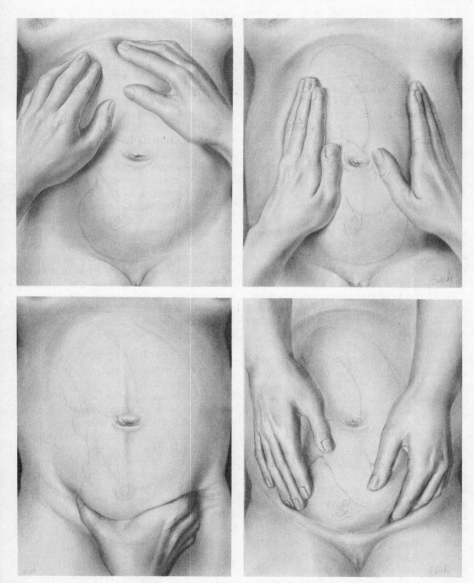

Fig. 83. Palpation: (*top, left*) first maneuver; (*top, right*) second maneuver; (*bottom, left*) third maneuver; (*bottom, right*) fourth maneuver.

carried downward along with the fingers. It will be found that the fingers of one hand meet no obstruction and can be carried downward well under Poupart's ligament; these fingers glide over the nape of the baby's neck. The other hand, however, usually meets an obstruction an inch or so above Poupart's ligament; this is the brow of the baby and is usually spoken of as the "cephalic prominence." This maneuver gives information of several kinds:

1. If the findings are as described above, it means that the baby's head is well flexed.

2. Confirmatory information is obtained about the location of the back, as naturally the back is on the opposite side from the brow of the baby, except in the uncommon cases of face presentation, in which the cephalic prominence and the back are on the same side.

3. If the cephalic prominence is very easily palpated, as if it were just under the skin, a posterior position of the occiput is suggested.

4. The location of the cephalic prominence tells how far the head has descended into the pelvis. This maneuver is of most value if the head has engaged and may yield no information with a floating, poorly flexed head.

Vaginal Examination

Vaginal examination is done by the physician and consists in identifying the fontanels and the suture lines of the fetal skull. During pregnancy the vaginal examination gives limited information concerning the position of the fetus because the cervix is closed. However, during labor, after more or less complete dilatation of the cervix, important information about the position of the baby and the degree of flexion of its head can be obtained.

Auscultation

The location of the fetal heart sounds, as heard through the stethoscope, yields helpful confirmatory information about fetal position but is not wholly dependable. Certainly, it never should be relied upon as the sole means of diagnosing fetal position. Ordinarily, the heart sounds are transmitted through the convex portion of the fetus, which lies in intimate contact with the uterine wall, so that they are heard best through the infant's back in vertex and breech presentations, and through the thorax in face presentation. In cephalic presentations the fetal heart sounds are heard loudest midway between the umbilicus and the anterior superior spine of the ileum. In general, in L.O.A. and L.O.P. positions the fetal heart sounds are heard loudest in the left lower quadrant. A similar situation applies to the R.O.A. and R.O.P. positions. In posterior positions of the occiput (L.O.P. and R.O.P.) often the sounds are heard loudest well down in the flank toward the anterior superior spine. In breech presentation the fetal heart sounds usually are heard loudest at the level of the umbilicus or above (see Fig. 97).

Roentgenograms

Roentgenograms are of particular value in diagnosis of fetal position in doubtful cases, particularly in obese women or in those with abdominal walls so rigid that abdominal palpation is difficult. In such situations the roentgenogram enables the physician to recognize the existence of conditions which might otherwise have escaped detection until late in labor. They give accurate information concerning position, presentation, flexion and descent of the fetal head (see Fig. 99).

SUGGESTED READING

Beck, Alfred C., and Rosenthal, Alexander: Obstetrical Practice, ed. 6, Baltimore, Williams & Wilkins, 1955.
Eastman, N. J.: Williams Obstetrics, ed. 11, New York, Appleton, 1956.
Greenhill, J. P.: Obstetrics, ed. 11, Philadelphia, Saunders, 1955.

The books listed above are among the standard American works on obstetrics. One of these, at least, will be found in any nurses' library and all in most medical libraries. The nurse will do well to augment her reading by consulting one or another of these volumes from time to time.

CONFERENCE MATERIAL

1. What would be your responsibility to a friend who is pregnant yet has not registered for delivery with either a doctor or a clinic?

2. How would you present the subject of human reproduction to a group of Girl Scouts or high school students?

3. What illustrative material and reference readings would you select for a group conference of young parents or those about to be married?

4. How would you go about looking up the costs of obstetric care in your community?

5. If a patient appealed to you to secure information about the best obstetric care in a certain city in the United States, how would you get this information for her?

6. What authentic sources are available for obtaining maternal and infant mortality statistics?

7. What is the status of the midwife in this country? How does this situation compare with other countries?

8. What forces are in operation to improve the maternity situation?

9. How can you stimulate the interest of a lay group in the community who are willing to give time and some financial support to help with an educational program for the less fortunate?

SELF-EXAMINATION QUESTIONS FOR THE STUDENT

After each unit of this book, some objectively scorable test questions are provided to aid you in making immediate *use* of the information and the knowledge that you have gained through studying each of these units. The questions are planned to enable you to see how some of the important facts function in the nursing care of patients and how knowledge of the facts enables you to (1) recognize, analyze and interpret the nursing needs of obstetric patients, (2) plan to meet these needs, (3) carry out the plan and (4) evaluate both the plan and the results.

These tests represent only a few sample instances where information, facts and principles presented in the units function in nursing care. If you are successful in these samples, you may be in many more instances, but you should not assume that success here guarantees success in all. Likewise, failure on many of these items does not necessarily mean complete lack of understanding, but it is a rather good indication that you need to restudy the unit more carefully.

Use these tests as a study device. After you believe that you have mastered the important points in the unit, fill out the objectively scorable test questions at the end of the unit. Think through each question and response carefully. Complete the entire unit test and then (and not until then) turn to the key on page 533, where you will find the right answers. See how many you had correct. Look up the answers to those that you answered incorrectly.

You will observe that many of the questions demand that you use your previously acquired knowledge of anatomy and physiology, bacteriology, chemistry, pharmacology, psychology, nursing arts and nutrition, together with obstetric nursing knowledge, for all nursing care demands the simultaneous functioning of facts and principles from many of these fields along with those of the special clinical field.

In some judgment and debatable questions the answer given in the key may conflict with the current practice in your institution or locality. Ask your teacher how she thinks you should score yourself on these points.

Since the purpose of these self-scoring tests is to aid you in learning, you will be defeating that purpose and penalizing yourself if you misuse them and look at the key before you have carefully thought through the question. *No one but you is interested in how well or how poorly you do on these tests.* When you have discovered how well or how poorly you have done, you will know better what and how much more to study.

Your teacher's evaluation of your ability to use the material presented in each unit may sample some of these and many other points presented in the unit. Your best preparation for your teacher's appraisal in class and on the ward is your own evaluation of your attainment and study in light of your accomplishment. But, more important, your best preparation for giving skilled professional nursing care to obstetric patients is to have a complete understanding of and ability to use the important facts and principles that relate to that care, an understanding that is largely within your own power to obtain through your own efforts.

Study Questions

UNIT ONE: HUMAN REPRODUCTION

Read through the entire question and place your answer in the parentheses.

1. Which of the following complications of pregnancy are responsible for the greatest toll in maternal mortality?
   a. Cardiac complications
   b. Toxemia
   c. Hemorrhage
   d. Infection
   e. Diabetes
   Select the number corresponding to the correct letters.
   1. A and B
   2. A, C and E
   3. B, C and D
   4. B, C and E   (___3___)

2. What improvement is believed to be the greatest single factor for decreasing maternal deaths during the past half century?
   a. Antepartal care
   b. Management of labor
   c. Analgesia during delivery
   d. Nursing care during delivery
   e. Care by the physician during delivery
   f. Care during the puerperium   (___A___)

3. A patient in the clinic, in the latter part of her pregnancy, reported to the nurse that she was suffering from backache and wanted to know the cause. What would be the most likely reason that the nurse could give her?
   a. The larger size of the fetus tires her more easily.
   b. Increased mobility of joints throws greater weight on surrounding muscles.
   c. She must have some abnormality in pelvic structures.
   d. The descent of the presenting part into the pelvic cavity prior to labor increases pressure against the sacrum.   (___b___)

4. In each of the following write the term or the phrase by which the pelvic measurement described is commonly called.
   a. Between the symphysis pubis and the depression below the fifth lumbar vertebra   a. (_ext conj_)
   b. From the lower margin of the symphysis pubis to the sacral promontory   b. (_diag. conj_)
   c. Between the lateral edges of the iliac crests   c. (_intercrist_)
   d. The posterior portion of the symphysis pubis to the promontory of the sacrum   d. (_true conj_)
   e. From the inner aspects of the ischial tuberosities   e. (_intertuber_ ischiadicum)

5. By using the letter or letters of the measurements described in Question 4 indicate:

  a. The one which must be estimated rather than measured directly   a. (———*b*———)

  b. The one which represents the most important diameter   b. (———*b*———)

  c. The one which represents the largest diameter   c. (———*a*———)

6. A patient's chart shows pelvic measurements of 11 cm. for the diagonal conjugate and 9.5 cm. for the true conjugate; therefore, the nurse caring for the patient in the labor room should anticipate that the patient might have:

  a. An easy, rapid delivery

  b. A delivery of reasonable duration

  c. A protracted labor with difficult delivery   (———*c*———)

7. To give adequate care to the patient during and after delivery, the nurse should fully understand the structure of the uterus. Which of the following are true of the uterus?

  a. Its muscular tissue is:

    1. Chiefly striated   3. Entirely striated

    2. Chiefly nonstriated   4. Entirely nonstriated

                                                   (———*4*———)

  b. Its muscle fibers are arranged to run:

    1. Circularly

    2. Longitudinally

    3. In all directions

    4. In three layers, the inner and the outer circularly, the other longitudinally

                                                     (———*3*———)

  c. Its blood is supplied directly from:

    1. Ovarian and uterine arteries

    2. Abdominal aorta and uterine arteries

    3. Internal iliac and ovarian arteries

    4. Internal iliac and uterine arteries   (———*1*———)

  d. Normally, it is:

    1. Attached anteriorly to the bladder wall

    2. Suspended freely movable in the pelvic cavity

    3. Suspended between the bladder and the rectum

    4. Attached posteriorly to the anterior wall of the sacrum   (———*2*———)

8. The perineum lies between the vagina and the rectum. This structure has:

  a. A single, strong elastic muscle

  b. A strong elastic tendon

  c. A tendon to which 5 muscles are attached

  d. Two strong muscles, the anal and the transverse perineal   (———*c*———)

9. Every effort is made to prevent the tearing of the perineum during childbirth. The chief hazard to the patient from laceration of the perineum would likely be:

  a. Incontinence

  b. Postpartal hemorrhage

  c. Perineal abscess

  d. Prolapsed uterus   (———*B*———)

10. A patient with small breasts in her first pregnancy was worried about her ability to feed her baby.
   a. The nurse could respond correctly to the patient by telling her that:
      1. She probably would be unable to feed her baby.
      2. The size of the breasts does not influence the amount of lactation possible.
      3. Mothers with small breasts usually have less difficulty feeding their babies.
      4. Her baby would be fed better by means of a formula.
                            (——2——)

   b. Milk is produced by the process of:
      1. Dialysis
      2. Osmosis
      3. Secretion   (——2——)
   c. The structures most directly involved in the production of milk are:
      1. Papillae
      2. Glands of Montgomery
      3. Acini cells
      4. Lactiferous sinuses
      5. Areola
      6. Lactiferous ducts   (——3——)

11. What are the ovarian hormones produced by the graafian follicle and the cells of the corpus luteum?
   a. Progesterone and gonadotropin
   b. Estrogen and progesterone
   c. Gonadotropin and FSH
   d. FSH and estrogen   (——B——)

12. A young mother-to-be told a nurse that she was sure that she would have a boy because her husband was such a strong, physically developed man. The nurse could respond correctly by saying:
   a. "It is the female cell which determines the sex of the child."
   b. "It is unlikely because there are more girls born than boys."
   c. "Physical strength does not influence the sex of the child."
   d. "You are probably right."   (——C——)

13. A patient expelled a fetus of 16 cm. prematurely. What would be the approximate age of the fetus?
   a. 2 months
   b. 3 months
   c. 4 months
   d. 5 months   (——C——)

14. Although the exact date of delivery cannot be predetermined, if a pregnant woman's last menstrual period began on September 10, the estimated due date would be nearest:
   a. May 6
   b. May 10
   c. June 10
   d. June 17   (——D——)

15. The only direct connection between the fetus and any other structure is through the umbilical cord. The umbilical cord contains which of these important structures?
   a. Umbilical artery
   b. Umbilical arteries
   c. Umbilical vein
   d. Umbilical veins
   e. Umbilical nerves
   f. Umbilical lymphatic duct
   g. Wharton's jelly

Select the number corresponding to the correct letters.
   1. A, D and F
   2. B, C and G
   3. C, E and G
   4. All of them   (——2——)

16. After a protracted labor and a difficult delivery, the mother, upon seeing the child, was shocked at the elongated appearance of the child's head. The nurse could correctly reassure the patient by saying:
   a. "The child's head is molded during delivery and will return to normal in a few days."
   b. "All newborn babies' heads are shaped this way."
   c. "The child's head shape was changed during delivery, and it will take six months for it to return to normal."
   d. "After the 'soft spot' closes the head will return to normal."   (——A——)

17. Indicate the abbreviations that might be used on a patient's chart to represent each of the positions and the presentations described:
   a. Back of head directed straight to the left   a. (—LOT—)
   b. Back of head directed toward the left side and the front quadrant of the pelvis   b. (—LOA—)
   c. Back of head directed toward the right side and the back quadrant of the pelvis   c. (—ROP—)
   d. Breech presentation, buttocks at the left back quadrant   d. (—LSP—)
   e. Face presentation, chin at the right front quadrant   e. (—RMA—)
   f. Transverse lie, shoulder is to the right of mother's pelvis, back is posterior   f. (—RADP—)

Note: The key to the correct answers to these questions is given on page 533.

UNIT TWO

Nursing in Pregnancy

ORIENTATION

The previous chapters, dealing with the anatomy and the physiology of the generative organs and the developing fetus, have been a foundation for the study of the human reproductive process. From a biologic point of view, pregnancy and labor represent the highest function of the female reproductive system and should be considered as a normal process. Nevertheless, medical supervision and care during pregnancy are essential to the health and the well-being of the mother and her infant throughout this period. The future health of the mother, as well as the foundation for the health, the growth and the development of her baby, are dependent upon adequate antepartal care. The doctor, the nurse, and all the members of the health team must assume the responsibility for the welfare of the family throughout the maternity cycle. The nurse, by means of her contacts with maternity patients in the home, the clinic and in the hospital, is able to appreciate the social, economic and emotional factors which influence the nursing needs of each individual patient and thus plan for care accordingly.

Since the maternity cycle extends throughout the 9-month period of pregnancy and the 6 weeks following, the student nurse misses the continuity in this complete picture in her practical experience. It may not be possible for the nurse to see the immediate results of this care, but she must be able to look ahead and aim for the results which can be obtained only by adequate antepartal care and good medical supervision.

During pregnancy, the mother has many emotional adjustments to make: sometimes fear, worries (financial as well as physical), apprehension and family difficulties or problems are present. These emotional disturbances in some degree or form accompany each pregnancy, whether it be the first or a subsequent one. Patients of all status have similar adjustments to make. The fact that delivery must be "faced," that there is no turning back or "changing the mind," can in itself sometimes create an overwhelming emotional crisis.

Each mother deserves the kind of antepartal care which will enable her to assume her full role as mother, wife and member of the community after her baby arrives. The obstetric nurse has unlimited opportunities to utilize health teaching in planning for and in providing care to meet the immediate and continuing nursing needs of her patients.

As we know it today, antepartal care developed into its present status through devious avenues of investigation and many bypaths of interrelated activity and work. The combined efforts of many groups have contributed to this achievement. The background of our present maternity situation is of interest both as a history and a story. (See Chap. 24, "History of Obstetrics," for background and development of antepartal care.)

CHAPTER SIX

Normal Pregnancy

PHYSIOLOGIC CHANGES OF PREGNANCY

By the physiologic changes of pregnancy are meant those alterations, both local and general, which affect the maternal organism as the result of pregnancy but subside at or before the end of the puerperium and leave the patient in practically the same condition in which she was before conception occurred. In other words, the physiologic changes of pregnancy are to be regarded as normal, inevitable and purely temporary; for they are present in varying degrees in every instance, and in the case of a physically healthy woman there should be no traces of them left after convalescence is complete. It must be remembered, however, that after pregnancy the uterus does not return to its normal nulliparous size, though it does return to a normal nonpregnant state. The adult parous uterus is slightly larger and weighs more than that of a woman who has never borne children (Chap. 3).

LOCAL CHANGES

Genitals

The uterus increases in size to make room for the growing fetus. Naturally, the enlargement of the uterus is the most striking change wrought by pregnancy and, moreover, is directly responsible for other important alterations. The growth of this organ in gestation is phenomenal. It increases in size from approximately 6.5 cm. long, 4 cm. wide and 2.5 cm. deep to about 32 cm. long, 24 cm. wide and 22 cm. deep. Its weight increases from 50 to 1,000 Gm. The small, almost solid organ which has a capacity of perhaps 2 cc. increases to become a thin-walled muscular sac capable of containing the fetus, the placenta and a large quantity of amniotic fluid. The tremendous growth is due partly to the formation of new muscle fibers during the early months of pregnancy, but principally to the enlargement of pre-existent muscle fibers which are 7 to 11 times longer and 2 to 7 times wider than those observed in the nonpregnant uterus (Fig. 84). Simultaneously, fibroelastic tissue develops between the muscle bands and forms a network about the various muscle bundles. This is of great importance in view of the function of the uterus in pregnancy and labor because it strengthens the uterine walls. During early pregnancy the hypertrophy of the uterus is probably.due to the stimulating action of estrogen on muscle fibers, but after the first trimester the increase in size is partly mechanical due to the pressure of

113

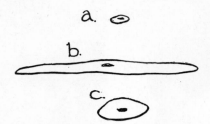

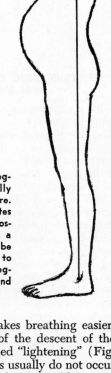

Fig. 84. (*Left*) Size of muscle cells. This illustrates the size of the muscle cells of the uterus (a) before pregnancy, (b) the changes in the size of these cells during pregnancy, and (c) in the puerperium (after Stieve).

the growing fetus (Fig. 85). The uterine wall thickens during the first few months of pregnancy from about 1 cm. to almost 2 cm., but thereafter it thins to about 0.5 cm. or less. By the end of pregnancy the uterus becomes a thin, soft-walled muscular sac which yields to the movements of the fetal extremities and permits the examiner to palpate the fetus easily.

The muscle fibers are arranged in three layers: the external hoodlike layer which arches over the fundus, the internal layer of circular fibers around the orifices of the fallopian tubes and the internal os and the figure-8 fibers in the middle layer which make an interlacing network through which the blood vessels pass. This latter group play an important role in childbearing and will be referred to particularly in the care of the mother during labor and after delivery, for when these muscle fibers contract they constrict the blood vessels.

Between the third and the fourth months of pregnancy, the growing uterus rises out of the pelvis and can be palpated above the symphysis pubis, rising progressively to reach the umbilicus about the sixth month and almost impinging upon the xiphoid process at the ninth month (Figs. 86-91). As the uterus becomes larger it comes in contact with the anterior abdominal wall and displaces the intestines to the sides of the abdomen. About two weeks before term, in most primigravidae the fetal head descends into the pelvic cavity. As a result, the uterus sinks to a lower level and at the same time falls forward. Since this relieves the upward pressure on the

Fig. 85. (*Right*) Pregnancy should and usually does improve posture. The diagram illustrates the correct standing posture showing that a straight line may be drawn from the ear to the ankle. During pregnancy "walk tall, stand tall and sit tall."

diaphragm and makes breathing easier, this phenomenon of the descent of the head has been called "lightening" (Fig. 92). These changes usually do not occur in multiparas until the onset of labor. By palpating the height of the fundus, experienced examiners can determine the approximate length of gestation.

Since the full-term pregnant uterus and its contents weigh about 12 pounds, a gravid woman may be likened to a person carrying a heavy basket pressed against the abdomen. Such a person will instinctively lean backward in order to maintain equilibrium. This backward

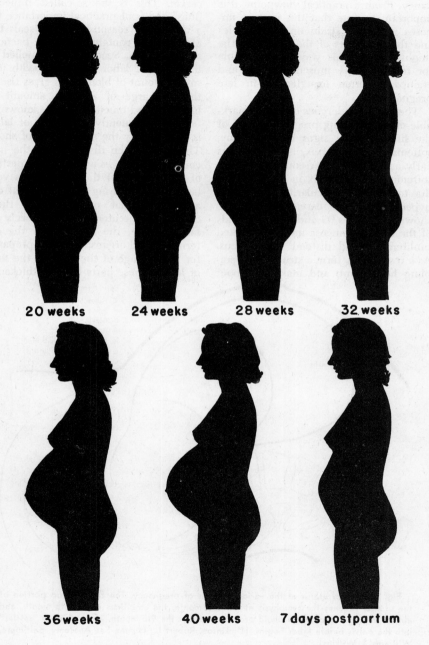

20 weeks **24 weeks** **28 weeks** **32 weeks**

36 weeks **40 weeks** **7 days postpartum**

Fig. 86. Changes in abdominal contour in pregnancy. Photographic
study of actual patient.

tilt of the torso is characteristic of pregnancy. From a practical viewpoint, it is important to note that this posture imposes increased strain on the muscles and the ligaments of the back and the thighs, and in this way is responsible for many of the muscular aches and cramps so often experienced in late pregnancy.

The cervix undergoes certain remarkable changes during pregnancy. One of the first physical signs of pregnancy, softening of the cervix, is apparent as early as a month after conception. The softening of the cervix in pregnancy is due to increased vascularity, edema and hyperplasia of the cervical glands. As shown in Figures 93 and 94, the glands of the cervical mucosa undergo marked proliferation and distend with mucus. As a result, they form a structure resembling honeycomb and make up about one half of the entire structure of the cervix. This is the so-called "mucous plug" and is of practical importance for a number of reasons. First, it seals the uterus from contamination by bacteria in the vagina. Second, it is expelled at the onset of labor and along with it a small amount of blood; this gives rise to the discharge of a small amount of blood-stained mucus, which is known as "show." Frequently, the onset of labor is heralded by the appearance of show. Third, since the discharge of the mucous plug removes a substantial portion of the interior of the cervix, it is very helpful in preparing for subsequent dilatation of that organ. While these changes in the uterus and the cervix are taking place, the vagina and the external genital organs are being prepared for the passage of the fetus at the time of labor. These parts become thickened

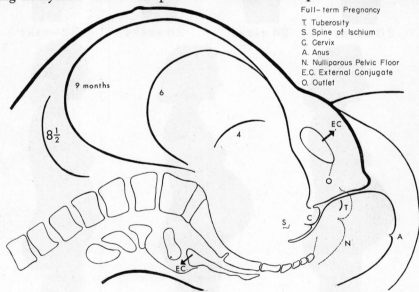

Fig. 87. Size of uterus at the various months of pregnancy. The fundus (top portion of the uterus) reaches the symphysis at the 3rd month, the umbilicus at the 6th month, and almost impinges upon the xiphoid process at about the 9th month, after which it "settles" into the pelvis before labor begins. (Dickinson, Robert L.: Human Sex Anatomy, Baltimore, Williams & Wilkins)

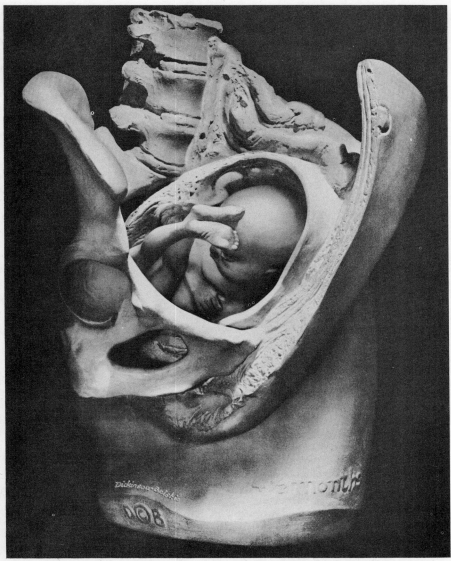

Fig. 88. Size and position of the fetus in the pelvis, at 4½ months. At about this time the mother first feels the fetal movements known as "quickening." (Dickinson-Belskie Birth Atlas Series, Maternity Center Association, New York)

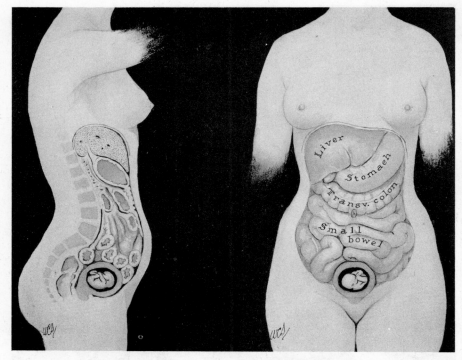

Fig. 89. Side and front views, showing the fetus at 4 months.

and softened, and their vascularity is greatly increased. This increase in the blood supply of the genital canal gives to the tissues a dark violet hue (Chadwick's sign), in contrast with the ordinary pink color of the parts, which is often described as a valuable sign of pregnancy. As the result of the succulence of the parts, the vaginal secretions may be considerably increased toward the end of gestation. The increased vascularity extends to the various structures in the vicinity, i.e., tissues in the perineal region, skin, muscle, and effects changes in preparation for labor.

As pregnancy advances there is a marked change in the position of the ovaries. Ovulation ceases during pregnancy. New follicles do not ripen, and only the single large corpus luteum can be found on one of the ovaries. The large

size of the corpus luteum of pregnancy is due mainly to the increased vascularity of the organ.

Abdominal Wall

The abdomen naturally enlarges to accommodate the increase in size of the uterus. The mechanical effect of this distention of the abdominal wall causes, in the later months of pregnancy, the formation of certain pink or slightly reddish streaks or striations in the skin covering the sides of the abdomen and the anterior and outer aspects of the thighs. These streaks are known as "striae gravidarum" and are due to the stretching, the rupture and the atrophy of the deep connective tissue of the skin (Plate 4, *left top and bottom*). They grow lighter after labor has taken place and finally take on the silvery whiteness

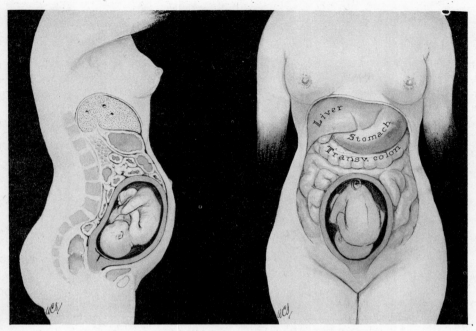

Fig. 90. Side and front views, showing the fetus at 6½ months.

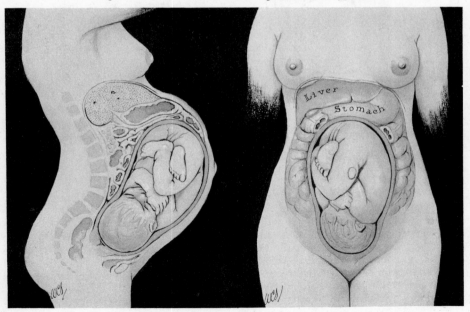

Fig. 91. Side and front views, showing the fetus at 9 months. Head not engaged.

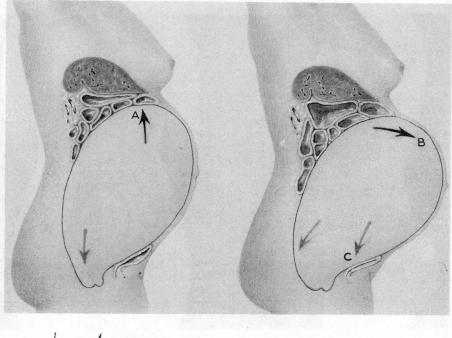

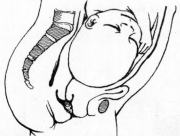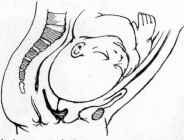

Fig. 92. The changes which take place in "lightening." (A) Pressure exerted on diaphragm before lightening. (B) Pressure relieved by falling forward of uterus. (C) Descent of head causes pressure on pelvic structures, particularly bladder.

of scar or cicatricial tissue. In subsequent pregnancies new pink or reddish lines may be found mingled with old silvery-white striae or striations. The number, the size and the distribution of striae gravidarum vary exceedingly in different women, and patients occasionally are seen in whom there are no such markings whatever, even after repeated pregnancies. As the striae are due solely to the stretching of the cutis, they are not peculiar to pregnancy but may be found in other conditions which cause great abdominal distention, such as the accumulation of fat in the abdominal wall or the development of large tumors of rapid growth.

Coincident with the uterine and abdominal enlargement, the umbilicus is pushed outward until, at about the seventh month, its depression is completely obliterated and it forms merely a darkened area in the smooth and tense abdominal wall. Later, it is raised above the surrounding integument and may project, becoming about the size of a hickory nut.

When the abdominal wall is unable to withstand the tension created by the enlarging uterus, the recti muscles become separated in the median line—so-called *diastasis.*

Breasts

Slight temporary enlargement of the breasts, causing sensations of weight and fullness, is noted by most women prior to their menstrual periods. The earliest breast changes of pregnancy are merely exaggerations of these changes. After the second month, the breasts

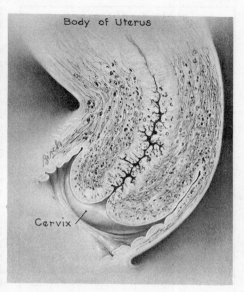

Fig. 93. Normal nonpregnant cervix.

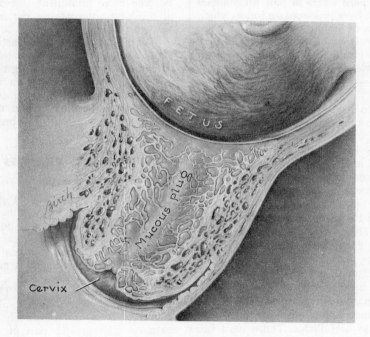

Fig. 94. Cervix at full term, showing mucous plug.

SOME IMPORTANT DEFINITIONS

Gravida: a pregnant woman.

Primigravida: a woman pregnant for the first time.

Primipara: a woman who has given birth to her first child. Usage is not uniform.

Multipara: a woman who has had two or more children.

Para I: a primipara.

Para II: a woman who has had two children (and so on up numerically, Para III, Para IV, etc.)

(The plural of these words is usually formed by adding "e," as "primigravidae.")

(The term *gravida* refers to a pregnant woman, regardless of the duration of pregnancy. In reference, it includes the present pregnancy. The term *para* refers to past pregnancies which have produced an infant which has been viable, whether or not the infant is dead or alive at birth. The terms *gravida* and *para* refer to pregnancies, not to fetuses.)

teenth century who described them very fully and, in summarizing, created a famous medical pun by saying, "They are, in fact, a constellation of miniature nipples scattered over a milky way" (Plate 4, *bottom right*). These glands of Montgomery result from hypertrophy of the sebaceous glands. In a few cases it is observed that patches of brownish discoloration appear on the normal skin immediately surrounding the areola. This is known as the "secondary areola" and is an almost certain sign of pregnancy, provided that previously the woman never has nursed an infant (Plate 5, *center right*). With the increasing growth and activity of the breasts, it is not surprising that a richer blood supply is needed, and to this end the blood vessels supplying the area enlarge. As a result, the veins beneath the skin of the breast, which previously may have been scarcely visible, now become more prominent and occasionally exhibit intertwining patterns over the whole chest wall.

The alterations in the breasts during pregnancy are directed ultimately to the preparation for breast feeding the baby. After the first few months, a thin viscous yellowish fluid may be expressed from the nipples by gentle massage. This is a watery precursor of breast milk called *colostrum*.

begin to become larger, firmer and more tender; a sensation of stretching fullness, accompanied by tingling both in the breasts and in the nipples, often develops, and, in many instances, a feeling of throbbing is also experienced. As time goes on, the nipple and the elevated, pigmented area immediately around it—the areola—become darker in color. The areola tends to become puffy, and its diameter, which in virgins rarely exceeds 1½ inches, gradually widens to reach 2 or 3 inches. Embedded in this areola lie tiny sebaceous glands which take on new growth with the advent of pregnancy and appear as little protuberances or follicles. These have been called "Montgomery's tubercles," after a famous Irish obstetrician of the nine-

GENERAL CHANGES
Weight Gain

The average total weight gain in pregnancy is about 24 pounds. During the first 3 months there may be a slight weight loss, or if weight is gained it is perhaps only a small per cent. About one half of the increment is gained in the second trimester and a similar amount in the last trimester. There are wide individual variations observed, however, even in completely normal patients. The greater part of this 24-pound increment is quite understandable, as shown by the following figures:

Baby	7 pounds
Placenta	1 "
Amniotic fluid	1½ "
Increase in weight of uterus	2 "
Increase in blood volume	1 "
Increase in weight of breasts	1½ "
	14 pounds

The remaining 10 pounds gained by the pregnant woman represent, in part, general accumulation of fat and, in part, the increased amount of fluid which tissues tend to retain at this time. Gains between 20 and 25 pounds are natural and in keeping with good health; usually they are lost after the baby is born.

Circulation

The total volume of blood in the body increases during pregnancy about 30 per cent. The minimal hematologic values for nonpregnant women apply to pregnant women, namely, 12 Gm. of hemoglobin, 3.75 million erythrocytes, 35 per cent of hematocrit. If there are adequate iron reserves in the body or if sufficient iron is supplied from the diet, the hemoglobin, the erythrocyte count and the hematocrit values remain normal during pregnancy.

An important aspect of this increase in blood volume relates to its effect on the heart. As a natural result of this change, the heart has more blood to pump through the aorta—about 50 per cent more blood per minute than it did prior to pregnancy. This augmented output of blood attains a peak at the end of the second trimester, then declines to the nonpregnant level at the last weeks of gestation. Immediately following delivery there is a sharp rise again. In women with normal hearts this is of no particular concern. However, in women with heart disease, this increase in the work which the heart has to do may add to the seriousness of the complication. The nurse can be of great help in the care of expectant mothers with heart disease, and it is well that she understand the underlying process by which pregnancy may aggravate the condition.

Palpitation of the heart is not uncommon; in the early months of pregnancy this is due to sympathetic nervous disturbance, and toward the end of gestation to the intra-abdominal pressure of the enlarged uterus.

Respiration

In the later months of pregnancy the lungs are subjected to pressure from the underlying uterus, and the diaphragm may be displaced upward as much as an inch. As a consequence, shortness of breath at that period is common. It might seem that this upward displacement of the diaphragm would decrease the capacity of the lungs, but a concomitant widening of the thoracic cage occurs which more than compensates for the other change. Actually, indeed, the pregnant woman breathes in much more air than the nonpregnant. This is necessary, since the mother is called upon to oxygenate not only her own blood but, by osmosis, that of her baby as well.

Digestion

The function of the digestive organs may be somewhat altered during pregnancy. During the early months the appetite may be diminished, particularly if nausea exists. Since the nutritional requirements to meet the needs of the mother's body and the growing fetus demand quality of the diet rather than an appreciable increase in the quantity of food ingested, this temporary manifestation should not produce injurious effects. As pregnancy advances and the digestive apparatus seems to become accustomed to its new conditions, the appetite is increased and may be voracious. Heartburn and flatulence may occur at this time, since the majority of pregnant women have a reduction in the total acidity of their gastric juice.

Also, the pressure from the diaphragm and the diminished tone may delay the emptying time of the stomach. Constipation is exceedingly common in pregnancy; at least one half of all gravid women suffer from this disorder. This suggests that the entire gastro-intestinal tract is limited by diminished tone and pressure of the growing uterus during gestation.

Skin

Striae gravidarum, which have already been discussed in relation to changes in the abdominal wall, often develop in the breasts, the buttocks and the thighs, presumably as the result of deposition of fat in those areas with consequent stretching of the skin. Certain pigmentary changes are also common, particularly the development of a black line running from the umbilicus to the mons veneris, the so-called *linea nigra* (Plate 4, *bottom left*). In certain cases, irregular spots or blotches of a muddy brown color appear on the face. This condition is known as *chloasma* or the "mask of pregnancy" (Plate 4, *top right*). These facial deposits of pigment often cause the patient considerable mental distress, but her mind may be relieved by the assurance that they will disappear after delivery. However, the increased pigmentation of the breasts and the abdomen never disappears entirely, although it usually becomes much less pronounced. All these pigmentary deposits vary exceedingly in size, shape and distribution and usually are more marked in brunettes than in blondes. Vascular spiders are minute, fiery-red elevations of the skin with branching legs coming out from the central body. They develop more often in white women, are of no clinical significance and will disappear. The skin changes may be associated with hypertrophy of the cortex of the adrenals.

In addition to the above skin changes, there is a great increase in the activity of the sebaceous and the sweat glands and of the hair follicles. The augmented activity of the sweat glands produces an increase in perspiration, an alteration which is helpful in the elimination of waste material.

Urinary System

The urine in pregnancy usually is increased in amount and has a low specific gravity. Pregnant women show a tendency to excrete dextrose in the urine. Although a reduction in the renal threshold for sugar is often associated with pregnancy, the presence of any sugar in the urine should always be reported to the physician. Lactosuria may be observed at times, especially during the latter part of pregnancy and the puerperium. It is of no significance, being due to the presence of milk sugar which is supposed to be absorbed from the mammary glands.

The ureters become markedly dilated in pregnancy, particularly the right ureter. This change apparently is due in part to the pressure of the gravid uterus on the ureters as they cross the pelvic brim and in part to a certain softening which the ureteral walls undergo as the result of endocrine influences. These dilated ureters, the walls of which have now lost much of their muscular tone, are unable to propel the urine as satisfactorily as previously; consequently, stasis of urine is common. Following delivery, the ureters return to normal within 4 to 6 weeks. The stretching and the dilation do not continue long enough to impair the ureter permanently unless infection has developed or pregnancies are repeated so rapidly that a subsequent pregnancy begins before the ureters can return to normal.

The bladder functions efficiently during pregnancy. The urinary frequency experienced in the first few months of pregnancy is caused by pressure exerted on the bladder by the enlarging uterus. This is observed again when "lightening" occurs prior to the onset of labor.

EFFECTS ON THE NERVOUS SYSTEM

The effect of pregnancy on the nervous system varies greatly; while many women escape nervous manifestations entirely, some patients present more or less altered mental and emotional characteristics, varying all the way from cravings for unusual foods, fretfulness and peevishness to rare instances of true psychoses. In exceptional cases the change is to the opposite extreme, and a woman who is ordinarily of an irritable disposition becomes exceedingly amiable and agreeable. The more unstable emotionally the patient is, the more likely is her nervous system to be affected by the strain of pregnancy.

ENDOCRINE CHANGES

Placenta

In Chapter 4 the placenta is considered simply as an organ designed to transmit nutritive substances from mother to fetus and waste products in the reverse direction. The placenta has another highly important function: it is one of the most important organs of internal secretion. The early chorionic villi of the implanted ovum secrete a hormone which finds its way into the mother's urine and makes possible the Aschheim-Zondek and the Friedman tests for pregnancy (pp. 132 and 133). This substance is called "chorionic gonadotropin" (meaning gonad-stimulating substance derived from the chorion). It permeates the tissues of the pregnant woman, of course, and is believed by some authorities to be responsible for many changes which take place in the organism during gestation. In addition to manufacturing this new hormone, the placenta takes over from the ovary the production of estrogen and progesterone and augments greatly the amount of those substances present in the body during gestation (p. 60). This increase in estrogen and progesterone is responsible for many important changes associated with pregnancy, such as the development of the breasts and the growth of the uterus. Estrogen, although stimulating breast growth and development, suppresses actual lactation; its removal from the body at delivery, therefore, by releasing this inhibiting force, plays a part in the onset of milk production. This relationship between estrogen and lactation is only one link in the very complicated but beautifully integrated endocrine chain which dominates pregnancy and in which the placenta plays a pre-eminent role.

Pituitary Body

The *anterior lobe* of this small gland located at the base of the brain has already been referred to as the "master clock" which controls the menstrual cycle. Its role in pregnancy is likewise very important. It secretes a number of hormones, one of which acts on the breasts, producing lactation (the lactogenic hormone, active only after placenta has been delivered) (see previous paragraph); another acts on the thyroid, another on the ovaries and still another on the growth process. The last is believed by some observers to be responsible for the rather coarse features which some pregnant women develop.

The *posterior lobe* of the pituitary secretes a substance which has a very strong stimulating effect on the uterine muscle, that is, an oxytocic hormone. This substance is widely employed in obstetrics to cause the uterus to contract after delivery and thereby diminish postpartal hemorrhage. It is usually referred to as "pituitary extract" or by the trade name Pitocin.

The pituitary body is thus another important link in the endocrine network of pregnancy. As a result of the far-reaching action of its hormones and of those of the placenta, many other endocrine glands show alterations. Thus, the thyroid tends to enlarge, and the parathyroid, the adrenal and the ovary develop characteristic changes.

SUGGESTED READING

Chesley, L. C.: Weight changes and water balance in normal and toxic pregnancy, Am. J. Obst. & Gynec. 48:565, 1944.

Gillespie, Edward Clark: Principles of uterine growth in pregnancy, Am. J. Obst. & Gynec. 59:949, 1950.

Holly, Roy G.: Anemia in pregnancy, Obst. & Gynec. 5:562, 1955.

Kerr, A., Jr.: Weight gain in pregnancy and its relation to weight of infants and to length of labor, Am. J. Obst. & Gynec. 45:950, 1943.

Nesbitt, R. E. L., Jr.: Prolongation of pregnancy; a review, Obst. & Gynec. Surv. 10:311, 1955.

Potter, Edith: Fundamentals of Human Reproduction, New York, McGraw-Hill, 1947.

CHAPTER SEVEN

Signs and Symptoms of Pregnancy

CLASSIFICATION OF SIGNS AND SYMPTOMS

The first visit of the modern expectant mother to her physician is usually prompted by the query, "Am I really pregnant?" Oddly enough, this is the one question which the physician may answer equivocally because even the most careful examination rarely will reveal clear-cut evidence of pregnancy until two menstrual periods have been missed, and occasionally the diagnosis may remain uncertain for a longer time. Some of the signs and symptoms of pregnancy can be recognized readily by the nurse, while others can be determined accurately only by one who has had a thorough medical or technical training.

Certain signs are absolutely indicative of pregnancy, but even these may be absent or lacking if the fetus has died in the uterus. Some so-called "positive" signs are not present until about the middle of gestation, and at that time the physician usually can make a diagnosis without them, by the "circumstantial evidence" of a combination of earlier and less significant symptoms.

The signs of pregnancy are usually divided into 3 groups, as indicated in the following classification:

A. Presumptive Signs
  1. Menstrual suppression
  2. Nausea, vomiting, "morning sickness"

3. Frequency of micturition
4. Tenderness and fullness of the breasts, pigmentation, etc.
5. "Quickening"
6. Dark blue discoloration of the vaginal mucous membrane (Chadwick's sign)
7. Pigmentation of the skin and abdominal striae
8. Fatigue

B. Probable Signs
  1. Enlargement of the abdomen
  2. Fetal outline, distinguished by abdominal palpation
  3. Changes in the uterus—size and shape and consistency (Hegar's sign)
  4. Changes in the cervix
  5. Braxton-Hicks contractions
  6. Positive pregnancy tests

C. Positive Signs
  1. Fetal heart sounds
  2. Fetal movements felt by examiner
  3. Roentgenogram—outline of fetal skeleton

PRESUMPTIVE SIGNS

Menstrual Suppression

In a healthy, married woman who previously has menstruated regularly, cessation of menstruation strongly suggests that impregnation has occurred. However, not until the date of the expected period has been passed by 10 days or more can any reliance be put on this symptom. When the second period is also missed, the probability naturally becomes stronger.

127

Although cessation of menstruation is the earliest and one of the most important symptoms of pregnancy, it should be noted that pregnancy may occur without prior menstruation and that occasionally menstruations may continue after conception. An example of the former circumstance is noted in certain Oriental countries, where girls marry at a very early age; here pregnancy frequently occurs before the menstrual periods are established. Again, nursing mothers, who usually do not menstruate during the period of lactation, often conceive at this time; more rarely, women who think they have passed the menopause are startled to find themselves pregnant. Conversely, it is not uncommon for a woman to have 1 or 2 periods after conception; but almost without exception these are brief in duration and scant in amount. In such cases the first period ordinarily lasts 2 days instead of the usual 5, and the next only a few hours. Although there are instances in which women are said to have menstruated every month throughout pregnancy, these are of questionable authenticity and are probably ascribable to some abnormality of the reproductive organs. Indeed, vaginal bleeding at any time during pregnancy should be regarded as abnormal and reported to the physician at once.

Absence of menstruation may result from a number of conditions other than pregnancy. Probably one of the most common causes of delay in the onset of the period is psychic influence; particularly fear of pregnancy. Change of climate, exposure to cold, as well as certain chronic diseases such as anemia, likewise may suppress the menstrual flow.

Nausea and Vomiting

About one half of pregnant women suffer no nausea whatsoever during the early part of pregnancy. About 50 per cent experience waves of nausea; of these perhaps one third experience some vomiting. "Morning sickness" usually occurs in the early part of the day and subsides in a few hours, although it may persist longer or may occur at other times. When this "morning sickness" occurs it usually makes its appearance about 2 weeks after the first missed menstrual period and subsides spontaneously 6 or 8 weeks later. Since this symptom is present in many other conditions, such as ordinary indigestion, it is of no diagnostic value unless associated with other evidence of pregnancy. When the vomiting is excessive, when it lasts beyond the fourth month, when it begins in the later months, or when it affects the general health, it must be regarded as pathologic. Such conditions are termed "hyperemesis gravidarum" or "pernicious vomiting" and will be discussed with complications of pregnancy in Chapter 18.

Frequent Micturition

Irritability of the bladder with resultant frequency of urination may be one of the earliest symptoms of pregnancy. It is attributed to the fact that the growing uterus stretches the base of the bladder so that a sensation results identical with that felt when the bladder wall is stretched with urine. As pregnancy progresses, the uterus rises out of the pelvis, and the frequent desire to urinate subsides. Later on, however, the symptom is likely to return, for during the last weeks the head of the fetus may press against the bladder and give rise to a similar condition. Although frequency of urination may be somewhat bothersome, both at the beginning and at the end of pregnancy, it never should constitute a reason for reducing the quantity of fluid consumed, which should be not less than 6 or 8 glasses a day.

Breast Changes

The breast changes of pregnancy have already been described (p. 121). In primigravidae (women pregnant for the first time) these alterations are helpful adjuncts in the diagnosis of pregnancy, but in women who have already borne children, particularly if they have nursed an infant within the past year, they naturally are of much less significance.

"Quickening"

This is an old term derived from an idea prevalent many years ago that at some particular moment of pregnancy life is suddenly infused into the infant. At the time this notion was in vogue, the first tangible evidence of intrauterine life lay in the mother's feeling the baby move, and the conclusion was only natural that the infant "became alive" at the moment these movements were first felt. As is reflected in the Biblical reference to "the quick and the dead," the word "quick" used to mean "alive" and the word "quickening" meant "becoming alive." Hence, our forebears were accustomed to say that when fetal movements were first felt, "quickening" or "coming to life" of the baby had occurred. We now know that the infant is a living organism from the moment of conception, but the old term "quickening" is still used in obstetric terminology, while among the laity "feeling life" is the common synonym. As used today, quickening refers only, of course, to the active movements of the fetus as first perceived by the mother.

Quickening is usually felt toward the end of the fifth month as a tremulous fluttering low in the abdomen. The first impulses caused by the stirring of the fetus may be so faint as to raise some doubt as to their cause; later on, however, they grow stronger and often become disturbingly active.

Many fetuses, although alive and healthy, seem to move about very little in the uterus, and, not infrequently, a day or so may pass without a movement being felt. Inability to feel the baby move does not mean that it is dead or

in any way a weakling but, in all probability, that it has assumed a position in which its movements are not felt so readily by the mother. Moreover, it is a well-established fact that the fetus sleeps in the uterus, and it seems likely that the periods of active movement and quiescence which the mother notices correspond to the phases of somnolence and wakefulness. Should 3 or 4 days pass without movements, the physician should be asked to listen for the fetal heart sounds. If these are heard, it means beyond doubt that the fetus is alive and presumably in good condition. It might seem that the sensations produced by the baby's movements would be so characteristic as to make this a positive sign of pregnancy, but, oddly enough, women occasionally misinterpret movements of gas in the intestines as motions of a baby and on this basis imagine themselves pregnant. Therefore, the patient's statement that she feels the baby move cannot be regarded as absolute proof of pregnancy.

Vaginal Changes

On inspection of the vagina, the physician is able to observe discoloration of the vaginal mucous membrane due to the influence of pregnancy. The mucosa about the vaginal opening and the lower portion of the anterior wall frequently becomes thickened and of a dark bluish or purplish congested appearance instead of its customary pinkish tint in the nonpregnant state. This sign, known as *Chadwick's sign*, is of no special value in women who have borne children; and, as it may be due to any condition leading to the congestion of the pelvic organs, it can be considered only as a presumptive sign of pregnancy.

Skin Changes

The changes in the skin which may accompany pregnancy, i.e., striae gravidarum, linea nigra, chloasma, pigmentation of the breasts, etc., have been referred to in the previous chapter.

These manifestations are often observed in pregnant women but vary exceedingly in different persons, often being entirely absent. The pigmentation changes in particular are often absent in decided blondes and exceptionally well marked in pronounced brunettes. As already mentioned, this pigmentation may remain from former pregnancies and cannot be depended upon as a diagnostic sign in women who have borne children previously.

Fatigue

During the early months of pregnancy the expectant mother becomes easily fatigued and experiences periods of lassitude and drowsiness. This frequently accompanies pregnancy and usually disappears after the first few months of gestation.

PROBABLE SIGNS
Abdominal Changes

The size of the abdomen in pregnancy corresponds to the gradual increase in the size of the uterus, which, at the end of the third month, is at the level of the symphysis pubis. At the end of the fifth month, it is at the level of the umbilicus, and toward the end of the ninth month at the ensiform cartilage (Figs. 86 to 91). Mere abdominal enlargement may be due to a number of causes, such as accumulation of fat in the abdominal wall, edema, or uterine or ovarian tumors. However, if the uterus can be distinctly felt to have enlarged progressively in the proportions stated above, pregnancy may properly be suspected.

Fetal Outline

After the sixth month, the outline of the fetus (head, back, knees, elbows, etc.) usually may be identified sufficiently well by abdominal palpation to justify a diagnosis of pregnancy. As pregnancy progresses, the outline of the fetus becomes more and more clearly defined. The ability to outline the fetus makes pregnancy extremely probable. In rare instances, however, tumors of the uterus may so mimic the fetal outline as to make this sign fallible.

Changes in the Uterus

Changes in shape, size and consistency of the uterus which take place during the first 3 months of pregnancy are very important indications. These are noted upon the bimanual examination which shows the uterus to be more anteflexed than normal, enlarged and of a soft, spongy consistency. About the sixth week, the so-called Hegar's sign, so named for the man who first described it, is perceptible (Fig. 95). At this time the lower uterine segment, or lower part of the body of the uterus, becomes much softer than the cervix. So soft does it become that in its empty state (for it has not yet become encroached upon by the growing embryo) it can be compressed almost to the thinness of paper. This is one of the most valuable signs in early pregnancy. Another valuable sign found on vaginal examination is "ballottement" (from the French "balloter," to toss up like a ball). During the fourth and the fifth months of pregnancy, the fetus is small in relation to the amount of amniotic fluid present; a sudden tap on the presenting part makes it rise in the amniotic fluid and then rebound to its original position and, in turn, tap the examining finger. When elicited by an experienced examiner, this response is the most certain of the probable signs.

Cervical Changes

Softening of the cervix usually occurs about the time of the second missed period. Although the nonpregnant cervix has a consistency approximate to the hardness of the tip of the nose, the pregnant cervix becomes softened and, when palpated, feels like the lips or like the lobe of the ear.

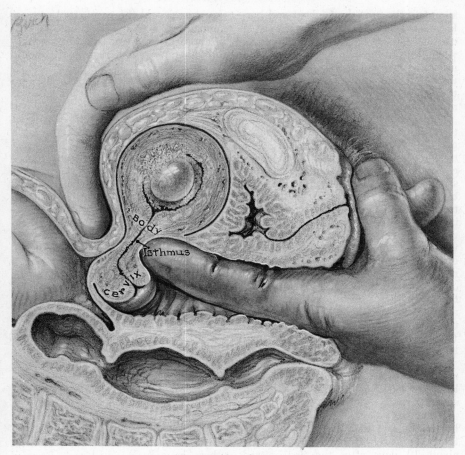

Fig. 95. Hegar's sign.

Braxton-Hicks Contractions

Uterine contractions begin during the early weeks of pregnancy and recur at intervals of from 5 to 10 minutes throughout the entire period of gestation. These contractions are painless, and the patient may or may not be conscious of them. They may be observed during the later months by placing the hand on the abdomen and during the bimanual examination. By means of these contractions the uterine muscles contract and relax, thereby enlarging in size to accommodate the growing fetus. These contractions are referred to as the Braxton-Hicks sign, after a famous London obstetrician of the last century who first described them.

Pregnancy Tests

Since the very dawn of civilization efforts have been made to devise a satisfactory test for pregnancy. The priest-physicians of ancient Egypt, in the earliest writings handed down to us, tell of a test then in vogue based on the seeming ability of pregnancy urine to stimulate the growth of wheat and barley seeds. The itinerant physicians of classical Greece employed similar tests, while, during the Middle Ages, the omniscient physician merely gazed at the urine and claimed in this way to be able to diagnose not only pregnancy but also many other conditions.

Today, interestingly enough, as in the tests of old, urine is used in a large number of tests for pregnancy. The tests are based on the fact that the early chorionic villi of the implanted ovum secrete a hormone, chorionic gonadotropin, which is excreted in the maternal urine. The method of its detection is dependent on the fact that urine containing this hormone, when injected into specific rodents and amphibia, produces readily visible changes on the rodent ovary and on the gonads of various amphibia. The tests, based on this fact, which are used most widely today are: (1) the Aschheim-Zondek test, (2) the Friedman test, (3) the Hogben test, (4) the American male frog and toad tests and (5) the Frank-Berman test.

The reactions of such tests are not of real diagnostic value unless two weeks have elapsed after the first missed menstrual period.

The great value of the endocrine tests lies in the fact that they become positive very early in pregnancy, usually about 10 days after the first missed menstrual period, sometimes even a few days earlier than this. If any of the tests have been carried out properly, the results are accurate in more than 95 per cent of cases. They are not, therefore, absolutely positive signs of pregnancy, but very nearly so.

If the diagnostic test for pregnancy is to be of value, the following procedure must be carried out. The patient is instructed to avoid drinking any fluids after the evening meal the night before the test in order to secure a concentrated urine specimen in the morning. She should void at bedtime and discard this urine. On arising the next morning, she should void the specimen to be examined into a clean, dry container. If it is impossible to send the specimen to the laboratory immediately, it should be kept cold.

Aschheim-Zondek Test. Five immature female white mice are injected with minute amounts of the urine specimen on 6 different occasions over a period of 2 days, each mouse receiving a total of 2.4 cc. of urine. Ordinarily, of course, the ovaries of these very immature animals (6 to 8 Gm. in weight) would be quiescent, but when the hormone is present in the urine injected, the follicles manifest very rapid development, so much so that several of them rupture or ovulate within a few days after the injection. Accordingly, if the urine of a pregnant woman has been injected into these animals, when the ovaries are inspected after a suitable interval (100 hours) they will reveal hemorrhagic follicles or corpora lutea. Even if only one mouse has an ovary which exhibits either a ruptured follicle and/or corpus luteum, the test is said to have a positive reaction. If the woman is not pregnant, the immature ovaries of the mice will remain in their quiescent condition and no points of follicle rupture will be seen—a negative test.

The Aschheim-Zondek test is the original endocrine test from which all others have been developed. From a practical viewpoint, the Aschheim-Zondek test has certain drawbacks: first, the difficulty of securing immature female mice of the correct weight for the procedure; second, the long 4-day wait before the result can be obtained; last, the many injections required by the procedure itself.

Friedman Test. In order to circumvent the difficulties of the Aschheim-Zondek test, Dr. M. H. Friedman, of the University of Pennsylvania, introduced an important modification of the test, using adult female rabbits instead of mice. Ten cc. of urine specimen is injected into the marginal vein of the rabbit's ear, and 24 hours later the animal is anethetized, the abdomen is opened, and the ovaries are inspected. The presence of ruptured follicles means that the test is positive.

For the reasons stated, the Friedman test is used in the United States much more widely than the original Aschheim-Zontek test and was long regarded as the standard laboratory test for pregnancy in this country, although now it has been superseded to a great extent by one or another of the frog tests. Its accuracy is about the same as the Aschheim-Zondek test.

Hogben Test. Another laboratory procedure which has gained wide popularity in the diagnosis of pregnancy is the South African toad or frog test, more properly called the Hogben test after the British physician who first described it in 1930. The test is based on the fact that female South African toads, when injected with the urine of a pregnant woman, extrude a large number of eggs within 8 to 12 hours. The particular toad employed in any given test is kept in a small glass aquarium with a black paper or cardboard beneath it, and, against this background, the myriad of eggs extruded (in the event the test is positive) are very plainly seen. The accuracy of this test is about the same as that of the Aschheim-Zondek and the Friedman tests, and it possesses the additional advantage that the result of a test can be ascertained much sooner than with the other procedures. It owes its popularity in part also to the fact that the toads are easier and more economical to keep than are mice or rabbits.

Male Frog Test. The American male frog is injected with a pregnant woman's urine. If the test produces positive results, spermatozoa will appear in the frog's urine and can be readily detected microscopically within 2 to 4 hours.

Male Toad Test. Two native species of the male toad have recently been employed as test animals in the same manner as the male frog.

Frank-Berman Test. This test has the advantage that results can be demonstrated within 8 to 24 hours. Two immature female rats (50 Gm. weight) are injected with urine. Pregnancy urine produces characteristic changes in the ovaries.

POSITIVE SIGNS

Although certain of the signs mentioned above—notably, the hormone tests, ballottement and palpating the fetal outline—are nearly positive evidences of pregnancy, they are not 100 per cent certain; errors in technic occasionally invalidate the hormone tests, while, on rare occasions, the other signs may be simulated by nonpregnant pathologic states. Using the term "positive" in the strict sense, there are only 3 positive signs of pregnancy, namely, the fetal heart sounds, fetal movements felt by the examiner and the x-ray outline of the fetal skeleton.

Fetal Heart Sounds

When heard distinctly by an experienced examiner, the fetal heart sounds can leave no doubt about the existence of pregnancy. Ordinarily, they become audible at about the middle of pregnancy, or around the twentieth week. If the abdominal wall is thin and conditions are favorable, they may become audible as early as the eighteenth week, but obesity or an excessive quantity of amniotic fluid may render them inaudible until a much later date. While the usual rate of the fetal heart is about 140 per minute, it may vary under quite normal conditions between 120 and 160. The use of the ordinary bell stethoscope, steadied by rubber bands, is entirely satisfactory (Figs. 96 and 97, left), but in doubtful cases the head stethoscope is superior, since the listener receives bone conduction of sound through the headpiece in addition to that transmitted to the eardrum (Fig. 97, right).

The nurse will find it advantageous to determine the fetal position by abdominal palpation before attempting to listen to the fetal heart tones, since ordinarily the heart sounds are best heard through the infant's back (see Chap. 5). Also, she will do well, while learning the characteristics of the fetal heart sounds, to accustom herself to place one hand on the maternal pulse and feel its rate at the same time that she hears the fetal heart tones through the stethoscope. Occasionally, the inexperienced attendant, particularly when listening high in the abdomen, may mistake the mother's heart sounds for those of the baby. Since the two are not synchronous (fetal 140, maternal 80), the method suggested above will obviate this mistake; in other words, if the rate that comes to your ear through the stethoscope is the same as the maternal pulse, it is probably the mother's heart beat; on the other hand, if the rates are different, it is undoubtedly the sound of the fetal heart.

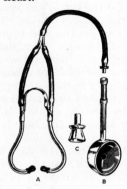

Fig. 96. Left stethoscope for use with interchangeable bells (A). Weighted bell used for auscultation of fetal heart sounds (B). Small bell used to determine mother's blood pressure (C). (J. Sklar Manufacturing Co., Long Island City, N. Y.)

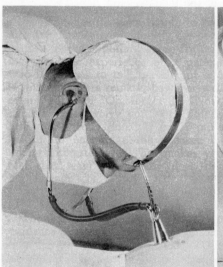 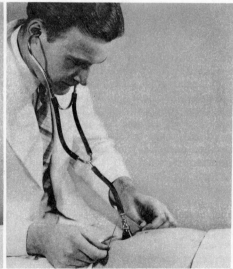

Fig. 97. (*Left*) Listening to fetal heart with ordinary stethoscope. (*Right*) Listening to fetal heart with head stethoscope. The head stethoscope gives bone conduction of sound in addition to otic (by ear) and in addition possesses the advantage that it can be used when hands are sterile.

Fig. 98. Normal
vertex position. (Bon-
ner, K. P.: Radiog-
raphy and Clinical
Photography, East-
man Kodak Com-
pany, Rochester,
N. Y.)

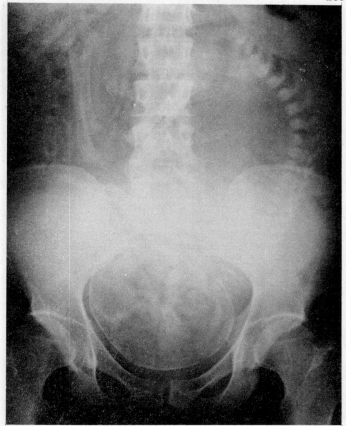

Two additional sounds may be heard in listening over the pregnant uterus: the funic souffle and the uterine souffle. Since the word "souffle" means a blowing murmur, or whizzing sound, the nature of these two sounds is similar, but their timing and causation are quite different. The word "funis" is Latin for umbilical cord, and, accordingly, the term funic souffle refers to a soft blowing murmur caused by blood rushing through the umbilical cord. Since this blood is propelled by the fetal heart, the rate of funic souffle is synchronous with the fetal heart. It is heard only occasionally, perhaps in one case out of every six. The funic souffle is a positive sign of pregnancy, but it is not usually so listed because almost always it is heard in close association with the fetal heart sounds. The uterine souffle is produced by blood rushing through the large vessels of the uterus. Since this is maternal blood, propelled by the maternal heart, it is synchronous with her heart rate. In other words, the rate of the funic souffle is ordinarily around 140 per minute (or the same as the fetal heart rate); that of the uterine souffle, near 80 (maternal heart rate).

Fetal Movements Felt by Examiner

As already noted, fetal movements

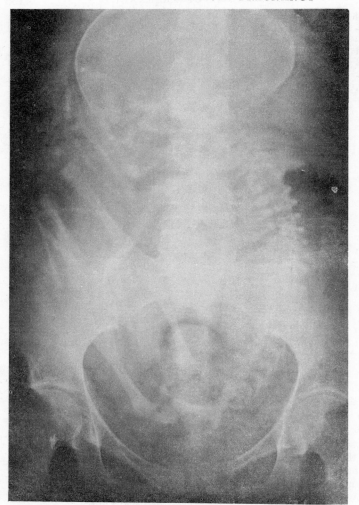

Fig. 99. Normal breech position. (Bonner, K. P.: Radiography and Clinical Photography, Eastman Kodak Company, Rochester, N. Y.)

supposedly felt by the patient may be very misleading in the diagnosis of pregnancy. However, when an experienced examiner feels the characteristic thrust or kick of the baby against his hand, this is positive evidence of pregnancy. Often this can be felt after the end of the fifth month.

Roentgenogram

A roentgenogram showing the outline of the fetal skeleton is, of course, undeniable proof of pregnancy. How early the fetal skeleton will show in the roentgenogram depends upon the thickness of the abdominal wall, the x-ray equipment and other factors. It has been demonstrated as early as the fourteenth week and is quite easily demonstrated, as a rule, after the twentieth week (Figs. 98-100).

SUGGESTED READING

Bruel, F.: Development of pregnancy

tests, Am. J. Obst. & Gynec. 63:591, 1952.

Foote, E. C., and Jones, G. E. S.: An evaluation of the Hogben pregnancy test, Am. J. Obst. & Gynec. 51:672, 1946.

Galloway, C. E.: The cervix in preg-

nancy, Am. J. Obst. & Gynec. 59:999, 1950.

Merkel, R. L.: A comparative study of chemical tests for the early diagnosis of pregnancy, Am. J. Obst. & Gynec. 60:827, 1950.

Salmon, U. J., Geist, S. H., Salmon,

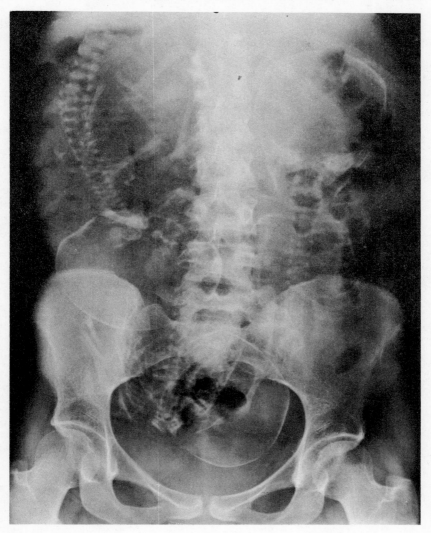

Fig. 100. Roentgenogram of triplets *in utero*. (Bonner, K. P.: Radiography and Clinical Photography, Eastman Kodak Company, Rochester, N. Y.)

A. A., and Frank, I. L.: A new six-hour test for pregnancy, J. Clin. Endocrinol. 2:137, 1942.

Saunders, C. B.: Frog test for pregnancy, Texas State J. Med. 42:375, 1946.

Schwartz, H. A.: A simple, accurate pregnancy test, Am. J. Obst. & Gynec. 59:213, 1950.

Weisman, A. I., Snyder, A. F., and Coates, C. W.: Use of the African clawed frog (*Xenopus laevis Daudin*) as a rapid diagnostic test for pregnancy, West. J. Surg. 50:557, 1942.

CHAPTER EIGHT

Antepartal Care

DEFINITION

The medical supervision and care given to pregnant women during the period between conception and the onset of labor is called antepartal care. The word antepartal is derived from the Latin word, *partus,* which means "before labor." In obstetric parlance the familiar adjective "prenatal" has been used more generally. Strictly speaking, the word prenatal means "before birth" and therefore includes the first and second stages of labor, a connotation which is not intended here. However, the reader will find these terms used interchangeably in current obstetric literature.

Good antepartal care aims to maintain the mother's health and peace of mind so that she may pass through pregnancy and labor with a maximum of mental and physical fitness. It aims further to ensure the optimum health of the mother and her baby and to increase her knowledge so that they may be kept healthy and happy after the delivery. This is accomplished through the combined efforts of the expectant parents, the obstetrician, the nurse and other members of the health team.

Antepartal care may be considered

the foundation for the normal development, the adequate growth and the good health of the baby. During this formative period the teeth, the bones and the various systems of the body have their beginnings, as well as the foundations for his future health. For the mother adequate antepartal care aids in stabilizing the daily health. As pregnancy advances, the demands of the fetus increase. Since individuals react differently to pregnancy, this supervision is of the utmost importance in detecting these reactions. This supervision not only helps to relieve discomforts and to prevent accidents and complications but also aids in ensuring a more rapid convalescence and continued good health.

THE IMPORTANCE OF PREVENTIVE CARE

Prior to the rise of present-day obstetrics, the physician usually had only one interview with his patient before he saw her in labor, and often at this interview he merely sought to compute the expected date of confinement. When he next saw her she might be in the throes of an eclamptic convulsion or striving vainly to overcome the resistance offered

139

by a contracted pelvis. It is in the prevention of such calamities as these that care and supervision of the pregnant mother have been found to be of such value. Indeed, antepartal care is an absolute necessity if a substantial number of women are to avoid disaster; and it is helpful to all.

From a biologic point of view, pregnancy and labor represent the highest function of the female reproductive system. As has been mentioned previously, this should be considered a normal process. But the numerous physiologic changes which occur in the mother's body during pregnancy (see Chap. 6) demonstrate that the borderline between health and illness is less distinctly marked during pregnancy than during the nonpregnant state. A slight variation in bodily function, which might be of but little significance if the woman were not pregnant, may be a warning signal of a potential pathologic condition in pregnancy which could seriously threaten the health of the mother or the child or both. Examples of such symptoms might be a weight gain of several pounds during one week or a persistent headache. Health supervision and teaching begun early in pregnancy are often the means of avoiding complications of pregnancy; and in the event that symptoms do occur, their early detection and prompt treatment may avert serious problems.

The importance of early and continued medical supervision during pregnancy cannot be overemphasized. If it were possible, care should begin as early as the patient conceives or perhaps even earlier than that, not only at the very beginning of her pregnant period, but ideally with her own mother's antepartal state, which likewise had everything to do with the patient's health. In recent years much has been accomplished through premarital and prepregnancy examinations to determine the patient's fitness for pregnancy. More and more physicians are offering

this care and encouraging this plan toward positive health.

MEDICAL CARE

Today the emphasis is on positive health, to determine the health status of those anticipating parenthood. Every patient should be under the care of her obstetrician during the entire period of her pregnancy. She should be seen as early in pregnancy as possible and at least every 4 weeks thereafter until the seventh month. Then she should make her visits every 2 weeks until the last month of pregnancy, during which time it is most important that she be seen every week. The therapy of all patients should be individualized. In the case of an expectant mother who has some abnormal condition, the visits should be spaced according to the demands of the situation. Each physician has his own system.

At the first examination the history of the patient is taken, then a general medical examination is carried out, and finally the obstetric examination, which includes an examination *per vaginam,* is given. The examination may be carried out according to the following outline.

The History

The name and the address of the patient, her age and parity and the date of the latest menstrual period are recorded, and the date of delivery is estimated. Inquiries are made regarding the family history, with special reference to any condition likely to affect childbearing, such as hereditary disease, tuberculosis or multiple pregnancy. The personal history of the patient is then reviewed not only in regard to previous diseases and operations but particularly in relation to any .difficulties experienced in previous pregnancies and labors, such as miscarriages, prolonged labor, death of infant, hemorrhage and other complications. Inquiry is then made into the history of the present pregnancy, especially in relation to nausea, edema of the

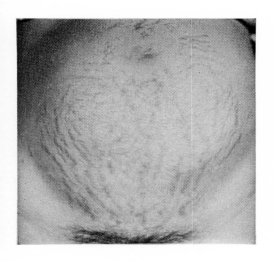

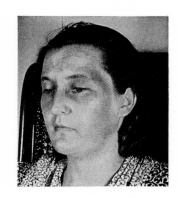

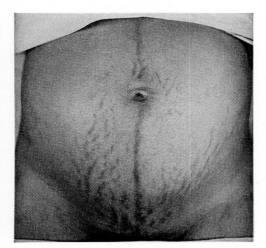

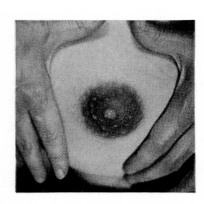

PLATE 4. (*Left, top*) Striae gravidarum.
(*Left, bottom*) Linea nigra and also striae gravidarum.
(*Right, top*) Mask of pregnancy (chloasma).
(*Right, bottom*) Montgomery's tubercles.

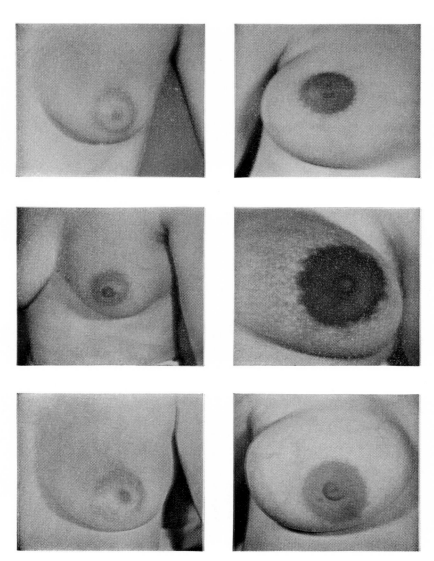

PLATE 5. (*Left, top*) Breast in nonpregnant blonde.
(*Right, top*) Breast in pregnant blonde, showing pigmentary changes.
(*Left, center*) Breast in nonpregnant brunette.
(**Right, center**) Breast in pregnant brunette, showing pigmentary changes
and marked secondary areola.
(*Left, bottom*) Breast in nonpregnant red-haired woman.
(*Right, bottom*) Breast in pregnant red-haired woman.

feet or the face, headache, visual disturbance, vaginal bleeding, constipation, breathlessness, sleeplessness, cramps, heartburn, lower abdominal pain, vaginal discharge, varicose veins, etc. Usually a suitable form for recording these particulars is employed. As a rule, obstetricians, hospital clinics and organizations have their own forms for recording these details.

General Medical Examination

The general medical examination includes weighing the patient, taking the blood pressure, inspecting the teeth and the throat and making an examination by auscultation and percussion of the heart and the lungs. Opportunity is taken at this time to inspect the breasts and the nipples, particularly in relation to their suitability for subsequent nursing. From an obstetric viewpoint, one of the important details of the general medical examination is the measurement of the blood pressure (Fig. 101). This is usually carried out first and always should be done when the patient is seen on subsequent visits. As will be explained subsequently, any substantial increase in blood pressure indicates one of the most serious complications in pregnancy—toxemia. A fact for the nurse to keep in mind is that any sudden or gradual rise in the systolic or

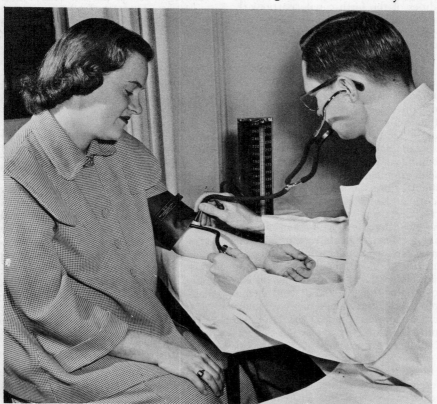

Fig. 101. The blood pressure is one indication of the expectant mother's state of health.

diastolic blood pressure is significant and may be alarming.

Obstetric Examination

The obstetric examination is comprised of 3 parts: (1) palpation and auscultation of the abdomen; (2) estimation of pelvic measurements; and (3) vaginal examination. Palpation and auscultation of the abdomen yield valuable information concerning the size and the position of the fetus. The great importance of careful pelvic measurements has already been emphasized, while the purpose of the vaginal examination (aside from its use in the diagnosis of pregnancy) is to rule out abnormalities of the birth canal (particularly those which might impede labor) and to take the diagonal conjugate measurement.

Laboratory Tests

The laboratory tests carried out in antepartal care are the urine examination, the blood test for syphilis, the estimation of the hemoglobin, tests for the Rh factor and blood type. At the first examination, the urine is tested for albumin and sugar and at all subsequent examinations for albumin. If the patient brings the specimen from home she should be instructed to collect a part of the first urine voided in the morning. The blood for the Wassermann or other serologic test for syphilis is usually obtained by venipuncture. A sufficient quantity of blood should be drawn at this time so that a portion may be employed for the Rh factor and hemoglobin estimation. Since many pregnant women develop anemia, the latter examination is highly important. A metabolism test is routine in the practice of some obstetricians.

If the test for the Rh factor shows the patient to be Rh negative, it may be necessary to check the husband. It is also a wise precaution for the doctor to have the husband's blood type.

Weight

The routine estimation of weight at regular intervals during pregnancy is an important detail of antepartal care. Any marked gain or loss in weight will be discussed by the obstetrician. At first the average gain in weight of the fetus is 1 Gm. daily; nine tenths of the weight is gained after the fifth month, and one half of the weight of the fetus is acquired during the last 8 weeks. It is to be expected that most pregnant women have an average gain in weight of between 20 and 25 pounds during pregnancy. In any excessive weight gain, or for a patient who is markedly overweight, one of the low caloric diets may be prescribed in an effort to control the weight. Weight gain should be considered in relation to the patient's general physical condition.

Return Visits

At return visits, careful inquiry is made into the general well-being of the patient, and questions are asked concerning any untoward signs and symptoms, such as edema of the fingers or the face, bleeding, constipation and headache. The patient is then weighed, her blood pressure is taken, and the urine is analyzed for albumin. An abdominal examination is usually carried out at this time. Abdominal, vaginal and rectal examinations should be done at regular intervals in order to determine that pregnancy is progressing at the expected rate and, following quickening, that the fetus is living. During these visits the patient should avail herself of the opportunity of asking the physician any questions which may be of concern to her.

Instructions to Patients

After the routine examination, the patient is instructed regarding diet, rest and sleep, daily intestinal elimination, proper exercise, fresh air and sunshine, bathing, clothing, recreation and dental care. It is usually possible and always desirable to assure the patient that the findings on examination were normal, and that she may anticipate an uneventful pregnancy followed by an uncomplicated delivery. At the same time, however, she is tactfully instructed regarding certain danger signals which demand immediate report to the physician. These symptoms are as follows:

1. *Vaginal bleeding, no matter how slight*
2. *Swelling of the face or the fingers*
3. *Severe continuous headache*
4. *Dimness or blurring of vision*
5. *Pain in the abdomen*
6. *Persistent vomiting*
7. *Chills and fever*
8. *Sudden escape of fluid from the vagina*

In addition to this detailed supervision, the patient needs an explanation of the changes that are taking place within her body. This intelligent instruction will give her greater reassurance and self-confidence. An understanding and sympathetic attitude will do much to buoy the patient's morale.

As the patient approaches full term, she should also be instructed about the signs and symptoms of oncoming labor, so that she may know when the process is beginning and when to notify the physician. At this time the physician will want to know the frequency of contractions and any other pertinent symptoms.

Most hospitals conduct routine tours of the maternity division for the registered maternity patients and their husbands. It is advisable to encourage the expectant parents to take advantage of this opportunity sometime during the pregnancy. Becoming familiar ahead of time with the surroundings where she will be delivered reduces the anxiety which may be experienced in going to a strange hospital for the first time after labor has begun. The details of the hospital admission routine should also be explained, so that she is familiar with this procedure before being admitted for delivery.

NURSING CARE
The Nurse in the Clinic

The nurse who is accustomed to caring for patients on the inpatient hospital service where she has rather continuous contacts with the same patient for days, or even weeks at a time, often finds the initial adjustment to the clinic service difficult because of the limited time the clinic schedule permits for contacts with each patient. During the patient's brief appointment period, the nurse must evaluate the present and continuing nursing needs of the individual and plan to meet these needs effectively. The nurse who recognizes and understands this problem of limited time will find the orientation period less frustrating and, as she becomes increasingly more skilled and learns to budget her time efficiently, will enjoy the satisfactions of giving care and guidance in this type of community service.

The clinic nurse devotes much of her nursing care to health teaching which the patient will utilize at home. This may be concerned with knowledge about physiology of childbearing, general hygiene, nutrition, etc. She teaches the mother how to maintain good health habits in daily living, interprets to her the reasons why these are important and suggests ways in which recommended changes can be made.

The initial contact with the patient is particularly important. The nurse can establish a productive relationship by the interest manifested and the pleasant professional manner in which she greets the patient. As the nurse makes the patient comfortable while waiting for her appointment with the physician, she may have an opportunity to find out about any new symptoms or problems that the mother may have and, in turn, report them to the proper person. The patient's problems are not always those of a physical nature. The nurse recognizes that emotional or social problems may interfere with the patient's ability to derive full benefit from medical services. It is the responsibility of the nurse to seek out ways in which the patient needs help, for to give comprehensive nursing care which will promote optimum health for the expectant mother it is not only necessary to care for her physical needs but also to recognize the psychological, social and economic factors which affect the pregnancy. In hospitals where the appointment system is used the waiting time for the patient is minimized. In others, the patient may have to wait longer periods. This waiting time may be utilized by providing the patient with reading material. Visual aids such as posters and charts may be both instructive and diverting. Through these contacts with patients, the nurse can also emphasize the importance of the patient's keeping her return appointment with the physician or the clinic.

The nurse has an opportunity to assist the physician with the physical examination and at the same time learn more about the patient's condition. She may be questioned afterward by the patient regarding her condition or may have to interpret the physician's instructions to make certain that they are understood. Often a patient is hesitant to discuss some matter with the physician because she considers it too trivial but may feel comfortable in talking about it with the nurse. In turn, the nurse may consider this a problem of some importance and, on reporting it to the physician, find that it has bearing on the course of treatment that he prescribes.

In a program which emphasizes family-centered service, the health problems of the individual patient and their relationship to other members of the family are of major importance. An ex-

ample of a situation might be the case of Mrs. Brown, the wife of a laborer and the mother of a small toddler and a 4-year-old boy. Her physician has advised her that she needs more rest in the course of the day. Her husband is at work, and the older boy is in nursery school until noon. In order to provide more rest for the mother, she needs help to make plans for the safety and care of the children during these rest periods, otherwise the physical rest would not accomplish its purpose. Even the consideration of meeting the nutritional needs for this family with a limited income may require guidance. It requires some knowlege of nutrition and entails extra planning in order that the meals supply the nutritional requirements for a pregnant woman, a father who performs hard physical labor and 2 small children.

The nurse in the clinic is alert to the patient's needs and thus may recognize a health problem, affecting either the patient or her family, which might be alleviated by a home visit. In such a situation she should see that a referral to the public health nurse is made through the proper channels. Real value may be derived from a visit in which the nurse is able to see the patient in her usual surroundings. For instance, if the patient has the problem of excessive weight gain and is not responding to clinic therapy, the public health nurse, visiting the patient in her home, may gain some insight into the basis of the problem during her visit. In her report back to the clinic staff she would relate information which would contribute to the medical management of this pregnancy. In another situation, if the clinic program is limited in educational opportunities, such as parents' classes and/or individual guidance, the public health nurse's visit to the home may be necessary to supplement the health teaching done in the clinic and to help the mother make preparations for herself and the new baby.

The Public Health Nurse

The extensive adoption of early antepartal care by various institutions, both lay and medical, is doing much to improve obstetric standards; and, in connection with this movement, the public health nurse has proved to be an invaluable asset. During the period before antepartal care was fully accepted, a case-finding program was a part of some organizations, i.e., the nurse would canvass the district for pregnant mothers. In recent years the demand for hospital deliveries has increased rapidly, so that the trend toward hospital care has exceeded the number of hospital beds to accommodate patients. Therefore, hospitals are not able to accept patients unless they register early in pregnancy. This has been a favorable contribution to early registration and, in larger cities especially, has resulted in more mothers getting adequate antepartal supervision early in pregnancy. In some isolated rural areas the public health nurse does case finding in the course of her usual activities and can assist the local practitioner in the antepartal care of maternity patients in the community.

In a well-organized clinic program the public health nurse is the intermediary between the physican and his patient. In localities where there is an interagency referral system, this is a valuable adjunct in the care of patients, especially when discriminatory reporting is utilized in the referral.

There can be no stereotyped routine followed by the public health nurse in her visits, since each one involves an individual patient in her own home setting. The visit should be based on what each patient needs or wants to know. Generally, such a visit includes giving the patient basic information about pregnancy, how to keep well during pregnancy, through practice of good hygiene and improved dietary habits, and teaching her how to make some of the necessary preparations for herself and her baby. She has many opportunities for family health supervision. In her observation of other children in the home the public health nurse may be the first person to notice a neglected orthopedic condition, to suspect a need for a chest roentgenogram or to observe a possible vision or hearing difficulty.

The most commonly recognized need is in the premature program in which public health nursing service is used to help the family prepare for the homecoming of the premature infant and to give constructive guidance accordingly.

In the analysis of this program, the nurse's records, through their content, accuracy and value, show the needs to be met. Antepartal care, then, consists of care and advice given by the physician, the complete co-operation on the part of the parents in carrying out this advice and conscientious follow-up on the part of the nurse. The combined efforts of many may be involved in the care of the pregnant mother: physician, dentist, nurse and social worker, each, in his own field, making a related contribution toward better health. "This pooling becomes possible if each member of the health team has a clear understanding of his own function, appreciates and understands the contribution of other professions represente ¹ on the team, knows something of the processes involved in the differing approaches, recognizes commonness of interest and skill, and has the intellectual and emotional capacity to enter into a team relationship."*

THE MEDICAL SOCIAL WORKER

In recent years the fact that the Social Service Department in the hospital constitutes an important part of the team of a hospital staff has been generally recognized. Previously, there were a few hospitals that appreciated

* Church, Gertrude M.: Understanding each other to achieve a common goal, Am. J. Nursing **56**:201, 1956.

this valuable asset, but today it is accepted as essential. The physical needs of the patient comprise only one of the many responsibilities carried by this department. The Social Service workers' function is to help people to meet problems which interfere with social functioning. In their professional role they are able to evaluate and alleviate the so-called social conditions. They make studies, visit homes and interview the patient, and perhaps other family members, to ascertain the physical and emotional needs of the family. All problems may seem overwhelming if the patient's physical condition is affected, and these problems, in turn, may interfere with the benefit she may derive from medical services. In addition, such a worker is the understanding counselor between the family and the patient during her hospital stay. In many hospitals the need for a social service referral is apparent when the patient is registered early in pregnancy. The social worker interviews the patient after the initial examination, and, from the physical and social findings, plans are made with the patient to meet her needs. Among the many problems encountered are placing of older children during the mother's hospital stay, arranging for a working housekeeper if the children are of school age and must be kept at home, planning for convalescent care for the mother and arranging for financial or material assistance.

In the care of the unmarried mother and the problem of illegitimacy there are many aspects to be considered. None of these patients fit into a typical category, and each patient reacts differently; some are apparently indifferent, others rather obviously are in a state of panic, still others exhibit a kind of silent withdrawal. The social worker tries to gain enough information so that she is able to offer guidance as to the sources of help available to the patient. These services should eliminate some of patient's worry and help her to make plans for herself and her baby. At the same time, the worker acknowledges the patient's right to form her plans and make her own decisions. Since these situations often involve the placing of the baby and plans for the re-employment of the mother, the social worker must know about the available approved nursing homes and the suitable employment agencies. Because some unmarried mothers are interested in having their babies adopted, she must be familiar with the legal aspects of adoption, as well as the reputable adoption agencies.

Every illegitimate pregnancy is not fraught with social problems. It must be remembered that in certain cultures illegitimacy does not carry the stigma which our society imposes. The infant is welcomed into the family very naturally, and the mother is not condemned as one who has broken a moral code. The community's interest may be incited if the children suffer because of lack of financial resources, and, therefore, assistance becomes necessary.

By her observation and experience, the social worker combines her efforts with other members of the health team to see the patient not only as an individual maternity patient but also as an important member of the family, and the family as an integral part of the community.

NUTRITION IN PREGNANCY

Much attention has been given to the diet of the pregnant mother in recent years since it has been proved that the improved nutritional status of the mother promotes not only her well-being but also that of her baby. An appropriate diet promotes the mother's health and provides essential building materials for the growth and development of her offspring.

The diet should be considered from the standpoint of quality rather than quantity. During the first part of pregnancy the daily energy requirements for the average pregnant woman should be about the same as usual, in the neighborhood of 2,300 calories a day, unless the mother's weight needs to be regulated. In the latter part of pregnancy the daily caloric intake would ordinarily be augmented because of the increased metabolic rate. The physician will prescribe specifically for each mother to meet her individual needs. The Food and Nutrition Board of the National Research Council recommends daily allowances of specific nutrients for pregnancy and lactation, as shown in Table 4.

During the early months the appetite may be poor, and there may be phases of dislike for certain foods. Then, later, there may be an increase in the desire for all food or certain types of food. This increase in appetite may have to be disciplined in accordance with the amount of food needed and the gain in weight of the individual. Sweets and high-calorie desserts, as well as the habit of frequent nibbling, should be avoided because of the interference with appetite for the more essential foods and the additional weight added by such foods. The so-called occasional

craving for unusual articles of food should be kept in mind; it may mean the lack of a certain element in the diet that the body seems to demand. Any desires of this nature may be granted with safety if they agree with the patient and are not exceptional in amount or content. If the diet supplies all the needs of the patient and the growing fetus, such cravings may not occur.

The Normal Diet

The physician will regulate the patient's diet according to her condition; but, as a rule, if her previous diet has been nourishing and well balanced, few changes will be necessary. There should be a relatively large proportion of fluids, including 1 quart of milk daily; proteins from meat, eggs and fish; dark, whole grain or enriched bread or cereal, a generous allowance of green, yellow and leafy vegetables; fruits, one of which should be citrus; and butter. Margarine labeled as containing at least 15,000 units of vitamin A per pound equals butter, except for vitamin D, obtainable in egg yolk, liver or in capsule form; in some brands of margarine vitamin D has been added.

TABLE 4. RECOMMENDED DAILY DIETARY ALLOWANCES*

NUTRIENTS	NONPREGNANT WOMAN (25 YEARS OLD, 5'4", 128 LBS.)	PREGNANT WOMAN (LATTER PERIOD)	LACTATING WOMAN	MAN (25 YEARS OLD, 5'9", 154 LBS.) MODERATELY ACTIVE
Calories	2,300	+300	+1,000	3,200
Protein (Gm.)	58	+ 20	+ 40	70
Calcium (Gm.)	0.8	1.5	2.0	0.8
Iron (mg.)	12	15	15	10
Vitamin A (I.U.)	5,000	6,000	8,000	5,000
Thiamine (mg.)	1.2	1.3	1.7	1.6
Riboflavin (mg.)	1.5	2.0	2.5	1.8
Niacin (mg.)	17	+ 3	+ 2	21
Ascorbic acid (mg.)	70	100	150	75
Vitamin D (I.U.)	+	400	400	+

* Recommended Dietary Allowances (Revised 1958), Publication 589, National Academy of Sciences, National Research Council, Washington, D. C.

Milk. Milk is nature's most nearly perfect food and is invaluable to the pregnant mother. It contains all the different kinds of mineral elements which are needed for fetal development. The high content of calcium and phosphorus in milk makes it almost indispensable for good growth of bone and teeth; it provides these minerals in exactly the correct proportions and in a digestible form which permits their complete utilization by both mother and fetus. It is not only an excellent source of protein or tissue-building material but also the most readily digested and easily absorbed of all food proteins. Milk is also rich in energy-providing values, so that 1 quart a day alone furnishes almost one fourth of the total energy requirements. Finally, milk contains some of the most important vitamins, particularly vitamin A, which increases resistance to infection and safeguards the development of the fetus (Fig. 102).

Due to the superb qualities of milk as such, an effort should be made to have the patient drink 2 glasses of milk a day. The remainder of the quart may be taken in some other form such as soup, cocoa, desserts, etc. Evaporated and whole dried milk, which have the same food value as the original milk,

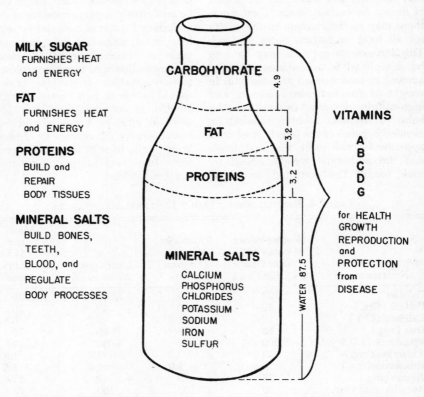

Fig. 102. Although milk varies somewhat with the breed of cow and the cow's food, the above chart gives a good idea of the reason why milk should be an important part of the diet in pregnancy. Milk is considered nonfattening because it supplies the largest portions of all needed proteins, minerals and vitamins with the fewest number of calories. (Maternity Consultation Service)

may be substituted for fresh cow's milk if that is not available.

For some patients, milk may be constipating or fattening or distasteful. If milk is found to be constipating, it is preferable to treat the constipation in some way other than by omitting the milk. Concerning the fattening effect of milk, the gain probably is due to the consumption of more food than is needed. If weight gain is excessive, the milk is not at fault, but the excess of foods such as bread, potatoes and desserts. These are the articles to be restricted and not the milk. If milk is distasteful, it may be disguised in other foods (soups, cereals, desserts). If the patient were made to realize the importance of this one article of food in relation to the development of this baby which she is anxiously anticipating, this sacrifice will be met willingly.

Skimmed milk or churned buttermilk might be substituted for whole milk. However, it would have fewer calories and less vitamin A per quart. Cultured whole milk (often used instead of churned buttermilk) has practically the same caloric value and vitamin content. American cheese may also be used as an occasional substitute. One ounce of cheese contains approximately the same minerals and vitamins as a large glass of whole milk.

Proteins. Meat, eggs and seafoods are high in protein, and during pregnancy the need for these foods is increased—not only to meet the mother's own demand but also to supply the elements needed by the fetus from conception to birth for the development of all the delicate and intricate systems of his body. These foods contain vitamins and valuable minerals, but their main value is in their amino acids or building stones, as they are sometimes called. Meat, eggs and fish contain complete proteins, proteins which have all the 10 amino acids which are necessary to maintain life and support growth.

Dark cereals and dark breads should replace the white varieties because they contain more vitamin B. Wheat contains one complete protein, but most cereals do not. When cereals are supplemented by milk they become adequate for growth as well as for maintaining life. Bread should be buttered as a means of increasing the vitamin A intake. The coarse cereals and the dark breads add roughage to the diet. Vitamin B and roughage both help to counteract constipation.

Vegetables. (Especially leaf, stem, green and yellow varieties.) These are also daily food necessities for the pregnant mother because they are rich sources of iron, calcium and several vitamins. It is desirable to include at least 2 or 3 of these each day, 1 should be raw. At mealtimes there is no reasonable limit to the amount of lettuce, tomatoes, celery, string beans, carrots, beets and asparagus which may be eaten, and by increasing the quantity of such foods to several times the amount ordinarily taken it is usually possible to satisfy the appetite without gaining abnormally in weight. Fresh frozen vegetables are a good alternate. Canned vegetables may be used if fresh are not available. If a good brand is obtained, the vitamin content is often higher than that of vegetables cooked at home. The careful preparation and cooking of vegetables will help to retain the maximum of vitamin and mineral content. Some vegetables contain several incomplete proteins which add to the total protein intake.

In addition to their value as nutrient agents, these vegetables deserve an important place in the diet as laxative agents, since their fibrous framework increases the bulk of the intestinal content and thereby stimulates the muscular, eliminative action of the intestines.

Fruits. Citrus fruits—oranges, lemons and grapefruit—are the best sources of vitamin C. Most of these fruits also supply vitamins A and B. Tomatoes are also an excellent source of vitamin C; the amount, however, must be twice that of the citrus fruits to supply the same amount of vitamin. The other fruits, both raw and cooked (prunes, apricots, etc.), contain important minerals (iron and copper) as well as vitamins. Fruits are important not only for their vitamins, but also they may be the means of stimulating a lagging appetite and counteracting constipation (see pp. 163 and 166). Fruit may be used in many ways—as juices, combination salads, additions to cereals or in-between-meal refreshments and desserts, such as gelatins and puddings. Fruits contain some incomplete proteins but only supplement the other proteins.

Fluids. Fluids should be taken freely, averaging 6 to 8 glasses daily. Water aids in the circulation of the blood, body fluids, and the distribution of mineral salts, as well as stimulating the digestion and the assimilation of foods. Fluids help to increase perspiration and to regulate elimination from intestines and kidneys. Tea and coffee may be included in the daily fluid quota if not found to be constipating or sleep-disturbing. Alcohol should be used sparingly, particularly if the mother must watch her weight, since beverages containing alcohol have a high caloric content. The use of alcohol by the pregnant woman has not shown a tendency to produce any pathologic changes in the mother or fetus, and no effect on the course of pregnancy or labor has been demonstrated.

Vitamins. Vitamins are the *live* elements in food and are essential to life. The best sources are the natural foods. In order to retain the vitamin value in foods they must be fresh, carefully prepared and not overcooked. During pregnancy and lactation the vitamin needs are increased, so it is apparent that a well-balanced diet containing all the vitamins is of first importance. Some physicians add vitamin preparations to the diet in order to assure meeting the adequate requirement.

Vitamin A is essential in the diet for the maintenance of body resistance to infection. Foods which are good sources of this vitamin include whole milk, fortified skimmed milk, dairy products containing butter fat, eggs, green leafy and yellow vegetables and liver.

The Vitamin B complex is essential to good nutrition. During pregnancy, thiamine (B_1) is necessary in increased amounts, as the fetus readily depletes the mother's reserve. Milk, eggs, lean meat and whole grain or enriched bread and cereal are good sources of thiamine. Riboflavin and nicotinic acid, absolute essentials in the diet, are found in such foods as meat, milk, eggs and green vegetables.

Vitamin C is necessary for the proper development of the fetus. Since an adequate reserve of this water-soluble vitamin is not stored in the body, an abundant supply of this vitamin is needed daily throughout pregnancy and lactation. Fresh citrus fruits, berries and green leafy vegetables (with the exception of lettuce) are foods which are a good source of vitamin C. These foods should be eaten raw as often as possible, since cooking destroys about half of their vitamin content.

Vitamin D is of great importance in safeguarding the mother and the fetus during pregnancy since it bears some relationship to calcium and phosphorus metabolism. Liver, eggs, fortified sweet milk and fish (particulaly Atlantic herring and mackerel) are food sources of vitamin D. Ordinarily, the diet does not supply this vitamin in sufficient amounts to meet the daily requirements for pregnancy and lactation recommended by the National Research Council. Particularly in localities where exposure to sunshine is limited, as in the northern part of the United States, the diet is usually supplemented by vitamin D preparations in the form of cod-liver oil or concentrates.

Minerals. Studies indicate that 13 or more mineral elements are essential for good nutrition. It is believed that if calcium, phosphorus, iron and iodine are provided in adequate amounts the others will also be present in sufficient quantities.

CALCIUM. Although two thirds of the calcium in the fetus is deposited during the last month of pregnancy, the mother's daily requirement of calcium is doubled during the entire course of pregnancy to prepare adequate storage for this demand. The principal foods from which calcium is obtained are cheese, eggs, oatmeal, vegetables and milk. A quart of milk alone supplies 1.2 Gm. of calcium.

PHOSPHORUS. This element is an essential constituent of all the cells and tissues of the body. Milk provides an abundant source of phosphorus. Actually, since phosphorus is an almost invariable constituent of protein, a diet which includes sufficient protein-rich foods, such as eggs, meat, cheese, oatmeal and green vegetables, will also provide an adequate amount of phosphorus.

IRON. The average American diet contains less than the recommended amount of iron to meet the requirements imposed by pregnancy. During the first two trimesters of pregnancy, iron is transferred to the fetus in moderate amounts, but during the last trimester, when the fetus builds up its reserve, the amount transferred is accelerated about 10 times. The diet should be balanced and nutritious as well as rich in iron-containing foods. It is believed that certain amino acids and vitamin C may be essential to normal iron absorption. If the daily diet contains egg yolk, lean meat (particularly liver), vegetables, fruit and whole grain cereals, the problem of anemia is less likely to occur. However, most physicians prescribe additional iron in the form of such preparations as ferrous sulfate and ferrous gluconate. These preparations should be administered 3 times a day, following the meals, to allow for maximum absorption and to eliminate much of the intolerance for iron which would occur if the daily prescription for iron were administered in one dose.

IODINE. Only very small amounts of iodine are needed for the health of the mother and the fetus. These are obtained very readily from seafoods and daily cod-liver oil. However, in certain localities around the Great Lakes and in the Northwest, the water supply and the vegetables grown are poor in iodine. This deficiency may be counteracted by the use of iodized salt, or the physician may prescribe small amounts of iodine.

Weight Control

Weight gain during pregnancy between 20 and 25 pounds is natural and in keeping with good health. Usually this weight is lost after the birth of the baby. However, increases in weight over 25 pounds are undesirable, for a number of reasons. First, they represent unnecessary poundage for the muscles of the legs and the back to carry about, and this suddenly imposed strain is a common cause of backache, pain in the legs and also easy fatigability. Second, certain serious complications of pregnancy, preeclampsia and eclampsia (see p. 392), are less common in patients whose weight increment is moderate. Third, if weight gain in pregnancy is excessive, it is likely to be a permanent acquisition, so that, if the expectant mother is interested in retaining her figure, she should also be interested in limiting weight gain at this time.

Obstetricians are emphasizing more and more the importance of weight control in pregnancy; some insist on as little as 15 pounds gain. If the patient's weight gain after the third month is of the order of 3 pounds a month it may be regarded as satisfactory, but if it exceeds 4 pounds a month, steps should be taken to control it. Here a nurse can be of the utmost help in advising expectant mothers about certain simple steps which may be taken, particularly in regard to the curtailment of certain nonessential foods.

Some of the specific suggestions which may be made are as follows.

1. The patient should be acquainted with the amazing fattening potentialities of certain common nonessential foods—foods which, in many people's minds, scarcely deserve that term at all, because most of them are likely to be regarded as mere snacks without appreciable effects on total caloric intake. Actually, these little extras taken between meals or at bedtime constitute one of the most common causes for excessive weight gain in pregnancy and at other times. Even a glass of ginger ale or Coca-Cola averages 100 calories. A chocolate bar approximates more than 300 calories. A single cocktail or highball runs 200 calories. A doughnut (without icing) plus a cup of cocoa yields 400 calories, while the average malted milk served at soda fountains contains some 500 calories. Pie à la mode approximates 600 calories. When it is recalled, as stated on page 146, that 2,300 calories per day is generally recognized as a satisfactory allowance for pregnancy—really, the uppermost limit—it is plain that these "little snacks" mentioned above loom tremendously large in relation to the total caloric allotment. They simply must be eliminated if the patient is gaining excessively. When hungry between meals, she may take the glass of milk scheduled for dinner, omitting it from her evening meal.

2. The patient should be reminded that the way in which a food is prepared may affect its caloric or fattening value almost as much as the nature of the food itself. Failure to heed this fact has resulted in many women gaining weight on diets which should cause them, theoretically at least, to lose. Perhaps the simplest way to show how the preparation of a food affects its caloric value is to be found in fried foods. Although the caloric content of a poached or boiled egg is about 80 calories and is so calculated in dietary lists, once that egg is fried, its caloric value jumps to around 120 calories because of the fat absorbed by the egg in cooking. A level tablespoon of fat, let it be emphasized, yields approximately 120 calories. In regard to soups and desserts, it is common knowledge that those made with milk are of much less caloric content than those made with cream, and that those made with skimmed milk are still lower. When flour or cheese in addition to cream is used, as in escalloped or au gratin dishes, the calories soar to unbelievable heights; in general, for this group of foods, the smoother and the more delicious the taste, the higher the caloric value.

The intrinsic caloric value of foods of the same type varies widely. Fruits show considerable variation according to their degree of sweetness. Canned fruit may be very high in calories because of the sugar in the syrup. Likewise, meats vary greatly in their caloric contents, lean meats being low and those with much fat in their substance being high. As an example of the latter, an average serving of linked country sausage may exceed 600 calories. To summarize this aspect of weight control in pregnancy, the patient should be reminded that fried foods invariably possess a high caloric content and must be curtailed or eliminated altogether; that milk, preferably skimmed milk, should be substituted for cream in preparing soups and desserts; and that lean meat rather than fatty meat must be chosen, and fresh fruit rather than canned.

3. The next suggestion to make to the patients is to substitute skimmed milk for the whole milk included in the recommendation about diet in pregnancy. This reduces forthwith the caloric content of the diet by about 300 calories—no small sum. Fat-free or skimmed milk contains the same nutrients as whole milk, except for fat and

vitamins A and D. However, fortified fat-free milk contains much greater amounts of these two vitamins than does whole milk. However, be sure that the patient is taking this quart of milk every day. It provides more proteins, minerals and vitamins for less calories (and money) than any other food; and skimmed milk contains, of course, as much protein and minerals (including calcium) as does whole milk.

4. The next suggestion is an easy one to carry out, namely, to substitute saccharin for sugar, not only in coffee or tea, but also for cereals and fruits. For cereals, it may be dissolved in the milk used over them, and to sweeten fruits it may be dissolved in a little water. Saccharin should not be cooked, as this makes it bitter.

5. The salt ordinarily added to foods in the kitchen should be reduced drastically or eliminated altogether. If there is any one substance which should be curtailed in any pregnancy, it is salt. First, the amount of salt consumed by the average person is far in excess of human requirements. Second, even if no salt were added to foods either in the kitchen or at the table, this mineral is distributed so widely in food materials that the likelihood of shortage would be exceedingly remote. Finally, there is a definite relationship between the amount of salt eaten and the amount of water retained by the body; that is, the greater the salt intake the greater the tendency of tissues to absorb water. The tissues of the pregnant woman manifest a particular avidity for water, as is evidenced by the tendency of the face and the fingers to become puffy, and if, superimposed on this tendency, there is an excess of salt in the diet, the tissues may become actually waterlogged, with dire consequences. It is a good rule to add no salt to the food at the table and, in the kitchen, to add a little less than one would like, this being the rule for any pregnant woman. As a substitute for flavor herbs, spices, pep-

per, paprika, vinegar, lemon juice, vanilla or almond extract may be suggested. In the case of excessive weight gain in pregnancy, it is quite possible that a still further reduction in salt, as recommended above, will reduce superfluous body water and cause a substantial weight loss. At first, this salt-poor diet may seem so bland and tasteless as to constitute something of a hardship; but it is surprising how quickly patients get used to it and after a few days, as a rule, do not object to it too much.

6. If the above recommendations do not serve to curtail weight gain, the patient should eliminate all desserts. For these, fresh fruits can be substituted, sweetened, if necessary, with saccharin water.

7. It may be necessary to remind the patient to take servings of average size and only one serving.

Because of the importance of the subject, the nurse must understand that it will not suffice simply to tell the patients to reduce their food consumption or to eat less fattening foods. Directions, to be effective, must be specific as well as rather comprehensive and should be reviewed with the patients in a sympathetic and understanding way. Above all, it must be emphasized that no curtailment is to be made in food essentials—doubly essential in pregnancy—such as milk, green and yellow leafy vegetables, proteins, minerals and vitamins.

If the simple suggestions listed above are not effective, the case is a special one, and the patient should be under the personal dietary supervision of her physician or a trained nutritionist.

GENERAL HYGIENE

Pregnancy should be a normal, happy, healthy experience for the pregnant woman. During the months preceding labor the physician will advise her as to her mode of life. He will usually encourage her to continue her usual habits with very little change, unless, of course, he finds that she has been leading an existence which is not conducive to healthy living.

Rest, Relaxation and Sleep

Because rest and sleep are so essential for health, the nurse must emphasize this detail in her teaching during the antepartal period. Pregnant women become tired more readily; therefore, the prevention of fatigue must be stressed very emphatically. The body is made up of various types of cells, each type with a specific function. Depletion of nerve-cell energy results in fatigue, and fatigue causes certain reactions in the body which are injurious. For all body processes, such as digestion, metabolism, working, playing and studying, our nerve-cell energy is utilized. Nature has made provision for some reduction in our normal energy without injury to health. Beyond this limit, the symptoms of fatigue are evidenced in irritability, apprehension, tendency to worry and restlessness. These symptoms are sometimes very subtle and misleading, but, in contrast, human beings are very conscious of tired muscles. It is more important to avoid fatigue than to have to recover from overfatigue. The pregnant woman should rest to prevent this fatigue. Rest and sleep replenish the cell energy. As Dr. Jastrow says of this code of rest and sleep, they "must be shaped according to the individual's nervous disposition, habits of life, age, and circumstances." If patients cannot sleep, they should attempt to rest. Rest is the ability to relax. Patients often need to learn how to relax. There is no code so variable, so necessarily adapted to the individual, as that of rest and sleep. The final test is whether the day's work is done with zest and energy to spare. The expectant mother should get as much sleep as she feels she needs. Some people need more than others. In addition to a good night's sleep, advise the mother to take a nap or at least to rest

for one half hour every morning and every afternoon. If this is not possible, advise her to lie down, if for only a few minutes, several times a day, in a well-ventilated room. It should be explained that rest means not only to lie down or perhaps to sleep, but also to lie down comfortably—to relax—to rest the body, the mind, the abdominal muscles, the legs and the back and to stretch out, and so make it easier for the heart to pump the blood to the extremities. During the last months of pregnancy, a small pillow used for support of the abdomen, while the patient lies on her side, does much to relieve the discomfort common during this period and adds materially to the degree of rest that the patient gets in a given time.

Suggest to the patient that, instead of standing, she sit whenever possible, even while doing her housework. Sitting to rest for other brief periods during the course of the day can be beneficial if the feet and the legs are elevated.

Often the so-called minor discomforts of pregnancy can be overcome by rest. Rest and the right-angle position (see Fig. 109) are advised for swelling, edema and varicosities of the lower extremities. Rest and the Sims' position (see Fig. 112) are advised for varicosities of the vulva and the rectum. Even for the more serious abnormalities, the simple aids included in "diet and rest" may help much until more specific orders from the obstetrician can be obtained. In such instances, the nurse must be aware of the mother's interpretation of "rest," and, if indicated, provide the necessary guidance to help the mother understand and plan for it.

Exercise

Outdoor exercise during pregnancy is usually very beneficial because it affords diversion in the sunshine and fresh air. However, for each individual patient the obstetrician must decide whether the customary exercise should be increased or diminished. There should be a difference in the amount of exercise for the early and late periods of pregnancy. When pregnancy is advanced, exercise may be limited in comparison with the amount advised previously. Exercise usually means diversion, and, of course, this phase is most important. Exercise also steadies the nerves, quiets the mind, promotes sleep and stimulates the appetite, all of which are valuable aids to the pregnant mother.

Walking in the fresh air is quite generally preferred to every other form of exercise during pregnancy, because it stimulates the muscular activity of the entire body, strengthens some of the muscles used during labor and is available to all women. Exercise of any kind should not be fatiguing; to secure the most beneficial results it should be combined with fresh air and sunlight, as well as periods of rest.

The woman who does her own housework needs little or no planned exercise from the physical viewpoint. However, she does need fresh air, sunshine and diversion. It is far better for the patient to be occupied than to sit idly, but standing for long periods of time should be avoided. Lifting heavy objects, moving furniture, reaching to hang curtains, any activity which might involve sudden jolts, sudden changes in balance which might result in a fall or the likelihood of physical trauma should be avoided. Dancing, swimming, horseback riding, tennis, golf and long climbs are all subjects that should be discussed with the obstetrician for his final decision. The pregnant woman who is accustomed to participating in certain sports and finds this an enjoyable form of recreation will usually be permitted to continue in moderation and at a mild pace if it proves harmless.

Employment

The same attitude of moderation should be maintained whether for work or play. Ideally, no work or play should be continued to the extent of even moderate fatigue. Jobs requiring moderate manual labor should be avoided if they must be continued over long hours, if they require delicate balance, or constant standing, or constant working on night shifts. Actually, the woman who has a "desk job" in an office often does less strenuous work than the average homemaker who does not go out to work. Nevertheless, positions which require the worker to sit constantly can be extremely tiring. Adequate rest periods should be provided for all pregnant women employed in such positions.

In some countries, the time of discontinuing routine jobs has been regulated by law, and the limits, although arbitrary, are generally from 6 to 8 weeks prior to the expected date of confinement.

During the war emergency, millions of women were engaged in war industries. Many women are still employed in various industries, and the problem of pregnancy for the working mother is a most important one. In order to safeguard the interests of expectant mothers so engaged, the following "Standards for Maternity Care and Employment of Mothers in Industry" have been recommended by the Children's Bureau of the U. S.

1. Facilities for adequate prenatal medical care should be readily available for all employed pregnant women; and arrangements should be made by those responsible for providing prenatal care, so that every woman would have access to such care. Local health departments should make available to industrial plants the services of prenatal clinics; and the personnel management or physicians and nurses within the plant should make available to employees information about the importance of such services and where they can be obtained.

2. Pregnant women should not be employed on a shift including the hours between 12 midnight and 6 A.M. Pregnant women should not be employed more than 8 hours a day nor more than

48 hours per week, and it is desirable that their hours of work be limited to not more than 40 hours per week.

3. Every woman, especially a pregnant woman, should have at least two 10-minute rest periods during her work shift, for which adequate facilities for resting and an opportunity for securing nourishing food should be provided.

4. It is not considered desirable for pregnant women to be employed in the following types of occupation, and they should, if possible, be transferred to lighter and more sedentary work:

a. Occupations that involve heavy lifting or other heavy work.

b. Occupations involving continuous standing and moving about.

5. Pregnant women should not be employed in the following types of work during any period of pregnancy, but should be transferred to less hazardous types of work.

a. Occupations that require a good sense of bodily balance, such as work performed on scaffolds or stepladders and occupations in which the accident risk is characterized by accidents causing severe injury, such as operation of punch presses, power-driven woodworking machines, or other machines having a point-of-operation hazard.

b. Occupations involving exposure to toxic substances considered to be extra hazardous during pregnancy, such as:

Aniline
Benzol and toluol
Carbon disulfide
Carbon monoxide
Chlorinated hydrocarbons
Lead and its compounds
Mercury and its compounds
Nitrobenzol and other nitro compounds
  of benzol and its homologs
Phosphorus
Radioactive substances and x-rays
Turpentine

Other toxic substances that exert an injurious effect upon the blood-forming organs, the liver, or the kidneys.

Because these substances may exert a harmful influence upon the course of pregnancy, may lead to its premature termination, or may injure the fetus, the maintenance of air concentrations within the so-called "maximum permissible limits" of State codes, is not, in itself, sufficient assurance of a safe working condition for the pregnant woman. Pregnant women should be transferred from workrooms in which any of these substances are used or produced in any significant quantity.

6. A minimum of 6 weeks' leave *before* delivery should be granted, on presentation of a medical certificate of the expected date of confinement.

7. At any time during pregnancy a woman should be granted a reasonable amount of additional leave on presentation of a certificate from the attending physician to the effect that complications of pregnancy have made continuing employment prejudicial to her health or to the health of the child.

To safeguard the mother's health she should be granted sufficient time off after delivery to return to normal and to regain her strength. The infant needs her care, especially during the first year of life. If it is essential that she return to work, the following recommendations are made:

a. All women should be granted an extension of at least 2 months' leave of absence after delivery.

b. Should complications of delivery or of the postpartum period develop, a woman should be granted a reasonable amount of additional leave beyond 2 months following delivery, on presentation of a certificate to this effect from the attending physician.

Diversion

Recreation is as necessary during pregnancy as it is at any other time in life. Labor must be anticipated, and the added responsibility of having a baby creates some concern for the mother. It is often beneficial to discuss with the mother some types of recreation which are most relaxing for her and perhaps make helpful suggestions. Consideration and understanding on the part of the husband, the family, the doctor and the nurse do much to relieve the mother's fears, anxieties and uncertainties. When husbands, in particular, understand more about all that is involved in their wives' pregnancies their helpfulness can be increased. If a "blue day" comes, the husband should make it his particular responsibility to provide a means of counteracting it. The nurse can also discuss with the father and the rest of the family ways in which they might help to make this period less of a strain. The husband cannot take over the innumerable discomforts that may be associated with pregnancy, but he can do a great deal to help his wife get the much-needed diversion. He can help her to secure the kind of social relaxation that she enjoys most. Good books, radios, music, movies, interest in sports, television, cards, sewing clubs, church functions, visiting, driving, walking and having friends come in are some of the means of providing relaxation and diversion. However, the mother should avoid crowds, chances of infection and all conditions likely to cause a sense of discomfort. Amusements, exercise, rest and recreation at proper intervals help to keep the pregnant mother well and happy in an environment conducive to her well-being and happy anticipation for the baby.

Traveling

This is perhaps a detail of antepartal care which most patients think very little about, unless they have a tendency to become nauseated or have had a previous miscarriage.

The restriction of travel to short trips had been a rule for maternity patients until World War II, when many women found it necessary to follow their husbands regardless of distance or modes of travel. It is now possible to apply the data compiled during that era to show that travel, almost regardless of distance and type of conveyance, has no deleterious effect on pregnancy.

The general advice given to a pregnant woman is to avoid any trip which will cause undue fatigue, since she is prone to tire easily. For traveling long distances the railway or airplane are safer and provide greater comfort. If travel is by private automobile, rest periods of 10 to 15 minutes should be planned at least every 2 hours. This not only avoids fatigue but also benefits the general circulation when one is able to stretch and walk about.

Although traveling is not usually contraindicated during pregnancy, the expectant mother should consult her physician concerning the advisability of extensive travel at any time during the period of pregnancy.

Care of the Skin

The skin may be more active during pregnancy, and there may be increased or decreased perspiration, resulting in irritation or dryness. Since the skin is one of the organs of elimination, bathing is obviously important, and baths should be taken daily because they are stimulating, refreshing and relaxing. They act not only as a tonic and general invigorator but also favor elimination through the skin as well. Elimination through the skin is thought to lessen the strain of elimination by the kidneys.

During pregnancy, showers or sponge baths may be taken at any time. The old idea that tub baths should be avoided because the wash water enters the vagina and thereby carries infection to the uterus is now believed to have little validity. There is only one objection to tub baths during the last trimester of pregnancy. At this period the heavy weight of the large abdomen may put the pregnant women off balance, thus making climbing in and out of the tub awkward. Therefore, the likelihood of her slipping or falling in the bathtub is increased. Chilling the body should be avoided. Cold baths, cold sponges and cold showers never should be taken unless approval has been given by the obstetrician.

Care of the Breasts

Special care of the breasts during pregnancy is one of the important prep-

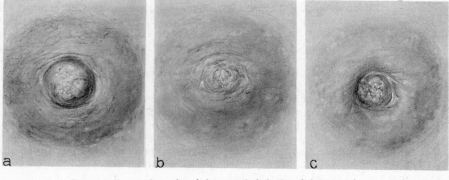

Fig. 103. Types of nipples. (a) Normal. (b) Flat. (c) Inverted.

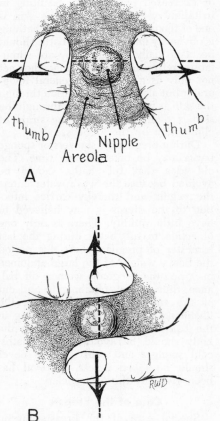

arations for breast feeding. During the antepartal period the breasts often have a feeling of fullness and weight. A well-fitted supporting brassière may relieve these discomforts. There may be sufficient secretion of colostrum from the nipples to necessitate wearing a pad to protect the clothing. The daily care of the nipples, and the reason for it, as well as the actual procedure, should be explained to the patient. Early in pregnancy the breasts begin to secrete, and this secretion often oozes out on the surface of the nipple and, in drying, forms fine imperceptible crusts. If these crusts are allowed to remain, the skin underneath becomes tender; if left until the baby arrives and nurses, this tender skin area is likely to crack. With this condition there is always a possibility of infection. Nipples that are kept clean and dry do not have a tendency to become sore or cracked.

Instruct the patient to wash her hands, and then bathe her breasts daily,

Fig. 104. A suggested treatment for inverted nipples. The thumbs are placed close to the inverted nipple, pressed firmly into the breast tissue, then gradually pushed away from the aerola. The strokes should be directed horizontally (A) and vertically (B) and be done 4 or 5 times in succession.

using a clean washcloth, soap and warm water. Begin each breast by washing the nipple thoroughly with a circular motion, making sure that any dried material has been removed, then gradually continue working away from the nipple in this fashion until the entire breast is washed. Rinse the breast in this manner and dry with a clean towel. The physician may advise the use of Massé nipple cream or some similar ointment in preparation of the breasts for the baby's nursing. This can be applied after the breasts are bathed. First, place a small quantity of cream on the thumb and the first finger, then grasp the nipple gently between the thumb and this finger and, with a kind of rolling motion, work the cream into the tiny creases found on the surface of the nipple. The position of the thumb and finger should be gradually shifted around the circumference of the nipple until a complete circuit has been made. This procedure should be limited to about 30 seconds on each breast.

If the patient's nipples are flat or inverted (Fig. 103), special care should be started in the fifth or six month of pregnancy, or earlier. Dr. J. B. Hoffman* has suggested a treatment which has proved to be helpful. With the thumbs placed close to the inverted nipple, press firmly into the breast tissue and gradually push the thumbs away from the areola. The strokes should follow an imaginary cross drawn on the breast (see Fig. 104) and be done 4 or 5 times in succession on awakening each morning. The nipple will assume an erect, projected position and then can be grasped as a unit and gently teased out a bit further. This should be done daily so that the nipples may be made more prominent for the baby to grasp. In extreme cases where the nipples are

* Hoffman, J. B.: A suggested treatment for inverted nipples, Am. J. Obst. & Gynec. 66:346, 1953.

badly inverted, the obstetrician will give instructions concerning the care needed.

Clothing

During pregnancy the clothes should be given the same or perhaps even a little more attention than at other times. The young mother who feels that she is dressed attractively and is well-groomed will reflect this in her manner. Her clothing should be practical, attractive and nonconstricting. Most women are able to dress in the manner to which they are accustomed in the nonpregnant state until the enlargement of the abdomen becomes apparent. Maternity specialty shops and department stores have made maternity fashions available, which has settled the problem of suitable clothing during pregnancy. Today designers and stylists are giving consideration to the pregnant mother's clothing so that she may dress attractively and feel self-confident about her appearance. The clothes are designed so that they are comfortable and "hang from the shoulders" to avoid any constriction; they are made in a variety of materials. The expectant mother should dress according to the climate and the temperature for her comfort.

Abdominal Support

Women who have been unaccustomed to wearing a girdle will scarcely feel the need of abdominal support, especially during the early months of pregnancy. Later, however, a properly fitted maternity girdle often gives the needed support to keep the mother from becoming fatigued. The natural softening of the pelvic joints which accompanies pregnancy and the increasing weight of the abdomen may encourage a change in posture to such a degree that severe backache results.

If the mother's abdomen is large, or if previous pregnancies have caused her abdomen to become lax or pendulous, a properly made and well-fitting maternity corset will give support and comfort. The purpose of the garment is for support, not to constrict the abdomen (see Fig. 105).

Breast Support

It is advisable that every pregnant woman wear a brassière that is well-fitted to support the breasts in a normal uplift position. Proper support of the breasts is conducive to good posture and thus helps to prevent backache (Fig. 106).

The selection of a brassière should be determined by individual fitting, influenced by the size of the breasts and the need for support. It is important to see that the cup is large enough and the underarm is built high enough to cover all the breast tissue. Wide shoulder straps will afford more comfort for the woman who has large and pendulous breasts. The size of the brassière is, again, a matter to be determined according to the individual being fitted, but usually this is about two sizes larger than that usually worn. The mother who is planning to breast feed will find it practical to purchase nursing brassières which can be worn during the latter months of pregnancy as well as during the postpartal period for as long as she is nursing her baby.

Garters

"Round garters" or any tight bands (rolled stockings, elastic tops on stockings) that encircle the leg tend to aggravate varicose veins and edema of the lower extremities and should be discarded in favor of suspender garters or some form of stocking supporters attached to an abdominal support (Fig. 107). It will be remembered that arteries have muscular tissue in their walls,

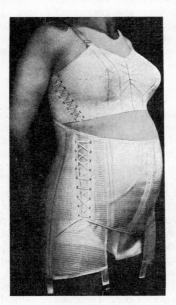

Fig. 105. Maternity corset and brassière. (Spencer, Inc., New Haven, Conn.)

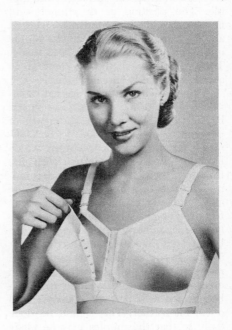

Fig. 106. Maternity brassière for use during and after the nursing period. Special construction allows for sanitary gauze over the nipples and convenient opening for nursing. (Maiden Form Brassière Co., New York)

while veins have little or none, so that arteries are able to resist pressure. The external veins lie close to the surface, while the arteries are embedded deeper in the tissues. Hence, any constriction of any extremity affects the veins far more than the arteries, and blood, which apparently meets with no obstruction whatever in its flow down the extremity through an artery, may on its return through the vein find at the point of constriction sufficient closure of the vessel to "dam it back" and so stretch the vein wall that a varicosity is formed. There is already a marked tendency toward this condition because the enlarged and constantly enlarging uterus tends to impede the return circulation from the lower extremities by compression of the great abdominal vessels, and round garters definitely tend to aggra-

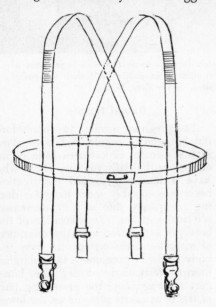

Fig. 107. Shoulder garters made of skirt belting, tape or ribbon, 1½ inches wide. The strap over the front should be attached to the belt far enough to the side to prevent pressure on the breasts.

vate the condition. Garters that encircle the leg never should be worn, even by growing children, for the tendency to varicosities is always present; and, when once formed, they never entirely disappear but later may lead to great discomfort.

Shoes

Expectant mothers should wear comfortable, well-fitted shoes. The postural changes which occur as the mother's abdomen enlarges may be aggravated by wearing high-heeled shoes, with resulting backache and fatigue. Low-heeled shoes should be worn during working hours. However, many women do not like to go out on the street without the usual high-heeled shoes. If they do not develop backache from the increased lordosis induced by the heels, and are able to maintain good balance, there is no real reason for insisting that they wear more practical but less welcome low-heeled shoes.

The nurse should remember that the height of the heel is but one consideration here, and that the support which the shoe gives the foot adds materially to the mother's comfort. Many of the flat-heeled and ballet-type shoes popular today give little or no support to the feet and thus may be the cause of fatigue and aching legs and backs. A simple method to check the support of a shoe can be done by placing the shoe flat on the floor, then, with the thumb, pressing down hard against the arch. If the shoe gives under this pressure, it indicates that it will give weak support to the foot.

Care of the Teeth

Good dental care is necessary because the teeth are important in relation to adequate mastication of food. This care need be little different during pregnancy from what is considered to be good, general mouth hygiene in any person who is not pregnant. The teeth should be brushed carefully on arising,

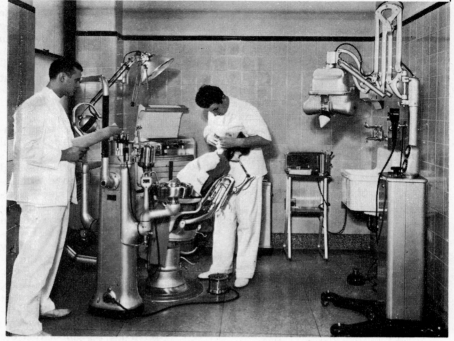

Fig. 108. Dental clinic as part of an obstetric service. Because of the importance of good dental care, some hospitals have a dental clinic in connection with their antepartal supervision. (Margaret Hague Maternity Hospital, Jersey City, N. J.)

after each meal and before retiring at night. An alkaline mouthwash may be used if desired. It is advisable for the expectant mother to visit her dentist at the very beginning of pregnancy and to follow his recommendations (Fig. 108). However, if he advises any extensive dental work to be done, the patient should consult her obstetrician.

The old saying, "For every child a tooth," based on a belief that the fetus takes calcium from the mother's teeth, has no real scientific basis. It should be carefully explained to the mother that an adequate diet during pregnancy will supply the baby with lime salts and other necessities in sufficient amounts to build his bones and teeth. Therefore, this old adage need not be true if proper attention is given to the care of the teeth and nutrition during pregnancy.

Bowel Habits

The pregnant woman who heretofore has adhered to regular habits of elimination usually experiences little or no change in the daily routine. Those who have a tendency toward constipation become noticeably more irregular during pregnancy due to (1) decreased physical exertion, (2) relaxation of the bowel in association with the relaxation of smooth-muscle systems all over the body, and (3) pressure of the enlarging uterus. Particularly during the latter part of pregnancy, the presenting part of the fetus exerts pressure on the lower bowel.

Personal habits of intelligent daily hygiene are the best resource that the expectant mother has to prevent constipation. The alleviation of this problem in modern society may be attributed to education, more reasonable bowel habits and greater latitude in physical exercise. During pregnancy the mother should pay close attention to bowel habits, drink sufficient quantities of fluid, eat fruits and other foods which add roughage to the diet and get reasonable amounts of daily exercise.

If these simple measures are not effective, the physician should be consulted about the problem. Harsh laxatives and enemas should be avoided unless the physician orders them specifically. He will probably prescribe some mild laxative. If this is a nonabsorbable oil preparation, such as mineral oil, it should be taken at bedtime. The mother should be advised that such medication taken at mealtime has the ability to dissolve and excrete the oil-soluble vitamins, such as vitamin A, and thus deprive her body of these vitamins which are necessary for good nutrition.

Constipation is conducive to the development of hemorrhoids and may be associated with the incidence of pyelitis. Aside from the discomfort associated with the passage of hard fecal material, this may injure the rectal mucosa and cause bleeding.

Douches

The vaginal douche, for so long considered by most married women to be a requisite of feminine hygiene, is unnecessary in most cases and should be kept at a reasonable minimum. During pregnancy, if it is indicated because of excessive vaginal secretion, the physician will prescribe the kind of douche and the frequency with which it is to be taken.

Specific instructions about douching should be given. The nurse will be able to give more intelligent guidance if she first learns from the patient about the available facilities at home (such as a bathtub), the patient's understanding of proper douching and the reasons for this treatment. It is well to remember that if a woman is not accustomed to douching she will need guidance in relation to purchasing the necessary equipment or improvising it.

The following precautions require emphasis:

1. *Hand-bulb syringes must be absolutely forbidden,* since several deaths in pregnancy from air embolism have followed their use. (See Suggested Reading.)

2. Plastic or hard rubber douche nozzles are preferable, since those made of glass may chip or break and injure the walls of the vagina.

3. The physician's order must be followed as outlined and the medicated solution prepared according to his instructions, i.e., the quantity of active ingredient and temperature (usually 108° F.), etc.

4. The bathtub should be scrubbed thoroughly before and after the treatment.

5. The external genitalia should be cleansed with soap and water before taking a douche to avoid transmitting bacteria into the vagina.

6. The douche bag should be placed no higher than 2 feet above the level of the hips in order to prevent high fluid pressure.

7. The nozzle should not be inserted more than 3 inches into the vagina.

For the most effective results, the patient should assume a reclining position with the knees flexed and the thighs slightly separated. The nozzle should be inserted carefully and rotated gently as the solution flows slowly and circulates in the vagina. This usually requires about 10 minutes.

Marital Relations*

The expectant mother should be under the guidance of a good physician from the time pregnancy is suspected. Great care especially should be taken

* Wood, L. F., and Dickinson, R. L.: Harmony in Marriage, New York, Round Table Press, p. 90.

to avoid excess in the sex relationship or to avoid it entirely at the period when menstruation would normally have taken place because of the greater liability of the wife to miscarriage at such times.

The husband is to realize that his wife is under nervous and emotional tensions which call for constant patience and sympathy on his part. If at this time a wife should feel a sudden and unexplained aversion to her mate, let both of them realize that it is an accompaniment of her condition rather than a real change in her attitude. Failing to realize this some young people have drifted into unpleasant and bitter experiences of misunderstanding and conflict entirely out of harmony with their love for each other. Sometimes this happens partly because the nature of the wife calls out all the more at this time, in a way which she may not fully understand, for the full sympathy and support of her husband. If he will help her through the early part of this period by unusual considerateness in every way he will be likely to find that health and happiness are improved, as her whole being meets the call of motherhood.

Smoking

While most obstetricians disapprove of excessive smoking in pregnancy, there is no reason for believing that a woman who smokes moderately, 10 cigarettes or less a day, need change her custom at this time. This subject should be discussed with the physician.

MINOR DISCOMFORTS

The so-called minor discomforts of pregnancy are the common complaints experienced by most expectant mothers, to some degree, in the course of a normal pregnancy. However, all mothers do not experience all of them, and, indeed, some mothers pass through the entire antepartal period without any of these discomforts. They are not serious in themselves, but their presence detracts from the mother's feeling of comfort and well-being. In many instances

they can be avoided by preventive measures, or entirely overcome by common sense in daily living once they do occur.

Frequent Urination

One of the first signs the young woman may notice to make her suspect she might be pregnant is the frequent desire to empty her bladder. This is caused by the pressure of the growing uterus against the bladder and will subside about the second or third month when the uterus expands upward into the abdominal cavity. Later, during the last weeks of pregnancy the symptoms will reoccur (see p. 209).

Nausea

Nausea and vomiting of mild degree, the so-called "morning sickness," constitute the most common disorder of the first trimester of pregnancy. For many years it has been thought that this condition has an emotional basis. In all life's encounters, there are probably few experiences which are at first more upsetting, mentally and emotionally, than the realization by a young woman that she is pregnant. At first there is the anxious uncertainty before she can be sure of the diagnosis. Then, there are numerous adjustments that have to be made and responsibilities that may seem to be overwhelming. Emotionally, the implications of pregnancy extend far back into her childhood, long before she met her husband. It is understandable that women who cannot adjust themselves to all these new circumstances could have problems. However, the whole cause of nausea and vomiting should not be attributed to the neurotic factor. Symptoms may be caused by physiologic changes of normal gestation.

Symptoms usually appear about the end of the fourth or sixth week and last until about the twelfth week. Nausea occurs in about 50 per cent of all pregnancies; of these, about one third experience some vomiting. Usually it occurs in the morning only, but a small percentage of patients may have nausea and vomiting throughout the entire day.

The typical picture of morning sickness starts with the patient's experiencing a feeling of nausea on arising in the morning. The mother is unable to retain her breakfast, but by noon she has completely recovered and has no further episodes until the next morning. This does not always occur in the morning but may happen in the afternoon or in the evening. In a small percentage of patients the nausea and vomiting may persist throughout the day and even be worse in the afternoon. With the majority of patients this problem lasts from 1 to 3 weeks and then suddenly ceases. There may be a slight loss of body weight but no other signs or symptoms.

Often this condition can be controlled and frequently it may be greatly relieved. Various "before breakfast" remedies are often used. If, one half hour before rising, the patient takes a dry piece of toast or a cracker, relief may be obtained. In some instances, sips of hot water (plain or with lemon juice), hot tea, clear coffee or hot milk have been tried, with successful results. However, the dry carbohydrate foods seem to be more effective. After taking any one of these "before breakfast" remedies, the patient should remain in bed for about one half hour; then she should get up slowly and dress slowly (meanwhile, sitting as much of the time as possible). After this she is usually ready for her breakfast.

Greasy foods, and those known to disagree with the patient, should be avoided in the diet. Other suggested remedies include eating an increased amount of carbohydrate foods during this period of disturbance or eating simple and light food 5 or 6 times a day instead of the 3 regular full meals. Unsweetened popcorn during the morning is sometimes advised. The patient may be helped by drinking sweet lemonade, about half of a lemon to a pint of water sweetened with milk sugar. Usually, after vomiting, the patient is quite thirsty, and it is not difficult for her to drink lemonade. Ginger ale or Coca-Cola in small amounts also are often most helpful. This nausea and vomiting, if once established, is difficult to overcome, and so it is especially desirable to prevent the first attack, or at least to control this condition as soon as possible after it develops. It must be remembered that if the patient is unable to retain most of her food her system is being depleted when the daily health should be maintained. Pregnancies may differ, and what may help one person may not benefit another. The "trial-and-error" method is often necessary to obtain results. If peristent vomiting develops, as it does with a small number of these patients, the condition is no longer considered a minor discomfort but then may develop into a serious complication. (See Chap. 18, Complications of Pregnancy.)

Heartburn

This is a neuromuscular phenomenon which may occur any time throughout gestation. As a result of the diminished gastric motility, which normally accompanies pregnancy, reverse peristaltic waves cause regurgitation of the stomach contents into the esophagus. It is this irritation of the esophageal mucosa which causes heartburn. It may be described as a burning discomfort diffusedly localized behind the lower part of the sternum, often radiating upward along the course of the esophagus. Although referred to as heartburn, it really has nothing to do with the heart. Often it is associated with other gastro-intestinal symptoms, of which acid regurgitation, belching, nausea and epigastric pressure are most troublesome. Nervous tension and emotional disturbances may be a precipitating cause. Worry, fatigue and improper diet may contribute to its intensity.

Little or no fat should be included in the diet. While fatty foods are especially aggravating in this disturbance, strangely enough, the taking of some form of fat, such as a pat of butter or a tablespoon of cream, a short time before meals, acts as a preventive, because fat inhibits the secretion of acid in the stomach. However, this will not help if the heartburn is already present.

Home remedies should not be used to relieve this condition. The physician usually will prescribe some alkaline preparation because it gives the best results. However, *sodium bicarbonate should not be used* because the sodium ion tends to promote water retention. It is important to make sure that the patient understands this point. Aluminum compounds, such as aluminum hydroxide gel, or this medication in tablet form with magnesium trisilicate, are medications which are equally effective.

Flatulence

This is a somewhat common and very disagreeable discomfort. Usually it is due to undesirable bacterial action in the intestines which results in the formation of gas. Eating only small amounts of food which are well masticated may prevent this feeling of distress after eating. Regular daily elimination is of prime importance, as is the avoidance of foods which form gas. Such foods as beans, parsnips, corn, sweet desserts, fried foods, cake and candy should be avoided. If these measures fail to relieve the condition, the physician should be consulted.

Constipation

This is not unusual during pregnancy. It is due largely to impaired peristaltic motion of the intestine caused by pressure from the gravid uterus. The patient should understand the importance of good bowel habits (see General Hygiene, p. 162), the influence of drinking adequate fluids and the appropriate diet in avoiding or alleviating this problem. Proper elimination cannot be emphasized too much, and daily regularity of

habit aids in preventing constipation. In mild cases of constipation a diet of fruits, vegetables, dark breads and coarse foods, with several glasses of water daily, may relieve the condition.

Enemas, laxatives or cathartics should not be used unless prescribed by the physician. Some obstetricians advise milk of magnesia or cascara for their patients. Cascara is easier to take in the pill form, but it seems to be less effective; when the fluid extract is given, the size of the dose and the frequency of its administration must be determined according to the individual patient's reactions. When the proper dosage has been determined, this drug is generally very satisfactory. The salines are usually reserved for the cases in which they are distinctly indicated, such as certain types of toxemia.

Simple measures, combined with a largely farinaceous diet, are ordinarily all that is necessary, and the obstetrician should be consulted before even these are used.

Diarrhea

Occasionally this occurs during pregnancy, and its onset should be reported at once to the physician. Milk boiled for 2 minutes may be recommended by the nurse, and the patient may be advised to rest. If diarrhea is allowed to persist, it may result in an abortion, either because of severe straining efforts or because of an extension of the existing intestinal contractions. In the latter months of pregnancy, diarrhea may cause premature labor.

Backache

Most pregnant women experience some degree of backache. As pregnancy advances, the woman's posture changes to compensate for the weight of the growing uterus. The shoulders are thrown back as the enlarging abdomen protrudes, and, in order to maintain the body balance, the inward curve of the spine is exaggerated. The relaxation of the sacro-iliac joints, in addition to the postural change, causes varying degrees of backache following excessive strain, fatigue, bending or lifting. The mother should be advised early in pregnancy how to prevent such strain through measures such as good posture and body mechanics in everyday living and avoidance of fatigue. Appropriate shoes worn during periods of activity and a supporting girdle may be helpful (see "Clothing," pp. 159 and 161, in General Hygiene).

A woman who has a pendulous abdomen, a weak abdominal wall which allows the uterus to fall forward, will experience severe back pain, in addition to a "drawing sensation" in the abdomen and general discomfort in walking or standing. The physician will prescribe measures to be taken here or for any persistent complaint.

Dyspnea

Difficult breathing or shortness of breath occasionally results from pressure on the diaphragm by the enlarged uterus and may be sufficient, in the last weeks of pregnancy, to interfere considerably with the patient's sleep and general comfort. Usually it is not a serious condition, but unfortunately it cannot be wholly relieved until after "lightening" (p. 209) (the settling of the fetus into the pelvic cavity with relief of the upper abdominal pressure) or after the birth of the baby, when it will disappear spontaneously. It is most troublesome when the patient attempts to lie down, so that her comfort may be greatly enhanced by propping her well up in bed with pillows. In this semisitting posture she at least will sleep better and longer than with her head low. It is well for the nurse to demonstrate how these pillows may be arranged comfortably so that the patient's back is well supported.

In patients with known heart disease, shortness of breath, especially of rather sudden onset, may be a sign of oncoming heart failure and should be reported at once to the physician.

Varicose Veins

Varicose veins or varices may occur in the lower extremities and, at times, extend up as high as the external genitals or even into the pelvis itself. A varicosity is an enlargement in the diameter of a vein due to a thinning and stretching of its walls. Such distended areas may occur at short intervals along the course of the blood vessel; they give it a knotted appearance. Varicosities generally are associated with hereditary tendencies and are enhanced by advancing age, pregnancy and activities which require prolonged standing. During pregnancy the pressure in the pelvis due to the enlarged uterus, which presses on the great abdominal veins, interferes with the return of the blood from the lower limbs. Added to this, any debilitated condition of the patient favors the formation of varicosities in the veins because of the general flabbiness and lack of tone in the tissues.

Naturally, the greater the pressure in the abdomen, the greater will be the tendency to varicose veins of the legs and the vulva. Therefore, any occupation which keeps a patient constantly on her feet, particularly in the latter part of pregnancy, causes an increase in abdominal pressure and so acts as an exciting factor.

The first symptom of the development of varices is a dull, aching pain in the legs due to distention of the deep vessels, and inspection will show a fine purple network of superficial veins covering the skin in a lacelike pattern. Later, the true varicosities appear, usually first under the bend of the knee, in a tangled mass of bluish or purplish veins, often as large as a lead pencil. As the condition advances, the varicosities extend up and down the leg along the course of the vessels, and in severe cases they may affect the veins of the labia majora, the vagina and the uterus.

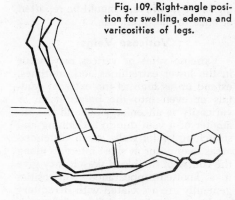

Fig. 109. Right-angle position for swelling, edema and varicosities of legs.

The treatment consists first and chiefly in the prompt abandonment, at the beginning of pregnancy, of round garters and all other articles of clothing that can cause pressure at any part of the body. If varicosities develop in spite of this precaution, the patient should be taught to take the right-angle position, that is, to lie on the bed with her legs extended straight into the air at right angles to her body, her buttocks and heels resting against the wall (Fig. 109). At first this position should be taken for from 2 to 5 minutes several times a day, and that will soon demonstrate what can be accomplished. For some patients this position is very uncomfortable at first; but if it is explained and the discomfort is therefore anticipated, the patient is less likely to discontinue the exercise. Late in pregnancy this position may be too difficult to assume because of pressure against the diaphragm.

In order to give support to the weak-walled veins, either an elastic stocking or elastic bandage is often recommended. The initial cost of elastic stockings is somewhat more than bandages, but they are easier to put on, have a neater appearance and longer useful life than bandages. The bandages should be applied spirally with firm even pressure, beginning at the foot and continuing up the leg above the varicosities (Figs. 110 and 111). The stocking or bandage should be removed at night and reapplied in the morning, after the legs have been elevated so that the vessels will be less dilated. The longer stocking or bandage is more satisfactory when the varicosities are above the knee. Either the elastic stocking or bandage is washable; indeed, washing helps maintain the original elasticity of these appliances.

Varicosities of the vulva may be relieved by placing a pillow under the buttocks and elevating the hips for frequent rest periods or by taking the elevated Sims' position for a few moments several times a day (Fig. 112). Patients suffering from this condition should not stand when they can sit, and they should not sit when they can lie down.

More important than the treatment of this condition is its prevention. Every pregnant woman should be advised to sit with her legs elevated whenever possible. And when the legs are elevated, care should be taken to see that there are no pressure points against the legs to interfere with the circulation, particularly in the popliteal space. Tight constricting garments, round garters, constipation, standing for long periods of time and improper amount of rest all tend to aggravate and also excite this condition.

A varicose vein in the vagina may rupture during the antepartal or intrapartal period, but this is rare. The hemorrhage is venous and can be controlled readily by pressure. The foot of the bed should be markedly elevated.

Hemorrhoids

Hemorrhoids, varicosities of the veins about the lower end of the rectum and the anus, may develop during the antepartal period and may cause rectal bleeding. On the other hand, they may become thrombosed or protrude through the anus. The little bumps and nodules seen in a mass of hemorrhoids are the distended portions of the affected vessels. Like varicosities in other areas, they are due to pressure interfering with return venous circulation and are ag-

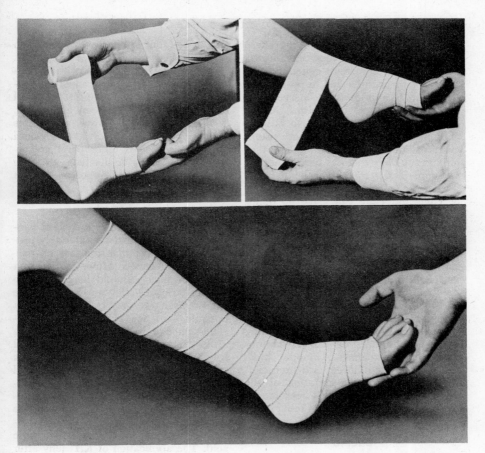

Fig. 110. (*Top*) The method of applying the Ace bandage for varicosities or edema of the legs, which are sometimes treated by the application of Ace Rubber-Elastic Bandage (Becton, Dickinson and Company) and Elastoplast Bandage (Duke Laboratories).

Fig. 111. (*Bottom*) The Elastoplast bandage is applied firmly, adjusting the stretch to produce the amount of compression desired, each turn overlapping to avoid gaps.

gravated by constipation. They often cause great distress to the pregnant patient and, due to pressure at the time of delivery, may cause great distress during the postpartal period.

The first step is treatment relieving the constipation. When internal hemorrhoids protrude through the rectum, they should be replaced carefully by pushing them gently back into the rectum. Usually the patient can do this for herself, after lubricating her finger with petrolatum or mineral oil, taking either the knee-chest position (see Fig.

196) or elevating her buttocks (Fig. 112) on a pillow. The application of an icebag, or cold compresses wet with witch hazel or Epsom salts solution, gives great relief. The physician may order tannic acid in suppositories, or compresses of witch hazel and glycerin. If the hemorrhoids are aggravated the first few days after labor, the same medications usually give relief. Surgery is seldom resorted to during pregnancy.

Cramps

Cramps are painful spasmodic muscular contractions in the legs. These cramps may occur at any time during the pregnancy but more generally during the later months due to pressure of the enlarged uterus on the nerves supplying the lower extremities. Other causes have been attributed to fatigue, chilling, tense body posture and insufficient calcium in the diet. A quart of milk in the daily diet has been generally recommended to meet the calcium needs during pregnancy. However, the studies of Page and Page can leave no doubt that large quantities of milk or dicalcium phosphate predispose to muscular tetany and leg cramps as the result of the excessive amount of phosphorus absorbed from these products (see Suggested Reading). Immediate relief may be obtained by forcing the toes upward and by making pressure on the knee to straighten the leg (Fig. 113). Rubbing the affected part also helps. Elevating the feet and keeping the extremities warm are preventives. Cramps, while not a serious condition, are excruciatingly painful for the duration of the seizure. If the husband has been taught the procedure for immediate relief much pain will be prevented.

Edema

Swelling of the lower extremities is very common during pregnancy and is sometimes very uncomfortable. It is especially prone to occur in hot weather. Often it may be relieved by a proper abdominal support or by resting frequently during the day. Elevating the feet or taking the right-angle position often gives much relief. If the swelling is persistent, the patient may have to stay in bed, but ordinarily this condition proves to be no more than a discomfort. However, as edema is one of the symptoms of toxemia, it never must be considered as a mere discomfort until all other suspicions have been eliminated.

When edema of the lower extremities is observed, careful investigation should be made to see if other parts are affected—the hands or the face, etc. The condition should be reported to the physician at once.

Vaginal Discharge

In pregnancy there is increased vaginal secretion, so that a moderately profuse discharge at this time has no particular significance. However, such a condition always should be brought to the obstetrician's attention, for a profuse yellow discharge may be regarded as a possible evidence of gonorrhea, especially when it is accompanied by such urinary manifestations as burning and frequency of urination. A smear may be taken, and the microscopic result may indicate whether or not definite treatment is necessary. If any discharge becomes irritating, the patient may be advised to bathe the vulva with a solution of sodium bicarbonate or boric acid. The application of K.Y. jelly after bathing often relieves the condition entirely. Instructing a patient to wear a perineal pad is sometimes all the advice that is needed. A douche never should be taken unless the obstetrician orders it.

A particularly stubborn form of leukorrhea in pregnancy is caused by the parasitic protozoan known as the *Trichomonas vaginalis*. It is characterized not

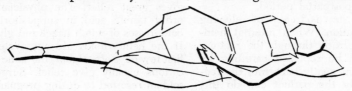

Fig. 112. Sims position for varicosities of vulva and rectum.

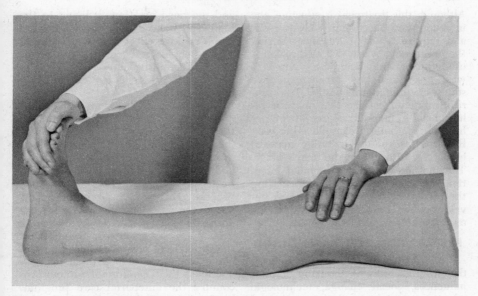

Fig. 113. Showing the nurse helping the patient during a leg cramp, forcing the toes upward while making pressure on the knee to straighten the leg.

only by a profuse frothy discharge, white or yellowish in color, but also by irritation and itching of the vulva and the vagina. The diagnosis is easily made by the physician by taking a small quantity of the fresh secretion and putting it under the microscope in a hanging-drop. Here the spindle-shaped organisms, somewhat larger than leukocytes, with whiplike processes attached, can be seen in active motion.

One form of treatment used in this condition is the vinegar douche (3 tablespoons of vinegar in 2 quarts of water), followed by the insertion of 1 Floraquin tablet into the fornix of the vagina. It is imperative that the expectant mother be given specific instructions about douching in pregnancy (see "Douches," p. 163, in General Hygiene).

Moniliasis, a yeast infection caused by the *Candida albicans,* is another common cause of profuse vaginal dis-charge. The organism is frequently present in the vaginal canal without producing symptoms, but during pregnancy the physical changes in the vagina produce conditions conducive to its development. It is characterized by white patches on the vaginal mucosa and a thick cottage cheeselike discharge which is extremely irritating, so that burning or pruritis are present. Even the external genitalia often become inflamed, and occasionally extensive edema is observed. Bleeding may accompany the other symptoms if the patches on the mucosa are removed in any way.

It is not necessary to treat patients in whom Monilia are found if signs and symptoms are not present. The most dependable drug used to treat this condition is aqueous solution of gentian violet, 1 per cent. Commercial preparations of gentian violet in the form of a gel are available for the patient to use.

Although this treatment is effective, the infection is stubborn and likely to recur and require repeated treatment during the pregnancy. When this medication is used the patient should be advised to wear a perineal pad because the dye stains clothing permanently. The *pruritis,* or itching of the skin, may be relieved to a marked degree if proper hygienic measures are employed to keep the area free of the irritating material being deposited upon the skin surface. The mother who has a monilial infection may transmit it to her infant during the process of the delivery. *Thrush* develops when the organisms attack the mucous membrane of the mouth.

PREPARATION FOR PARENTHOOD

Childbirth in modern society reflects the progress brought about by cultural influences, social change, technologic advances and, above all, the progress of medicine. The concept of family-centered care which prevails in all health services today could have no more appropriate application than with the beginning of a new life in the family unit. Having children is no longer the mother's responsibility alone; it is a joint undertaking of both parents. From the moment of conception, when the baby begins his existence, the husband is encouraged to begin to assume his responsibility as a father. A helpful, understanding and sympathetic husband can do much to make the pregnancy an experience which will contribute to the foundation of a more enriched family life.

Preparation for parenthood actually begins with the mother's own birth or earlier, as was stated in the beginning of this chapter, and its development is influenced by an accumulation of her experiences through infancy, childhood, adolescence and maturity. The father's feelings and attitudes are influenced in like manner by his previous experiences. The addition of courses in sex education

and marriage and family living to the high school and college curriculums has had a positive effect on the attitudes of young people. In recent years much has been accomplished also through premarital and prepregnancy examinations and counseling.

The emphasis placed on "education" of parents for childbirth has stimulated them to attend antepartal classes which, in part, has further helped to dispel misunderstandings or lack of knowledge and increase the understanding of childbirth as a normal physiologic body process. This is not an entirely new approach. In Manchester, during the 18th century, Dr. Charles White wrote a book which concerns instructions for the supervision of mothers during pregnancy and how to help them in labor and make them comfortable. In our own country the antepartal care programs have influenced the formation of preparation classes which have contributed toward good antepartal care.

Classes

Today there are definite courses offered for mothers and fathers in preparation for childbearing. These classes are included as a part of the programs of the Visiting Nurse Associations, Red Cross Chapters, many State Departments of Health, hospitals and private organizations such as the Maternity Center Association in New York City. Some of these classes are given for expectant mothers or fathers alone, in others the parents attend classes together. In the latter group, the classes aid the parents in their mutual appreciation of the value of antepartal preparation and tend to promote the idea of sharing parenthood. The goals set for the parents in any of these classes are similar, namely, to gain increased knowledge about childbearing and to gain increased understanding of ways to promote and maintain optimum health through the practice of good health habits in daily living.

Several disciplines may be represented in teaching any one group of classes, so that those who teach may be nurses, obstetricians, pediatricians, nutritionists, health educators and, in some courses which include exercise classes, physical therapists. Material related to the physiology of pregnancy and labor, general hygiene and the care of the mother during pregnancy, labor and the puerperium is included, as well as that related to the baby. All of the class content is approved by a medical council or advisory board, but the details of the classes are usually worked out by nurses to suit the conditions under which the courses are conducted.

The classes are attended by individuals from various social, cultural and economic groups, each with his or her own needs and desires. Those who teach must use care to be realistic about their teaching and never forget that although the teacher has set up objectives for the students (in this case, the parents), she must help the parents attain the goals which they have set up for themselves. For instance, a mother who has the satisfaction of appetite as her goal for family nutrition considers that if her family is not hungry they are well fed. This goal may astound the nutritionist or the nurse who sees the importance of planning well-balanced meals. In this instance, the job of health teaching requires the application of sound educational principles in order not to destroy the mother's goal with one fell swoop. The nurse's teaching can be most effective if she first identifies their common goals, then, gradually, as she teaches, begins to change the mother's objective without undermining her security.

Conventional-Type Program

This is the most widely used program. It is planned to serve everyone in the community and places its emphasis on a general kind of "education for childbirth." The course usually includes the physiology of childbearing, general hygiene, preparations for the baby and the care of the mother and her baby after the delivery.

Natural Childbirth

Childbirth as a normal or natural process has received increasing emphasis during the past decade. The reader will develop more understanding of this broad concept of maternity care from the writings of Read, Thoms and Goodrich (see Suggested Reading).

The interpretation of "labor" as "pain" has been held by women from time immemorial, with the result that today many women still approach childbirth in dread of an ordeal. Much of the misunderstanding, fear and apprehension can be overcome by understanding gained from education. This is no simple way to a painless or easy childbirth, but a means to enable a woman to gain more self-understanding, to help herself in labor and to increase her self-confidence.

Increasing emphasis has been placed on the fact that there is an "emotional labor" which is as definite and important as its physical counterpart. There can be no doubt that the attitude of a woman toward her confinement has a considerable influence on the ease of her labor. This fact was stressed for many years by the British obstetrician, the late Dr. Grantly Dick Read, and has been endorsed by various groups in this country, notably the Maternity Center Association of New York and by Drs. Thoms and Goodrich of New Haven and others. Dr. Read emphasized certain psychological aspects of labor—that "fear is in some way the chief pain producing agent in otherwise normal labor." The neuromuscular mechanism by which fear exerts a deleterious effect on labor is obscure, but the general validity of Read's contention is in keeping with common clinical knowledge. The mother builds up a state of tensions because she is frightened, and these tensions create an antagonistic effect on the muscular activity of normal labor, with resulting pain. The pain causes more fear, which further increases the tensions, and so on until a vicious circle is established. Rather unfortunately, certain overzealous people inferred that a spontaneous delivery during which the mother is conscious is of psychological importance to her. The connotation of "painless childbirth" was also injected here, an interpretation which is not accurate.

The family-centered approach to maternity care, which is a fundamental part of the natural-childbirth program, is not basically different from that practiced when deliveries were conducted at home with the father present. But changes are apparent. The current trend to have babies born in the hospital has the advantage of increased safety provided by improved medical technics and modern obstetric practice. For so long women approached childbearing without any real understanding of what to expect or, for that matter, without much knowledge of the anatomy and the physiology of their reproductive organs. The majority of husbands were included insofar as they were present in the household, but were not actually made to feel that they were really participating in the event. The natural-childbirth program provides an opportunity to help both parents gain more knowledge and the satisfaction from mutual participation. The program of education during pregnancy is designed to eliminate fear. Facts which concern the anatomy and the physiology of childbearing and the appropriate care of the mother are taught. The mother not only learns how labor progresses but also is helped to gain an understanding of the sensations likely to accompany labor and the methods to work co-operatively with them. The exercises which are included are designed for the muscles which will be used in labor, as well as those which will promote the general well-being of the body. In the performance of any skill, the individual is more efficient if the muscles involved are in the best condition. The exercises are not strenuous and, for the most part, are ones which will contribute to improved posture, body balance, agility and increased strength and endurance. The mother learns breathing technics which will aid her ability to relax in the first stage of labor, and technics which will help her to work effectively with muscles used in the delivery. To enable the parents to meet better the needs of their baby after he is born, information about his growth and development is also included in these classes.

An important consideration throughout the program is "to help the mother help herself," so that her pregnancy will be a healthy happy experience, and at the time of labor she will be better able to participate actively in having her baby. In former days when mothers often were given heavy sedation they were unable to appreciate this satisfying experience.

The encouragement and support of those about her are particularly important to the expectant mother, especially during labor. Every modern obstetric aid for the mother's safety and comfort is at her disposal. It should be emphasized that the proponents of natural childbirth have never claimed that labor should be conducted without anesthetic aids or that it can be made devoid of pain (Thoms). The response to pain is individual, and if the mother and/or the physician decides that some assistance in the form of medication is necessary, it is readily available. It would be rather incongruous to suggest that any program would reject medical advances which have made such important contributions to obstetrics. However, many mothers who are "prepared" for natural childbirth often are reluctant to accept any form of medication, feeling that it is rather a personal blow to their integrity. In such a case, the mother needs help to understand that this will not detract from her experience, but rather will enhance it. She may need help to remember that the physician is the one person capable of making the final decision as to what is best for her and her baby. The use of medication should not be a criterion in the consideration of "how well the mother did" during labor and delivery. The real measure of success can be determined only by the satisfactions which the mother derives from being able to co-operate with the natural processes of labor to the best of her ability. The new infant is really the important entity and, after he is born, should be the mother's chief concern, not an elaboration of her physical feats.

The results of the program "Training for Childbirth," at the Grace New Haven Community Hospital (University Service), are interesting, informative and convincing. This program was started in 1947. In addition to the usual antepartal program, they emphasize the education of the mother, the use of certain exercises primarily aimed at relaxation and the importance of sympathetic continuous attention and care (support) during labor. Dr. Thoms graciously gave his permission to print the following exercises taught in the clinical program (Figs. 114-120).

THE EXERCISES*

In the following pages the exercises are explained. A copy of this explanation, including the illustrations, is given to each woman at the first exercise class.

EXERCISE No. 1—BREATHING. Lie on your back (on a blanket or a pad on the floor, or on a bed that does not sag), with the legs bent at the knees and the feet flat on the floor or the bed.

Type 1 (Abdominal Breathing). With the mouth closed, breathe gently in and out, keeping as relaxed as possible. Let the abdominal wall rise with each breath taken in and drop down with each outgoing breath.

If you find this difficult at first, place your hands gently on each side of the

* Make certain that the bladder is empty before practicing any of the exercises.

abdomen, with the arms and the elbows at rest on the floor or the bed, and imagine that you are raising and lowering your hands as you breathe and move your abdomen (Fig. 114).

This is to be practiced every day until it can be done rapidly or slowly and to any depth. Aim at allowing one half minute for taking in a breath and raising the abdominal wall and one half minute for letting the breath go and lowering the abdominal wall. With practice you may be able to take longer.

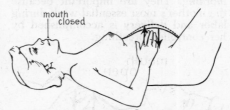

Fig. 114. Abdominal breathing.

Type 2. There is an inverted V (like this: Λ) made by the ribs in the front of your chest. Take in a deep breath with the mouth closed and try to open the inverted V wider by pushing the ribs on either side of your chest farther apart. Place the palms of the hands on either side of the ribs with arms and elbows at rest on the bed or the floor and practice moving the hands in and out as the chest moves with this breathing. Do this both slowly and rapidly, varying the rhythm, for a period of 2 or 3 minutes at least 4 times daily (Fig. 115).

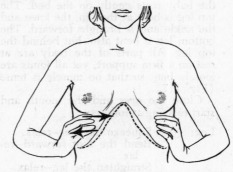

Fig. 115. Costal breathing.

Type 3 (Panting). With the mouth open, breathe in and out, lifting up the sternum, or breast bone, and letting it fall again. This breathing is compared with the panting of a dog—rapid short breaths with the mouth open, using the top of the chest only. Similarly, the hands can be placed lightly on the chest and moved up and down as you pant (Fig. 116).

These breathing exercises can be done on the bed before you go to sleep at night or before you get up in the morning. They are important because the mother's most essential work during labor and delivery is accomplished by her controlled breathing.

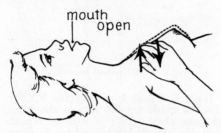

Fig. 116. Panting.

EXERCISE No. 2—RELAXATION. Lie on either side, on the floor or the bed, with your head on one pillow, the neck bent slightly forward, and the pillow at an angle for best support.

Place the under arm behind the back, with the elbow and the wrist slightly bent, and the top arm bent forward to lie at rest on the pillow or on the bed. The back is slightly bowed forward, and the baby rests gently on the bed. The top leg is bent at the hip, the knee and the ankle and is brought forward. The bottom leg is bent also, but behind the top leg. All parts of the body are at rest on a firm support, yet all joints are loosely bent so that no muscle is tense (Fig. 117).

Close the eyes and the mouth and start relaxing as follows:

Leg: Squeeze the toes—relax.
         Bend the foot forward—relax.
         Straighten the leg—relax.
         Tighten the hip—relax.
Other leg: Same.

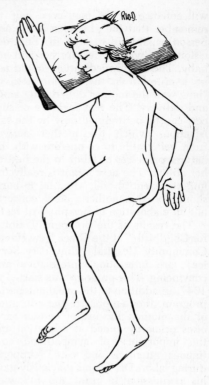

Fig. 117. Relaxation.

Arm: Make a fist—relax.
        Straighten the elbow—relax.
        Tighten the shoulder—relax.
Other arm: Same.
Face: Screw it up—relax.
        Let the facial muscles relax as thoroughly as possible.
Breathing: Breathe regularly and as slowly as possible, moving the abdomen forward and backward, as you have been practicing in Exercise No. 1 on abdominal breathing.
        Think *only* of breathing in and out; your mind will be at peace, and usually sleep will follow.

After you have learned the relaxation in steps, try relaxing suddenly and instantly so that you will be able to use controlled relaxation during the first stage of labor.

Important: After such complete relaxation, a sudden upright position occasionally may bring slight dizziness. Bring the slowed circulation to normal for activity by moving the feet and the hands, stretching, turning over, and sitting up gradually.

EXERCISE NO. 3—CONTRACTION AND RELAXATION OF THE PELVIC FLOOR MUSCLES. Lie on the back with the legs crossed at the ankles and the knees straight.

a. Squeeze together the muscles of the two buttocks, or where you sit, as you count to 5 slowly—1, 2, 3, 4, 5.
b. As you count, press your thighs together at the back and count on to 7—6, 7.

Try not to hold your breath during the two exercises above.

c. While doing *a* and *b* try to contract your anus (back passage) by tucking it further in toward your pelvis as if you were trying to keep from having a bowel movement. As you do this, count on to 10— 8, 9, 10.

When these contractive exercises are completed, relax these muscles slowly, then repeat the exercise in the 3 steps *a, b,* and *c* 4 or 5 times.

When the exercise is properly done you will feel the "drawing in" sensation as you practice, first only in your anus, then gradually also in your vagina, or birth canal, and finally to the front, up into the region of the uterus. *Relax very slowly!*

A pregnant woman should have good posture and carry her baby well supported gracefully.

EXERCISE NO. 4—POSTURE. *Squatting.* Stand with the feet flat, about 24 inches apart, and squat. Rest the arms on the knees. If you find this difficult, practice squatting by holding lightly to some heavy article of furniture until you can balance yourself (Fig. 118).

Pelvic Rocking, Lying Down. Lie on the back with the knees bent and the feet flat on the bed or floor.

a. Push both hands under the lower back to make sure of a hollow, then arch the back. At the same time relax the muscles in the lower abdominal wall and push the abdomen up.
b. Pull the hands out and flatten the back so that there is no space between the back and the floor or the bed. At the same time, tighten the lower abdominal muscles and the muscles of the buttocks (Fig. 119).

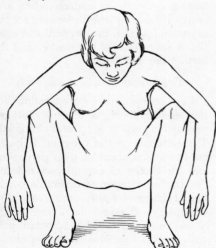

Fig. 118. Squatting.

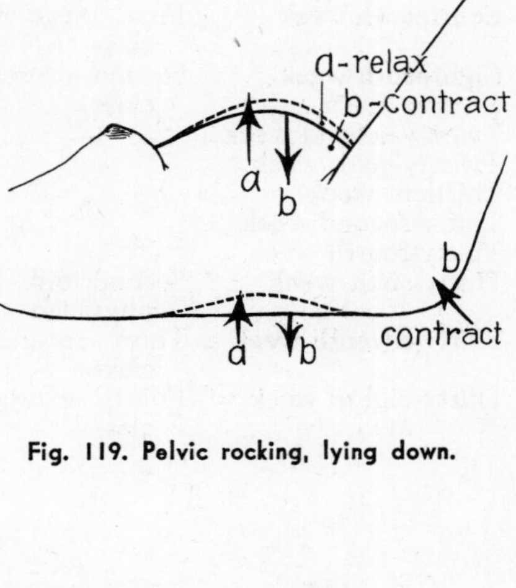

Fig. 119. Pelvic rocking, lying down.

Pelvic Rocking, Standing. Stand with the feet about 6 inches apart but parallel, and the toes pressed into the floor.

a. As before, make a hollow in the back. Relax the lower abdominal muscles and bring the abdomen forward.
b. Then straighten up the back. Tense or tighten the muscles in the lower abdomen and in the buttocks (Fig. 120).

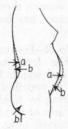

Fig. 120. Pelvic rocking, standing.

After practicing *a* and *b* until *b* is easier, open out the chest for full chest breathing, lift the head in "proud" position, and walk carrying your baby. with good support.

Schedule. The average normal prenatal patient makes her first visit to the clinic in the sixth week of pregnancy. At that time her history is taken, physical and laboratory examinations are made, and instructions are given in the hygiene of pregnancy. The remaining prenatal checkups take place according to the following schedule:

Tenth week . . . . First talk by
physician
Fourteenth week . . . . . First exercise
class
Eighteenth week . . . . . Second exercise
class
Twenty-second week
Twenty-sixth week
Thirtieth week
Thirty-second week
Thirty-fourth week
Thirty-sixth week . . . . Second talk by
physician
Thirty-seventh week . . Third exercise
class
Thirty-eighth week . . . Fourth exercise
class

Any time after the thirty-second week, the four classes for fathers- and parents-to-be are given at weekly intervals, usually in the evening. This course is given every two months. A member of the pediatric staff attached to the nursery sees each prenatal patient at some regular visit to acquaint her with the plans for care in the hospital for the coming infant.

As Dr. Thoms says, "We recognize that fear and anxiety play a large part in the creation of tension, which has undesirable effects, but we do not place undue emphasis on this aspect. We prefer to think of our program in a broad sense as being directed toward childbirth with understanding and support rather than childbirth without fear."

Satisfactory results in connection with natural childbirth are aided by such factors as attaining good physical health and emotional stability; learning about the baby's development during the antepartal period; understanding the muscular processes that take place during labor and delivery; preparing for labor by attending classes where supervised exercises are practiced and perfected; having sympathetic understanding and "support" during labor; planning for the postpartal period, the physical and emotional adjustment of the mother and the care of the new baby.

Psychoprophylactic Childbirth

Psychoprophylactic preparation for painless childbirth is a somewhat less permissive version of natural childbirth. The rationale of the program is based on Pavlov's concept of pain perception and his theory of conditioned reflexes, i.e., the substitution of favorable conditioned reflexes for unfavorable ones. For example, most women have been conditioned since childhood to associate pain with certain functions of the reproductive organs, such as with menstruation and child-bearing. To disprove such beliefs, repeated emphasis is placed on the fact that normal contractions of the uterus need not be any more painful than those of other organs of the body, such as the bladder or the bowel. The teaching in this program consists of combating the fears associated with pregnancy and childbirth by instructing the pregnant woman about the anatomy and the neuromuscular activity of the reproductive system and the mechanism of labor. Nutrition and general hygiene are included during the course. Simple exercises which strengthen the abdominal muscles and relax the perineum are taught, and proper breathing technics to help the process of labor are practiced. These breathing technics differ from the ones taught in the natural-childbirth classes.

The core of this program is the abolition of fear through knowledge, preparation for labor by education and exercise and peace of mind during labor through cheerful skilled attendance and the creation of a familylike environment.

The psychoprophylactic method and natural childbirth without fear, as practiced by Read or by Thoms, have in fact the following 3 points in common: (1) Fear enhances the perception of pain but may diminish or disappear when the parturient knows about the physiology of labor. (2) Psychic tension enhances the perception of pain but the parturient may more easily relax if childbirth takes place in a calm and agreeable atmosphere and when good human contacts are established between her and the nursing personnel. (3) Muscular relaxation and a specific type of breathing diminish or abolish the pains of labor.*

Psychoprophylactic-childbirth programs have not been introduced widely into this country but are used more in Russia, parts of China and in various sections of Europe.

* de Watteville, P. H.: The use of obstetrical analgesia at the maternity hospital of Geneva, Am. J. Obst. & Gynec. **73**:473, 1957.

PREPARATIONS FOR THE BABY

Layette

The baby's layette and equipment are of real interest to all parents—in fact, interesting to the majority of people. The cost of the layette should be in keeping with the individual economic circumstances. The entire layette can be purchased ready-made or can be made at home quite inexpensively. Much or little may be spent in its preparation, but nurses who are teaching parents should know the reasons why certain types of clothes and equipment are preferable. In the selection of clothing the following points should be considered: comfort; ease in laundering; ease in putting on and taking off; and very light in weight. The new baby's skin is easily irritated by wool. Any clothing which comes in contact with the infant's skin should be made of soft cotton material. Knitted materials have the advantage of ease in laundering and sufficient stretch quality to allow for more freedom in dressing the baby. Garments that open down the length and fasten with ties or grippers are easier to put on. Ties or grippers are not only less difficult to fasten than buttons but also are more desirable from the standpoint of safety. The geographic location and climate of the year will greatly influence the selection of the infant's clothing. Size 1 shirts and gowns are recommended, since the infant grows rapidly in the first 6 months and quickly outgrows his garments. It is well to remember that his clothing should not inhibit his normal activities. The complete outfit of clothes that the baby wears should not weigh more than 12 to 16 ounces.

The mother should be advised to prepare a very simple layette. As she sees how fast her baby grows and what he will need, the additional items can be secured. The complete layettes which can be purchased often contain unnecessary items and are usually costly. Also, many of the articles may be received as baby gifts. Therefore, it is wise to choose only those things which are necessary for immediate use.

Layette necessities are:

5 or 6 shirts
3 to 4 dozen diapers (if diaper service
    is not used)
4 receiving blankets
3 nightgowns or kimonos
6 diaper pads (11" x 16")
2 waterproof protectors for under diaper
    pads
2 afghans or blankets ⎰
1 bunting ⎱ (if climate is cold)
2 to 4 soft towels (40" x 40")
2 to 4 soft washcloths

Nursery equipment should consist of:

basket, bassinet or crib
mattress (firm, flat and smooth)
mattress protector (waterproof)
sheets or pillowcases for mattress
chest or separate drawer
cotton crib blanket
bathtub
diaper pail
toilet tray—equipped
absorbent cotton—or cotton balls
baby soap (bland, white, unscented)
rustproof safety pins
soap dish
bath apron (for mother)
table, for bath or dressing
chair (for mother)

Additional suggestions for layette and equipment are:

sacques
sweaters
kimonos
crib blankets
crib spreads
bibs
clothes drier
chest of drawers
nursery stand
footstool
diaper bag (for traveling)
disposable diapers
nursery light
carriage

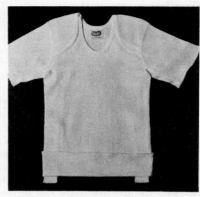

Fig. 121. The pull-over or slip-on type shirt. The shoulder treatment permits the neck to be opened the full width of the garment when it is slipped on. The pin tab allows the diaper to be pinned to something of a more durable nature than the knitted shirt itself. (The Vanta Company, Inc., Stoughton, Mass.)

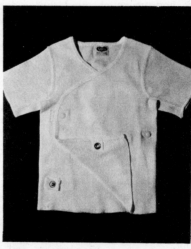

Fig. 122. The double-breasted shirt may be fastened with the conventional side-ties or with snap-fasteners placed on tabs (as shown above). (The Vanta Company, Inc., Stoughton, Mass.)

Some further suggestions in relation to the selection of specific items are as follows:

Shirts, gowns, etc. The sleeves

should have roomy armholes, such as the raglan-type sleeve. If the pull-over-type garments are used, the neck openings should be so constructed that they are large enough to be put on easily from over the feet or the head (Figs. 121 and 122).

Diapers. Of the several varieties of diapers available, birds-eye or gauze diapers are the most popular. The selection of diapers should be considered from the standpoint of their comfort (soft and light in weight), absorbency and washing and drying qualities. The mother who plans to use the services of a commercial diaper service should have a dozen diapers of her own.

Receiving blankets. These should be made of flannelette 1 yard square.

This square is used to fold loosely about the baby. If properly secured, the baby may lie and kick and at the same time keep covered and warm. In the early weeks these squares take the brunt of the service and in this way save the fine wool covers from becoming soiled so quickly.

Afghans or blankets. These should be of very lightweight cotton or wool material (Fig. 123). The temperature and the weather will determine the amount of covering needed.

Sheets. Crib sheets are usually 45″ x 72″ and are available in muslin, percale and knitted cotton materials. The knit sheets are practical for bottom sheets and do not need to be ironed. Pillowcases are very usable for the carriage or

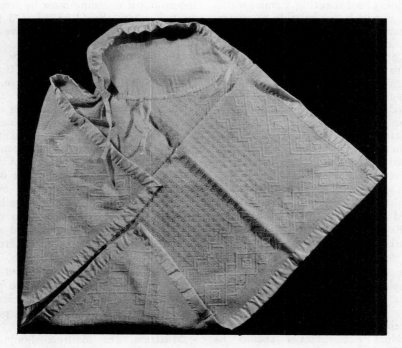

Fig. 123. An afghan converted into a practical bunting by sewing a piece of silk into one corner with shirr strings so that it can be drawn into a hood. (Zabriskie: Mother and Baby Care in Pictures, Philadelphia, Lippincott)

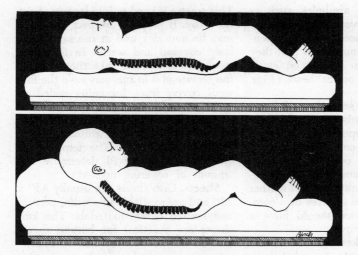

Fig. 124. This illustration shows what happens to a baby's sensitive spine when the mattress of his bed is too soft to support his back, or when a pillow is used. Babies should have a firm mattress to lie on and they should not be propped up with a pillow. (*Trained Nurse and Hospital Review*)

the basket mattress. Receiving blankets may be used for top sheets.

Waterproof sheeting. *Various* waterproof materials are suitable to protect the mattress and to be used under the pads. Even though the mattress may have a protective covering, it is necessary to have a waterproof cover large enough to cover the mattress completely—something that can be removed and washed. (Waterproof material should not be dried in the sun.)

Waterproof pants. These offer protection for special occasions. If the plastic variety is used they should not be tight at the leg or the waist. For general use, a square of protective material such a Sanisheeting or a cotton quilted pad should be used under the baby next to the diaper.

Bath apron. This is a protection for both mother and baby and may be made of plastic material covered with terry cloth.

Nursery Equipment

In choosing the equipment, again the individual circumstances should be taken into consideration. Expense, space and future plans all influence the selections. Most nurseries are planned for

the satisfaction of the parents. Eventually the baby's room becomes the child's room; and if economy must be considered, furniture should be selected that will appeal to the child as he grows and develops.

The baby's room. Preferably, the baby should have his own room. If this is not feasible, a quiet airy place, out of drafts, may be selected.

Bed. The baby should have his own bed. This may be a basket, a bassinet or a crib. The trimming on the basket or bassinet should be such that it can be removed easily and laundered. A bed may be improvised from a box or a bureau drawer, placed securely on a sturdy table or on chairs which are held together with rope. Many parents may have a carriage that may be used as a bed. However, after about the first 2 months, the baby will need a crib. The crib should be so constructed that the bars are close enough together to prevent the baby's head from being caught between them. If it is painted, a paint "safe for babies" should be used.

Mattress. The mattress should be firm (not hard) and flat (Fig. 124). All mattresses, including the waterproof-covered, should be protected by a waterproof sheeting to prevent the mattress from becoming stained and from absorbing odors. The waterproof sheet is easily washed and dries quickly.

Netting. This will be needed for the carriage, the basket or the crib during the insect season. If the Kiddie-Koop is used, it is screened to protect the baby from insects and animals.

Bathtub. The enamel tub is safe and easy to keep clean.

Bathtub table. The table on which the tub is placed for the baby's bath should be of convenient height (Fig. 204). A kitchen table, or other sturdy table without wheels, may be used for this purpose.

Mother's chair. The chair should also be a convenient height and comfortable for the individual mother.

Diaper pail. It should be large enough for the day's supply of soiled diapers. It may also be used for boiling the diapers.

Toilet tray. This tray should be prepared and ready for use immediately after the delivery of the baby (Fig. 125).

PLANS FOR AFTER-CARE OF MOTHER AND BABY

It is always a relief to the mother and her husband when the plans for delivery and the arrangements for the period following have been completed. The parents should make some provision for the mother to be free from other responsibilities until she has regained, in part at least, her physical strength and until lactation has been established.

The nurse should make an effort to include the father when discussing the details of the mother's care. Often it is

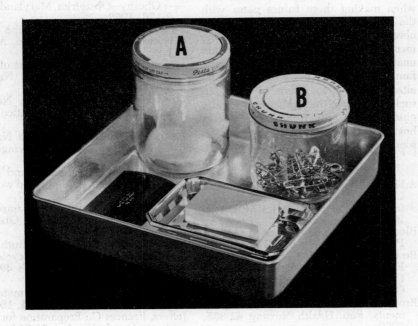

Fig. 125. Improvised toilet tray for baby. A household tray or baking pan and miscellaneous jars may be utilized. Comb has fine teeth with smooth rounded edges. Soap dish contains mild, white, unscented soap. (A) Jar for clean absorbent cotton. (B) Jar for safety pins.

with his help that his wife gets the full care she needs and that the doctor and the nurse wish her to have (see Chap. 9).

Return to Employment

The expectant mother who is employed may desire to know how early she may return to work after the baby is born. Following delivery, 6 weeks are needed for the obstetrician to determine whether or not the reproductive organs are returning to their approximate normal size and position. Accordingly, no commitments should be made until the baby is from 6 to 8 weeks old. At the time of the postpartal examination, the obstetrician will discuss with the patient her future plans. It always must be kept in mind that the mother-child relationship during the first 6 years of a child's life is most important, and when making these future plans with the mother, this fact must not be ignored because of interest in re-employment. There are, of course, certain unavoidable circumstances within some family units which leave the mother no alternative but to return to work. In such a situation, the mother may require guidance not only from her physician but also from the nurse and the medical social worker to help her plan for this.

SUGGESTED READING

A.M.A., Council on Pharmacy and Chemistry: Current status of therapy in nausea and vomiting, J.A.M.A. 160: 208, 1956.

Block, Babette: The unmarried mother, Pub. Health Nursing 43:375, 1951.

Bowes, Anna, and Church, Charles: Food Values of Portions Commonly Used, ed. 8, Philadelphia, College Offset Press, 1956.

Brooks, Ethel G.: Union health departments, Pub. Health Nursing 42:335, 1950.

Burke, Bertha S., and Kirkwood, Samuel B.: Problems and methods in nutrition services for pregnant women, Am. J. Pub. Health 40:960, 1950.

Cavanagh, William V.: The effectiveness of a hospital birth control clinic, Am. J. Obst. & Gynec. 59:883, 1950.

Cole, Miriam L.: Classes that mothers like, Pub. Health Nursing 43:442, 1951.

Corbin, Hazel: A rose is a rose is a rose, Briefs 19:2, 1955.

Darby, W. J., et al.: The Vanderbilt cooperative study of maternal and infant nutrition, Obst. & Gynec. 5:528, 1955.

DeLee, Sol T., and Duncan, Iva: Training for natural childbirth, Am. J. Nursing 56:48, 1956.

deWatteville, P. H.: The use of obstetrical analgesia at the Maternity Hospital of Geneva, Am. J. Obst. & Gynec. 73:473, 1957.

Donnell, H. C., and Glick, S.: The nurse and the unwed mother, Nursing Outlook 2:249, 1954.

Eastman, N. J.: Expectant Motherhood, ed. 3, Boston, Little, 1957.

——: Obesity—Obstetrics, Maryland M. J. 2:176, 1953.

Field, Minna: The nurse and the social worker on the hospital team, Am. J. Nursing 55:694, 1955.

Fitzhugh, Mabel L.: Is this part of your antepartal program?, Am. J. Nursing 50:742, 1950.

Goodrich, Frederick W., Jr.: Natural Childbirth, New York, Prentice-Hall, 1950.

Heardman, Helen: A Way to Natural Childbirth, London, Livingstone, 1954.

Hesseltine, H. C.: Obstetric and gynecologic problems of employed women, Obst. & Gynec. 5:431, 1957.

Hirst, Donald: Dangers of improper vaginal douching, Am. J. Obst. & Gynec. 64:179, 1952.

Hunscher, Helen, Leverton, Ruth, and Cederquist, Dena: The life cycle and its diet, J. Home Economics 49:101, 1957.

Jackson, Edith: New trends in maternity care, Am. J. Nursing 55:584, 1955.

Jeffers, Frances C.: Preparation for marriage, Am. J. Nursing 51:514, 1951.

Kirkwood, S. B.: Complete maternity care, Am. J. Pub. Health 46:1547, 1956.

——: An experiment in maternal and

infant care, New England J. Med. **256**:596, 1957.

Lesser, M., and Keene, V.: Nurse-Patient Relationships in a Hospital Maternity Service, St. Louis, Mosby, 1956.

Leverton, Ruth: Food Becomes You, Lincoln, Nebr., Univ. Nebraska Press, 1952.

Literature on Class Outlines from State Departments of Health.

Macy, I. G., and Mack, H.: Implications of nutrition on the life cycle of woman, Am. J. Obst. & Gynec. **68**:131, 1954.

Mullane, D. J.: Varicose veins of pregnancy, Am. J. Obst. & Gynec. **63**:621, 1952.

Murphy, Patricia: Expectant mothers organize for natural childbirth, Am. J. Nursing **56**:1298, 1956.

Nurse's Guide for Teaching Maternal Nutrition, New York State Dept. of Health, 1955.

Page, E. W., and Page, E. P.: Leg cramps in pregnancy, Obst. & Gynec. **1**:94, 1953.

Peck, Elizabeth, and Carney, Ruth: Guidance programs for new mothers, Am. J. Nursing **51**:184, 1951.

Read, Grantly Dick: Childbirth Without Fear (Rev.), New York, Harper, 1953.

——: Introduction to Motherhood, London, Heinemann, 1950.

Scholten, Paul: The premarital examination, J.A.M.A. **167**:1171, 1958.

Stone, Abraham: Marriage counseling today and tomorrow, Marriage & Family Living **12**:39, 1950.

Thoms, Herbert: A consideration of childbirth programs, New England J. Med. **255**:860, 1956.

——: Preparation for childbirth programs, Obst. & Gynec. Surv. **10**:1, 1955.

——: Training for Childbirth, New York, McGraw-Hill, 1950.

Thoms, Herbert, and Roth, L. G.: Understanding Natural Childbirth, New York, McGraw-Hill, 1950.

Understanding natural childbirth, Briefs **20**:28, 1956.

U. S. Children's Bureau: Infant Care, Washington, D. C., 1955.

——: Prenatal Care, Washington, D. C., 1949.

Worrell, Kathryn E.: The maternal and child health consultant in the hospital program, Pub. Health Nursing **42**:329, 1950.

Young, Leontine: Out of Wedlock, New York, McGraw-Hill, 1954.

Zabriskie, Louise: Mother and Baby Care in Pictures, ed. 4, Philadelphia, Lippincott, 1953.

CHAPTER NINE

The Mental Hygiene of Pregnancy

LEO KANNER, M.D.

Director, Children's Psychiatric Service, the Johns Hopkins Hospital, Baltimore, Md.; Associate Professor of Psychiatry, the Johns Hopkins University School of Medicine

INTRODUCTION

Human pregnancy is a biologic event and an emotional experience. It begins with the relationship between two people and ushers in a new relationship between them and their offspring. The nature of the biologic event depends on anatomic and physiologic conditions; the nature of the emotional experience is determined by the mother's attitude toward herself, her husband and her child. The physical hygiene of pregnancy is directed primarily toward the mother's body; the mental hygiene of pregnancy addresses itself to her as a thinking, feeling and behaving individual.

It is true of all branches of medicine that a physician's or nurse's attention should not be limited exclusively and impersonally to the functions and the ailments of the patient's body. The need for sympathy and understanding has been emphasized since the days of Hippocrates. The combination of professional competence and humane interest in the patient has been rightly extolled as the ideal attribute of persons who make themselves responsible for the health of human beings.

The nature of childbearing is such that medical contacts with the parturient mother extend over a period of approximately a whole year. For nearly 12 months, the obstetrician and the obstetric nurse take over the guidance of an adult woman, supervise her nutrition, regulate her activities, answer her questions, clear up her puzzlements, advise her about the handling of the baby when it comes and generally chart her conduct during the 24 hours of the day. This offers ample opportunity to become acquainted with the mother's personality, the circumstances of her environment, her attitudes and opinions, her outlook on life and the degree of her emotional stability. It is not too difficult to sense and spot genuine happiness over the pregnancy, resentful rebellion against it, stunned acceptance of the conception as an unexpected decree of destiny or disturbing apprehension regarding the outcome.

The present can rarely be understood without reference to the past. Obstetrics cannot possibly dispense with a thoroughgoing evaluation of the patient's past history. Verbal reports, clinical examination and laboratory tests are indispensable as a preparation for the adequate physical hygiene of pregnancy. Needed information is thus obtained about factors of pelvic formation, miscarriages and stillbirths, cardiac illness, tuberculosis, syphilis and other conditions which existed before the recent conception and may complicate the course of events and influence the direction of obstetric procedure.

Analogously, a true appreciation of mental health during pregnancy can be obtained only by the ability to trace the mother's present attitudes to those personal experiences which have helped to shape them. In one sense, it is relatively easy to become familiar with such experiences and their effects, because no special or elaborate equipment is required. In another sense, such a study is extremely difficult and complex. Few people are inclined to disclose their most intimate feelings unless they are reasonably assured that the listener has the maturity, the tactfulness and the honest desire to understand, to guard confidences and to alleviate perplexities and anxieties.

THE MOTHER'S ATTITUDE TOWARD HER PREGNANCY

Under ordinary circumstances, the discovery of a woman's pregnancy is a happening which is welcome to her and to her husband. It is a source of rejoicing or at least of tranquil acceptance. The temporary discomforts, restrictions and changes of appearance which go with gravidity are awaited and borne with good nature. Even if there is some fear of the delivery, it is richly counterbalanced by the wish to have the baby, the gentleness of husband, relatives and friends, the full confidence in the physician and the nurse, the knowledge of good health and of satisfactory progress of the pregnancy and the ever-shortening distance from the moment of childbirth.

Such an attitude of positive and gratifying anticipation of motherhood, which is the essence of good mental hygiene, is usually predictable because it is based on a definite constellation of fortunate factors.

1. The mother herself has had a happy childhood and thereby has come to think of a family with children as something desirable and enjoyable. Her vision of a family unit is one of reciprocal satisfactions. Having experienced the benefits of parental fondness, she is prepared to give affection as she has received it.

2. The mother is secure in her relationship with her husband. The child comes to her as the result of intimacy with a man whom she loves and of whose love she is certain. She has no doubt about the safe and unperturbed continuity of her marriage.

3. The mother is not harassed by the drudgeries and the worries which arise from material insecurities, such as the husband's unemployment or protracted hospitalization, poor housing conditions or severe illness of one of her children.

Luckily, this combination of circumstances prevails often enough to deserve being regarded as the average, ordinary mental state of a mother at the onset of pregnancy. If it exists, her medical guides may look forward with a feeling of relief to the likelihood of freedom from untoward psychological complications. There is ground for the same sense of relief as that which obtains when, at the end of a thorough physical examination, the findings warrant a favorable prediction of the course of the biologic process.

However, departures from these healthy preliminary conditions are not at all uncommon. They can and should be studied, diagnosed and treated with the same care, knowledge and interest as are the major and minor deviations from bodily health and comfort. The principal directions of an unwholesome maternal attitude toward pregnancy present themselves to the knowing observer in the form of two disturbing psychological complexes: (1) fear of the delivery and of the fate of the child to be delivered; and (2) rejection of the child to be delivered.

Fear

Helene Deutsch, whose work on the psychology of women has received great acclaim, wrote in the volume devoted to motherhood: "That great power in human psychic life, *fear,* whatever its nature, certainly has a considerable influence on the emotional course of pregnancy."

A pregnant woman may be beset by two types of fearful anticipations, which often run concurrently: (1) fear for herself; and (2) fear for the baby.

The Mother's Fear for Herself. Every expectant mother knows that there will be pain, hospitalization or at least confinement in bed, perhaps the administration of an anesthetic, and a revolutionary physical change at the end of the pregnancy road. The whole procedure of childbirth, however normal it may turn out to be, must impress her as a sort of surgical intervention to which she will have to submit and from which there is no possible escape. There is hardly a human being who is entirely devoid of fear of an operation. The astounding progress of medicine and preventive hygiene has greatly reduced the actual dangers; also it has reduced, but not entirely eliminated, the dread. Statistics have shown a marked decline in maternal mortality, but this fact does not remove from the individual woman the anxiously perplexing question: What if it gets *me?* In the not too distant past many more women have lost their lives in pregnancy, labor and soon after birth than it is pleasant to contemplate. Even though conditions have improved tremendously and there is good reason for the expectation of further improvement, the public is still held in awe by the experiences gathered in centuries. Pregnant women's fear of death is therefore understandable and not at all unusual. It has been emphasized by

every author who has ever written about the mental hygiene of pregnancy.

There are many possible reactions to fear; some of them are flight, shrinking, avoidance of danger, stupefied inactivity, panic and bravery. No soldier, not even the most courageous, has ever gone into battle without being afraid; when we speak of "fearlessness" on such occasions, we do not refer to absence of fear but the conquest of fear. The conquest is successful if it is prompted and aided by a consistent motive. A pregnant woman is not unlike a soldier with regard to her attitude toward anticipated dangers. When there is an eager desire for a child, when security has been built up by the same kind of confidence in the people important to the mother which brave soldiers have in their commanders and buddies, then the motive is strong enough to conquer fear to the point that it is not even realized. The more the motive has been weakened by anxiety, insecurity and unhappiness, the less strength will the mother have to subdue her fear of childbirth, the more will the manifestations of her dread come to the fore.

The Mother's Fear for the Child. Pregnancy is in many respects a journey into the unknown. There are justified uncertainties about the expected baby's gender, appearance and general endowment. Uncertainty is a breeder of fear, particularly if previous experiences and orientations have tended to select some special areas of apprehension. Nobody can prophesy the future destiny of a human embryo even with approximate definiteness. But a mother to whom life has been good, who is thrilled by the prospect of having a child, who has fortified herself with a reasonable degree of optimism in all other respects, does not go around imagining all or any of the possible misfortunes which may befall her child. If, however, there is a background of anxiety, then the memory of dire happenings, pseudoscientific notions and folk beliefs may contrive to introduce torturing visions of impending disaster. There are three types of maternal fears for the baby which occur with special frequency.

1. Fear of losing the baby is apt to arise if the pregnancy has been preceded by spontaneous abortions, miscarriages or stillbirths; if previous pregnancies have been, or the present gestation is, accompanied by pathologic complications; or if these things have happened to relatives or close friends.

2. Fear of heredity is based on the layman's vague and frequently distorted interpretations of the results of scientific research. No real scholar has ever claimed that a child's personality development is merely an inherited repetition of some progenitor's antics, that traits are handed down as trinkets are, or that statistics can be applied to individuals. But this is exactly what "heredity" means to many people. As a result, anxious parents consult their respective genealogic trees and, finding an uncongenial ancestor hanging from one of the branches, worry themselves sick in the expectation of similar propensities in the baby-to-come. It can be said with considerable assurance that fear of heredity has caused at least as much mental anguish as heredity itself ever did.

3. Superstitious fears are found not only among the lowly and ignorant; they sometimes seem to be too powerful to be squelched even by a college diploma. The idea of mysterious prenatal influences which are said to "mark the baby" is still prevalent in many quarters. The notion is still abroad that a mother's experiences during her pregnancy will in some fashion shape the baby's fate. If she looks wistfully at a handsome child, the beauty will communicate itself to the embryo in her womb. She must be careful to keep her glances off ugliness and misshapen features or her baby may grow up to be ugly and misshapen.

Klein, Potter and Dyk collected many samples of such misconceptions. A few quotations may serve as illustrations. One mother thought that if one craved expensive out-of-season food the baby might have a birthmark, but if the same food were in season the baby would not be marked. Another believed that if she had a permanent wave during her pregnancy she might be electrocuted. One young woman, convinced that her own small hemangioma was caused by the fact that her mother had eaten strawberries while carrying her, feared that her child might be "marked by a mouse seen on a stove."

Rejection

Not all children arrive in this world because they have been wanted by their parents. The number of unplanned and unwanted pregnancies in our civilization is truly appalling. Statistics cannot possibly reach the annual total of illegally induced abortions, because every effort is made by the participants to keep them under the cover of secrecy. The unquestionably high figure is augmented by numerous unskillful attempts which do not succeed in destroying the child, who therefore comes into existence as an "unsuccessful abortion." This is a tragic state of affairs, both because of the interference with human life and because of the circumstances and the mental attitudes leading to the interference.

However, rejection of the pregnancy does not always end in the drastic ejection of the embryo from the uterus and from life. It often expresses itself more or less subtly in the parental attitude toward the unwanted pregnancy. It is not too unusual to hear rejecting mothers speak of the conception as an "accident" and describe their feelings at the time of the discovery as a "shock."

Therefore, maternal rejection results in one of three clearly circumscribed reactions: (1) illegal abortion, (2) unsuccessful attempt at abortion, (3) a nonaccepting attitude toward the pregnancy.

It is not easy for the average healthy person to comprehend the fact of a woman's repudiation of her own off-spring. Maternal rejection is indeed a very complex phenomenon anchored deeply in the mother's personality and relationships formed over a long period of time. What seems to be solely a matter of her feelings limited to *bearing and borne* has its origins in her own childhood and adolescence, her sexual orientation, her way of facing and adjusting to life in general. Of course, nurses cannot be expected to undertake the specifically psychiatric task of delving into the details or even the essentials of every pregnant woman's life history and its meaning to her. Nevertheless, there are several typical situations, ascertainable without too much difficulty, which play a prominent part in the immediate etiology of maternal rejection.

Socially unsanctioned, "illegitimate" conception is one of the most easily recognized sources of maternal resentment. The child so borne may unfortunately learn that he will be a permanent reminder of his mother's misstep, will either precipitate a "forced marriage" or be a hindrance in the consideration of future matrimonial aspirations, will raise the difficult problem of support, may estrange her from her relatives and friends and may thoroughly alter her status in society. All this naturally makes for an unhappy state of mind. Nevertheless, illegitimate pregnancy is not always synonymous with rejection. In certain ethnic groups—segments of our Negro population, for instance, in which some circles have a tolerant attitude toward babies born out of wedlock —such pregnancies are often accepted by the mothers with far greater ease than is generally the case.

Unplanned, "accidental" pregnancies are often resented because of economic distress. There already are too many mouths to be fed out of a meager budget. The mother already has her hands full, cooking, cleaning, laundering and taking care of her older children. Under such circumstances, the newcomer may be viewed chiefly as an added expense and burden. The husband's displeasure with the addition to the family may further aggravate the resentment.

The mother's feelings about her husband and her marital happiness determine to a considerable extent the degree of her acceptance or rejection of her pregnancy. If dissensions and incompatibilities have led to disillusionment and raised the specter of eventual dissolution of the marriage, it is extremely difficult to look forward to the birth of a child with unmixed pleasure and equanimity. This is equally true of pregnancies which, though planned and premeditated, have been entered into with ulterior motives, in which the genuine desire for a child figures much less than the purpose which his existence is intended to serve. Children sometimes are conceived as part of a scheme to keep the husband (or wife), to appeal to the marital partner's sense of responsibility, to satisfy the family's clamor for an heir to the name. If the mother finds that the disclosure of her pregnancy has not reduced her husband's alcoholism, gallivanting, lack of ambition or indifference toward her, then the child's coming has failed to accomplish the major purpose for which it was designed and therefore is resented as a bad investment.

Our culture has departed healthily and progressively from the idea that childbearing is a woman's only function and fulfillment. Women have embarked fruitfully on many occupations which had not been open to them previously. Many women come to matrimony and motherhood from the ranks of stenographers, salesgirls, nurses, teachers, factory workers, entertainers and waitresses. Some continue working while married until some time during the first pregnancy. Few people realize that the transition from a busy vocational life, from participation in group activities (office, store, hospital, school, factory, restaurant, etc.), and from a variety of interests and associations to quiet domesticity, change and narrowing of duties, and limitation of contacts with people, calls for major adjustments of routine and attitudes. Stable mothers, happily married, have gained a great deal from their jobs, which had given them an opportunity for personal enrichment, the satisfaction of having had a fling at life before their domestication and practice in dealing with human beings. The new experience of pregnancy is enjoyed because the mother obtains a richer biologic and psychological gratification from motherhood than she has obtained from her job, because she wants a child or children from the man whom she loves.

However, if the marriage turns out to be emotionally and economically disappointing, often there is a compensatory toying with the idea of returning to the former occupation and associates. Then comes the first pregnancy, which is either "accidental" or desired as a means of cementing a brittle husband-wife relationship and giving to the mother a new content in life. With it, however, comes a realization of finality. The child's expected arrival is looked upon with mixed feelings as a trap and a promise of something more precious than a job. This constant swaying between acceptance and rejection creates many quandaries which complicate the mother's attitude toward her pregnancy. I have heard a sizable number of mothers report how, under such conditions, they had felt "trapped," "hemmed in," "confined" or "cooped up" during pregnancy and how, in their night dreams and daydreams, they were not pregnant and were happily back at their jobs.

Though matrimonial unhappiness is one of the oustanding immediate factors in the etiology of maternal rejection, there are many other elements which color the picture in individual instances. A few specific examples may suffice.

Mrs. A. conceived immediately after marriage. A vivacious friend of hers, whose defiance of local bigotry had caused the neighbors' tongues to click for years, had given premature birth to a child seven months after her wedding; the whole community had raised suspicious eyebrows and cast aspersions. Mrs. A., who was pathetically dependent on the opinions of other people, lived throughout her pregnancy in dread that her child might come prematurely and arouse similar suspicions. She began to resent her pregnancy as coming "too soon." The combination of fear and rejection created an urgent psychiatric problem, caused her to attempt an abortion and almost wrecked the marriage.

Mrs. B. avowedly did not want children. Her husband likewise did not wish to "be bothered." They got along well for ten years. Their relatives and friends did not approve of their childlessness. They pointed out that, being people of wealth and standing, it was their "duty" to have children. They finally yielded when Mrs. B. decided that, having reached her thirties, she should "hurry up" if she was to have any children at all. But, once pregnant, she felt very bad and hated the child from the moment she discovered her pregnancy. She hated her advisers and blamed her husband for submitting to their dictates.

Mrs. C. was kept despotically under the thumb of her domineering mother, who consented to her marriage at 19 years on the condition that, being "too young," she promise not to have any children for several years. Mrs. C. was in love with her husband, who was anxious to become a father before his anticipated departure for the Pacific combat zone. When Mrs. C.'s mother learned about the pregnancy, she reproached her daughter, kept reminding her of the broken pledge, and finally refused to speak to her for several weeks. Matters were aggravated by the fact that, after the husband's departure, Mrs. C. was enticed by her mother to live in her house. Worried about her husband, made to feel guilty by her mother who ascribed recurrent headaches to her daughter's "disobedience," Mrs. C. was driven to despair. She came to accept her mother's endlessly repeated verdict that she should not have become pregnant so soon and looked on her pregnancy as an irreparable mistake destined to be a permanent reminder of her filial disloyalty.

Effect of Fear and Rejection

Fear and rejection, the principal obstacles in the path of good mental health in pregnancy, may be damaging in a variety of ways. An attitude of dread of the things to come and a revulsion against that which has become inevitable are obviously not conducive to comfort and composure.

However, it should be pointed out from the start that mild fear and resentment which are not too deeply rooted in the mother's personality can often be handled by her satisfactorily without too much interference with her equanimity. She is ready to seek and accept from her physician or nurse enlightenment with regard to her apprehensive puzzlements. She is able to overcome the first "shock" of the discovery of her pregnancy and to adjust to, or at least compromise with, the new situation.

A different picture obtains when strong emotional conflicts are at play, when the mother is the victim of powerful unconscious crosscurrents and when the pregnancy is complicated by fundamental personality difficulties.

It is well known that psychological distress has marked effects on one's ordinary physiologic functions. Everybody is familiar with headache, stomach ache and backache which obtrude themselves as "body protests" against emotional conflicts, even though no organic pathology can be demonstrated in the head, the stomach or the back.

Pregnancy is accompanied by a number of physical discomforts on a biologic basis. Nausea and vomiting are among the most frequent and most disturbing. Certainly enough momentous changes are taking place in the mother's somatic condition to explain nausea as a physiologic by-product of the pregnancy. Nevertheless, there are several features which have convinced obstetricians that emotional influences play a significant part in the picture.

1. Nausea, with or without vomiting, is not universal. It has been estimated that in about one third of all pregnancies it is either absent or so mild and fleeting that it constitutes no problem. This has rightly raised the question why identical bodily processes cause severe vomiting in one woman and barely a trace of nausea in another. The search for an answer to this question has led to the observation that the mother's personality and attitudes could be correlated with the degree of severity of the vomiting.

2. This assumption was strengthened by the fact that emotional factors were found to alleviate or aggravate the nausea. There were many instances during the war in which the husband's furlough put a stop to an expectant woman's nausea. A young, "accidentally" impregnated primipara became nauseated as soon as she had discovered the fact. Her husband had a poorly paid job at the time. Her nausea was very disturbing for several weeks but ceased abruptly when her husband was offered a well-paying position.

3. The milder forms of nausea are usually restricted to the early part of pregnancy. This indicates that nausea has a tendency to fade away when there has been a psychological as well as somatic adjustment to the condition.

4. Excessive or pernicious vomiting

seems to respond to psychotherapeutic measures at least as well as to other efforts.

Aside from nausea and vomiting, pregnancy is by its very nature associated with other discomforts, which stable mothers take in their stride. Fear-ridden and rejecting mothers tend to be disturbed by them to a much greater extent. When the pregnancy as such is resented, the necessary changes of routine, the temporary limitation of social activities or the disruption of employment are equally unwelcome. This attitude often results in poor co-operation with the regimen which has been mapped out by the physician and the nurse. Individual behavior differs in accordance with personalities.

One woman will not only follow recommendations anxiously but also be exasperating in her demands for the constant and undivided attention of the nurse, her husband, her relatives and everybody else. Her self-spoiling, for-ever-complaining and dissatisfied demeanor will calculate to surround her with people expected to cater to her hypochondriac whining or nagging. It is possible, though not certain, that some pregnant women's peculiar appetite for strange and not easily obtainable food items may have an unconscious basis in this type of self-indulgence.

Other women may go out of their way to disregard recommendations. They may continue scrubbing floors, rushing up and down the stairs or—in socially different settings—riding on horseback beyond the time when such strenuous activities are permissible. Their poor mental hygiene may cause them to neglect the essentials of physical hygiene. This devil-may-care or leave-me-alone attitude sometimes poses major problems to the obstetric nurse.

THE MOTHER'S ATTITUDE TOWARD LABOR

Dershimer has called attention to the great facility of childbirth among primitive peoples. Many ethnologists were amazed at the easy labor in civilizations less complex than our own. Deutsch wrote: "In some tribes, the whole confinement period is a matter of minutes. The young mother immediately bathes herself and the newborn infant in the nearest river and returns to her interrupted work as though nothing had happened. If a woman is suddenly seized with labor pains while traveling on land or by water, she resumes her journey immediately after delivery and continues on her way until she reaches her destination."

From this one might—a little too hastily, perhaps—infer that such bliss can be bought for the price of ignorance only. For it is true that primitive woman has not had the day of delivery calculated and marked for her on the calendar; she has not been enlightened about the process of parturition; and she has utter faith in the protective magic of her amulets. But this is not the whole story by far. There are many other primitive tribes, equally untutored, in which there is considerable agitation, kindled by all sorts of rituals, in connection with childbirth. Furthermore, precipitate deliveries occur in our culture as well as in any other. The psychology of labor and delivery is not too well known as yet to afford satisfactory explanations for differences in duration, intensity of pain and psychosomatic relationships in different cultures.

We are on safer ground when we consider differences among individual women in our own midst. We can understand that a stable, well-adjusted mother accepts the confinement as a hoped-for climax, at the end of which comes the coveted reward—the baby. The pain is felt as strongly by her as by any other woman in labor but is tolerated with a determination which keeps the goal in mind. It is recognized as a transition, demanded by Nature, to something that has been eagerly desired. There may be fear similar to that which is felt immediately before a surgical operation. But a stable person, though afraid, submits to the operation because she keeps in mind the goal of relief from the illness which has necessitated the surgeon's intervention. To a woman in good mental health, labor represents not only a first step toward the full restoration of her usual physical adequacy but also the welcome realization of imminent fulfillment.

But long-term anxiety, reinforced by rejection, makes labor appear as something like the painful signing of a contract into which a person has been pushed against her will. Or, if the analogy of an operation may again be resumed, delivery under those circumstances may be compared with a major surgical procedure from which the patient, instead of looking forward to relief, expects lifelong suffering and unpleasantness. Such an attitude rarely appears in undisguised form. No mother can afford to admit even to herself that she does not want her child. The closer the baby's arrival is at hand, the less can the mother's conscience allow her to wish the baby out of the way. There is no such thing as a "maternal instinct," but there is definitely a need for protection against the "unnatural" feelings of rejection. This protection is supplied by an unconscious mechanism called *ambivalence*.

Ambivalence is a fundamental human trait which makes it possible to love and hate the same person simultaneously, to want and not to want a child at the same time. When love and desire predominate, as they do in emotionallly healthy mothers, any coexisting negative feelings are weak and negligible and hardly ever come to the surface. But when there is resentment and rejection, the mother has the face-saving need for strengthening and emphasizing whatever positive feelings she has for the baby. The matrimonially unhappy

mother discovers that the child, conceived against her wishes, will, after all, be everything that is left to her to live for. She begins to feel guilty about ever having felt an aversion toward the pregnancy and is determined to make up for this when the child arrives.

All these sentiments and attitudes, some of which are intricately embedded in the mother's unconscious, are a significant part of her mental status during labor. It has been said that they may even influence the vigor of uterine contractions, but this, though quite possible, still remains to be demonstrated.

Some obstetricians, realizing the role of fear in labor, have tried to devise methods intended to alleviate the fear. In England, Read, convinced that much of the labor pain is attributable to tension produced by fear, worked out an obstetric regimen intended to keep the mother free from fear and pain by appropriate instruction, preparation and assistance. He described his method in a book entitled *Childbirth Without Fear*. Though in individual cases this may prove to be a helpful contribution to obstetric technic, Read did not pay sufficient attention to the basic mechanisms of the emotional conflicts which are at the bottom of a mother's tensions and fears.

THE MOTHER'S ATTITUDE TOWARD THE NEWBORN

People differ in their attitudes even toward inanimate possessions. One woman will treat her new set of furniture casually. Another will keep dusting and polishing it almost incessantly. A third will have spots and scratches on it in no time. Casualness, obsessiveness and negligence are expressions of personality and, when present, are applied to all phases of living.

A new baby certainly means much more than a new set of furniture. A woman's whole biography, the sum total of her philosophy of life, the background of her attitudes and relationships, her past and her vision of the future are reflected in her mode of adjustment to motherhood and to the newborn. Furthermore, a baby is, unlike a set of furniture, sensitive to the manner in which he is treated. The realization of an infant's responsiveness to affection or lack of affection has been one of the most significant discoveries made by students of human development. Many people are still skeptical when they are confronted with evidences of this discovery. Are not proper nutrition and physical hygiene all that a baby needs? What can he possibly know of his mother's worries or satisfactions? Indeed, he "knows" nothing about them. But he "senses" and responds to a tense or relaxed attitude, a personal or impersonal approach, genuine acceptance or dutiful subjection to regulations.

A series of studies in the past decade brought clinical proof of these observations. Babies reared for the first two or three years in orphanages under ideal hygienic and nutritional conditions, but without attention to their emotional needs, were found to be severely damaged psychologically. The emotional deprivations had lasting results which showed themselves in behavior deviations, character defects and intellectual deficit. By contrast, control groups reared in foster homes during early infancy achieved a much more satisfactory life adjustment and did far better in intelligence and personality tests.

An infant's need for maternal affection is now recognized as an undisputed scientific fact, as is the need for food and shelter. A loved child is a happy and secure child. An unloved child is unhappy, insecure and riddled with anxieties.

Rejected children are unloved children. A rejecting attitude is apt to push the mother into one of several sets of practices which are harmful to the child's mental hygiene as well as her own. There are, in our civilization, three

principal types of maternal behavior in response to the rejection of her baby: open hostility and neglect, perfectionism and overprotection.

Open Hostility and Neglect

Abandonment and desertion are the extreme forms of such behavior. They are, in a sense, postpartal "abortions"; the baby is tossed out of its mother's existence. But the tossing is sometimes done in a much subtler and more refined form which, though sanctioned by convention, still deprives the baby of a mother. There is no fondling and cuddling. The bottle takes the place of the breast. The mother returns as soon as possible to her work or social functions and leaves the care of her child to relatives or governesses. I have known working mothers who went to see their boarded babies once a week, mainly in order to pay for the board. I have known socialite mothers who had their babies brought to them for a few minutes' inspection "by appointment."

Perfectionism

Ambivalence plays an important part after childbirth, as it has played during pregnancy and labor. The inability to accept a child is coupled with a desire for the ability to accept him. The rejecting mother, justifying her feelings on the basis of the child's imperfections (no "perfect" human has ever existed), goes out of her way to assure the child's acceptability by trying to make him perfect. These are usually mothers who have long had a tendency to obsessive perfectionism, who scrub (or have the maid scrub) the floor until it sparkles, who live by the clock and make a fetish of orderliness and regularity. The baby must be made to fit into this scheme. All sorts of books on child rearing and child psychology are consulted and all but memorized. The advice of doctors and nurses is taken and carried out far too literally. If the baby does not comply with the desired ideal of perfection, the impatient mother resorts to coercion. Psychiatrists have learned that many difficulties of personality development have their origin in forced feeding and coercive bowel training in early infancy. Force and restraint lead to meek submission, listless withdrawal or rebellious negativism. All of these reactions are signs of frustration of a child who, being human, cannot live up to the demanded standards of perfection.

Overprotection

Some mothers cannot stand the thought that they have resented the pregnancy and the baby's coming. The mother's unsolved conflicts over her own unhappy childhood, matrimonial disillusionment or disrupted career are, after all, not the poor baby's fault. There is a feeling of remorse about the rejection. This feeling is compensated and overcompensated by a determination to sacrifice everything to the baby, to center on him all attention and energy every moment of the day. The child is wrapped in a heavy blanket of overprotection and oversolicitude.

Overprotection is not always the result of rejection. A woman who has lost one or more children through miscarriage, stillbirth or illness, a mother of an only child incapable of having more children because of hysterectomy, a woman whose child has come to her after a long period of childlessness may come to feel that she must be perpetually on guard lest something disastrous befall the child. Her overprotection of the baby is not an expiation for a rejecting attitude but an overdose of mothering and, figuratively speaking, the constant pulling at an uncut umbilical cord.

Regardless of the psychological origin of maternal overprotection, the result is unmerciful "spoiling" of the child. While the neglected or coerced child lives in an emotional refrigerator, the overprotected child lives in a heated oven in which mother love becomes smother love. Maturation and gradual emancipation are made impossible; whenever the child attempts to make use of his newly acquired abilities, he is pushed back into the oven. The mother is alarmed if he cries or if he does not cry, if he wants more food or less food than she believes that he should have, if his stools are softer or harder than she thinks they should be.

Neglect, perfectionism and overprotection are poor substitutes for genuine, natural maternal affection. They indicate emotional difficulties in the mother and create profound emotional difficulties in the infant. A sustained atmosphere of warmth, equally removed from refrigerator and oven, is a sign of good mental health of the parent and the safest guarantee of an infant's wholesome personality development.

THE PSYCHOSES OF PREGNANCY

In rare instances, the mother's emotional conflicts have been so deeply intrenched that they cannot be solved by neurotic mechanisms. The ordinary psychopathologic escapes and defenses, such as neglect, perfectionism and overprotection, are insufficient to keep the mother's personality functioning, even though the function be inadequate. The unconscious conflicts then become so overwhelmingly powerful that a major psychosis results. Estimates about the frequency of psychoses of pregnancy vary widely; they range from 1 in 400 pregnancies to 1 in 1,000 pregnancies.

Puerperal psychoses, with very few exceptions, have their onset after the birth of the child, usually between the first and the fourteenth day following the delivery. Apparently, even though there may have been symptoms of emotional discomfort during the period of gestation, the psychotic break does not come until the process of childbirth has been completed. It is then that the need for new adaptations which confront the mother finds her pathetically unprepared. Psychoses occur in primiparae and multiparae with almost the same frequency. Acute psychotic episodes have been known to repeat themselves in subsequent pregnancies.

There is no specific puerperal psychosis. Its general nature and symptoms may vary considerably. It usually takes the form of one of the two principal types: schizophrenia or manic-depressive psychosis. Recent studies have made it certain beyond question that neither mode of mental collapse is brought about by the pregnancy as such. Childbirth is a strong precipitating factor rather than the actual cause. It is mainly the agent which, shortly after the baby's arrival, tends to disintegrate a personality structure which has long been held together rather loosely and falls apart under the impact of the incisive psychobiologic experience of parturition. Toxic and infectious elements undoubtedly contribute to and hasten the process of disorganization.

The onset is characterized by a noticeable change of general demeanor. Sleeplessness, irritability, anxiety, excessive sadness or excitement, talkativeness, suspiciousness, preoccupation with trivialities and tense agitation should make one very cautious and mindful of psychotic developments. Once the clinical features have established themselves, their recognition presents no difficulty even to a lay person. Regardless of the type of the psychotic condition, antagonism toward the husband, hostility to the baby and concern over sexual matters are encountered with great frequency. The pathologic attitude toward the child may express itself in a variety of ways. The mother develops an amnesia for the birth of her child; she refuses to believe that the baby is her own; she has the delusional conviction that the baby is dead; she shrinks from contact with the baby because of the tormenting apprehension that she may harm him; she even may actually attempt to kill the baby.

Whenever there is the slightest suspicion of psychotic development, the nurse should immediately inform the physician in charge of the patient. He, in turn, will make immediate provisions for psychiatric care.

THE NURSES'S CONTRIBUTION TO THE MENTAL HYGIENE OF PREGNANCY

Psychiatry has gained important insights into the psychology and the psychopathology of pregnant women. In the great majority of instances psychiatrists are not, and need not be, consulted. This does not mean, however, that in our day and age every pregnant woman should not receive the benefits of existing knowledge. All branches of medicine are now availing themselves of the modern achievements of psychiatry and mental hygiene. Obstetricians, dealing as they do with women who are pregnant, guiding them for a period of almost a whole year, perceiving the great variety of marital and parent-child relationships, have been especially alert in this respect. If proof of this were necessary, one could point to Menninger's questionnaire, the answers to which bespeak great interest and understanding, and to Baker's work, which was carried out at the invitation and under the auspices of the Obstetrical Clinic of the Johns Hopkins Hospital.

The psychiatrically oriented and informed obstetrician and the obstetric nurse are the ideal mental hygienists of pregnancy. The nurse, without being a psychiatrist, can contribute a lion's share to the emotional well-being of the mother and to the baby's wholesome start in life. For this purpose, she needs three major attributes: (1) the ability to understand; (2) the ability to listen; (3) the ability to guide.

The Ability to Understand

Adequate information is one of the first prerequisites. As everywhere else in science, there are a few basic facts which must be learned before any sort of understanding can be reached. Furthermore, a nurse needs this knowledge not only for the sake of her own enlightenment but also in order to be able to impart it to her patients. Hall and Mohr recorded the types of questions which expectant mothers ask of their mentors in the course of pregnancy. The most frequently recurring questions were about physical care during pregnancy, the initial needs of the child, heredity and "marking." Some of these questions indicate in themselves the presence of quandaries and apprehensions and a desire for clarification.

The Ability to Listen

Patient, sympathetic listening is one of the greatest assets of anyone who tries to help human beings. People who have problems appreciate nothing more than an opportunity to pour out their troubles. The very act of verbalizing one's perplexities, of trying to hold them before oneself, of setting them forth before someone else, often affords great relief and helps the complainant to gain a better perspective regarding her complaints. There is nothing more frustrating than the experience of a patient who is anxious to talk herself out and is shut off with a remark, however well meant, such as: "Oh, forget it," "Now, don't let that worry you," or "This is just your imagination." It is far more helpful to encourage the speaker by asking interestedly: "What makes you feel that way?", or "Why does this bother you?"

The Ability to Guide

There is a great difference between guidance and direction. Inexperienced, insecure or tactless people often have a tendency to parade their authority and their better knowledge. Advice is given in terms of: "Do as I tell you," and "Take it or leave it." Such an approach does not invite willing co-operation. Patients want to be guided, not

bullied. Guidance includes readiness to explain one's directions and to make them acceptable. The aim is voluntary compliance through insight, not blind obedience through intimidation.

Understanding, listening and guidance are the cornerstones of the nurse's positive contribution to the mental hygiene of pregnancy. Without them, mothers will shy away from an otherwise most efficient nurse. They will, and should, shrink back if, having reached out for psychological help, they find that their plea is not recognized or is handled clumsily.

The first contact between the expectant mother and the obstetric nurse should be made an occasion for the establishment of a cordial mutual relationship. In this first interview, the pregnant woman should be helped to feel that she has acquired a sympathetic friend to whom she can talk about herself without hesitation. If there is economic distress, the nurse ought to be sufficiently familiar with the communal resources to be able to advise the family about possibilities of applying for and obtaining the necessary financial assistance.

The expectant mother's fears about herself and the baby-to-come should not be dismissed lightly with some indifferent phrase. When the mother has been allowed to reveal the nature and, as far as she can, the sources of her apprehension, she can be reassured by the nurse's explanations based on her better knowledge of the facts. Superstitious fears can thus be dispelled; erroneous notions about heredity and antepartal influences can thus be corrected. There will always be a greater or lesser degree of anxiety about the delivery, especially in primiparae and in mothers whose earlier pregnancy or pregnancies have been aggravated by unpleasant complications. In such instances, no amount of reasoning or disputing will succeed in removing the residual fear, but the mother can be helped to accept and adjust to the fear, much as a brave soldier accepts and adjusts to the fear of impending battle. She will be helped particularly by being allowed to live a normal and active life as long as this is possible. Activity is the best prophylaxis against brooding. Though a reasonable amount of rest is needed and highly desirable, modern obstetricians are rightly not in favor of inactivity and inertia during pregnancy. Eastman, discussing "The abuse of rest in obstetrics," wrote: "In whatever class of society, unoccupied life is not conducive to the health of the expectant mother." In view of the experiences with employed pregnant women in both world wars in this country and in England, Eastman felt that "it seems to have been clearly established that it is just as safe, with certain reservations, for pregnant women to work in industrial plants as it is for them to work at home."

The nurse often has an opportunity to contribute to the mental hygiene of the expected baby's older sibling. Profound jealousies among brothers and sisters are created sometimes by the improper preparation of a child for the arrival of a new baby. The existing child, who has had all the attention of his parents, suddenly and unexpectedly finds that an unannounced intruder is occupying his place and, by the very nature of things, seems to be monopolizing his mother's time. Prudishness or ignorance of the possible effects keeps many parents from introducing the new situation to the child gradually and in a manner which would help him to welcome, instead of jealously resenting, the new baby. The nurse can enlighten the family about the best means to prepare the child and bring home to them an understanding of his emotional needs for continued attention and show of affection.

There is little that a nurse can do about the fundamental mechanisms of maternal rejection. Rejection, as we have seen, involves deep-rooted uncon-scious conflicts which cannot be solved on a conscious level. Nevertheless, even then it helps the mother if she can voice her feelings in the presence of an understanding listener who, by her sympathetic attitude, can at least relieve her of some of her guilty feeling and anxiety. Besides, as Menninger stated, many "prospective parents can accept consciously an unwanted pregnancy with few, if any, manifestations of rejection," especially if they have a chance to discuss their failings with someone who has insight into their emotional attitudes.

Even though the basic background of rejection is beyond the nurse's scope, she can do much to alleviate some of its most disturbing effects, namely, those of perfectionistic coerciveness and overprotection. In fact, she can be a key figure in the task of parent education.

We have emerged but recently from an era in which physicians and psychologists alike not only sanctioned parental perfectionism but also imposed on mothers rigid rules and regulations which invited obsessiveness. Even then, the average mother, using common sense, did not allow herself to become a mechanized robot to whom the rules were more important than the baby. But insecure mothers, unable to rely on their own resources, inclined to punctiliousness, binding themselves to thou-shalts and thou-shalt-nots, developed a habit of rearing their children "by the book." The psychological school of behaviorism preached the gospel of impersonal "conditioning." Earlier pediatrics tried to cultivate addiction to the clock, a prescribed number of ounces, standard weight charts and calculation of calories. She was considered a good mother who never departed an iota from all these commandments. The sooner and the more persistently she started with toilet training, the higher was her efficiency rating in the eyes of her environment.

The past two decades witnessed a

wholesome rebellion against this enthrallment of mother and child. The discovery—or rediscovery—of the character-shaping value of maternal warmth, affection, naturalness and personal handling of the baby initiated a trend toward recognition of "the rights of infants." A baby is no longer regarded as something like a machine to be oiled, cleaned, purged of refuse and immobilized by the clock. He is looked upon as a human being on the way to form relationships with other human beings, relationships which depend on the attitudes of the people closest to him as much as the health of his body depends on proper nutrition, shelter and cleanliness.

This by no means indicates an abandonment of principles and rules based on such principles, but it does indicate an abandonment of obsessive enslavement to rules. It introduces the emphasis on *enjoyment* of the baby whose care is made a pleasure rather than a succession of chores. It was found that, unless there are physical obstacles, breast feeding makes for a happier contact between mother and child than bottle feeding. It was learned that patient and not too precocious bowel training is far better for the mental hygiene of the child than coercive bowel training. It has been established that occasional picking up and fondling, far from resulting in the dreaded "spoiling," builds in the child a sense of security and of being accepted and loved.

A mother who had reared two children well found herself "accidentally" pregnant again. The discovery was a "shock" to her. Remembering that her two children occasionally refused their spinach and sometimes did not obey her promptly, she made up her mind to rear her third child "scientifically." She lived up to every rule. The child was kept in her crib, was never picked up except to have the diapers changed. Nutrition, ventilation and everything else pertaining to physical welfare were perfect. Yet the baby, who was well endowed, failed to relate herself to her environment. She lived "in a world of her own." When I saw her at the age of five years, she was completely withdrawn and, in her schizophrenic aloneness, gave the impression of an idiotic child. This girl, who had been reared "perfectly," became a tragic victim of this type of perfection.

An obstetric nurse could have saved this child by helping the mother to recognize the grave hazards of impersonal perfectionism. Pregnancy and puerperium are the best time for implanting healthy methods of child rearing. It cannot be emphasized strongly enough that the obstetric nurse, in conjunction with the obstetrician, can do more than any other professional person to engender wholesome attitudes in parents toward their children. The work can then be taken up by pediatricians. Psychiatrists are not called into play until something has gone wrong. It is their job to study the causes of the damage and to communicate these causes to the natural mental hygienists of childhood—obstetricians, pediatricians and public health nurses.

SUMMARY

The mental hygiene of pregnancy, extending over a period of almost a year, is concerned with the emotional health of the expectant mother, the baby-to-come and sometimes the children already present. The mother's fear for herself and the baby and a rejecting attitude toward pregnancy and the child are the most powerful obstacles to emotional well-being. Rejection can manifest itself through neglect, perfectionistic coercion or overprotection. The public health nurse can do much to prevent mental difficulties by her understanding, ability to listen and tactful guidance, by dispelling pseudoscientific and superstitious fears and, above all, by helping the mother to institute adequate methods of child rearing. Such an orientation places the nurse in the front line of mental hygiene.

SUGGESTED READING

Bowlby, John: Maternal Care and Mental Health, Geneva, World Health Organization, 1952.

Caplan, Gerald: The mental hygiene role of the nurse in maternal and child care, Nursing Outlook 2:14, 1954.

——: Preparation for healthy parenthood, Children 1:171, 1954.

——: Psychological aspects of maternity care, Am. J. Pub. Health 47:25, 1957.

Dershimer, F.: The influence of mental attitudes in childbearing, Am. J. Obst. & Gynec. 31:444, 1936.

Deutsch, H.: Psychology of Women, Vol. II: Motherhood, New York, Grune & Stratton, 1945.

Eastman, N. J.: The abuse of rest in obstetrics, J.A.M.A. 125:1077, 1944.

Hargreaves, G. R.: The mental hygiene aspects of pregnancy, Child-Family Digest 14:92, 1956.

Kartchner, Fred D.: A study of the emotional reactions during labor, Am. J. Obst. & Gynec. 60:19, 1950.

Klein, H. R., Potter, H. W., and Dyk, R. B.: Anxiety in Pregnancy and Childbirth, New York, Hoeber, 1950.

Newton, Niles: Maternal Emotions, New York, Hoeber, 1955.

Parks, John: Emotional reactions to pregnancy, Am. J. Obst. & Gynec. 62:339, 1951.

Pheshette, Norman, et al.: A study of anxieties during pregnancy, labor, the early and late puerperium, Bull. New York Acad. 32:436, 1956.

Straus, Barbara: Mental hygiene in pregnancy, Am. J. Nursing 56:314, 1956.

Wooten, Betty: A psychosomatic approach to maternity care, Pub. Health Nursing 44:493, 1952.

CONFERENCE MATERIAL

1. What opportunities are available for teaching in the antepartal clinic while the patients are waiting their "turn" for examination?

2. How would you assist the mother with arrangements for the care of her children during the time that she is in the hospital? What organizations provide such care in your community?

3. For the antepartal patient who never has had any hospital experience, how would you introduce her to the antepartal clinic and prepare her for the complete physical examination?

4. How would you include the father and the other children in helping with the preparations for the new baby and the care of both the mother and the baby after delivery?

5. In discussing antepartal care with parents, how would you explain the relationship of diet to the baby's development from the time of conception until his birth?

6. In regard to the danger signals of pregnancy, how could you present these to an apprehensive patient without creating undue alarm?

7. What are the reasons for stressing the importance of completing the preparations for delivery by the seventh month of pregnancy?

8. What sources would you consult to find out which states in the United States require premarital and antepartal examinations for syphilis?

9. What type of referral system is used when it is necessary for the patient to consult other services or organizations?

Study Questions

UNIT TWO: NURSING IN PREGNANCY

Read through the entire question and place your answer in the parentheses.

1. Below are some signs, symptoms and conditions commonly associated with pregnancy. Those which the patient might notice and describe in the first trimester of pregnancy are:
   A. Amenorrhea
   B. Enlargement and tenderness of breasts
   C. Enlargement of uterus
   D. Frequent micturition
   E. Goodell's sign
   Select the number corresponding to the correct letters.
   1. A and C
   2. A, B and D
   3. B, D and E
   4. All of them   (____2____)

2. A. In pregnancy, morning sickness is most common during which of the following periods?
   1. First month
   2. First 6 weeks
   3. Sixth to twelfth week
   4. First 4 months
   5. Eighth to sixteenth week   (____3____)
   B. A nurse should suggest to the patient who complains of morning sickness that she might overcome this discomfort by using remedies to help:
   1. Emptying the stomach.
   2. Washing the stomach.
   3. Eating 6 small meals instead of 3 per day.
   4. Digestion of fats.   (____3____)

3. A pregnant woman seen for the first time in the antepartal clinic has a hemoglobin of 70 per cent. The nurse should understand that this condition is:
   A. A true anemia
   B. Caused by increased blood volume
   C. Dangerous to baby's development
   D. Predisposing to postpartal hemorrhage   (____B____)

4. The nurse in the obstetrician's office should instruct the patient regarding the collection of the specimen for the Aschheim-Zondek test by telling the patient to:
   A. Save the first voided specimen in the morning.
   B. Withhold fluid intake during the night and bring in the first voided specimen in the morning.
   C. Report to the laboratory in the morning for a blood specimen.
   D. Take a warm voided specimen to the laboratory.   (____B____)

5. Though the pregnant woman is usually advised to include a quart of milk in her diet daily, which of the following, if any, would justify the omission of milk?
A. Milk makes her constipated.
B. She is gaining weight too rapidly.
C. She is not gaining fast enough and needs more concentrated foods.
D. Milk causes a feeling of fullness, decreasing her appetite for other foods.
E. Milk causes heartburn.
F. None of the above; milk should not be omitted.   (———*F*———)

6. The most essential foods in a 2,300-calorie diet for a pregnant woman are:
A. High in carbohydrate, low in protein
B. High in protein, low in carbohydrate
C. High in protein, low in fat
D. High in fat, low in protein   (———*C*———)

7. The nurse in the antepartal clinic will encourage the pregnant woman to see her dentist at the earliest convenience because:
A. Each baby causes the mother to lose one tooth.
B. Bone development of the baby requires calcium.
C. Foci of infection should be removed early in pregnancy.
D. The increased carbohydrate needed in pregnancy is detrimental to sound teeth.   (———*C*———)

8. What instruction should the clinic patient be given concerning the care of her breasts during pregnancy?
A. A brassière should:
   1. Not be worn
   2. Be worn snugly enough to support and lift up the breasts
   3. Be worn snugly enough to press the breasts flat against the chest wall
   4. Be worn snugly enough to apply constant firm pressure toward the midline   (———*2*———)
B. Special care of the nipples should begin:
   1. As early as pregnancy is confirmed
   2. Between the third and fourth month
   3. Between the sixth and seventh month
   4. At the beginning of the ninth month   (———*3*———)

9. The exercises developed by Dr. Thoms at Yale included in the program of "Natural Childbirth":
A. Have as the central purpose:
   1. Teaching the patient how to relax
   2. Informing the patient of physiologic changes of pregnancy
   3. Developing intra-abdominal space for uterine enlargement   (———*1*———)
B. In addition to the exercises given, the pregnant patient needs during labor:
   1. Sympathetic care
   2. Heavy sedation
   3. Understanding of the progress of labor   (———*3*———)
C. Which week of pregnancy should the nurse begin to teach these exercises in the antepartal clinic?
   1. Sixth
   2. Tenth
   3. Fourteenth
   4. Thirty-sixth   (———*3-*———)

10. A. If the pregnant woman complained of painful, swollen veins in the legs, the nurse would understand that the condition would be likely to be due to:
1. Infection of the blood-vessel wall
2. Toxins accumulating in the blood
3. Pressure against the veins in the pelvis
4. Pressure directly against the walls of the arteries
5. Force of gravity   (——3——)
B. To remedy this condition, the nurse would expect that the patient would be advised that she should:
1. Refrain from wearing restricting clothing around the legs or the abdomen
2. Refrain from wearing a corset
3. Lie down each day for an hour's rest
4. Apply an Ace bandage, starting above the source of obstruction
                                                       (——1——)

11. The nurse teaching parents' classes should stress the importance of which one of the following?
A. Husbands doing the housework for their wives during the period of pregnancy
B. The idea of sharing responsibility in parenthood
C. The causes of invalidism during pregnancy
D. The moral responsibility of being parents   (——B——)

12. If a woman 6 months pregnant asked if she should or should not wear a corset, in your opinion the patient should be advised:
A. To avoid wearing any corset
B. To adjust her regular corset loosely
C. To wear a corset that will keep the uterus from rising too high in the abdomen
D. To wear a corset that will firmly support the lower portion of the abdomen and back
E. To wear a corset that will not disclose her condition.   (——D——)

13. The reason that pregnant women are warned against wearing high-heeled shoes from the seventh to the ninth month is:
A. To avoid additional backstrain
B. To increase venous pressure in the legs
C. To allow freer movement in taking daily exercises
D. To dress themselves according to current styles   (——A——)

14. The expectant mother who is employed as a stenographer should be advised that:
A. Rest periods are unnecessary if the job requires only "desk work."
B. Part-time employment should be requested after the fourth month of pregnancy.
C. A position which requires moderate manual labor would be more advantageous because it affords physical exercise.
D. Employment should be discontinued if the work causes moderate fatigue.
                                                       (——D——)

15. The clinic nurse would expect the pregnant patient to be advised to get in touch with her doctor *immediately* as soon as she observed which of the following?
A. Abdominal pain
B. Bleeding with bright blood
C. Blood-streaked mucus
D. Chills and fever
E. Constipation
Select the number corresponding to the correct letters.
   1. A, B and D
   2. B, C and E
   3. C, D and E
   4. All of them   (———/———)

16. In teaching the pregnant woman how to take a vaginal douche prescribed by the physician, the following should be emphasized:
A. A hand-bulb syringe is satisfactory if the mother is accustomed to using it.
B. The medicated solution must be prepared according to the physician's instructions.
C. The external genitalia should be cleansed with soap and water before taking a douche.
D. The douche may be taken while sitting on the toilet if the douche bag is placed no higher than 2 feet above the level of the hips.
E. The douche nozzle should be inserted gently into the vagina as far as it will go.
Select the number corresponding to the correct letters.
   1. A and B
   2. B and C
   3. B, D and E
   4. All of them   (———2———)

17. During her first visit to the clinic, the mother confides to the nurse that she is afraid to have a baby. The most appropriate response of the nurse might be:
A. "Modern obstetrics makes having a baby so safe that you have absolutely nothing to fear."
B. "Perhaps if you discussed this with a psychiatrist he could help you to overcome this feeling."
C. "Many women feel this way, so I wouldn't be concerned about it if I were you."
D. "I can understand that you might feel this way. What is it, in particular, that you are worried about"?   (———D———)

Note: The key to the correct answers to these questions is given on page 533.

UNIT THREE

Nursing During Labor and Delivery

ORIENTATION

The subject of labor deals with a period which is the climax of the entire maternity cycle. To attempt to understand this phenomenon and to gain some appreciation of its immediate reactions, the nurse must have a knowledge of obstetrics which has been discussed to this point, in addition to those understandings which are necessary in order to meet the nursing needs of all patients. Labor is an event which has extraordinary significance for the pregnant woman. Therefore, during this transition period, the nurse must try to understand the mental as well as the physical adjustments which the mother is having to make. Every measure which is essential to providing for the safety, comfort and welfare of the mother must be considered. It must be remembered that the course of labor and the quality of care the mother receives during her childbearing experience may influence markedly the future health of both the mother and her infant.

CHAPTER TEN

Phenomena of Labor

DEFINITIONS

By labor is meant the series of processes by which the products of conception are expelled from the mother's body (Fig. 126). Childbirth, travail, accouchement, confinement — all are names for the same process. The word "delivery" refers, as a rule, to the actual birth of the baby.

PREMONITORY SIGNS OF LABOR

During the last few weeks of pregnancy, a number of changes indicate that the time of labor is approaching. Particularly in primigravidas, "lightening" occurs about 10 to 14 days before delivery. This alteration is brought about by a settling of the fetal head into the brim of the pelvis, often to such a degree that the lowest part of the occiput is at the level of the ischial spines (Figs. 127 and 128). This may occur at any time during the last 4 weeks, but occasionally does not eventuate until labor has actually begun. Lightening may take place suddenly, so that the expectant mother arises one morning entirely relieved of the abdominal tightness and diaphragmatic pressure that she had experienced previously (Fig. 92). But the relief in one direction is often followed by signs of greater pressure below, such as shooting pains down the legs, an increase in the amount of vaginal discharge and greater frequency of urination due to pressure on the bladder. In mothers who have

had previous children, lightening is more likely to occur after labor begins.

For a varying period before the establishment of true labor, the patients will often suffer from so-called "false labor," and the nurse should be able to distinguish between this and effective uterine contractions. False contractions may begin as early as 3 or 4 weeks before the termination of pregnancy. They are merely an exaggeration of the intermittent uterine contractions which have occurred throughout the entire period of gestation but are now accompanied by discomfort. They occur at decidedly irregular intervals, are confined chiefly to the lower part of the abdomen and the groin and do not increase in intensity, frequency and duration. The discomfort is rarely intensified if the mother walks about and may even be relieved if she is on her feet. Examination by the physician will reveal no changes in the cervix. The signs which accompany true labor contractions present a contrasting picture. True labor contractions usually are felt in the lower back and extend in girdlelike fashion from the back to the front of the abdomen. These contractions have a definite rhythm and gradually increase in frequency, intensity and duration. In the course of a few hours of true labor contractions a progressive effacement and dilatation of the cervix would be apparent.

Another sign of impending labor is pink "show." After the discharge of the

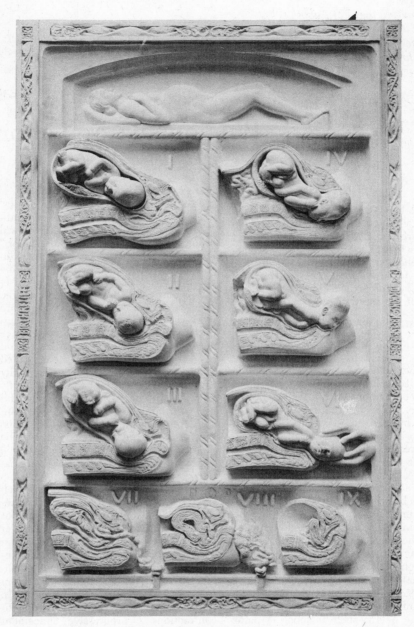

Fig. 126. "The Birth Relief." This distinguished sculptured relief depicts the orderly progression of labor with a vertex presentation from the moment of descent of the fetal head into the true pelvis through the delivery of the placenta. (The late Robert Latou Dickinson, M.D., famous obstetrician, gynecologist and artist, and Abram Belskie, artist and sculptor.)

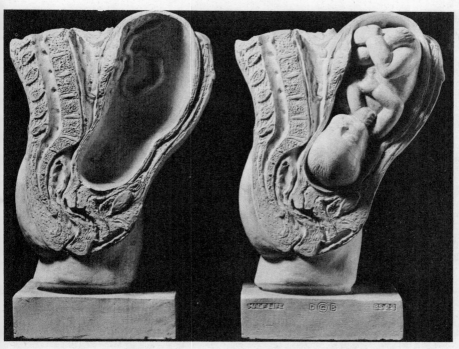

Fig. 127. Full-term pregnancy, showing median section of the abdomen and pelvis in the erect position. (Dickinson-Belskie models, Cleveland Health Museum, Cleveland)

mucus plug which has filled the cervical canal during pregnancy, the pressure of the descending presenting part of the fetus causes the minute capillaries in the mucous membrane of the cervix to rupture. This blood is mixed with mucus and therefore has the pink tinge. The nurse should understand that pink show is simply the appearance of a small amount of blood-tinged mucus, and that any substantial discharge of blood should be reported to the physician.

Occasionally, rupture of the membranes is the first indication of approaching labor. It used to be thought that this was a grave sign, heralding a long and difficult labor, but present-day statistics show that this is not true, and that rupture of the membranes is often followed by labors which are even shorter than the average. Nevertheless, the physician should be notified at once; under these circumstances, he will usually advise the patient to enter the hospital immediately. After the rupture of the membranes there is always the possibility of a prolapsed cord if the presenting part does not adequately fill the pelvic inlet. This might occur if the infant presents as a footling breech, or by the shoulder, or in the vertex presentation when the fetal head has not descended far enough into the true pelvis prior to the rupture of the membranes (see Fig. 258).

CAUSE OF ONSET OF LABOR

Regardless of species, whether the

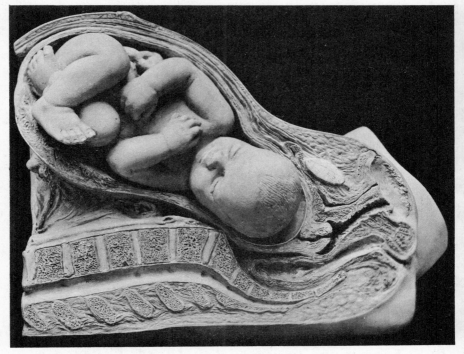

Fig. 128. Before labor, showing the uterus relaxed with the cervix closed, and a thick pelvic floor. (The following series of pictures are reproductions of the models made by Robert L. Dickinson, M.D., and Abram Belskie, Sculptor. They were reproduced for teaching purposes in the *Birth Atlas* published by the Maternity Center Association, New York.)

fetus weighs 2 Gm. at the end of a 21-day pregnancy, as in the mouse, or whether it weighs 200 pounds at the end of a 640-day pregnancy, as in the elephant, labor regularly begins at the right time for that particular species, namely, when the fetus is mature enough to cope with extra-uterine conditions but not yet large enough to cause mechanical difficulties in labor. The process responsible for this beautifully synchronized and salutary achievement is obscure. Nevertheless, countless theories have been advanced to explain the phenomenon. Among them may be mentioned increased irritability of the uterus as the result of greater distention, growing distention of the lower uterine struc-

tures with pressure on the surrounding nerves and the influences of hormones.

UTERINE CONTRACTIONS

In all languages, the word for the uterine contractions of labor has been interpreted the same, namely, "pain." Alone among normal physiologic muscular contractions, moreover, those of labor can be painful. The duration of these contractions ranges from 45 seconds to 1 minute and a quarter, averaging about 1 minute. Each contraction presents 3 phases: a period during which the intensity of the contraction increases (increment), a period during which the contraction is at its height (acme), and a period of diminishing

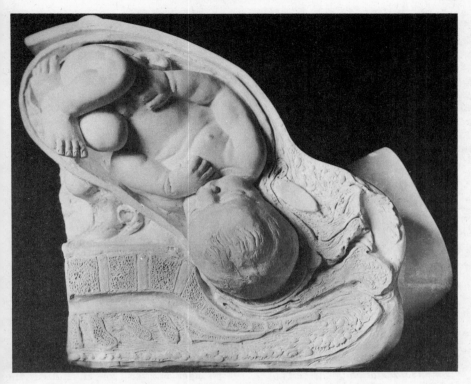

Fig. 129. First stage of labor. The rhythmic contractions of the uterus aid the progressive effacement and dilatation of the cervix, as well as the descent of the infant.

intensity (decrement). The increment, or crescendo phase, is longer than the other two combined. The contractions of the uterus during labor are intermittent, with periods of relaxation between, resembling in this respect the systole and the diastole of the heart. The interval between contractions diminishes gradually from about 10 minutes early in labor to about 2 or 3 minutes in the second stage. These periods of relaxation not only provide rest for the uterine muscles and for the mother but also are essential for the welfare of the fetus, since unremitting contractions may so interfere with placental functions as to produce fetal distress as a result of lack of oxygen. Another characteristic of

labor contractions is that they are quite involuntary, their action being not only independent of the mother's will but also of extra-uterine nervous control. In other words, uterine action in labor, like that of the heart, is under control of nerves located within the organ itself. Today, it is believed that the manifestations of suffering are more often influenced by mental and emotional reactions than by the physical condition.

THE THREE STAGES OF LABOR

The process of labor is divided, for convenience of description, into 3 distinct stages.

The first stage of labor, or the dilating stage, begins with the first true

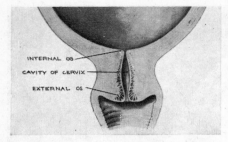
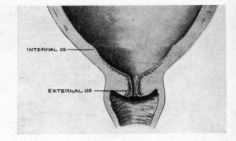
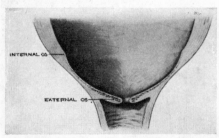
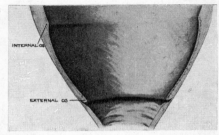

Fig. 130. Cervix in primagravida. (*Top, left*) At beginning of labor; no effacement or dilatation. (*Top, right*) About one half effaced, but no dilatation. (*Bottom, left*) Completely effaced, but no dilatation. (*Bottom, right*) Complete dilatation. (Bumm)

labor contraction and ends with the complete dilatation of the cervix.

The second stage of labor, or the stage of expulsion, begins with the complete dilatation of the cervix and ends with the delivery of the baby.

The third stage of labor, or the placental stage, begins with the delivery of the baby and terminates with the birth of the placenta.

The First Stage of Labor

In the beginning of the first stage, the contractions are short, slight, are 10 or 15 minutes or more apart and may not cause the patient any particular discomfort. She may be walking about and between contractions is generally quite comfortable. Early in the first stage, the discomfort is usually located in the small of the back, but, as time goes on, it sweeps around, girdlelike, to the anterior part of the abdomen. The contractions recur at shortening intervals, every 3 to 5 minutes, and become stronger and last longer. Indeed, the contractions which precede and accompany full dilatation are often of excruciating severity. At this time, furthermore, there is usually a marked increase in the amount of show due to rupture of capillary vessels in the cervix and the lower uterine segment. The average duration of the first stage in primigravidas is about 12½ hours; in multiparas, about 7½ hours.

As the result of the uterine contractions, two all-important changes are wrought in the cervix during the first stage of labor—*effacement* and *dilatation* (Fig. 129).

Effacement is the shortening of the cervical canal from a structure 1 or 2 cm. in length to one in which no canal at all exists, but merely a circular orifice with almost paper-thin edges. As may be seen in Figure 130, the edges of the internal os are drawn several centi-

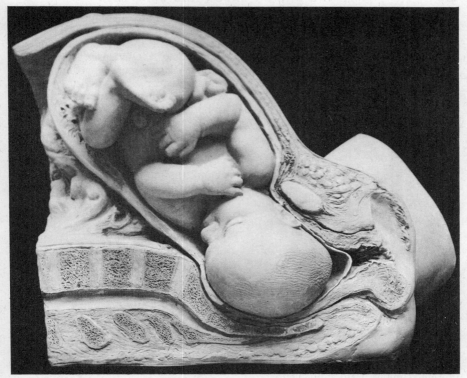

Fig. 131. Full dilatation: cervix high, head deep in birth canal, membranes intact.

meters upward, so that the former cervical mucosa becomes part of the lower uterine segment and lies parallel with and contiguous to the chorion membrane. Effacement may be compared with a funneling process in which the whole length of a moldable tube (the cervical canal) is converted into a very large, flaring funnel, with only a small circular orifice for an outlet. In primigravidas, effacement is usually complete before dilatation begins, but in multiparas it is rarely complete, dilatation proceeding, as a rule, with rather thick cervical edges. Synonymous with effacement are the terms "obliteration" and "taking up" of the cervix.

Dilatation of the Cervix. By this is meant the enlargement of the external

os from an orifice a few millimeters in size to an aperture large enough to permit the passage of the fetus—that is, to one with a diameter of about 10 cm. When dilatation has reached this figure, it is said to be complete. Although the forces concerned in dilatation are not well understood, several factors appear to be involved. In the first place, the muscle fibers about the cervix are so arranged that they pull upon its edges and tend to draw it open. In the second place, the uterine contractions make pressure on the bag of waters and this, in turn, burrows into the cervix in pouchlike fashion, exerting a dilating action (Fig. 131). This is usually called the hydrostatic pressure of the bag of waters. In the absence of the bag of

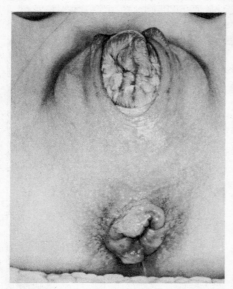

Fig. 132. Extreme bulging of perineum showing patulous and everted anus.

waters, the pressure of the presenting part against the cervix and the lower uterine segment has a similar effect.

It should be noted that the dilatation of the cervix in the first stage of labor is solely the result of uterine contractions which are involutary. In other words, there is nothing that the mother can do, such as bearing down, which will help the slightest in expediting this period of labor. Indeed, bearing-down efforts at this stage serve only to exhaust the mother and cause the cervix to become edematous.

The Second Stage of Labor

The contractions are now severe and long, lasting 50 to 70 seconds and occurring at intervals of 2 or 3 minutes. Rupture of the membranes usually occurs during the early part of this stage of labor by a gush of amniotic fluid from the vagina. Sometimes, however, they rupture during the first stage and occasionally, as already indicated, be-

fore labor begins. In rare instances, the membranes fail to rupture, and the baby is born with the intact amniotic sac surrounding it. Obviously, in such cases the membranes must be artificially ruptured at once, for otherwise the infant will drown. In some rare cases the baby is born in a "caul," which is a piece of the amnion which sometimes envelops the baby's head. Superstitious parents consider this to be a good omen.

During this stage, as if by reflex action, the muscles of the abdomen are brought into play; and when the contractions are in progress the patient will strain, or "bear down," with all her strength so that her face becomes flushed and the large vessels in her neck are distended. As a result of this exertion she may perspire profusely. During this stage the mother directs all her energy toward expelling the contents of the uterus.

Toward the end of the second stage, when the head is well down in the vagina, its pressure causes the anus to become patulous and everted (Fig. 132), and often small particles of fecal material may be expelled from the rectum at the occurrence of each contraction. This condition must receive careful attention to avoid contamination. As the head descends still further, the perineal region begins to bulge, and the skin over it becomes tense and glistening. At this time the scalp of the fetus may be detected through a slitlike vulvar opening (Fig. 133). With each subsequent contraction the perineum bulges more and more, and the vulva becomes more dilated and distended by the head, so that the opening is gradually converted into an ovoid and at last into a circle. With the cessation of each contraction the opening becomes smaller, and the head recedes from it until it advances again with the next contraction.

The contractions now occur very rapidly, with scarcely any interval between. As the head becomes increasingly visi-

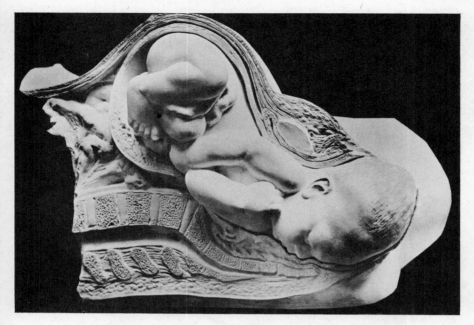

Fig. 133. Second stage of labor. "Caput," or top of infant's head, begins to appear through the vulvar opening.

ble, the vulva is stretched further and finally encircles the largest diameter of the baby's head. This encirclement of the largest diameter of the baby's head by the vulvar ring is known as "crowning." The physician now supports the tissues surrounding the perineum and delivers the head between contractions. One or two more contractions are normally enough to effect the birth of the baby.

Whereas in the first stage of labor the forces are limited to uterine action, during the second stage two forces are essential, namely, uterine contractions and intra-abdominal pressure, the latter being brought about by the bearing-down efforts of the mother. (The force exerted by the mother's bearing down can be likened to that used in forcing an evacuation of the bowels.) Both forces are essential to the successful spontaneous outcome of the second stage of labor, for uterine contractions without bearing-down efforts are of little avail in expelling the infant, while, conversely, bearing-down efforts in the absence of uterine contractions are futile. As explained in Chapter 12, "Conduct of Normal Labor," these facts have most important practical implications.

In its passage through the birth canal, the presenting part of the fetus undergoes certain positional changes which constitute the mechanism of labor. These movements are designed to present the smallest possible diameters of the presenting part to the irregular shape of the pelvic canal, so that it will encounter as little resistance as possible. The mechanism of labor consists of a combination of movements, several of which may be going on at the same time. As they occur, the uterine contractions bring about important modifications in

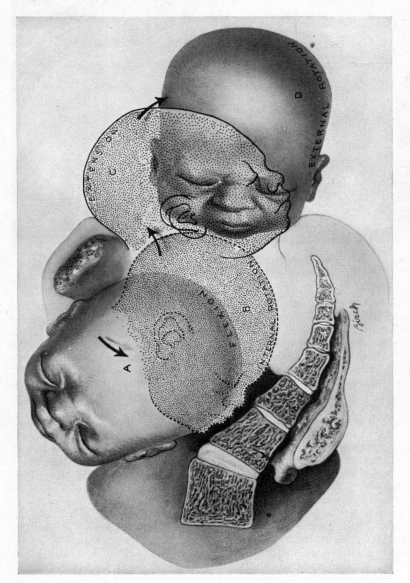

Plate 6. L.O.A. Positional changes of head in passing through birth canal.

the attitude or habitus of the fetus, especially after the head has descended into the pelvis. This adaptation of the baby to the birth canal, as descent takes place, involves the four processes called flexion, internal rotation, extension and external rotation (Plate 6).

For purposes of instruction, the vari-

ous movements will be described as if they occurred independently of one another.

As previously stated, in the primigravida, engagement usually occurs during the last weeks of pregnancy, but in the multipara it ordinarily does not take place until after labor has begun. When

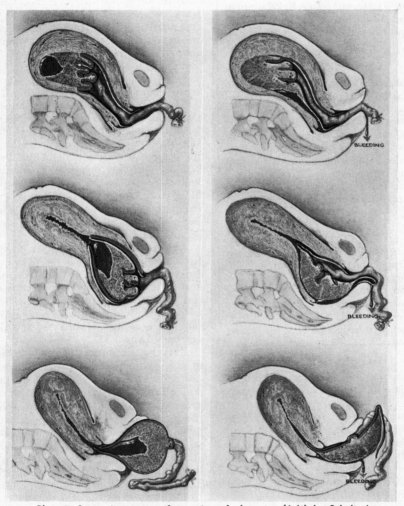

Plate 7. Successive stages of extrusion of placenta: (*left*) by Schultze's mechanism; (*right*) by Duncan's mechanism.

SUMMARY OF MECHANISM OF LABOR *

FIRST STAGE— DILATING STAGE

Definition. Period from first true labor contraction to complete dilatation of cervix.

What Is Acommplished? Effacement and dilatation of cervix.

Forces Involved. Uterine contractions.

SECOND STAGE— EXPULSIVE STAGE

Definition. Period from complete dilatation of cervix to birth of baby.

What Is Accomplished? Expulsion of baby from birth canal—facilitated by certain positional changes of fetus: descent, flexion, internal rotation, extension, external rotation and expulsion.

Forces Involved. Uterine contractions plus intra-abdominal pressure.

THIRD STAGE— PLACENTAL STAGE

Definition. Period from birth of baby through birth of placenta.

What Is Accomplished? (a) Separation of placenta; (b) expulsion of placenta.

Forces Involved. (a) Uterine contractions; (b) intra-abdominal pressure.

the biparietal diameter of the infant's head is within the pelvic inlet, engagement is said to have occurred.

Descent. The first requisite for the birth of the infant is descent. In primigravidas, because engagement is frequently deep at the onset of labor, further descent does not necessarily begin until the second stage of labor sets in. In multiparas, on the other hand, descent begins with engagement. In either event, once having been inaugurated, descent is inevitably associated with the various movements of the mechanism of labor.

Flexion. Very early in the process of descent, the head becomes so flexed that the chin is in contact with the sternum, and, as a consequence, the very smallest anteroposterior diameter (the suboccipitobregmatic plane) is presented to the pelvis.

Internal Rotation. As seen in Chapter 2, the head enters the pelvis in the transverse or diagonal position. When it reaches the pelvic floor, the occiput is rotated and comes to lie beneath the symphysis pubis. In other words, the sagittal suture is now in the anteroposterior diameter of the outlet (Fig 14). Although the occiput usually rotates to the front, on occasion it may turn toward the hollow of the sacrum. If anterior rotation does not take place at all, the occiput usually rotates to the direct occiput posterior position, a condition known as persistent occiput posterior. Since this represents a deviation from the normal mechanism of labor, it will be considered in Chapter 19, under "Abnormal Fetal Positions."

Extension. After the occiput emerges from the pelvis, the nape of the neck becomes arrested beneath the pubic arch and acts as a pivotal point for the rest of the head. Extension of the head now ensues, and with it the frontal portion of the head, the face and the chin are born (Fig. 134).

External Rotation. After the birth of the head, it remains in the anteroposterior position only a very short time and shortly will be seen to turn to one or another side of its own accord. When the occiput originally has been directed toward the left of the mother's pelvis, it rotates toward the left tuberischii, and in the opposite direction when it originally has been toward the right. This is known as external rotation and is due to the fact that the shoulders of the baby, having entered the pelvis in the transverse position, undergo internal rotation to the anteroposterior posi-

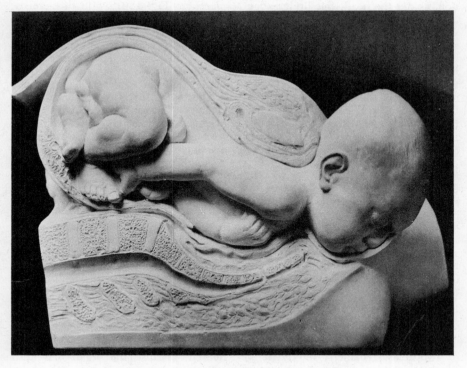

Fig. 134. Head extends upward; pelvic floor retreats.

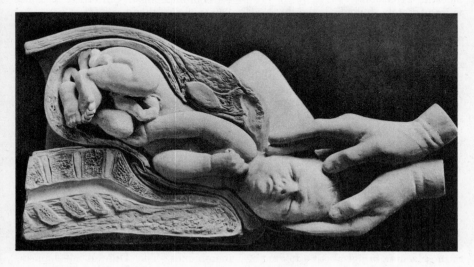

Fig. 135. Birth of shoulders: rotating to accommodate to birth passage.

tion, as did the head; this brings about a corresponding rotation of the head which is now on the outside. The shoulders are born in a manner somewhat similar to that of the head. Almost immediately after the occurrence of external rotation, the anterior shoulder appears under the symphysis pubis and becomes arrested temporarily beneath the pubic arch, to act as a pivotal point for the other shoulder (Fig. 135). As the anterior margin of the perineum becomes distended, the posterior shoulder is born, assisted by an upward lateral flexion of the infant's body. Once the shoulders are delivered, the infant's body is quickly extruded (expulsion) because of its relative size.

The average duration of the second stage of labor in primigravidas is an hour and a quarter, and in multiparas about 30 minutes or less. Sometimes 2 or 3 contractions suffice for the completion of the period of expulsion.

The Third Stage of Labor

The third stage of labor is made up of two phases, namely, *the phase of placental separation* and *the phase of placenta expulsion.*

Immediately following the birth of the infant, the remainder of the amniotic fluid escapes, after which there is usually a slight flow of blood. The uterus can be felt as a firm globular mass just below the level of the umbilicus. Shortly thereafter, the uterus relaxes and assumes a discoid shape. With each subsequent contraction or relaxation the uterus changes from globular to discoid shape until the placenta has separated, after which time the globular shape persists.

Placental Separation. As the uterus contracts down at regular intervals on its diminishing content, the area of placental attachment is greatly reduced. The great disproportion between the reduced size of the placental site and that of the placenta brings about a folding or festooning of the maternal surface of the

placenta (Fig. 136); with this process separation takes place. Meanwhile, bleeding takes place within these placental folds, and this expedites separation of the organ. The placenta now sinks into the lower uterine segment or upper vagina as an unattached body.

The signs which suggest that the placenta has separated are: (1) the uterus becomes globular in shape and, as a rule, firmer; (2) it rises upward in the abdomen; (3) the umbilical cord descends 3 or more inches farther out of the vagina; and (4) a sudden gush of blood often occurs. These signs usually occur within 5 minutes after the delivery of the infant.

Placental Expulsion. Actual expulsion of the placenta may be brought about by bearing-down efforts on the part of the mother if she is not anesthetized. If this cannot be accomplished, it is usually effected through gentle pressure on the uterine fundus by the physician after he has first made certain that the uterus is hard. This should never be attempted when the uterus is relaxed, because the organ may turn inside-out and result in one of the gravest complications of obstetrics, so-called "inversion" of the uterus (see Chap. 19).

The extrusion of the placenta may take place by one of two mechanisms. First, it may become turned inside-out within the vagina and be born like an inverted umbrella with the glistening fetal surfaces presenting. This is known as Schultze's mechanism and occurs in about 80 per cent of cases. Second, it may become somewhat rolled up in the vagina, with the maternal surface outermost, and be born edgewise. The latter is known as Duncan's mechanism and is seen in about 20 per cent of deliveries (Plate 7). It is believed that the Schultze's mechanism signifies that the placenta has become detached first at its center, and usually a collection of blood and clots is found in the sac of membranes. The Duncan mechanism, on the other hand, suggests that the placenta has separated first at its edges, and it is in this type that bleeding usually occurs at the time of separation.

The contraction of the uterus following delivery serves not only to produce placental separation but also to control uterine hemorrhage. As the result of this contraction of the uterine muscle fibers, the countless blood vessels within their interstices are clamped shut. Even then,

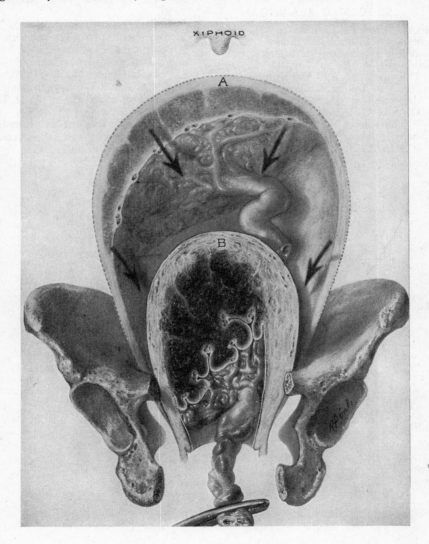

Fig. 136. (A) Area of placental attachment before birth of baby. (B) Greatly reduced area of placental attachment after birth of baby. Note folding or festooning of placenta brought about by the reduced area of attachment. (Ischia and pubic bones cut away for clarity.)

a certain amount of blood loss in the third stage is unavoidable, the average being about 250 to 300 cc. It is one of the aims of the conduct of labor to reduce this bleeding to a very minimum.

SUGGESTED READING

Beck, Alfred C., and Rosenthal, Alexander: Obstetrical Practice, ed. 6, Baltimore, Williams & Wilkens, 1955.

Caldwell, W. E., Moloy, H. C., and D'Esopo, D. A.: A roentgenologic study of the mechanism of the engagement of the fetal head, Am. J. Obst. & Gynec. 28:824, 1934.

——: The role of the lower uterine soft parts in labor, Am. J. Obst. & Gynec. 37:618, 1939.

Davis, M. Edward, and Sheckler, Catherine E.: DeLee's Obstetrics for Nurses, ed. 16, Philadelphia, Saunders, 1957.

Eastman, Nicholson J.: Williams Obstetrics, ed. 11, New York, Appleton, 1956.

Javert, Carl T., and Hardy, James D.: Measurement of pain intensity in labor and its physiologic, neurologic, and pharmacologic implications, Am. J. Obst. & Gynec. 60:552, 1950.

Lull, Clifford, and Kimbrough, Robert: Clinical Obstetrics, Philadelphia, Lippincott, 1953.

Redman, T. F.: Descent of presenting part in pregnancy and labor, Am. J. Obst. & Gynec. 66:607, 1953.

CHAPTER ELEVEN

Analgesia and Anesthesia In Labor

From the time of early civilizations the pains and the tortures endured by women in childbirth have been related in the historical records. It was not until the middle of the 19th century that medical science introduced anesthesia to relieve this pain. Two important pioneers who made important contributions in the use of anesthesia in obstetrics were Sir James Y. Simpson, of Edinburgh, and his contemporary in this country, Dr. Walter Channing, of Boston. A knowledge of the historical development of pain relief used in obstetrics will assist the nurse to gain an increased understanding of modern practices utilized in this approach to providing the mother with more comfort during labor. In addition, she will find that this study provides fascinating reading material. Space will not permit an adequate discussion here, thus the student is advised to pursue it in appropriate texts. (See Suggested Reading and Chapter 24, History of Obstetrics.)

TYPES OF PAIN RELIEF

Pain relief in labor may be of two main types: (1) *obstetric analgesia* and (2) *obstetric anesthesia.*

By *obstetric analgesia* is meant the administration of certain drugs during the first and second stages of labor, prior to the actual birth of the baby, for the purpose of relieving the discomfort caused by labor contractions.

By *obstetric anesthesia* is meant the administration of certain drugs for the total obliteration of pain and sensation during the procedure of delivery of the infant, the placenta and perineal repair, if required.

In modern obstetric practice various technics may be utilized for pain relief in labor. No one method should be employed universally for all women. In this country, Demerol or one of the other synthetic narcotics, in combination with scopolamine and/or one of the drugs such as Phenergan, is most commonly used to achieve systemic analgesia and amnesia. Systemic anesthesia is produced by the inhalation of anesthetic gases (nitrous oxide, cyclopropane, ethylene) or volatile anesthetics (ether, chloroform) or by the intravenous infusion of thiopental sodium (Pentothal Sodium). Regional anesthesia may be produced by spinal or caudal anesthesia, or by local infiltration of the tissues concerned with an anesthetic solution such as procaine. Certain technics, such as continuous caudal, may be used for both obstetric analgesia and anesthesia. When regional anesthetics are used the patient is awake, but painful sensation is abolished in the areas concerned. Inhalation or intravenous anesthetics, of course, produce unconsciousness.

GENERAL PRINCIPLES

The proper psychological preparation of the expectant mother in the care she receives throughout her pregnancy and labor is an indispensable basic sedative. A women who is carefree, unafraid and

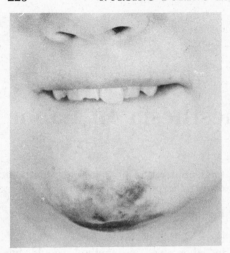

Fig. 137. This patient chipped off her right front tooth and bruised her chin when under analgesic and amnesic drugs, as the result of throwing herself against a radiator near the bed. Patients receiving such medications during labor must never be left unattended, even for a moment.

possessed of complete confidence in her obstetrician and nurses usually enjoys a relatively comfortable first stage of labor and requires a minimum of medication. This wholesome attitude toward parturition must be assiduously fostered at all times as an essential phase of pain relief.

When any form of pain relief is administered in labor, the safety of two patients, the mother and her infant, is the most important consideration. When prescribing analgesic medication, the physician's judgment is influenced by many factors, such as the length of gestation; the mother's emotional behavior; her response to pain; her previous obstetric and anesthetic experiences; and, of course, the frequency, intensity and duration of uterine contractions and the general character of the labor. Analgesia should not be initiated too soon. One rule should be absolute: such medica-

tion should never be started until positive proof exists that the cervix is showing progressive effacement and dilatation. In general, primigravidas should not be given analgesic medication until the contractions are strong and regular and the cervix is 3 to 5 cm. dilated; in multiparas the cervix should be 4 to 6 cm. dilated. If the medication is administered before good labor is established, the drugs may appreciably retard the progress of labor or even stop it. On the other hand, when medication is started somewhat later than the optimal time, the efficacy of the analgesia is diminished as a rule, especially in rapid multiparous labors. These drugs may also affect the infant's respirations at birth if sufficient time has not elapsed for their metabolism and excretion prior to the birth of the baby. It is important that the drugs exert little effect on the uterine contractions, otherwise not only will the progress of labor be impeded but also, after the delivery, if the uterine contractions are suppressed, postpartal hemorrhage may occur.

Any mother in labor should be in a single room if possible, but particularly when drugs are administered to promote obstetric analgesia. When the drugs administered will produce systemic analgesia, the environment should be conducive to rest, that is, free from such forms of external stimuli as bright lights and noises, even conversation. The room should be quiet and dimly lighted, though light enough to permit the nurse in attendance to observe the signs of progress of labor, as well as the mother's general condition.

Before administering the drugs, the nurse should give the patient certain explanations about the therapy so that she understands what is happening and particularly that the darkened quiet environment will enhance the effect of the medication. At this time the patient should be encouraged to empty her bladder. This not only contributes to her immediate comfort but also often avoids the necessity of catheterization if she is not able to void later on in labor. In addition, this is a preventive measure to avoid postpartal urinary retention. The fetal heart tones are taken now, and again after the medication is administered. In the latter instance, only sufficient time should elapse to permit absorption of the medication, which, of course, would be dependent on the route of administration utilized. Most physicians advocate that patients receive nothing by mouth after analgesia is started.

Patients under any form of analgesia require constant and meticulous attention. The nurse must be alert to the signs which indicate progress of labor even more carefully now since the mother is sedated, particularly those signs which herald the second stage of labor. Also, if left alone, a patient may throw herself against the wall or out of bed, or may vomit and aspirate the gastric contents. Numerous injuries and a few deaths are on record as a result of such negligence. Figure 137 illustrates the results of an accident which occurred when the patient was under sedation. Similarly, conduction anesthesia demands meticulous attention to the blood pressure and anesthetic levels if safety is to be achieved.

Before any agent is administered to produce general anesthesia, false teeth, chewing gum or any other foreign object must be removed from the mouth, because these may be swallowed or aspirated when the patient loses consciousness. Because vomiting is likely to occur during the induction of anesthesia and during the emergence from the anesthetic state, an emesis basin and towels must be within easy reach. During the entire period of unconsciousness after returning from the delivery room, the patient should lie on her right side, with or without a slight degree of Trendelenburg position, with the neck extended. This position augments drain-

age of vomitus should emesis occur and at the same time helps prevent obstruction of respiration due to relaxation of the tongue. To prevent further interference with respiration until the patient awakens, and until the danger of the tongue slipping back is eliminated, the lower jaw should be supported by pressure against the mandible.

OBSTETRIC ANALGESIA

"Twilight Sleep." The first medication used to produce amnesia in labor was a combination of morphine and scopolamine. Introduced in Germany during the early years of this century, this method of producing "a state of clouded consciousness" met with widespread public interest in the United States about 1918, under the name of "Twilight Sleep." Although it is now seldom employed, it is of great historical interest because the delicate balance between amnesic and depressive drugs that it utilized forms the basis of many modern technics.

Morphine and other opium derivatives are less frequently used in labor today because of the marked depression that these narcotics cause on the maternal and fetal respiratory centers and on uterine contractions. Since these drugs readily cross the placenta, an infant born before the drugs are metabolized and excreted suffers the effects of respiratory depression and at birth may be slow to breathe. However, morphine is a most valuable drug and in specific instances may be the drug of choice, as in the case of uterine inertia. Here it affords a means of giving the patient a much needed rest, the so-called "morphine rest." (See Chap. 19, Complications of Labor.)

Narcotic Amnesia

The most commonly employed method of obstetric analgesia used in this country today is a combination of drugs to produce narcotic amnesia of everything which occurred throughout labor. Scopolamine, a drug which produces amnesia, is used in combination with an analgesic agent, such as Demerol, or a hypnotic, such as a barbiturate.

Scopolamine, an alkaloid of belladonna, is a parasympathetic depressant drug with a diversant action on the central nervous system. The action of this drug provides several advantages for the mother in labor (such as its ability to counteract respiratory depression). However, the real aim in using such a drug as scopolamine is to produce forgetfulness or amnesia (Greek for "without memory") and thus obliterate the memory of whatever events occurred when under its influence, not to provide for actual pain relief. If the patient is without pain, as in the periods between contractions, the drug acts as a depressant and causes fatigue, drowsiness and sleep. However, prior to sedation, the drug may produce restlessness, excitement, hallucinations and delirium; and these manifestations are most likely to occur in the presence of pain. For this reason an analgesic drug is given with scopolamine to forestall this kind of stimulation during the period of uterine contractions. A woman thus medicated may shriek, make grimaces and show other evidences of pain, but on awakening from the effects of the drug will remember nothing about her labor and will vow that she has experienced no discomfort whatsoever. Unfortunately, this will not be the case if the person in attendance refreshes the mother's memory with an account of the events which have taken place.

The average adult dose of scopolamine is 0.4 mg. ($\frac{1}{150}$ gr.) to 0.6 mg. ($\frac{1}{100}$ gr.), the initial dose usually ordered being 0.4 to 0.45 mg. Subsequent doses in decreasing amounts, i.e., 0.3 mg., 0.2 mg., may be prescribed to follow at 30-minute to 2-hour intervals. When an analgesic drug, such as Demerol, is given in conjunction with this, it may be given with the initial dose of

scopolamine and repeated in 4 hours, if necessary, in a somewhat lesser dose. The dosage schedule for sedation must always be individualized according to the progress of labor and the individual patient's needs. However, the total amount of scopolamine given within a 24-hour period should be limited to 1.5 mg.

Meperidine hydrochloride (Demerol) is a synthetic compound which resembles morphine in its analgesic properties and atropine in its antispasmodiclike effects. Hence, in labor it not only relieves pain but is believed to exert also a relaxing effect on the cervix and so expedite dilatation. It is usually administered intramuscularly in dosages of 50 to 100 mg., with repetition of the dosage in a few hours if necessary. The total dose in any 8-hour period should not exceed 200 mg. A moderate sedative effect is produced, the patient usually sleeping between contractions but awakening when spoken to. Demerol, used alone, does not cause excitement or disorientation, but rather a mental state of well-being. The effect of Demerol on the respiratory center is decidedly less depressing than morphine. However, many authorities feel that it crosses the placental barrier and has more effect on the fetus than previously thought.

Demerol alone produces analgesia but not amnesia. If amnesia also is desired, scopolamine may be used in conjunction with it. Like morphine, Demerol is included under the Harrison Act, and its distribution and sale are governed by the regulations of the Federal Bureau of Narcotics.

Barbiturates. Since about 1934, derivatives of barbituric acid, usually in combination with scopolamine, have become increasingly popular for obstetric analgesia. Barbiturates are hypnotics and produce relaxation from tension and absence of fear but are not in themselves analgesic. Some of the more commonly employed are Nembutal (pentobarbital sodium), Amytal Sodium and Seconal Sodium. These three drugs are very similar in their action, but Amytal Sodium is likely to be the choice of the doctor when labor gives prospects of being prolonged, because its effect is more enduring than the other two. As an example of the technic employed in barbiturate analgesia, the following program is one which might be carried out when this form of pain relief is desired.

If the patient complains of discomfort and the cervix is effaced and 3 to 4 cm. dilated:

Amytal sodium or Nembutal or Seconal } 0.3 Gm. (5 grains) by mouth

In 20 minutes:
Scopolamine 0.3 or 0.4 mg. ($\frac{1}{200}$ to $\frac{1}{150}$ grain) by hypodermic.

One hour after initial dose:
Scopolamine 0.1 or 0.2 mg. ($\frac{1}{600}$ to $\frac{1}{300}$ grain), depending on condition of patient.

Repeat scopolamine 0.1 mg. ($\frac{1}{600}$ grain) hourly if necessary, but maximum dosage should not exceed 1.0 mg. ($\frac{1}{60}$ grain).

Barbiturate may be repeated every 4 hours in 0.1 Gm. doses.

Patients with kidney diseases should not be given barbiturates, since the confused state produced may persist for many hours thereafter due to delayed elimination.

Paraldehyde. This pungent-smelling liquid is favored by a few obstetricians as an analgesic and amnesic agent. It may be administered by mouth or by rectum. The average dose of paraldehyde is from 10 to 15 cc., depending on the weight of the patient, and may be repeated in about 6 hours or supplemented by other drugs. When paraldehyde is given orally it must be prepared so as to disguise the objectionable taste, for example, with sugar and chipped ice or with port wine and a little water. For rectal administration it should be mixed with 25 or 30 cc. of olive oil. The effect is similar to that produced by the bar-

biturate-scopolamine program described above.

Inhalation Analgesia

The intermittent, brief inhalation of *nitrous oxide, ether, trichlorethylene* or *chloroform* ("analgesia a la reine") may also be administered with contractions for analgesia. (See Obstetric Anesthesia, p. 232.)

It is usually the nurse's responsibility to administer oral, subcutaneous or intramuscular medications in providing nursing care for the patient receiving obstetric analgesia. Unless the nurse has had special training in a school of anesthesia, it is highly undesirable to have her master technics for administration of anesthesia, and she should not be expected to assume responsibility for administering obstetric inhalation analgesia or anesthesia. Knowledge of anesthetic drugs and their desired and untoward effects is necessary in order for her to perform her professional role as an obstetric nurse. Only in an emergency, however, and under the direction of a physician, may she administer anesthetic agents. In such a situation the physician assumes full responsibility for the anesthesia.

OBSTETRIC ANESTHESIA

The most commonly employed methods of obstetric anesthesia are inhalation of narcotic gases or volatile anesthetics, intravenous anesthesia with a soluble barbiturate, and regional anesthesia, such as local infiltration, spinal or caudal. The continuous caudal technic provides both analgesia in the first and second stages of labor and anesthesia for delivery.

Regional Anesthesia

Local Infiltration. The injection of local anesthetic agents such as procaine, Metycaine and the like may be employed to desensitize the area of the perineum for a spontaneous delivery, or, in the event of an operative deliv-

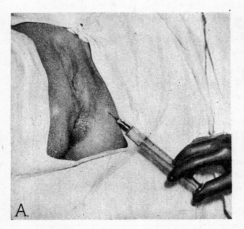
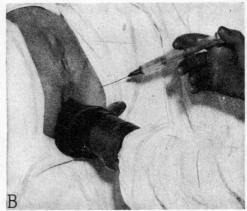

Fig. 138. Local infiltration anesthesia for episiotomy. (A) Intradermal wheals raised over ischial tuberosities. (B) Index finger in rectum for palpation of ischial spines and infiltration of internal pudic nerves. Infiltration of perineal fibers of the ilioinguinal nerves and posterior cutaneous femoris nerves completes the procedure. (Eastman: Williams Obstetrics, ed. 11, New York, Appleton)

ery, to block the pudendal nerves in order to produce more profound anesthesia of the area supplied by these nerves. This technic is usually of no value for analgesia during labor and is not begun until the delivery is imminent, when it can be administered by the obstetrician. After the mother is prepared and draped for delivery, the injection is made first to the right and then to the left of the fourchet, using the needle in a fan-shaped manner and following the lower border of the vulva on each side (see Fig. 138).

When the *pudendal block* is to be accomplished, a No. 20 spinal needle 10 cm. long, attached to a 10- or 20-cc. Luer syringe, is passed first just below and beyond the ischial spine. Solution is then injected to anesthetize the internal pudendal nerve. The needle is partially withdrawn, then inserted laterally toward the tuberosity of the ischium, where more solution is injected. The needle is again withdrawn in the same manner and inserted to infiltrate

the labia. The entire procedure is repeated on the opposite side. In a few minutes, perineal muscles are relaxed and the skin of the perineum becomes anesthetized.

When one considers an anesthetic agent from the standpoint of safety for both mother and her infant, local infiltration of the tissues has manifold advantages. First of all, there is practically no anesthetic mortality. Since the uterine contractions are not impaired, the progress of the mother's labor is not retarded, and after the delivery the effect of the anesthetic agent will not cause uterine relaxation and thus excessive bleeding. And since there is no direct effect of the anesthetic on the infant, it is protected from asphyxia.

Continuous Caudal. At the lower end of the sacrum and on its posterior surface, there is an opening resulting from the nonclosure of the laminae of the last sacral vertebra. It is screened by a thin layer of fibrous tissue. This opening is called the sacral hiatus and leads to a space within the sacrum known as the caudal canal or the caudal space. This space is really the lowermost extent of the bony spinal canal. Through it a rich network of sacral nerves pass downward after they have emerged from the dural sac a few inches above. The dural sac separates the caudal canal below from the spinal cord and its surrounding spinal fluid.

By filling the caudal canal with a suitable anesthetic solution, pain sense in the sacral nerves is abolished, and anesthesia of the pelvic region is produced.

When the patient is in good labor and the cervix is 5 cm. dilated in the multipara (preferably 7 to 8 cm. in primipara), caudal analgesia may be started. By the addition of anesthetic solution through the caudal catheter at appropriate intervals, the desired effect can be maintained throughout labor (anesthesia for delivery).

To insert the catheter, the obstetric patient is placed on her side in a modified Sims' position, with the upper leg well flexed at the hip and knee joints and the lower leg extended. The sacral and coccygeal area is cleansed with an antiseptic solution. The area is surrounded with sterile towels or a sterile drape. The physician, of course, wears sterile gloves for the procedure since it requires surgical aseptic technic. After the pliable needle or fine plastic catheter has been inserted into the caudal space, a test dose of 8 cc. of the local anesthetic solution, such as Metycaine 1.5 per cent, Pontocaine 0.15 per cent, Xylocaine 1 per cent or Nesacaine 3 per cent, is injected. When 5 minutes have elapsed, the test for spinal anesthesia is made to be assured that the drug has not been injected into the subarachnoid space. Only after this is the patient given the obstetric dose of 20 to 30 cc. of medication which will block the afferent nerve supply from the uterus and usually provide anesthesia to the tenth thoracic dermatone.

At first the patient experiences a sense of fullness along the distribution of the sciatic nerve in one or both legs, which may cause temporary discomfort. About 15 minutes after the injection, relief is obtained from the abdominal discomfort of uterine contractions, and in about 20 minutes the analgesia should be complete. One observes the lower extremities for pronounced vasodilatation and cessation of sweating as one of the first effective signs. The great toe and the ball of the foot are the first parts to develop vasomotor block, thus this area is the first to become pink, warm and dry. The heel will be the last to show these signs. The effect may be unilateral at first, and some minutes may elapse before it affects the other side, or the physician may have the patient lie on the unaffected side to encourage diffusion of the anesthetic agent. The nurse should remember that the physician should be consulted before changing the patient's position to one side or the other during this early stage of analgesia. After anesthesia has been well established, there is usually no contraindication to changing the patient's position so long as the pliable needle or plastic catheter is protected. If the procedure is successful, the patient experiences no pain whatsoever in labor and is not conscious of either uterine contractions or of perineal distention, except for some minor degree of pressure.

Provided that the maternal systolic blood pressure does not fall below 100 mm. Hg., with resulting fetal hypoxia, a continuous caudal has the advantage of exerting the least possible effect on the infant, because it does not cross the placental barrier in significant pharmacologic doses. This factor is an advantage to the premature infant particularly, as well as the fact that caudal analgesia tends to retard rapid and forceful labor and enables the physician to perform an easy, controlled delivery. It also lessens the strain of labor for mothers handicapped with heart disease, pulmonary tuberculosis, acute respiratory infections or diabetes.

One of the chief hazards of caudal is that it causes a fall in the maternal blood pressure. This can be controlled by alertness and prompt action on the part of the attendant. The physician may prescribe a vasopressor drug, such as ephedrine, if it is indicated, but often merely the elevation of the patient's legs, perhaps only temporarily, or turning the patient on her side and relieving uterine pressure on the inferior vena cava will restore the blood pressure to normal.

In addition to its tendency to produce hypotension, other disadvantages of continuous caudal are (1) it increases the rate of forceps deliveries, (2) it may prolong labor, and (3) if the anesthetic level reaches above T 10 there is a marked increase in uterine atony. It would be contraindicated in the case of shock or hemorrhage because of its vasodilator tendencies and, for the same reason, should be used cautiously in toxemia. Any infection of the skin over the sacral area, in particular, would likewise be a contraindication for its use.

This type of anesthesia requires hospital facilities and is more demanding on the time and the skill of the medical staff, so that in many smaller hospitals it is not feasible to employ it.

Continuous caudal analgesia was introduced in the autumn of 1942 by Dr. Robert A. Hingson and Dr. Waldo B. Edwards, of Staten Island, N. Y. It was received with wide acclaim and at the present writing is employed in many hospitals.

Spinal Anesthesia. Spinal anesthesia, as used in obstetrics, falls into two major divisions. The first is a semiterminal type of anesthesia which is employed for the latter part of labor and delivery and is provided by low dosage of a hyperbaric solution. The second is a terminal type and is administered either by the single-dosage method or

the continuous technic; its largest field of employment is in cesarean section. Although minute doses of spinal anesthesia can be given to provide pain relief throughout labor, this technic is difficult and, by and large, unsatisfactory. Too often labor is stopped by spinal anesthesia.

Low-Dosage Hyperbaric Spinal (Saddle Block). This form of anesthesia is one of the most popular in the United States today. Nearly all the local anesthesia agents have been used in saddle-block anesthesia. By the addition of glucose to the solution of Pontocaine or other anesthetic agent, localization and concentration of the drug in the conus of the dural sac are facilitated. Inasmuch as this anesthetic is of short duration, it is necessary to time its administration properly, and delivery should be anticipated within an hour or so following the onset of anesthesia.

Inhalation Anesthesia
Volatile Anesthetics

Ether, chloroform and *trichlorethylene* are volatile anesthetic agents which are used for obstetric analgesia and anesthesia. These substances cross the placenta readily and are capable of producing narcosis in the fetus. From the standpoint of the mother, ether and chloroform inhibit uterine contractions and thus increase the possibility of excessive bleeding both during and following the delivery. These two compounds are better suited to anesthesia for delivery and do not lend themselves to obstetric analgesia. On the other hand, trichlorethylene should *not* be used for anesthesia.

The inhalation of the volatile anesthetics is contraindicated when upper respiratory infection or pulmonary disease exists and, of course, after the patient has had a full meal. This type of anesthesia is also contraindicated in the presence of prematurity or when, for other reasons, one expects possible fetal hypoxia.

Ether. Because of the slowness of its action, the margin of safety is greater with ether than with any other inhalation anesthetic, and with careful administration it is relatively safe even in the presence of severe cardiac or hypertensive disease. At the present time, when modern apparatus is employed, ether is administered by the closed circuit or semiclosed circuit technic, so that it is possible to administer an adequate amount of oxygen simultaneously and to complement or supplement nitrous oxide or ethylene anesthesia when deeper anesthesia is needed or desired (see Fig. 139).

Ether may also be administered by the open-drop method, using a wire mask covered with gauze and a can of ether (Fig. 140). A bent safety pin is put through the cap of the ether can to make a dropper; or a small V-shaped incision is made lengthwise in the cork which comes with the ether can, and after a 1-inch wick of gauze is inserted into this crevice, it is inserted into the can. When the can is tilted, ether will drop off the gauze wick. Some anesthetists prefer to administer ether from a small glass bottle, prepared with the cork and wick, to permit visualization of the amount of ether in the container. When ether is dropped on a mask placed over the patient's nose and mouth, care must be taken to permit an adequate mixture of air to maintain oxygen re-

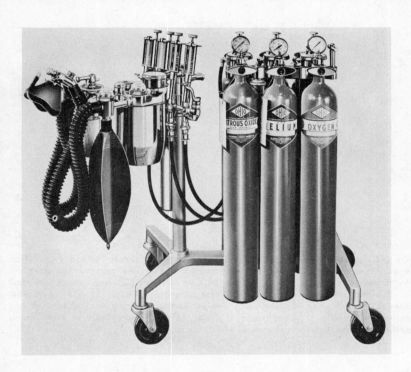

Fig. 139. Circle filter anesthesia apparatus. With this type of machine any combination or mixture of gases can be administered to the patient. (Heidbrink Division, Ohio Chemical & Surgical Equipment Co., Madison, Wis.)

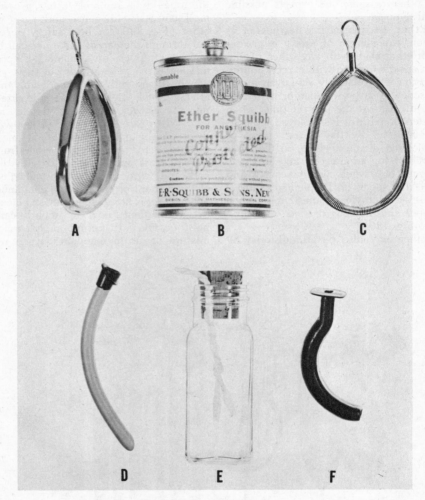

Fig. 140. Equipment for administration of ether by the open-drop method. (A) Bottom view of wire mask, showing metal retaining-ring which holds the gauze on the mask and prevents the gauze from touching the skin. (B) Can of ether. (C) Top view of wire mask covered with a few layers of gauze. (D) Nasopharyngeal airway. (E) Glass bottle for dispensing "drop" ether, demonstrating one method of utilizing an incised cork and gauze wick in a bottle. (F) Oropharyngeal airway. (These airways should be available for immediate use when any form of general anesthesia is administered.)

quirements and prevent any hypoxia. The hypoxia can be averted if oxygen flowing at 4 liters is administered simultaneously through a small rubber catheter placed under the mask. The use of an improvised cone made from newspaper covered with cloth is not advised. Even with the wire mask there is an additional "dead space" of 60 cc., i.e., space filled with the exhaled air and carbon dioxide. When the paper cone is used the air exchange is hindered, and the volume of this "dead space" is increased to about 200 cc. Since there is an inadequate supply of fresh air to supply oxygen demands, the patient rebreathes carbon dioxide. In order to avoid irritation from open-drop ether, care should be exerted that none of the liquid ether touches the skin or the conjunctiva. The face should be anointed with petrolatum and the eyes protected with Vaseline gauze or a towel. When the eyes are covered with a towel it must be ascertained that the lids completely cover the eyes at all times during anesthesia, otherwise a corneal abrasion will result from the irritation of the towel. After this preparation, the mask is held slightly above the patient's nose and mouth, and a few drops of ether are poured onto the mask. This will acclimate the patient to the pungent odor of ether and will help to prevent a coughing attack due to the irritating effect of ether on the laryngeal mucous membrane. Then the mask is lowered to the patient's face, covering her nose and mouth, and, as the patient tolerates the increasing concentration of the ether vapor, the rate of flow of the drops of ether is slowly increased. The increased flow of the drops of ether should never reach a point where it becomes a steady flow of the liquid. In addition, care must be exercised to distribute the flow of ether drops evenly about the mask so that it does not concentrate in one spot. This diffuse saturation of the mask will hasten vaporization of the liquid ether and will cause a steady, even increase

in the concentration of ether vapor under the mask. If the patient does not tolerate the rate of flow of ether during this stage of induction of anesthesia, the anesthetist should reduce the rate. At times it is proper to remove the mask and permit the patient to have a few breaths of fresh air until she breathes normally. When respirations are again normal, the anesthetist may slowly reapply the mask to the face and then slowly start to drop ether again. As long as the patient remains conscious she is in Stage 1, the analgesia stage of anesthesia.

About 5 to 10 minutes after the start of ether anesthesia, the patient loses consciousness and enters Stage 2, the excitement stage of anesthesia. During Stage 2 the patient may become violent, cry out, pull at the restraints and attempt to get off the delivery table. The respirations are irregular in depth and rate, and muscle tonicity is increased. For this reason the nurse should refrain from touching the patient at this time and await the anesthetist's signal before doing so. Meanwhile, the anesthetist carefully continues with the rapid flow of ether to hasten the patient's entry into Stage 3, the surgical stage of anesthesia. However, during periodic episodes of apnea, which may occur due to irregular respirations, the mask should not be oversaturated with ether. Such oversaturation with ether will inhibit the vaporization of the liquid ether (by preventing an adequate exchange of air through the wet mask) and will also cause some retention of carbon dioxide by the patient. When the respirations again regain their regular rate and rhythm, the patient is in Stage 3. At this point one must be careful not to permit the patient to "lighten" in depth of anesthesia and slip back into Stage 2. If this should occur, it will be noticed that the patient starts swallowing, and unless the anesthesia is deepened immediately, the swallowing will be followed by vomiting. If the patient should unavoidably vomit, her head should be turned to the side and the table put into slight Trendelenburg position. In addition, the vomitus should be sucked out of the patient's mouth by adequate suction via either the oral or the nasal route. The finesse with which the anesthetist carries the patient through the first two stages of anesthesia into the surgical stage of anesthesia is very important. Frequently, this determines the "smoothness" of the anesthesia and influences the occurrence of complications both during and after anesthesia.

It should be remembered that in the period following the delivery the mother is often unconscious. During ether narcosis, her face should be slightly flushed, but never pale or cyanotic; her respiration should be deep, possibly stertorous, but never irregular; and her pulse should be full, of good quality, fairly rapid, but never intermittent. At this time, excessive uterine bleeding may occur due to the direct effect that ether has on the uterine musculature.

Chloroform. In 1847, Sir James Y. Simpson's famous experiment with chloroform convinced him that this anesthetic was far stronger and better than ether and a means to afford painless delivery. But Simpson's discovery was met with tremendous opposition on all sides. The clergy rebelled against his work and defamed him as a heretic and blasphemer for his attempt to ease the suffering which women had experienced since time immemorial. Their attacks were based on the Bible, with such verses as "In sorrow thou shalt bring forth children" (Gen. 3:16). But Dr. Simpson, also a student of the Bible, was able to refute their charges with such quotations from the Scriptures as "And the Lord God caused a deep sleep to fall upon Adam, and he slept; and he took one of his ribs, and closed up the flesh instead thereof" (Gen. 2:21).

ANALGESIA À LA REINE. In 1853, when Queen Victoria's eighth child was born, she was given momentary inhalations of chloroform with each labor contraction. It proved to be a highly efficacious means of pain relief, and since that time the method has been known as "Queen's anesthesia" or *anesthesia à la reine*. Actually, the procedure does not produce complete anesthesia but simply diminishes the intensity of the discomfort and may be best regarded as a form of analgesia.

Chloroform is now considered to be too toxic a drug for common use and is rejected by most of the large American hospitals. Nevertheless, it is still used in some rural areas when the mother is a normal healthy parturient. This agent must be preserved in tight, light-resistant containers, otherwise decomposition will occur, forming toxic phosgene gas. In the liquid state, chloroform will produce severe irritation and burns of the skin and the conjunctiva, so care must be exercised to ensure that none of the liquid, or objects moistened with the liquid chloroform, touches the skin or the conjunctiva. Before administering chloroform, the patient's face should be anointed with petrolatum and her eyes protected by the instillation of a drop of castor oil, in addition to being shielded with a towel, as previously described for protection during administration of open-drop ether. The chloroform is administered 10 to 15 drops per minute by the open-drop method. The mask should be supported at least 2 or 3 fingerbreadths from the face. At no time should the mask encircle the nose and the mouth tightly because chloroform must be given with high concentrations of oxygen or fresh air. Under no circumstances should towels be placed around the mask when giving chloroform.

Chloroform is pleasant to take, rapid in action and in recovery, and rarely gives rise to nausea. For the mother, on the other hand, it may be dangerous unless handled with care. It must never be "pushed"—that is, anesthetic action must never be hastened by pouring the chloroform on rapidly or by lowering the mask to the face. Nor should it be continued to the point of complete anesthesia, since the prolonged administration of chloroform anesthesia (for the repair of laceration, for instance) may give rise to myocardial damage. For the latter reason, chloroform is used less frequently than formerly. In giving chloroform the following danger signals should be watched for: pallor; shallow, jerky respirations; weak pulse; cyanosis, and deep, stertorous respiration (the last a sign that complete anesthesia has been produced). Should breath holding occur, the mask should be removed instantly, otherwise the patient may suffer from cardiac arrest due to the massive concentration of the drug inhaled with the next respiration.

Epinephrine and Pituitrin should *never* be used in conjunction with chloroform anesthesia because ventricular fibrillation may result. If any of these signs develop, the anesthetic should be discontinued at once.

Trichlorethylene (Trilene). For the past 10 years, Trilene has been used extensively as an obstetric analgesic in Great Britain, and only quite recently has been used for this purpose in the United States. This drug should *not* be used to achieve anesthetic levels. Trilene has an advantage in that it can be self-administered with simple inhalers which, when properly regulated, carry a high degree of safety. The Duke Inhaler is such an adjustable device. When first administered, the concentration should be low, and the patient then instructed to breathe with her mouth open and the mask loosely applied. Once she is accustomed to the odor of Trilene, which is not objectionable, the concentration may be raised to the desired level, about 0.65 per cent. The apparatus is attached by a wrist strap, and the analgesia is self-administered. No one should try to hold the mask over the patient's face. If the mask does not fall, it should be removed when the patient loses con-

sciousness. Satisfactory analgesia is obtained in 15 seconds. When excessive amounts of Trilene are inhaled, bradycardia may result; thus the nurse should be alert to changes in pulse and respiratory rates.

Trilene should not be used with Pituitrin or its derivatives, sympathomimetic amines, i.e., certain drugs which have a response resembling the effect produced by stimulation of the sympathetic nervous system, or epinephrine. The nurse should be familiar with this fact since she is most frequently called upon to administer drugs at the time of the delivery. Also, it should never be used with soda lime, the agent used in some types of anesthesia machines to absorb carbon dioxide, because when Trilene comes in contact with soda lime it decomposes into dichloracetylene, a respiratory irritant and highly explosive gas, and phosgene, a very toxic and poisonous gas.

Gas Anesthetics

Nitrous oxide and *cyclopropane* are two anesthetic gases widely used in current obstetric practice. They should always be administered by a physician or a specially trained nurse anesthetist and restricted to use where adequate apparatus is available. Although these anesthetic agents are safe in the hands of the skilled practitioner, in the hands of the inexperienced they may suddenly become dangerous to both mother and her infant.

Nitrous oxide in combination with oxygen is used for pain relief in labor when deep relaxation is not required. The concentration is of extreme importance. For the purposes of analgesia and anesthesia, nitrous oxide should never exceed 80 per cent concentration (frequently referred to as 80-20, meaning 80 per cent nitrous oxide and 20 per cent oxygen), a concentration which has little effect on the uterine activity. Too low a concentration of oxygen will cause asphyxia neonatorum in the fetus, and such asphyxia may cause irreparable damage to the higher centers of the infant's brain.

Once the cervix becomes fully dilated, nitrous oxide may be administered intermittently for pain relief during contractions. When the patient indicates that a uterine contraction has begun, the mask is placed over her nose and mouth and she is encouraged to take 3 deep breaths of a high flow 80-20 mixture of nitrous oxide and oxygen, or 1 breath with lower concentration of nitrous oxide and a higher concentration of oxygen if it will suffice. As soon as the contraction is over, the mask is removed until the next one begins. The mother should not lose consciousness but will be relieved of the discomfort of the contraction. This method of intermittent pain relief may be continued until the head crowns, when the anesthetic may be deepened to facilitate the control of the infant's head, and for the performance of episiotomy, if it is necessary. When the infant's head is born, the nitrous oxide is shut off temporarily, and the mother is given oxygen until the cord has been clamped.

One cannot overemphasize the importance of keeping an almost constant check on the fetal heart tones when nitrous oxide is administered to the mother in labor. It is not only the nurse's responsibility to listen to the fetal heart tones almost constantly but also to inform both the obstetrician and the anesthetist of her findings.

Cyclopropane. This highly explosive substance is the most potent of the anesthetic gases and is particularly advantageous in cases where rapid induction with good relaxation is desired because of tumultuous labor. Cyclopropane may be administered with a higher concentration of oxygen than the other anesthetic gases, which one would assume to be of benefit to the unborn infant. However, if the mother's respiratory center is depressed, the oxygen saturation in the maternal arterial blood

will be diminished because of her diminished respirations, and thus the oxygen concentration in the infant's arterial blood will also be decreased. In addition, if cyclopropane is administered to the mother for a prolonged period of time the fetal respiratory center will be depressed.

Uterine contractions are not decreased when the concentration of cyclopropane given is maintained at a low level, but they are rapidly abolished as this level is increased. For this reason, when cyclopropane is given for a prolonged period, excessive uterine bleeding may occur.

Cardiac irregularities in the mother may occur when pituitary extract or certain vasopressors are given during the administration of cyclopropane anesthesia. As in the case when either Trilene or chloroform is given to the mother, such drugs as Pituitrin or Pitocin, epinephrine and those drugs which have a sympatheticlike action or mimic sympathetic nervous system response (sympathomimeticamines) should not be used in conjunction with cyclopropane. The nurse should be familiar with this principle, since she may be given a verbal order to administer the oxytocic drug at the time of delivery.

Because of the explosion hazard, every protection should be used to protect the mother as well as the hospital personnel. Cyclopropane is usually administered with the closed system machine and with continuous flow of the gas. In 1954, Dr. Robert Hingson perfected a small, lightweight, portable machine, the Western Reserve Miniature Anesthesia Machine and Resuscitator, which may be used to administer either pure oxygen or a mixture of cyclopropane and helium with oxygen (Fig. 141).

Intravenous Anesthesia

Thiopental Sodium (Pentothal Sodium). Intravenous Pentothal, one

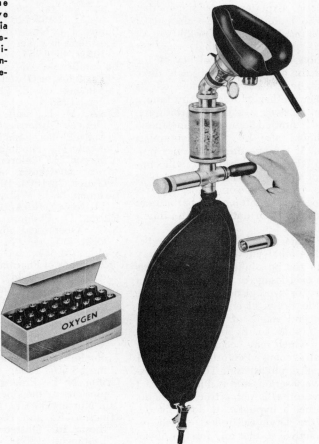

Fig. 141. The Western Reserve Miniature Anesthesia Machine and Resuscitator. (Continental Hospital Industries, Inc., Cleveland, Ohio)

of the soluble barbiturates, may be used to produce anesthesia for rapid spontaneous deliveries, for uncomplicated outlet forceps deliveries or to induce anesthesia for the extraction of an infant by cesarean section. It may also be indicated in some cases of toxemia, when convulsive seizures are anticipated; in certain neurologic diseases, such as epilepsy; or in neuropsychiatric problems, when the patient is psychotic. This technic requires the skills of a competent physician anesthesiologist and, there-

fore, cannot be employed by the inexperienced or "occasional" anesthetist.

Recent studies have shown that within 5 minutes after the introduction of Pentothal Sodium into the mother's circulation there is an equalization of barbiturate in the mother's and the infant's blood. Therefore, when the use of the drug is elective, the anesthesia should not be started until the patient has been fully prepared and draped and the obstetrician is ready to start the delivery immediately after induction of anesthesia. Experience has shown that with the limitation of the amount of drug (a maximum dosage of 200 mg. of 2 or 2½ per cent Pentothal) used for induction and to aid expediency on the part of the operating obstetrician, there are very few, if any, deleterious effects on either mother or infant. Any time a mother receives a soluble barbiturate, such as Pentothal Sodium, for anesthesia she should also be given continuous oxygen. If the anesthesia becomes prolonged, then the anesthetist will supplement it with another agent, such as nitrous oxide or cyclopropane, and repeat doses of the intravenous barbiturate will not be given until after the infant is delivered.

The major disadvantages of intravenous Pentothal anesthesia for delivery are (1) the possibility of *fetal narcosis* due to overdosage of the drug, delay in delivery or synergistic action with the analgesic drugs given during the first and second stages of labor; (2) *fetal hypoxia* due to hypotension in the mother which may occur as a result of the intravenous Pentothal; and (3) *maternal laryngospasm*. The latter hazard is very serious and is due to the fact that Pentothal is not a true anesthetic, but rather a hypnotic. It does not depress the laryngeal reflex, which remains active, so that any foreign object such as saliva or mucus can cause a severe episode of laryngospasm. Another factor to consider is that there is also a rectal reflex which, when stimulated, will cause laryngospasm. In this instance, the passage of the head through the birth canal is apparently adequate stimulus to initiate this reflex.

SUGGESTED READING

Apgar, V., *et al.*: Comparison of regional and general anesthesia in obstetrics, J.A.M.A. **165**:2155, 1957.

Bonica, J. J.: Obstetric analgesia and anesthesia in general practice, J.A.M.A. **165**:2146, 1957.

Bookmiller, M. M., and Bowen, G. L.: Textbook of Obstetrics and Obstetric Nursing, ed. 3, Philadelphia, Saunders, 1958.

Davis, M. E., and Sheckler, C. E.: DeLee's Obstetrics for Nurses, ed. 16, Philadelphia, Saunders, 1957.

Duncan, C., Hindman, J., and Mayberger, H.: Chloroform as an obstetrical anesthesia, Am. J. Obst. & Gynec. **72**:1004, 1956.

Eastman, N. J.: Williams Obstetrics, ed. 11, New York, Appleton, 1956.

Ellison, G., Philpott, N., and Simpson, G.: Obstetrical anesthesia, Am. J. Obst. & Gynec. **74**:283, 1957.

Faddis, M. O., and Hayman, J. M.: Textbook of Pharmacology for Nurses, ed. 5, Philadelphia, Lippincott, 1959.

Flowers, C. E., Jr.: Increasing the safety of obstetrical anesthesia, Bull. Maternal Welfare, **2**:9, 1955.

——: Trilene; an adjunct to obstetrical anesthesia and analgesia, Am. J. Obst. & Gynec. **65**:1027, 1953.

Frohman, I. P.: Demerol, Am. J. Nursing **53**:567, 1953.

Griffin, N. L.: Preventing fires and explosions in the operating room, Am. J. Nursing **53**:809, 1953.

Hingson, R., and Hellman, L.: Anesthesia for Obstetrics, Philadelphia, Lippincott, 1956.

Lock, F. R., and Greiss, F. C., Jr.: The anesthetic hazards in obstetrics, Am. J. Obst. & Gynec. **70**:861, 1955.

National Fire Protection Association: Recommended Safe Practice for Hospital Operating Room (Bulletin No. 56), The Association, 60 Battery-March St., Boston 10, Mass.

Read, G. D.: Childbirth Without Fear, ed. 2, New York, Harper, 1953.

Thoms, H.: Training for Childbirth, New York, McGraw-Hill, 1950.

CHAPTER TWELVE

Conduct of Normal Labor

Since the vast majority of deliveries in this country are now conducted in hospitals, in this chapter we shall discuss only the institutional management of normal labor. Actually, the principles and the methods of examinations involved in the conduct of labor in the hospital and in the home are identical, the only modifications necessary for home delivery being in such matters as equipment, positioning of the mother in bed and anesthesia. Once the nurse thoroughly understands the principles of aseptic technic and has learned to utilize this knowledge in the care of mothers in labor in a hospital, only a little ingenuity is required to adapt it to the circumstances encountered in most homes.

ADMISSION TO THE HOSPITAL

In modern obstetric practice the expectant mother has visited her physician or attended the hospital prenatal clinic at stated intervals during her pregnancy and has been instructed by the physician or the nurse as to what she can anticipate when she comes to the hospital to have her baby. If this is the mother's first hospital experience, it will be much easier for her if she has been told about the necessary preliminary procedures,

such as vulvar and perineal preparation, the methods of examination employed to ascertain the progress of labor and the usual routines exercised for her care in the course of labor. The mother should be advised to come to the hospital at the onset of labor, for after labor progresses these activities are more difficult to carry out and are much more distressing to the patient. The preparation for delivery will of necessity vary, since every hospital has its own admission procedure. The nurse must understand, particularly in reading the present chapter, that many details may be accomplished in a number of ways. Very few hospitals employ precisely the same technic in preparing a mother for delivery. Actually, the differences are in details only, the objectives being the same everywhere, namely, asepsis and antisepsis, together with careful observation of the mother for any deviations from the normal.

After greeting the patient, the nurse ascertains her general condition, that is, the frequency of her contractions, their duration and intensity, the amount and character of show and whether the membranes have ruptured or are intact. At this time it is expedient to learn when the first signs of labor became apparent to the mother and the description of uterine contractions from that time. Since the mother's emotional status often has bearing on her physical labor, it is wise to be continuously alert to her behavior—whether she is unduly apprehensive or if she is relatively relaxed and calm. The nurse should report these findings to the physician as soon as possible. Although the nurse should avoid any outward display of rush or hurry, she should proceed with the admission as quickly as possible. In order to avoid tensions or alleviate anxiety on the part of the patient, the nurse should always explain unfamiliar procedures and be assured that the mother understands the reasons for them before she proceeds. While waiting for the physician, the nurse will take the temperature, pulse, respirations, blood pressure and listen to the fetal heart tones. In preparing the patient for examination, she should be encouraged to void, not only to facilitate the physician's examination but also for the collection of the admission urine specimen. Patients in labor should use a bedpan or a commode, because it is important that the physician should have available for the examination whatever material may be passed per vagina, as well as the urine specimen. If the patient is in labor the doctor will probably order such procedures as shaving and cleansing of the vulva, and unless the labor is progressing too rapidly, a soap-and-water enema. The admission bath is rarely a routine procedure. Most patients have sufficient warning at the onset of labor to enable them to bathe prior to coming to the hospital. When a bath is deemed desirable, the type used will depend to some extent on the facilities of the hospital. The types usually given are the shower and the sponge bath. The hand spray may be used as an improvised shower when the shower stall is not available.

Vulvar and Perineal Preparation. The aim in shaving and washing the

vulva should be to cleanse and disinfect the immediate area about the vagina and to prevent anything contaminated from entering the birth canal. During labor, pathogenic bacteria ascend the birth canal more readily, and every effort should be made to protect the mother from intrapartal infection. In some hospitals a sterile gauze sponge or a folded towel is placed against the introitus to prevent contaminated matter, such as hair or soapy fluid, from entering the vagina during the preparation procedure. In addition, when performing any task which requires the attendant's face to be directly over the vulva, a clean, dry face mask covering the nose and the mouth may be worn to eliminate contamination from a possible source of infection (the nasopharynx).

In most hospitals the pubic and the vulvar hair are lathered prior to shaving to facilitate the procedure and make it more comfortable for the patient. An ordinary safety razor is used, and, beginning at the mons veneris, with the direction of the stroke being from above downward, the area of the vulva and the perineal body is shaved. The nurse should stretch the skin above each downward stroke and permit the razor to move smoothly over the skin without undue pressure. When the entire area anterior to an imaginary line drawn through the base of the perineal body has been shaved, the patient can be turned to her side to enable the nurse to complete the shaving of the anal area. With the upper leg well flexed, the anal area is lathered and shaved, again with a front-to-back stroke. It must always be remembered that anything which has passed over the anal region must not be returned near the vulvar orifice.

The solutions as well as the technics used in cleansing the genitals will vary in different hospitals, but sterile water with soap is probably the most commonly employed. More recently, pHisoHex has come into popular usage. A little of this antibacterial liquid cream, used with water and applied to the area with friction, creates a lather and cleanses the skin. On repeated use, it develops cumulative bacteriocidal and bacteriostatic properties.

When washing the genitals, the surrounding areas should be thoroughly cleansed first, using a sterile sponge for each area and gradually working in towards the vestibule. The strokes must be from above downward and away from the introitus. Special attention should be paid to separating the vulvar folds in order to remove the smegma which may have accumulated in the folds of the labia minora and/or at the base of the clitoris. Finally, the region around the anus is cleansed. It should be emphasized here again that a sponge which has passed over the anal area must not be returned near the vulvar orifice but should be discarded immediately. The patient is instructed not to touch the genitals lest she infect herself.

IS THE PATIENT IN LABOR?

Since the nurse is with the patient more constantly than the doctor, she will be expected to report on the general character of the labor contractions, the appearance of show and any other symptoms. First comes the question—Is the patient actually in labor? While this is occasionally a difficult problem to settle, usually a decision can be reached on the grounds of the following differential points between true and false labor:

TRUE LABOR

Contractions
    Occur at regular intervals
    Intervals gradually shorten
    Intensity gradually increases
    Located chiefly in back
    Intensified by walking
Show is usually present
Cervix becomes effaced and dilated

FALSE LABOR

Contractions
    Occur at irregular intervals
    Intervals remain long
    Intensity remains same
    Located chiefly in abdomen
    Walking has no effect; often relieves
No show
Cervix usually uneffaced and closed

ESTABLISHMENT OF THE NURSE-PATIENT RELATIONSHIP

With emphasis now placed on the importance of seeking adequate medical supervision early in pregnancy to ensure maximum physical and emotional health, the majority of expectant mothers are acquainted with doctors and nurses long before labor begins.

But for many a young mother in labor, admission to a maternity hospital may mark her first acquaintance with hospitals as a patient. Her immediate reaction may be one of strangeness, loneliness and homesickness, particularly if her husband is not permitted to stay with her in the labor room. Moreover, not a few of these young patients enter labor thoroughly afraid of the whole process. This may be attributed in part to the fact that the mother's preparation for childbearing has been limited. In such situations where the young woman has been reared in an environment fraught with the mysteries of childbirth and old wives' tales, this fear is understandable. Accordingly, it is one of the first responsibilities of the nurse to recognize that, in addition to the physical manifestations, there are social, economic and emotional factors which influence each mother's pregnancy and thus have bearing on her individual needs for care. The nurse who is cordial, empathic and interested in the welfare of her patients establishes good rapport with relative ease and, without prying, secures information which will enable her to gain greater insight into the individual's nursing needs. Regardless of the amount of preparation for this event, every mother deserves encouragement that tends to inspire assurance during labor. Her discomfort should never be minimized, but attention should be directed to the fact that progress is being made, that this is the usual course of events, and that if she can work co-operatively with her labor it will be a great help to her. The nurse must be constantly alert to symptoms associated with the progress of normal labor. At the same time, she should be a vigilant watcher for any sign which may point to abnormal developments. For instance, an increase in pulse rate, a rise in temperature, excessive bleeding, changes in the character of uterine contractions, passage of meconium or alterations in the fetal heart sounds are changes which the physician must be informed about at once. Accordingly, the nurse is counted upon to be the zealous guardian of both the mental and the physical welfare of the patient in labor.

EXAMINATIONS IN LABOR

General. The pulse, respirations and temperature are taken, as previously stated, and are repeated every 4 hours. In cases in which there is fever, or in which labor has lasted more than 24 hours, it is desirable to repeat these observations every 2 hours. The blood pressure is recorded by either the physician or the nurse and is repeated every hour; in cases of toxemia of pregnancy, this may be done more frequently, according to the physician's instructions. As soon as possible after admission, a complete examination of the heart and the lungs is carried out by the physician to make certain that there are no conditions present which might contraindicate the type of analgesia or anesthesia to be used.

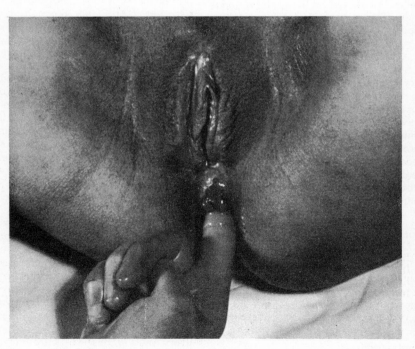

Fig. 142. Rectal examination, showing flexion of thumb of the gloved hand to prevent contamination of the vulva.

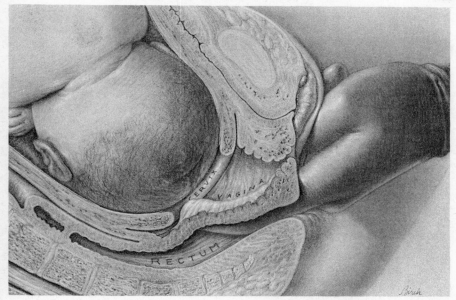

Fig. 143. Rectal examination, showing how the examining finger palpates the cervix and the infant's head through the rectovaginal septum.

Abdominal. The abdominal examination is similar to that carried out in the antepartal period, comprising estimation of fetal size and position and listening to the fetal heart sounds.

Rectal. The majority of the examinations during labor are abdominal and rectal; vaginal examinations are performed only for special reasons. It was previously thought that rectal examinations were much safer than vaginal examinations, since they reduced the risk of carrying pathogenic bacteria from the introitus and the lower vagina to the region of the cervix and the lower uterine segment. Studies and general experience show that this supposed advantage of rectal examinations over vaginal examinations has been greatly exaggerated. Nevertheless, rectal examinations do have the advantage of not requiring preliminary disinfection on the part of the physician or the patient.

For either rectal or vaginal examina-

tion the patient should lie on her back with her knees flexed. The nurse should drape the patient so that she is well protected, but with the perineal region exposed. In making a rectal examination the index finger is used, the hand being covered by a clean but not necessarily sterile rubber glove. As shown in Figure 142, the thumb should be fixed into the palm of the hand, because otherwise it may enter the vagina and introduce infection. The finger is anointed liberally with a lubricating jelly and introduced slowly into the rectum. The cervical opening usually can be felt as a depression surrounded by a circular ridge (Fig. 143). The degree of dilatation and the amount of effacement are noted. Very often the membranes can be felt bulging into the cervix, particularly during a contraction. The level of the fetal head is now ascertained and correlated with the level of the head as being a certain number of centimeters above or be-

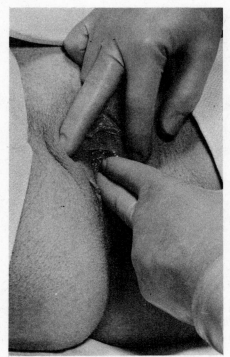

Fig. 144. Vaginal examination.

Vaginal. The mother is prepared for vaginal examination by cleansing the vulvar and perineal region in a manner similar to that used in preparation for delivery. (Some hospitals also use sterile drapes.) The physician scrubs his hands, as for an operation, and dons sterile gloves. Before introducing his fingers into the vagina, he takes care to separate the labia widely in order to minimize possible contamination of his examining fingers if they should come in contact with the inner surfaces of the labia and the margins of the hymen. Then the index and the second fingers of the examining hand are gently introduced into the vagina (Fig. 144). Vaginal examination is more reliable than rectal, since the cervix, the fontanels, etc., can be palpated directly with no intervening rectovaginal septum to interfere with tactile sense. Ordinarily, the vaginal examination is employed only when rectal examination is unsatisfactory or when the physician suspects that it is not yielding complete information.

CONDUCT OF THE FIRST STAGE

The first stage of labor (dilating stage) begins with the first symptoms of true labor and ends with the complete dilatation of the cervix. The physician examines the patient early in labor and sees her from time to time throughout the first stage but may not be in constant attendance at this time. In normal labor his examinations (fetal heart, rectal, etc.) will show that the baby is in good condition and that steady progress is being made. Furthermore, the rate of progress will often give some indication as to when delivery is to be expected. Since the physician is usually unable to be with the mother constantly during this stage, he must rely on the nurse not only to safeguard the welfare of mother and fetus but also to notify him concerning the progress of labor.

Support During Labor. As already emphasized, an attitude toward the

low the ischial spines. After the completion of the examination the rectal glove is cleansed and boiled, and the examiner's hands are washed.

The frequency with which rectal examinations are required during labor depends on the individual case; often one or two such examinations are sufficient, while in some instances more are required. The nurse who stays with the mother constantly will find that she becomes increasingly skillful in her ability to follow the progress of labor to a great extent by careful evaluation of subjective and objective symptoms of the mother, i.e., the character of the uterine contractions and the show, the progressive descent of the area on the abdomen where fetal heart sounds are heard, the mother's over-all response to her physical labor, etc.

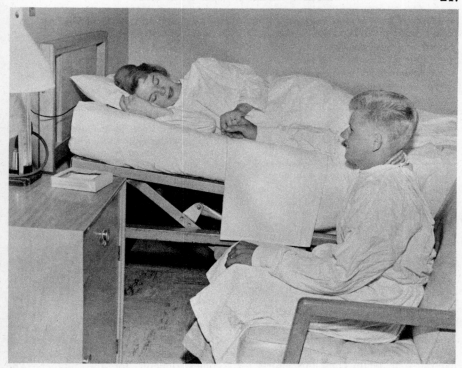

Fig. 145. The expectant parents share the experience of labor together. The husband's presence in the labor room gives his wife comfort and support and, in addition, helps him to feel he has a more vital role in participating with his wife in the delivery of their child. (MacDonald House, The University Hospitals of Cleveland)

mother in labor which combines cheerfulness, empathy and encouragement is equally as important as the nurse's ability to interpret the progress of labor and to perform certain technical procedures skillfully. The cheerful, home-like environment of the modern labor room undoubtedly is conducive to putting the patient more at ease, but this in itself is not enough. Once labor is well established, the mother should not be left alone. The morale of women in labor is sometimes hopelessly shattered, regardless of whether or not they have been prepared for labor during pregnancy, if they are left by themselves over long periods of time. At this time the mother is often more sensitive

to the behavior of those about her, particularly in relation to careless remarks which might be dropped in conversation. The nurse will recognize that her own anxieties in the situation may be communicated to the patient. It is well to remember that comments made in the corridor outside the patient's room may be overheard and contribute to her uneasiness. Laughter may also be interpreted by the patient in the light that she is being laughed at (although it may be about something entirely different). The process of labor and the forthcoming delivery will produce normal anxieties which are no more than a healthy anticipation or apprehension of the events to come. Most pa-

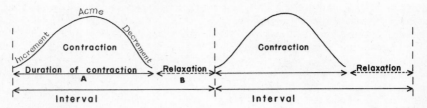

Fig. 146. The interval and the duration of uterine contractions. The frequency of contractions is the interval timed from the beginning of one contraction to the beginning of the next contraction. The interval consists of two parts: (A) the duration of the contraction and (B) the period of relaxation. (The broken line indicates an indeterminate period since this time (B) is usually of longer duration than the actual contraction (A).)

tients tolerate their contractions much better if they can be told the kind of progress that is being made and assured that they are doing a good job working with labor.

The mother who has attended antepartal classes in preparation for "natural childbirth" is usually better prepared for labor but, nevertheless, needs to be coached in utilizing technics which will enable her to co-operate with the natural forces of labor. She should not be encouraged to begin conscious efforts for relaxation when labor first begins because it is not necessary, and the concentration, when contractions are mild, has a tiring effect. At this time the patient usually prefers to move about the room and frequently is more at ease sitting in a comfortable chair. If hospital policy permits the husband to be in the labor room, his presence can be a valuable asset because of the support this gives his wife. Not only does this benefit the mother but also helps the father to feel that he has a more vital role in participating with his wife in the labor and the delivery of their child (Fig. 145).

When the "prepared" mother begins to mind her labor she may need help to get into a comfortable position and to relax. During the contractions she should be coached as necessary in doing diaphragmatic breathing. Regardless of how diligently the mother has practiced the various breathing and relaxing technics during pregnancy, or the level of her understanding about the physiology of labor, the situation is changed somewhat for her by active labor. Each mother may react in a slightly different way, for each is an individual. Some analgesic medication may be required for the mother's comfort after good labor is established (see p. 226). The nurse may observe in time that as the transition approaches, diaphragmatic breathing becomes difficult for the mother. The mother herself is aware that "her diaphragm won't co-operate." Encouraging her to change to rapid, shallow costal breathing with these contractions is usually easier and more effective.

Uterine Contractions. The term "pains" has been associated with uterine contractions of childbirth since time immemorial. One finds this term of reference still in common usage, so that even today many young women approach childbirth with fear of pain. It is no easy task to dispel this age-old fear, but throughout the childbirth experience a conscious effort must be made to instill a wholesome point of view in the mother. The nurse should avoid the use of the word "pain" whenever possible because of the very connotation of the word, and it is hoped that she will never use it in reference to uterine contractions.

The frequency, the duration and the

intensity of the contractions should be watched closely and recorded. The frequency of contractions is timed from the beginning of one contraction until the beginning of the next contraction. The duration of a contraction is timed from the moment the uterus first begins to tighten until it relaxes again (Fig. 146). The intensity of a contraction may be mild, moderate or strong at its acme. Since this is a relative factor, it is difficult to interpret unless one is at the mother's bedside. For the sake of description, one might say that during a mild contraction the uterine muscle becomes somewhat tense, during a moderate contraction the uterus becomes moderately firm, and during a strong contraction the uterus becomes so firm that it has the feel of woody hardness, and at the height of the contraction the uterus cannot be indented by pressure of the examiner's fingers.

When the mother first becomes aware of the contractions they may be 15 to 20 minutes apart and lasting perhaps 20 to 25 seconds. Since these are of mild intensity, she usually can continue with whatever she is doing, except that she is alert to time the subsequent contractions to have specific information to give the physician when she calls him. If this is her first pregnancy, he may advise her to wait until the contractions are 5 to 10 minutes apart before coming to the hospital (depending on the other signs of labor). However, if she is a multipara, she will more than likely be told to come to the hospital as soon as a regular pattern of contractions is established (again, depending on other criteria).

As labor progresses the character of the contractions will change (see Chap. 10, Phenomena of Labor). The contractions will become stronger in intensity, last longer (duration of 45 to 60 seconds) and come closer together (frequency of every 2 to 3 minutes). The only effective method the nurse can employ to time contractions is by keep-ing her finger tips lightly on the fundus. In this manner she is able to detect the contraction as it begins, by the gradual tensing and rising forward of the fundus, and feel the contraction through its 3 phases until the uterus relaxes again. The inexperienced nurse can get some idea of how a contraction will feel under her finger tips if she feels her own biceps contract. First, the forearm should be extended and the finger tips of the hand on the opposite side placed on the biceps. Then, the arm is gradually flexed until the muscle becomes very hard, held a few seconds and then gradually extended. This should take about 30 seconds to simulate a uterine contraction. It is not reliable to ask the mother to let you know when contractions begin, because often she is unaware of it for perhaps 5 or 10 seconds, sometimes even until the contraction reaches its acme. It is important for the nurse to observe the rhythm of the contractions and be assured that the uterine muscle relaxes completely after each contraction. As the labor approaches the transition, the contractions will be very strong, last for about 60 seconds and occur at 2-to-3-minute intervals. If any contraction lasts longer than 70 seconds and is not followed by a rest interval with complete relaxation of the uterine muscle, this should be reported to the physician immediately because of its implications for both the mother and her infant (see Chap. 19, Complications of Labor).

Since during the first stage of labor the uterine contractions are involuntary and uncontrolled by the patient, it is futile for her to "bear down" with her abdominal muscles because this only leads to exhaustion. The mother who has been prepared for "natural childbirth" has been schooled in breathing technics, such as diaphragmatic breathing or rapid shallow costal breathing, and with coaching from her husband or her nurse is usually able to accomplish conscious relaxation. With the "unprepared" mother, it would be futile to attempt to teach her these specific breathing technics when she is in labor, nor would it be desirable. But the nurse can help this mother to relax by encouraging and coaching her to keep breathing slowly and evenly and not to hold her breath. Most mothers in labor want to co-operate, and the calm, kind but firm guidance of an interested nurse can do much to help the mother to utilize her contractions effectively.

Show. This mucoid discharge from the cervix is present after the discharge of the mucus plug. As progressive effacement and dilatation of the cervix occurs, the show becomes blood tinged due to the rupture of superficial capillaries. The presence of an increased amount of bloody show (blood-stained mucus, not actual bleeding!) suggests that rather rapid progress may be taking place and should be reported immediately, particularly if associated with frequent severe contractions.

A perineal pad should not be worn during labor because of the nature of the vaginal discharge. The tenacious mucoid discharge frequently comes in contact with the anus and could easily be smeared about the external genitalia and vaginal orifice when the patient moves about the bed or adjusts the pads. A quilted pad placed under the mother's buttocks serves very well to absorb material discharged from the vagina. This pad should be changed frequently to keep the mother clean and dry.

Fetal Heart Tones. The behavior of the fetal heartbeat in labor is of great importance. When taking the fetal heart sounds, one should listen and count for 1 full minute in order that any irregularity or slowing may be detected. As already explained, the fetal heart rate normally is between 120 to 160 beats per minute, except during and immediately after a uterine contraction when it may fall to as low as 100 to 110. It may be difficult to hear the sounds dur-

ing a contraction because the uterine wall is tense and, in addition, it is more difficult for the mother to lie still during this period. But it is particularly important to listen at this time since these observations inform the listener how the fetus reacts to the contraction. Provided that the infant is in good condition, if the fetal heart rate has slowed but returns to its normal rate within 10 or 15 seconds immediately following the contraction, it is usually not significant. But if it slows and remains so following the contraction, or is slow to return to its normal rate, this is significant of fetal distress. If the infant is in distress, either because of insufficient oxygen or due to an abnormal degree of pressure on the head or the cord, the fetal heart rate is constantly slow or fluctuating and may fall below 100. Occasionally this slow rate is accompanied by the passage of meconium, another sign indicative of fetal distress. It must be remembered that unless the membranes have ruptured the meconium will not be apparent. Any unusual observations must be reported to the physician promptly so that measures can be instituted before permanent damage is done to the infant.

Repeated auscultation of the fetal heart sounds constitutes one of the most important responsibilities in the conduct of the first and second stages of labor (see Chap. 6, Normal Pregnancy). During the early period of the first stage of labor, the nurse should record the fetal heart rate every hour, and once good labor is established every half hour, or even more often if indicated. During the second stage of labor it should be done every 5 or 10 minutes.

Immediately following the rupture of membranes, the fetal heart sounds should be checked immediately, regardless of whether they rupture spontaneously or are artificially ruptured by the physician. Any indication of fetal distress from pressure on the umbilical cord could thereby be detected. Passage of meconium-stained amniotic fluid in a vertex presentation suggests fetal distress, but this does not have the same significance when the breech is the presenting part.

Temperature, Pulse and Respiration. The pulse in normal labor is usually in the 70's or the 80's and rarely exceeds 100. Sometimes the pulse rate on admission is slightly increased because of the excitement of coming to the hospital, but this returns to normal shortly thereafter. A persistent pulse rate over 100 suggests exhaustion or dehydration. The temperature and respirations should also be normal. If there is an elevation of temperature over 37.2° C. or 99° F. (orally), or the pulse and respirations become rapid, the physician should be notified. The temperature should be recorded every 4 hours, or more frequently if indicated. On the other hand, the pulse and respirations should be taken every hour.

Blood Pressure. The blood pressure should be recorded every hour during labor. During the first stage of labor there is little change in blood pressure between contractions, but during contractions an average increase of 5 to 10 mm. Hg. may be expected. For this reason the blood pressure readings should be taken between the contractions. Any unusual recordings of either systolic or diastolic pressure should be reported immediately.

Fluid and Food Intake. The practice here varies greatly among different physicians and in different institutions. Therefore, the wishes of the physician in charge should be ascertained before proceeding. In general, it is customary to urge the mother to take water or clear fluids, such as tea with sugar, during the early phase of the first stage of labor, but she should not be given solid or liquid foods because their digestion is delayed during labor. Evidence that the powers of digestion are impaired at this time is demonstrated by the fact that it is not unusual for nausea and/or vomit-

ing to occur near the end of the first stage of labor. It may be necessary to administer a general anesthetic for the delivery, so that if the patient takes fluid or food shortly before delivery, vomiting and consequent difficulties may occur. On the other hand, in a prolonged labor, it is most important to maintain adequate fluid and caloric intake in order to forestall dehydration and exhaustion, in which case the physician may find it desirable to administer intravenous glucose solutions.

Bladder. The patient should be asked to void at least every 3 or 4 hours. The mother in labor often attributes all of her discomfort to the intensity of uterine contractions and therefore is unaware that it is the pressure of a full bladder which has increased her discomfort. In addition to causing unnecessary discomfort, a full bladder may be a serious impediment to labor (Fig. 147) or the cause of urinary retention in the puerperium. If the distended bladder can be palpated above the symphysis pubis, and the patient is unable to void, the physician should be so informed. Not infrequently he will order catheterization in such cases. Various technics are used, all designed at maintaining strict asepsis. One technic, illustrating the use of sterile tissue forceps to hold the catheter, is shown in Figure 148.

Analgesia. (See Chap. 11, Analgesia and Anesthesia.) Before administering the medication prescribed to promote analgesia, the nurse should inform the mother that she is going to give her medication which will make her more comfortable and help her in labor. She should encourage the mother to try to rest and assure her that she will not be left alone. It is wise to tell her also that you will remain quietly at the bedside and keep conversation at the very minimum in order for her to get the maximum benefit from the medication. Her bladder should be emptied prior to administering the drugs, and the fetal heart

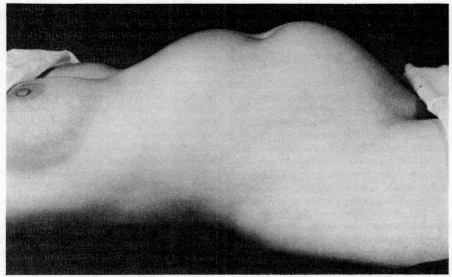

Fig. 147. Dystocia due to bladder distention. The tremendously distended bladder is plainly seen in the photograph. This patient was sent to the hospital after 3 days of ineffectual labor at home. The cervix had been dilated, it is believed, for 24 hours, yet no progress had been made. Catheterization of the greatly distended bladder yielded 1,000 cc. of urine. Following this, the infant's head descended at once and delivery was easy. (Eastman: Williams Obstetrics, 11th edition, New York, Appleton)

tones and the mother's vital signs should be recorded before and after such medication is given. Once analgesic therapy has been instituted, the mother should not receive fluids or food by mouth and should remain in bed. The environment should be conducive to rest, the room quiet and darkened but with sufficient light to permit accurate observation of the patient. The progress of labor must be observed even more carefully now that the mother is sedated, and she must *never* be left unattended. Particularly if scopolamine has been administered, the mother may become extremely restless during uterine contractions. If she throws herself around the bed her movements should be guided to protect both mother and her baby, but she should never be restrained. The policies of some hospitals permit the use of protective equipment,

such as siderails, when indicated. Even with such equipment the mother should not be left alone, for she may have a precipitate delivery unattended, injure herself on the siderails during the restlessness accompanying a contraction or fall out of bed.

Signs of Second Stage. There are certain signs and symptoms which herald the onset of the second stage of labor which should be watched for carefully. These are as follows: (1) The patient begins to bear down of her own accord; this is caused by a reflex when the head begins to press on the perineal floor. (2) There is a sudden increase in show, usually more blood tinged. (3) The patient thinks that she needs to defecate. This symptom is due to pressure of the head on the perineal floor and consequently against the rectum.

(4) The membranes rupture, with discharge of amniotic fluid. This, of course, may take place at any time but occurs most frequently at the beginning of the second stage. (5) The perineum begins to bulge and the anal orifice to dilate. This is a late sign, but if 1, 2, 3 and 4 occur, it should be watched for with every contraction. Only rectal or vaginal examination (or the appearance of the head) can definitely confirm the suspicion. Emesis at this time is not unusual.

In order to spare the mother a hurried trip to the delivery room and permit adequate time to cleanse and drape her properly for the delivery without unnecessary rush, the nurse should report promptly any or all of these symptoms which she observes. If these signs are overlooked, a precipitate delivery may occur without benefit of medical attention. In general primigravidas should be taken to the delivery room when the cervix is fully dilated and multiparas when it is 7 or 8 cm. dilated.

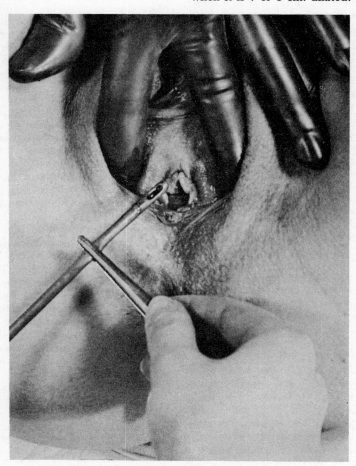

Fig. 148. Technic of catheterization, showing use of 6-inch
sterile tissue forceps to insert catheter.

CONDUCT OF THE SECOND STAGE

The second stage of labor (expulsion stage) begins with the complete dilatation of the cervix and ends with delivery of the baby. The complete dilatation of the cervix can be confirmed definitely only by rectal or vaginal examination. However, the nurse often is able to make a nursing diagnosis on the basis of her observations of the progress of labor, particularly if she correlates these findings with knowledge of the mother's parity, the speed of any previous labors, the pelvic measurements, etc., noted in the antepartal record. Although the general rule regarding the optimal time for taking a mother to the delivery room has been stated, it must be remembered that, in addition, the physician will be guided in his decision to give such an order by factors such as the station of the presenting part and the speed with which labor is progressing. If on examination of a primigravida, the physician finds the cervix to be fully dilated but the presenting part of the fetus only descended to the level of the ischial spines (mid pelvis), he undoubtedly will want the mother to remain in the labor room to permit the forces of labor to bring about further descent of the fetus before taking the mother to the delivery room. During this period, he may want the patient to exert her abdominal forces and "bear down." In most cases, bearing-down efforts are reflex and spontaneous in the second stage of labor, but, occasionally, the mother does not employ her expulsive forces to good advantage, particularly if she has had caudal analgesia. The nurse will be asked to coach and encourage the mother in this procedure. The thighs should be flexed on the abdomen, with hands grasped just below the knees when a contraction begins. Instructions should be given to take a deep breath as soon as the contraction begins and, with her breath held, to exert downward pressure exactly as if she were straining

at stool. Pulling on the knees at this time, as well as flexing the chin on the chest, is a helpful adjunct. The effort should be as long and sustained as possible, since short "grunty" endeavors are of little avail. If, at this time, the mother is in the delivery room but her legs as yet have not been put up in stirrups or leg holders, she can be coached in the same manner. In most hospitals the delivery tables have firmly attached hand grips which can be adjusted in position so that the mother can reach them comfortably to pull against. Her legs should be flexed so that simultaneously she can push her feet against the table. At the end of each contraction the mother is assisted to put her legs down and encouraged to rest until the next contraction begins. Usually, these bearing-down efforts are rewarded by increased bulging of the perineum, that is, by further descent of the head. The patient should be informed of such progress, for encouragement is all-important. In certain cases it may be undesirable for the mother to bear down, thus the nurse should not encourage the mother to do so without the physician's request.

Muscular cramps in the legs are common in the second stage because of pressure exerted by the baby's head on certain nerves in the pelvis. To relieve these cramps the leg should be straightened and the foot flexed by exerting pressure upward against the ball of the foot until the cramp subsides (see Fig. 113). Meanwhile, the knee should be stabilized with the other hand. These cramps cause excruciating pain and must never be ignored.

Good obstetric care during the second stage of labor demands the closest teamwork among physician, nurse and anesthetist. By previous understanding, or more often by established hospital routine, each has his or her own responsibilities in the delivery room, and, if the best interests of the mother and her infant are to be fulfilled, the

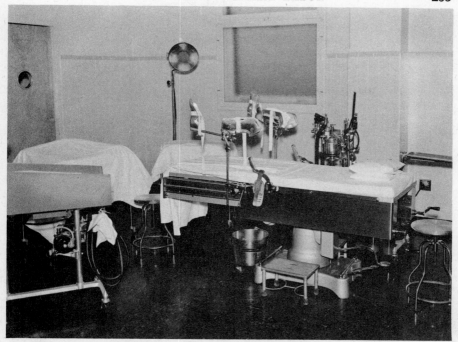

Fig. 149. Delivery room. The instrument table and the double-bowl solution stand are "set up" and covered with sterile drapes. The delivery table, with removable knee crutches, is composed of 2 adjoining sections. The resuscitator is at the left. The anesthesia machine is on the far side of the delivery table. (MacDonald House, University Hospitals of Cleveland)

responsibilities of each must be carried out smoothly and efficiently.

Preparation of the Delivery Room. There are no two hospitals in which the set-up of a delivery room or the procedure for delivery are precisely the same, and this is one phase of the nurse's work which she must learn wholly from actual observation and experience in her own institution. Nevertheless, she can obtain a general idea of the main equipment used from Figures 149 and 150.

The delivery table is designed so that its surface is actually composed of two adjoining sections, each covered with its own mattress. This permits the patient to lie in the supine position until it is desired to put her legs up into stirrups, that is, put her in the lithotomy position. At this time, the table is "broken" by a mechanical device. The retractable or lower end of the table drops and is rolled under the main section of the table, giving ready access to the perineal region. Or, if it is desired to deliver the patient in the dorsal recumbent position, the lower portion of the table can be allowed to remain in place.

The instrument table opposite the foot of the delivery table contains the principal sterile supplies and instruments needed for normal delivery, including, among other articles, towels, sponges, catheter, solutions, basins and the "cord set." The cord set is a group of instruments used for clamping and cutting the umbilical cord, namely, 2 hemostats, a

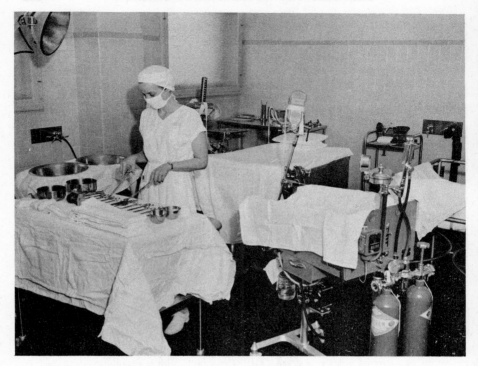

Fig. 150. Delivery room setup. The sterile table and the solution stand are uncovered, showing the arrangement of linen, instruments and equipment. The resuscitator is draped with a sterile receiving blanket, ready for the infant. The delivery table is "broken" as it would be after the mother's legs have been placed in the knee crutches. (The delivery table has a mechanical device which drops the lower, retractable end and rolls it under the main section of the table.) The infant's crib is at the far right. For illustrative purposes the major equipment for delivery has been grouped together. (MacDonald House, University Hospitals of Cleveland)

pair of scissors and a cord tie or clamp. More instruments are often included because it may be necessary for the physician to perform an episiotomy or to repair lacerations (p. 278). Additional instruments frequently included are 2 hemostats, 2 Allis clamps, 1 mouse-tooth tissue forceps, 2 sponge sticks, 1 vaginal retractor, 2 tenaculae, 1 needle holder, assorted needles and a pair of obstetric forceps.

A double-bowl solution stand or basin rack is generally used to hold the basins, one for wet sponges and the other for

the placenta. Emergency · instruments, a crib and a resuscitator, such as the Kreiselman (see Fig. 263), which provides heat in addition to mechanical suction and oxygen equipment, are part of standard delivery room equipment. Even if the infant does not require resuscitation, the resuscitator affords him a warm, protected environment, and it is a convenient place in which to give him care. To facilitate the delivery, all equipment should be in readiness at all times.

Asepsis and Antisepsis. Of prime

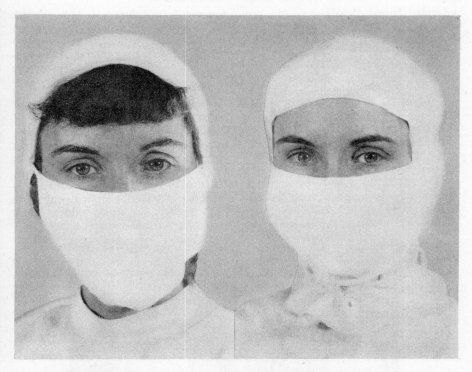

Fig. 151. (*Left*) *Incorrect* method of wearing cap. Bacteria, hairs and other infectious particles can readily fall from exposed hair and contaminate sterile fields. (*Right*) *Correct* method of adjusting cap so that *all* hair is covered.

importance in the conduct of the second stage are strict asepsis and antisepsis throughout. To this end, everyone in the delivery room must wear a clean cotton uniform, cap and mask, and those actually participating in the delivery are in sterile attire. Masking must include both nose and mouth. Caps should be so adjusted as to keep *all* hair covered (Fig. 151). Persons with colds or those who have had recent respiratory infections should not be permitted in the delivery room. If the nurse scrubs to assist the doctor, the strictest aseptic technic must be observed. The hands should be disinfected as carefully as for a major surgical operation. Scrubbing the hands should be started sufficiently early so that full time may be allotted, as well as to don gown and gloves. Figure 152 shows the correct method of donning gloves so that the exterior of the glove never is touched by the ungloved hand. Even after scrubbing the hands they are not considered sterile.

Transfer of the Mother to the Delivery Room. When the physician deems the birth to be imminent he will ask that the mother be transferred to the delivery room and prepared for delivery. If the mother is awake she should be told what is happening and be informed in advance about any procedure. This kind of support is not only reassuring to her but also enables her to co-operate more fully. It should be remembered, however, that the sound of several voices at one time can be confusing, so if the physician is coaching or instructing the mother it is well for the nurse not to try to participate or interfere at that time.

If spinal anesthesia is to be administered, the patient is turned on her side for the administration, unless it is a saddle block, in which case she is assisted to a sitting position on the side of the delivery table, with her feet supported on a stool and her body leaning forward against the nurse. Although this takes only a few minutes, the mother undoubtedly will be extremely uncomfortable due to the severity of the contractions at this time and should be given emotional as well as physical support. If the mother is to receive general anesthesia she lies supine on the table. As has been previously stated, anesthesia should be administered only by a qualified physician or a nurse anesthetist. This entire subject is discussed in Chapter 11, Analgesia and Anesthesia.

During the time the anesthesia is being administered, the circulating nurse can uncover the sterile tables, check the resuscitator and attach a sterile suc-

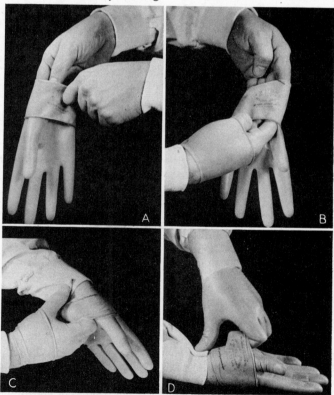

Fig. 152. Method of putting on sterile gloves so that the exterior of the glove never is touched by the ungloved hand.

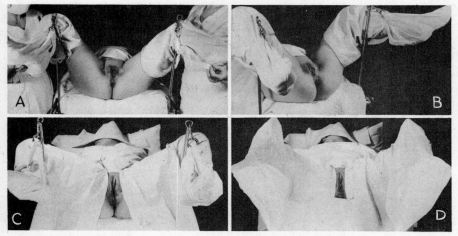

Fig. 153. (A) Raising legs simultaneously into stirrups. (B) Legs in stirrups. These are rods with heel stirrups; many hospitals, however, prefer metal knee crutches, as shown in Fig. 149. The patient's buttocks must be brought well down to the edge of the delivery table. (C) Three sterile towels have been applied. (D) Draping completed by covering sterile towels with sterile delivery sheet. The sheet contains "pillowcaselike" inserts to encase legs and stirrups in addition to aperture for delivery.

tion catheter and oxygen mask, and perform other duties for which she is responsible.

Before elevating the mother's legs into the stirrups, cotton flannel boots which cover the entire leg should be put on. The mother's hands should be secured with wrist straps which allow some limited movement but prevent her from reaching up to touch the sterile drapes after they are applied (an important point to explain to her, since mothers often complain about being "strapped down").

In putting the legs of the patient up into stirrups or leg holders, care should be used not to separate the legs too widely or to have one leg higher than the other. Both legs should be raised or lowered at the same time, with a nurse supporting each one. Failure to observe these instructions may result in straining the ligaments of the pelvis, with consequent discomfort in the puerperium.

With the patient in the lithotomy position, the nurse carries out the procedure for cleansing the vulva and surrounding area. If the delivery is to be conducted with the mother in the recumbent position, this may be carried out with the knees drawn up slightly and the legs separated. Then, the physician, who meanwhile has scrubbed his hands and donned sterile gown and gloves, drapes the patient with towels and sheets appropriate for the purpose (Figs. 153 and 154).

After the patient has been prepared for delivery, catheterization, if done, is carried out by the physician. Sometimes it is difficult to catheterize a patient in the second stage of labor, since the infant's head may compress the urethra. If the catheter does not pass easily, force should never be employed.

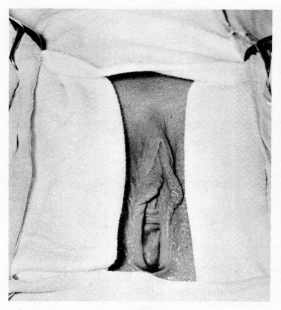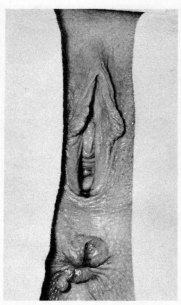

Fig. 154. Proper draping for delivery showing appropriate placement of sterile towels, one of which covers the anus. (The Johns Hopkins Hospital, Baltimore, Md.)

Fig. 155. Scalp of the infant detected through a slitlike vulvar opening as the perineal region begins to bulge and the skin over it becomes tense and glistening. Pressure of the descending head causes the anus to become patulous and everted. For purposes of showing changes which take place in the anus the lower towel has been removed from this photograph and the succeeding ones of this series, but this is for illustrative purposes only. (The Johns Hopkins Hospital, Baltimore, Md.)

As the infant descends the birth canal, pressure against the rectum may cause fecal material to be expelled. The physician will employ sponges (as a rule soaked with saline solution) to remove any fecal material which may escape from the rectum. As soon as the head distends the perineum to a diameter of 6 or 8 cm., the physician will often place a towel over the rectum and exert forward pressure on the chin of the baby's head while the other hand exerts downward pressure on the occiput (Figs. 155-159). This is called Ritgen's maneuver, and allows the physician to control the egress of the head; it also favors exten-

sion so that the head is born with the smallest diameter presenting. The head is usually delivered between contractions and as slowly as possible (Fig. 160). All these measures (control of head by Ritgen's maneuver, extension and slow delivery between contractions) help to prevent lacerations. If a tear seems inevitable, an incision which is called an episiotomy may be made in the perineum. This will not only prevent lacerations but also will facilitate the delivery (see p. 278). Immediately after the birth of the infant's head, the physician passes his finger along the occiput to the infant's neck in order to feel

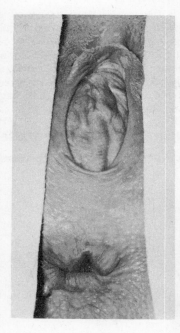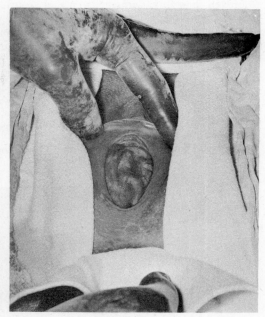

Fig. 156. Appearance of the infant's head with subsequent contractions. The vulva becomes more dilated and distended by the infant's head so that the opening is gradually converted into an ovoid. (The Johns Hopkins Hospital, Baltimore, Md.)

Fig. 157. Control of the progress of the head to preserve the perineum from tearing. (The Johns Hopkins Hospital, Baltimore, Md.)

whether a loop or more of umbilical cord encircles it. If such a coil is felt, it should be gently drawn down and, if loose enough, slipped over the infant's head. This is done to prevent interference with the infant's oxygen supply which could result from pressure of his shoulder on the umbilical cord. If the cord is too tightly coiled to permit this procedure, it must be clamped and cut before the shoulders are delivered; then the infant must be extracted immediately before asphyxiation results. As shown in Figure 161, the anterior shoulder is usually brought under the symphysis pubis first and then the posterior shoulder is delivered, after which the remainder of the body follows without particular mechanism (Figs. 162 and 163). The exact time of the baby's birth should be noted. The infant usually cries immediately, and the lungs become expanded; about this time the pulsations in the umbilical cord begin to diminish. The physician will usually defer clamping the cord until this occurs, or for a minute or so if practicable, because of the marked benefit of the additional blood to the infant. Using sterile instruments, the cord is cut between the 2 Kelly clamps which have been placed a few inches from the umbilicus, then the tie or umbilical clamp is applied. The tie, a sterilized linen tape ligature, is usually applied about an inch from the abdomen, with care to secure it tight enough to prevent bleeding, without its cutting into the cord (Figs. 164 and 165). A second ligature may be applied for further protection if it is desired, or if it is necessary because of any bleeding. There are several types of umbilical clamps, such as the Kane, the Zeigler and the Hesseltine, which are used extensively in many institutions (Fig. 166). With these, the possibility of hemorrhage is minimized.

The first 15 minutes after the infant's birth is the most hazardous period of life, when more infants succumb than during any subsequent time. The responsibility for much of the care during this period is delegated to the nurse, so that the physician may devote his attention to the mother during the third stage of labor (see p. 270 and Chap. 15).

CONDUCT OF THE THIRD STAGE

The third stage of labor (placental

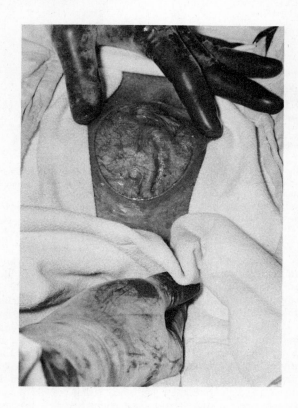

Fig. 158. Farther advanced extension of the head. The left hand is used to prevent sudden expulsion of the head as it crowns, while pressure on the infant's chin through the perineum by the right hand expedites extension and delivery. This is Ritgen's maneuver. (The Johns Hopkins Hospital, Baltimore, Md.)

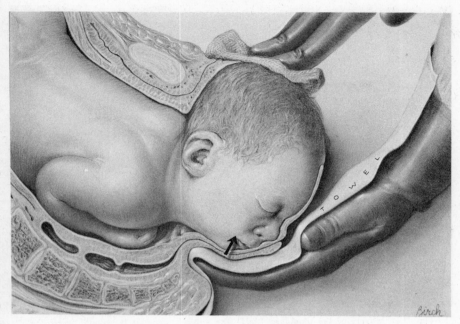

Fig. 159. Ritgen's maneuver, as it appears in median section. Arrow
shows direction of pressure.

stage) begins after the delivery of the
baby and terminates with the birth of
the placenta. Immediately after delivery
of the infant, the height of the uterine
fundus and its consistency are ascertained. The physician may do this by
palpating the uterus through a sterile
towel placed on the lower abdomen, but
it is a duty which is often delegated to
the nurse, at least while the physician is
engaged in clamping and cutting the
umbilical cord. The nurse may do so by
placing her hand on the abdomen *under*
the sterile drape. The uterus should be
held very gently with the fingers behind
the fundus and the thumb in front. So

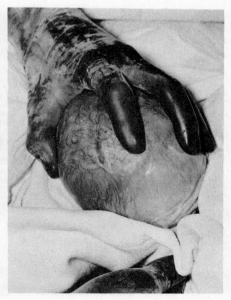

Fig. 160. Birth of the head. The full
hand is used to control the progress with
emergence of the forehead and face. (The
Johns Hopkins Hospital, Baltimore, Md.)

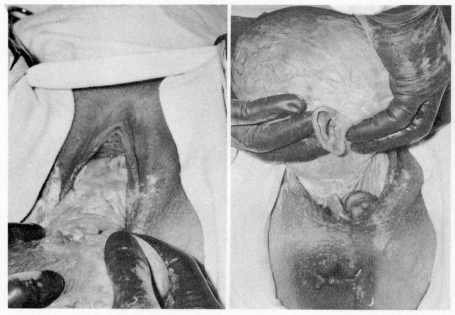

Fig. 161. Delivery of the shoulders. (*Left*) The anterior shoulder is brought under the symphysis pubis. (*Right*) Delivery of the posterior shoulder. (The Johns Hopkins Hospital, Baltimore, Md.)

long as the uterus remains hard and there is no bleeding, the policy is ordinarily one of watchful waiting until the placenta is separated; no massage is practiced, the hand simply resting on the fundus to make certain that the organ does not balloon out with blood. Since attempts to deliver the placenta

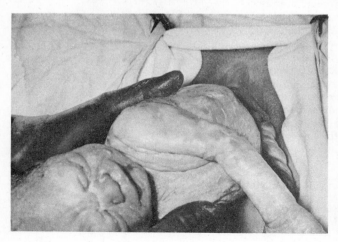

Fig. 162. Delivery of the infant's body. (The Johns Hopkins Hospital, Baltimore, Md.)

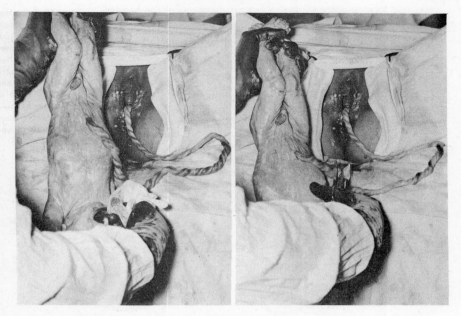

Fig. 163. Upon delivery the infant is held in the head down position to promote drainage of secretions from the respiratory passage. Mucus is gently wiped from the infant's face, then suctioned from the nostrils and the mouth with an ear bulb syringe or other suction device. *Note* there is no traction on the cord which is still attached to the placenta. (The Johns Hopkins Hospital, Baltimore, Md.)

Fig. 164. The cord is cut between the two Kelly clamps which have been placed a few inches from the umbilicus. (The Johns Hopkins Hospital, Baltimore, Md.)

prior to its separation from the uterine wall are not only futile but may be dangerous, it is most important that the signs of placental separation be well understood. If the responsibility of "guarding" the fundus is delegated to the nurse, she should watch for signs of placental separation and report such to the physician. The signs which suggest that the placenta has separated are as follows:

1. The uterus rises upward in the abdomen; this is due to the fact that the placenta, having been separated, passes downward into the lower uterine segment and the vagina, where its bulk pushes the uterus upward.

2. The umbilical cord protrudes 3 or more inches farther out of the vagina, indicating that the placenta also has descended.

3. The uterus changes from a discoid to a globular shape and becomes, as a rule, more firm.

4. A sudden trickle or spurt of blood often occurs.

These signs are sometimes apparent within a minute or so after delivery of the infant, usually within 5 minutes. When the placenta has certainly separated, the physician first ascertains that the uterus is firmly contracted. He then may ask the patient, if not anesthetized, to "bear down," and the intra-abdominal pressure so produced may be adequate to expel the placenta (Fig. 167). If this

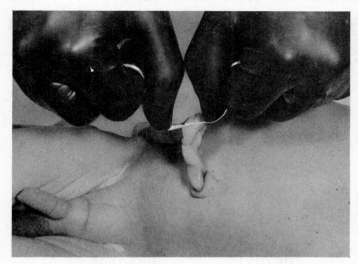

Fig. 165. Tying umbilical cord. Note that knuckles are kept together. This gives a better controlled tie and is a safeguard against jerking and tearing the cord in case one hand should slip. (*Bottom*) Square knot: first and second steps in tying.

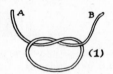

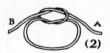

fails or if it is not practicable because of anesthesia, the physician, again having made certain that the uterus is hard, exerts gentle pressure downward with his hand on the fundus and, employing the placenta as a piston, simply moves the placenta out of the vagina. This procedure, known as placental "expression," must be done gently and without squeezing (Fig. 168). It never should be attempted unless the uterus is hard, otherwise the organ may be turned inside-out. This is one of the gravest complications of obstetrics and is known as "inversion" of the uterus (p. 446). The physician carries out a careful inspection of the placenta to make sure that it is intact (Fig. 169); if a piece is left in the uterus, it may cause subsequent hemorrhage.

Pituitary extract and/or ergonovine, or their derivatives, may be administered at the physician's request to increase uterine contractions and thereby minimize bleeding. These agents are employed widely in the conduct of the normal third stage of labor, but the timing of their administration differs greatly in various hospitals. These oxytocics are not necessary in most cases, but their use is considered ideal from the viewpoint of minimizing blood loss and the general safety of the mother.

The Oxytocics. Ergonovine is an alkaloid of ergot. It is a powerful oxytocic, i.e., it stimulates uterine contractions and exerts an effect which may persist for several hours. When administered intravenously the uterine response is almost immediate, and within a few minutes after intramuscular or oral administration. This response is sustained in character with no tendency toward relaxation and so is ideal for the prevention and the control of postpartal hemorrhage. This drug will cause an elevation of blood pressure. More recently a semisynthetic derivative of

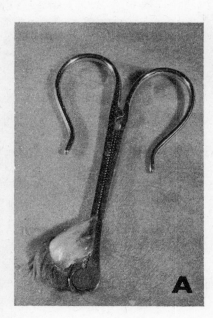

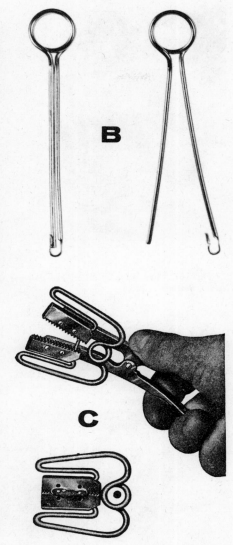

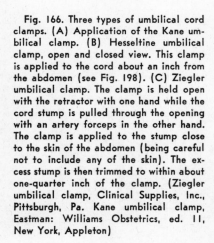

Fig. 166. Three types of umbilical cord clamps. (A) Application of the Kane umbilical clamp. (B) Hesseltine umbilical clamp, open and closed view. This clamp is applied to the cord about an inch from the abdomen (see Fig. 198). (C) Ziegler umbilical clamp. The clamp is held open with the retractor with one hand while the cord stump is pulled through the opening with an artery forceps in the other hand. The clamp is applied to the stump close to the skin of the abdomen (being careful not to include any of the skin). The excess stump is then trimmed to within about one-quarter inch of the clamp. (Ziegler umbilical clamp, Clinical Supplies, Inc., Pittsburgh, Pa. Kane umbilical clamp, Eastman: Williams Obstetrics, ed. 11, New York, Appleton)

ergonovine, methyl ergonovine tartrate, has been widely employed because it possesses several advantages over the parent drug. Usually called by its trade name, Methergine, it has the ability to produce stronger and longer contractions and is less likely to cause elevation of the blood pressure. Both drugs when given intravenously may cause transient headache and, to a lesser extent, temporary chest pain, palpitation and dyspnea. These side-effects are less likely to occur

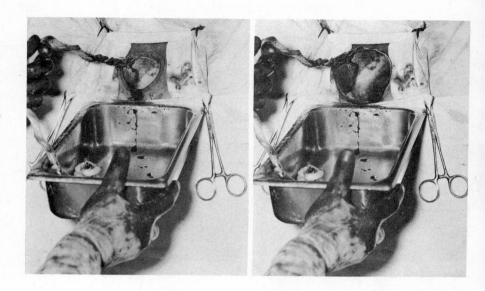

Fig. 167. Third stage of labor. The delivery of the placenta. (The Johns Hopkins Hospital, Baltimore, Md.)

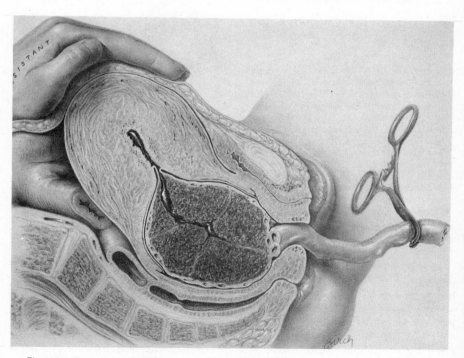

Fig. 168. Expression of placenta is usually done by the physician, if necessary, but *on his instructions* may be done by an assistant. The *uterus must be hard* if this is attempted. Note that the uterus is not squeezed.

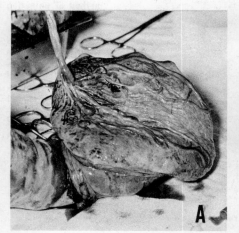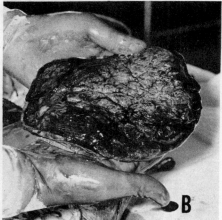

Fig. 169. Inspecting the placenta: (A) the fetal side, (B) the maternal side. (The Johns Hopkins Hospital, Baltimore, Md.)

with intramuscular administration of the drugs.

Posterior pituitary extract is another agent which, like ergonovine, causes a marked contraction of the uterus. However, the response of the uterus to posterior Pituitrin resembles that of ergonovine for only the first 5 or 10 minutes, then normal rhythmic contractions of amplified degree return, with intermittent periods of relaxation. In obstetric practice today, the oxytocic fraction separated from posterior pituitary extract, usually referred to by the trade name Pitocin, is widely used because it does not possess the strong vasopressor and antidiuretic effects of Pituitrin, both of which are highly undesirable for the obstetric patient.

On the obstetrician's order, the nurse administers the oxytocic intramuscularly, intravenous medications being administered by a physician. The average intramuscular doses of these drugs are as follows: posterior pituitary extract, 10 units or 1 cc.; Pitocin, 10 units or 1 cc.; ergonovine, 0.2 mg. (1/320 gr.) or 1 cc.; and Methergine, 0.2 mg. (1/320 gr.) or 1 cc. One method used at the Woman's Clinic of The Johns Hopkins Hospital is as follows: Pitocin, 10 units (1 cc.), intramuscularly, immediately after the birth of the baby, followed by Methergine, 0.2 mg. (1 cc.), intramuscularly, immediately after the delivery of the placenta.

Constant massage of the uterus during the period after the delivery of the placenta is unnecessary and undesirable. However, if the organ shows any tendency to relax it must be massaged immediately with firm but gentle circular strokes until it contracts effectively in order to prevent blood loss.

After the delivery has been completed, the drapes and the soiled linen under the mother's buttocks are removed and the lower end of the delivery table is replaced. The mother's legs are lowered from the stirrups simultaneously, and after a sterile perineal pad is applied, she should be covered with a

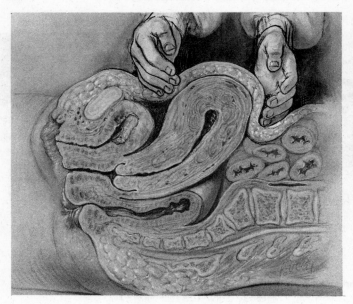

Fig. 170. Proper method of palpating fundus of uterus during first hour after delivery to guard against relaxation and hemorrhage. The right hand is placed just above the symphysis pubis to act as a guard, meanwhile the other hand is cupped around the fundus of the uterus.

blanket to avoid chilling. She is now ready to be transferred to her own bed.

If the mother is awake at this time she will be eager to have a closer look at her baby and hold it, if this is possible.

The first hour following the delivery is a most critical one for the mother. It is at this time that postpartal hemorrhage is most likely to occur as the result of uterine relaxation. Thus, it is mandatory that the uterus be watched constantly throughout this period by a competent nurse who keeps her hand more or less constantly on the fundus and at the slightest sign of diminishing contraction massages it, to make sure that it does not relapse and balloon with blood (Fig. 170). Not only is it important for the nurse to be constantly alert to the condition of the mother's uterus but also to any abnormal symptoms related to her general condition.

IMMEDIATE CARE OF THE INFANT

As soon as the infant is born, measures should be taken to promote a clear air passage before the onset of respirations.

Often, as the head is delivered, it is necessary to wipe the mucus and fluid from the infant's nose and mouth before he has a chance to gasp and aspirate with this first breath. From the moment of delivery the infant should be kept in the head-down position until his upper respiratory passage is cleared of mucus, amniotic fluid, etc. A small rubber bulb syringe, or a soft rubber suction catheter attached to a mechanical suction or mouth aspirator, should be used promptly to suction the oropharynx and remove fluids which may be obstructing the airway. If there seems to be much mucus present, the physician will hold the infant up by his ankles to encourage more mucus to drain from the throat. "Wiping of mucosal surfaces of the palate and posterior pharynx with gauze should be avoided, since its rough texture leads to abrasions and the development of thrush."*

* Special Committee on Infant Mortality of the Medical Society of the County of N. Y.: Resuscitation of newborn infants, Obst. & Gynec. 8:17, 1956.

The baby may not "cry" at once, but he usually gasps or cries after the mucus has been removed, as he now needs oxygen by way of the lungs, since the accustomed supply was cut off when the placental circulation stopped. If crying has to be stimulated it must be done with extreme care. As the infant is being held in the head-down position to promote the drainage of mucus from the respiratory passages, gentle rubbing of the infant's back is usually sufficient stimulus to initiate crying. And, in the act of crying, mucus is forced from the nose and the throat, thus enabling the infant to be better able to breathe. "A host of external irritants should be mentioned only to be condemned. These include spanking the soles of the feet, spanking the buttocks, forcible rubbing of the skin along the spine, the alternating hot and cold tubbing of the infant, and dilatation of the anal sphincter. The external irritants mentioned are not only obsolete, but are in many instances shocking to the tender infant. They are dangerous and unnecessary."*

A sterile receiver should be available for the physician to wrap around the infant until it can be placed in a warm crib. It must be remembered that any room is much cooler than the mother's body, and the infant should never be

Op. cit., p. 351.

exposed to chilling. As soon as the physician has clamped and cut the cord, he usually places the infant in a heated crib or resuscitator (previously draped with a sterile receiver to avoid contaminating his gloves) so that he may devote his attention to the mother during the third stage of labor. As mentioned previously, even for the infant who requires no resuscitation, the resuscitator affords a warm protected environment for the infant and, in addition, a convenient place for the nurse now to proceed with the infant's care. If a circulating nurse is responsible for the infant's care in the delivery room, she will have cleansed her hands thoroughly with some agent such as pHisoHex or surgical soap in preparation, preferably while the physician is delivering the infant's head. After she draws the receiver around the infant to protect him from chilling, her first consideration is in relation to the infant's breathing and color. It may be necessary to suction further mucus from the oropharynx and, if the infant's color appears dusky, to administer oxygen by mask at a flow not exceeding 4 liters. The gentle patting and rubbing with the receiving blanket to dry the infant's body usually acts as an additional stimulus.

Care of the Cord. In some hospitals no dressing is applied after the cord has been clamped or ligated and cut; in

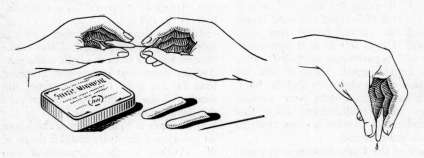

Fig. 171. (*Left*) Silver nitrate 1 per cent solution for the care of the eyes of newborn babies; needle puncture of wax ampule. (*Right*) Showing how to manipulate the ampule in administering the drug. (Eli Lilly and Company)

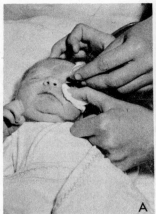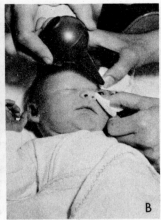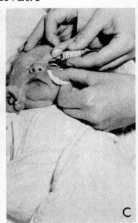

A   B   C

Fig. 172. Photographs showing 2 different methods of prophylactic treatment of the newborn infant's eyes for protection against ophthalmia neonatorum:

1. *Silver nitrate prophylaxis.* (A) Instillation of 2 drops of silver nitrate 1 per cent solution from a wax ampule into the conjunctival sac of each eye. (B) After the medication has diffused over the entire conjunctiva (2 minutes), the conjunctival sac of each eye is gently flushed with sterile distilled water or normal saline solution to remove the excess silver nitrate.

2. *Bactericidal ointment prophylaxis.* (C) Instillation of an approved bactericidal ointment. A half inch strip of the ointment is applied across the conjunctival sac of each eye and should diffuse over the entire conjunctiva. No irrigation is used following this treatment.

others, a sterile plain gauze dressing is applied around the cord stump and secured with a binder, which is removed at appropriate times (Figs. 201-202). Regardless of the technic employed, it is imperative that frequent inspection be done to note any signs of bleeding and that strict aseptic precautions be utilized in caring for the cord stump. The method of leaving the cord stump exposed has proved to be very satisfactory. If it is left free, it apparently dries and separates more quickly than when kept covered. There is also less irritation of the abdomen and the back, which sometimes results from a moist binder. Some pediatricians think that the abdominal muscles become stronger by not being bound.

Care of the Eyes. As soon as the cord is cared for and the infant's respirations are well established, the eyes should receive prophylactic treatment for protection against ophthalmia neonatorum

(see Chap. 21, Disorders of the Newborn). This treatment is so important that at the present time the use of a silver preparation is mandatory by statute in the majority of states. If silver nitrate is to be used (Credé method), it should be supplied in *wax ampules* containing silver nitrate 1 per cent solution, especially prepared for eye instillation (Fig. 171).

Instilling drops in the infant's eyes is more easily accomplished if the nurse shades the eyes from the light while putting the drops first in one eye, allowing time for the baby to recover from the shock and the smarting before she puts the drops in the other eye. One of the best methods is to draw down the lower lid gently and carefully instill 2 drops of the solution in the conjunctival sac, using great care not to drop it on the cornea. After 2 minutes, when it will have diffused itself over the entire conjunctiva, the lids should again be held apart and the conjunctival sac of each eye flushed gently with normal saline solution or sterile distilled water to remove any excess silver nitrate (Fig. 172). The nurse must take especial precautions against allowing any contamination of the eyes and against dropping any silver solution upon the face. Silver nitrate prophylaxis may cause signs of irritation, such as redness, edema or discharge, but these manifestations are transient and in no way cause permanent damage if the silver nitrate solution used is in correct concentration.

Recent research has resulted in the adoption of penicillin by many doctors as prophylaxis for the baby's eyes. The methods used have been intramuscular injections and the local instillation of an aqueous solution or ointment. At present, the most practical and effectual is the ointment preparation, penicillin ophthalmic ointment, 100,000 units per Gm. It is easy to instill into the conjunctival sac and it is economical, the cost being about the same as that of the silver nitrate ampules. As with the instillation of silver nitrate solution, the nurse must use extreme gentleness in applying the ointment and must apply a strip of it across the entire sac. The recommendation has been made that, where necessary, statutes and board of health regulations be changed to permit in hospital practice the instillation of an approved bactericidal ointment when the doctor prefers it as a prophylaxis against ophthalmia neonatorum.

Identification Methods. Some method of identification of the newborn is applied before the cord is cut or before the baby is removed from the delivery room. There are several satisfactory methods in use. Some hospitals use the linen tapes marked with the mother's name and hospital number, fastening one to the baby's arm or ankle and the other to the mother's wrist. The identification beads are made up with the mother's surname and initials and sealed with a lead bead. This bracelet or anklet

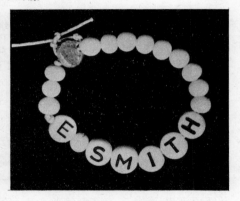

Fig. 173. Identification method, using strand of beads. If surname is at all common use initial of mother's first name also, as shown above. The beads must be sealed around baby's wrist or ankle before he leaves the delivery room.

is applied before the baby leaves the delivery room (Fig. 173). The pliable plastic bracelet or anklet has space for the mother's name and initials as well as a permanent lock which has to be cut to be removed.

The palmprint and footprint method of identification consists of a stainless procedure made on chemically treated sensitized paper. It is designed to take the palmprints or footprints of the baby and the thumbprint of the mother at the time of delivery and may be repeated at the time of discharge from the hospital. It is a simple, quick and permanent method.

The following editorial comment presents the recommendations of the American Hospital Association.

Mix-ups involving two or more babies are quite rare in hospital nurseries, but they still can happen. In one state alone in a period of 18 months eight mix-ups or alleged mix-ups occurred. When such a mix-up, alleged or actual, does occur, a torrent of unfavorable publicity is unloosed and the parents concerned may be haunted by a lifetime of doubt about their child. The confusion sometimes

OHIO DEPARTMENT OF HEALTH
DIVISION OF VITAL STATISTICS
CERTIFICATE OF LIVE BIRTH

Reg. Dist. No._____
Primary Reg. Dist. No._____

Registrar's No. _____

Birth No. 134 -

1. PLACE OF BIRTH	2. USUAL RESIDENCE OF MOTHER (Where does mother live?)
a. COUNTY	a. STATE b. COUNTY
b. CITY, VILLAGE, OR LOCATION	c. CITY, VILLAGE, OR LOCATION
c. NAME OF HOSPITAL OR INSTITUTION (If not in hospital or institution, give street address)	d. STREET ADDRESS
d. IS PLACE OF BIRTH INSIDE CITY LIMITS? YES ☐ NO ☐	e. IS RESIDENCE INSIDE CITY LIMITS? YES ☐ NO ☐ f. IS RESIDENCE ON A FARM? YES ☐ NO ☐

CHILD

3. NAME (TYPE OR PRINT)   First   Middle   Last

4. SEX	5a. THIS BIRTH SINGLE ☐ TWIN ☐ TRIPLET ☐	5b. IF TWIN OR TRIPLET, WAS CHILD BORN 1ST ☐ 2D ☐ 3D ☐	6. DATE OF BIRTH MONTH DAY YEAR

FATHER

7. NAME First Middle Last	8. COLOR OR RACE
9. AGE (At time of this birth) YEARS	10. BIRTHPLACE (State or foreign country)	11a. USUAL OCCUPATION	11b. KIND OF BUSINESS OR INDUSTRY

MOTHER

12. MAIDEN NAME First Middle Last	13. COLOR OR RACE

14. AGE (At time of this birth) YEARS	15. BIRTHPLACE (State or foreign country)	16. PREVIOUS DELIVERIES TO MOTHER (Do NOT include this birth)
		a. How many OTHER children are now living?	b. How many OTHER children were born alive but are now dead?	c. How many fetal deaths (fetuses born dead at ANY time after conception?)

17. INFORMANT'S NAME OR SIGNATURE

18. MOTHER'S MAILING ADDRESS	19. DATE SEROLOGIC TEST FOR SYPHILIS

I hereby certify that this child was born alive on the date stated above.	19a. SIGNATURE	19b. ATTENDANT AT BIRTH M. D. ☐ D. O. ☐ MIDWIFE ☐ OTHER (Specify)
	19c. ADDRESS	19d. DATE SIGNED

20. DATE RECD. BY LOCAL REG.	21. REGISTRAR'S SIGNATURE	22. DATE ON WHICH GIVEN NAME ADDED BY (Registrar)

FOR MEDICAL AND HEALTH USE ONLY
(This section MUST be filled out)

23. LENGTH OF PREGNANCY WEEKS	24. WEIGHT AT BIRTH LB. OZ.	25. LEGITIMATE Yes ☐ No ☐	26. CONGENITAL MALFORMATION Yes ☐ No ☐

Fig. 174. Certificate of live birth used by Ohio State Department of Health. Similar forms are used by other cities and states.

arises because two mothers in a hospital at the same time have the same surname; it sometimes arises because a single identification becomes detached from the baby; or it may even arise because parents get to wondering after they leave the hospital how the attendants maintained the identity of the babies. Sometimes the confusion is easily straightened out, and sometimes it leads to giving the wrong baby a harmless prescription; only rarely does it lead to an actual exchange of babies. The American Hospital Association has long been aware of this problem, and, because it has been found that photographs, footprints, handprints, and fingerprints are adjuncts but cannot yet be considered reliable as the sole means of identifying the newborn infant, the Association has urged the adoption of a standard operating procedure that if applied would reduce mix-ups to the vanishing point.

The main features of this procedure are as follows: (1) Each baby should be marked in the delivery room with two items of identification. (2) The identification items should show the mother's full name, date and time of birth, and some correlation with the mother, such as her fingerprint or number. (3) Each time the baby comes to the mother, the mother should be informed that it is her responsibility to identify her baby by the marking. (4) When the baby and mother are discharged, one of the bands should be removed, preferably by the mother, and, after the mother has properly identified her baby, the removed identification should then be pasted to the baby's chart. The mother should acknowledge in writing that this is how her baby was marked, and that she identified it as hers. The leaflet that gives the full procedure in detail has been available since December, 1949. Once established as a routine, this procedure, far from being a burden, would prevent a type of mistake that would otherwise be easy to make but is nonetheless inexcusable.*

As already discussed in Chapter 1, the registration of the infant's birth is a legal responsibility. It is mandatory that a birth certificate, such as that shown in Figure 174, be filled out on every birth and submitted promptly to the local registrar.

After the Delivery. After caring for the infant, the nurse will continue to assist the physician with the care of the mother and her infant. If the mother is awake she may be anxious to have her baby brought near so that she may see it at close range. If she is drowsy it may be better to wait until she is more alert. The nurse will be governed by each mother's response at this time. Some mothers want to touch their babies; others are eager to hold their babies at this time, and if this is sanctioned by the physician, there is no reason why it should not be permitted for a brief period. In this instance, the nurse should be careful to keep her hand under the infant for support and added protection should this be necessary because of the mother's excitement in her first contact with her newborn.

If the infant is well wrapped and warm he may be kept in a crib at the mother's side until the mother leaves the delivery room. He should be kept in Trendelenburg position to promote the drainage of mucus, and on his side to

* *Editorial Comment:* Identification of the newborn infant, J.A.M.A. **162:**44, 1956.

avoid aspiration of this mucus. The nurse should observe the infant at frequent intervals to make sure that he is breathing properly, that the mouth and the nose are free from mucus and that there is no bleeding from the cord. Because this period may be a critical one for the infant, many hospitals have facilities, such as a receiving nursery, on the labor and delivery division where the infant is transferred at this time. This not only provides closer supervision and care for the infant but also permits the nurse in the delivery room to devote her undivided attention to the mother.

Baptism of Infant. If there is any probability that the infant is in imminent danger and may not live, the question of baptism should be considered in cases where the religion of the family is Roman Catholic; this also applies to some of the other denominations of the Christian church. This is an essential duty and means a great deal to the families concerned, and thoughtfulness in this matter will never be forgotten by them. (It is to be understood that such baptism would be reported to the family.)

The following simple instructions were given by the late Rev. Paul L. Blakely, S.J., Ph.D.

The Catholic Church teaches that in case of emergency, anyone may and should baptize. What is necessary is to make the intention of doing what the Church wishes to do and then to pour the water on the child (the head by preference) saying at the same time, "I baptize thee in the name of the Father and of the Son and of the Holy Ghost." The water may be warmed if necessary but it must be pure water and care should be taken to make it flow. If there is any doubt whether the child is alive or dead, it should be baptized, but conditionally; i.e., "If thou art alive, I baptize thee," etc.

On page 281 of the Book of Common Prayer of the Protestant Episcopal Church, it is stated: "In cases of extreme sickness, or any imminent peril, if a Minister cannot be procured, then any baptized person present may administer holy Baptism, using the foregoing form" (the same form which is used by the Roman Catholic Church).

EMERGENCY DELIVERY BY THE NURSE

In the course of labor, one occasionally encounters the so-called *precipitate delivery*, a rapid spontaneous delivery in which the infant is born without adequate preparations on the part of the physician or the nurse, sometimes even without benefit of their immediate care. This may occur in certain multiparous women, particularly if the soft parts of the pelvis offer little resistance, if the contractions are unusually strong and forceful or if the mother does not experience painful sensations during labor and thus has inadequate warning that the delivery is approaching. The mother, of course, may suffer lacerations of the tissues as the result of tumultuous labor. The infant is endangered because, in its rapid progress through the birth canal, it may suffer cerebral trauma; or the umbilical cord may be torn in the process of the delivery. In addition, if the mother is unattended, the infant may be in jeopardy from lack of care during the first few minutes of life.

Whether the nurse is caring for a mother in the hospital labor room, making a home visit or involved in some emergency situation, it is well for her to be prepared for a precipitate delivery. It seldom happens that the nurse is alone with her patient in the hospital when the delivery is imminent; but knowing what to do in such a situation, in the event that the physician is not present, is advantageous for all concerned. In the excitement which may ensue, the nurse's concern for the immediate safety of the mother and the baby usually demands all of her attention. The nurse who is consistently conscientious about applying principles of asepsis and antisepsis will automatically apply them in this instance, to the best of her ability. Usually there is inadequate time for proper cleansing of the vulva, or scrubbing her own hands and donning sterile gloves, or draping the mother, all of which would be ideal. However, a clean delivery area should be maintained, and, if time and facilities permit, the nurse's hands should be cleansed. The mother will be so involved in having her baby that little else concerns her, but the nurse is ever conscious of her patient's general condition and will give her the physical and emotional support necessary.

Delivery of the Head. As the head distends the perineum at the acme of a contraction, gentle pressure is exerted against the head to control its progress and thereby prevent undue stretching of the perineum. This kind of *control* applied to the descending head during each contraction will prevent its sudden expulsion through the vulva, reducing the possibility of consequent complications. *The head must never be held back.* The mother should be encouraged to pant during the contraction to deter bearing down efforts on her part, particularly as the head, which will be supported by the nurse, is being delivered. Whenever possible, the infant's head should be delivered between contractions.

Rupture of the Membranes. If the membranes have not ruptured previously, they may remain intact until they appear as a smooth, glistening object at the vulva. If they protrude they may rupture with the next contraction. But if the membranes have not ruptured previously before the head is delivered, they must be broken and removed immediately (by nipping them at the nape of the infant's neck) to prevent aspiration of fluid when the infant takes its first breath.

Precautions Concerning the Cord. As soon as the head is delivered, the nurse should feel for a loop or loops of cord around the neck and, if found, gently remove it (see p. 261).

Delivery of the Infant's Body. After external rotation of the head, which is usually spontaneous, there is no occasion for haste in the delivery of the body. Gentle downward pressure with the hands on either side of the head may be exerted to direct the anterior shoulder under the symphysis pubis, then reversed upward in order to deliver the posterior shoulder over the perineum. The infant's body will now follow easily and quickly and should be supported as it is born.

Immediate Care of the Infant. As soon as the face appears, mucus and fluids should be wiped from the nose and the mouth. Then, after the infant is born, if he does not cry spontaneously, or if there seems to be mucus in the respiratory passages, the infant should be held up by his ankles to encourage the mucus to drain from his nose and mouth. In doing this, care must be exercised to avoid any traction on the umbilical cord and, at the same time, to prevent the infant's head from pressing down against the bed. Drainage of mucus is stimulated when the infant cries but can be encouraged by "milking the trachea," i.e., with the forefinger, stroking the neck from its base toward the chin. Further stimulation by gentle rubbing of the back may stimulate breathing.

Care of the Cord. There is no hurry to cut the cord, so this should be delayed until proper equipment is available. It is a good plan to clamp the cord after pulsations cease (but not imperative at the moment) and wait for the physician to cut the cord after he arrives. One must always bear in mind that sterile conditions must exist for the cord-cutting procedure, otherwise the infant's safety is jeopardized. Also, the technic for applying the cord tie or umbilical clamp must be assiduously carried out to prevent bleeding from the umbilical stump (see p. 261).

Delivery of the Placenta. When signs of placental separation are apparent, the mother can be asked to bear down with the next contraction to deliver the placenta. Since the danger of hemorrhage is always to be guarded against, the fundus should be massaged after the delivery of the placenta if there is the slightest tendency toward relaxation of the uterine muscles.

When the infant is breathing satisfactorily he can be placed on his side across his mother's abdomen (with his head kept low to promote postural drainage and his body covered to prevent chilling). This accomplishes several things: the mother is given her baby, she can touch him and is usually enthralled by the close physical contact with him; the warmth of the mother's body prevents the infant from being chilled; and the pressure exerted on the uterus by the weight of the infant helps it to contract.

One must remember to proceed slowly and carefully throughout the delivery. The nurse's reaction to the situation undoubtedly will be transferred to the mother, so if the nurse remains poised and unfaltering, the mother is more likely to do so.

LACERATIONS OF THE BIRTH CANAL

During the process of a normal delivery, lacerations of the perineum and the vagina may be caused by rapid and sudden expulsion of the head (particularly when it "pops" out), the excessive size of the infant and very friable maternal tissues. In other circumstances they may be caused by difficult forceps deliveries, breech extractions or contraction of the pelvic outlet in which the head is forced posteriorly. Some tears are unavoidable, even in the most skilled hands.

Perineal lacerations are usually classified in 3 degrees, according to the extent of the tear.

First-degree lacerations are those

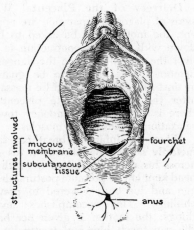

Fig. 175 A. First-degree tear.

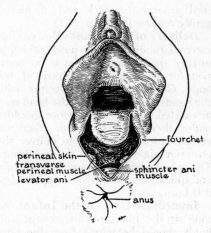

Fig. 175 B. Second-degree tear.

which involve the fourchet, the perineal skin and the vaginal mucous membrane without involving any of the muscles (Fig. 175 A).

Second-degree lacerations are those which involve (in addition to skin and mucous membrane) the muscles of the perineal body but not the rectal sphincter. These tears usually extend upward on one or both sides of the vagina, making a triangular injury (Fig. 175 B).

Third-degree lacerations are those which extend completely through the skin, the mucous membrane, the perineal body and the rectal sphincter (Fig. 175 C). This type is often referred to as a complete tear. Not infrequently these third-degree lacerations extend a certain distance up the anterior wall of the rectum.

First- and second-degree lacerations are extremely common in primigravidas, thus being one of the reasons why episiotomy is widely employed. Fortunately, third-degree lacerations are far less common. All 3 types of lacerations are repaired by the physician immediately after the delivery to ensure that the perineal structures are returned approxi-

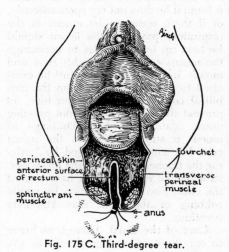

Fig. 175 C. Third-degree tear.

mately to their former condition. The technic employed for the repair of a laceration is virtually the same as that used for episiotomy incisions (see p. 280), although the former is more difficult to do because of the irregular lines of tissue which must be approximated.

EPISIOTOMY AND REPAIR

An episiotomy is an incision of the

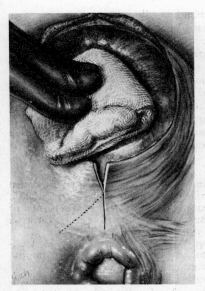

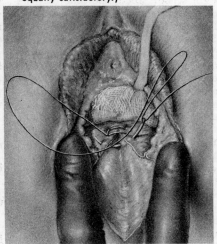

(Technic employed at the Johns Hopkins Hospital. Many other methods are equally satisfactory.)

Fig. 176. Episiotomy. Showing lines of incision for median and mediolateral episiotomy.

Fig. 177. Episiotomy. "Tail-sponge" in vagina to occlude bleeding, continuous suture in vaginal mucosa.

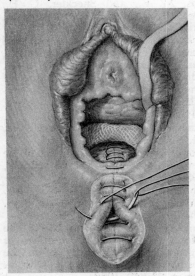

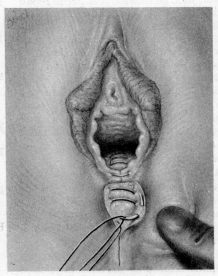

Fig. 178. Episiotomy. After the levator ani muscle has been united by two or more sutures (shown tied and cut), the fascia covering the muscle is sutured. Note the "tail-sponge."

Fig. 179. Episiotomy. After suturing to the lowermost angle of the fascia, the round needle is replaced by cutting needle and the running suture continued upward in subcuticular fascia.

perineum made to facilitate delivery. The incision is made with blunt-pointed straight scissors about the time that the head distends the vulva and is visible to a diameter of several centimeters. The incision may be made in the midline of the perineum—a median episiotomy. Or it may be begun in the midline and directed downward and laterally away from the rectum—a mediolateral episiotomy (Fig. 176). In the latter instance the incision may be directed to either the right or to the left side of the mother's pelvis.

As the infant's head distends the vulva, if a laceration seems to be inevitable, the physician undoubtedly will choose to incise the perineum rather than allow that structure to sustain a traumatic tear. This operation serves several purposes:

1. It substitutes a straight, clean-cut surgical incision for the ragged, contused laceration which is otherwise likely to ensue; such an incision is easier to repair and heals better than a tear.

2. The direction of the episiotomy can be controlled, whereas a tear may extend in any direction, sometimes involving the anal sphincter and the rectum.

3. It spares the baby's head the necessity of serving as a "battering ram" against perineal obstruction; if prolonged, this "pounding" of the infant's head against the perineum may cause brain injury.

4. The operation shortens the duration of the second stage of labor.

In view of these several advantages of episiotomy, many physicians employ it routinely in the delivery of the primigravida.

There are many equally satisfactory methods utilized by different physicians for episiotomy repair. The suture material ordinarily used is a fine chromic catgut, either 00 or 000. The technic employed at the Johns Hopkins Hospital is shown in Figures 177 through 179.

A round needle and continuous suture is used to close the vaginal mucosa and fourchet, then laid aside while several interrupted sutures are placed in levator ani muscle and fascia. Then the continuous suture is again picked up and used to unite the subcutaneous fascia. Finally, the round needle is replaced by a large, straight cutting needle and the running suture continued upward as a subcuticular stitch.

SUGGESTED READING

Adams, M.: Appraisal of a newborn infant, Am. J. Nursing 55:1336, 1955.

Bloxsom, A.: Posture requirements of the newborn infant, Am. J. Obst. & Gynec. 74:186, 1957.

Crisp, W. E., and MacDonald, R.: Control of pain following episiorrhaphy, Obst. & Gynec. 1:289, 1953.

Davidson, H. H., Hill, J. H., and Eastman, N. J.: Penicillin in the prophylaxis of ophthalmia neonatorum, J.A.M.A. 145:1052, 1951.

Davis, M. E., and Sheckler, C. E.: DeLee's Obstetrics for Nurses, ed. 16, Philadelphia, Saunders, 1957.

Dieckmann, W. J., et al.: The placental stage and postpartum hemorrhage, Am. J. Obst. & Gynec. 54:415, 1947.

Duchman, S., et al.: The importance of gravity in delayed ligation of the umbilical cord, Am. J. Obst. & Gynec. 66:1214, 1953.

Eastman, N. J.: Williams Obstetrics, ed. 11, New York, Appleton, 1956.

Editorial Comment: Identification of the newborn infant, J.A.M.A. 162:414, 1956.

Fitzhugh, M. L., and Newton, M.: Muscle action during childbirth, Phys. Therapy Rev. 36:805, 1956.

Forman, J. B., and Sullivan, R. L.: The effects of intravenous injections of ergonovine and Methergine on the postpartum patient, Am. J. Obst. & Gynec. 63:640, 1952.

Gold, E. M., et al.: Principles for improving patient care in the hospital labor and delivery suite, J.A.M.A. 146:1459, 1951.

Goodrich, F. W., Jr.: Modern obstetrics

and the nurse, Am. J. Nursing **57**:586, 1957.

——: Natural Childbirth, New York, Prentice-Hall, 1950.

Hamra, M. L.: Congenital dysplasia and dislocation of the hips, Am. J. Nursing **56**:1276, 1956.

Heardman, H.: A Way to Natural Childbirth, Baltimore, Williams & Wilkins, 1948.

Hesseltine, H. C.: Simple, safe and economical cord clamp, Am. J. Obst. & Gynec. **33**:884, 1937.

Hogan, A.: Bomb born babies, Pub. Health Nursing **43**:383, 1951.

Judd, G. E.: Management of labor in reference to prevention of perinatal mortality, J.A.M.A. **156**:1474, 1954.

Kantor, H., and Miller, D.: The urinary bladder during labor, Am. J. Obst. & Gynec. **58**:354, 1949.

Kelley, A. J.: Care of the unmarried mother, Obst. & Gynec. **7**:218, 1956.

La Salvia, L. A., and Steffen, E. A.: Delayed gastric emptying time in labor, Am. J. Obst. & Gynec. **59**:1075, 1950.

Lesser, M. S., and Keane, V. R.: Nurse-Patient Relationships in a Hospital Maternity Service, St. Louis, Mosby, 1956.

Mack, H. C.: Back to Sacajawea, Am. J. Obst. & Gynec. **69**:933, 1955.

Newton, N.: Maternal Emotions, New York, Hoeber, 1955.

Ormsby, H.: Prophylaxis of ophthalmia neonatorum, Am. J. Nursing **57**:1174, 1957.

Owen, R. E., and Denman, L. G.: Experiences in childbirth, Am. J. Nursing **51**:26, 1951.

Prystowsky, H.: Is the danger of vaginal examination in labor overestimated? Am. J. Obst. & Gynec. **68**:639, 1954.

Ratcliff, J. D.: Birth, New York, Dodd, 1951.

——: Surviving the first day, Today's Health, pp. 24-26, Sept., 1952.

Read, G. D.: Childbirth Without Fear (rev.), New York, Harper, 1953.

Roth, L. G.: Natural childbirth in a general hospital, Am. J. Obst. & Gynec. **61**:167, 1951.

Silver nitrate endorsed, Sight-Saving Rev. **25**:101, 1955.

Special Committee on Infant Mortality of Medical Society of the County of New York: Resuscitation of Newborn Infants, Assoc. for Aid of Crippled Children (1956), 1790 Broadway, New York 19, N. Y.

Speck, G.: Childbirth with dignity, Obst. & Gynec. **2**:544, 1953.

Statement of American Academy of Pediatrics: Oxygen for newborn infants, J.A.M.A. **161**:1275, 1956.

Thoms, H.: Training for Childbirth, New York, McGraw-Hill, 1950.

Thoms, H., and Billings, W.: A consideration of childbirth programs, New England J. Med. **552**:860, 1956.

Thoms, H., and Roth, L. G.: Understanding Natural Childbirth, New York, McGraw-Hill, 1950.

Thoms, H., and Wiedenbach, E.: Support during labor, J.A.M.A. **156**:3, 1954.

Van Blarcom, C.: Obstetrical Nursing (rev. by E. Ziegel), ed. 4, New York, Macmillan, 1957.

Wrieden, J.: The unmarried obstetrical patient, Hospitals **30**:26, 1956.

CONFERENCE MATERIAL

1. A mother who is contemplating the delivery of her first child is worried for fear that she may not get her own baby if another infant is born at the same time she is delivered. How would you reassure this mother concerning the identification methods for newborn infants?

2. An 18-year-old mother having her first baby is admitted to the hospital in early labor. It is obvious from her behavior that she has had no preparation for this experience and is frightened and apprehensive. What specific measures would you include in your nursing plan for her care?

3. An unwed mother goes into labor, having made no arrangements for the care of her 2-year-old girl and her 12-year-old boy. What resources could you suggest in this situation? What is the responsibility of hospital and community agencies in this case?

4. How do the public health organizations and hospitals in your community

help the patient and her family to prepare for the delivery?

5. Why is prophylaxis for the eyes of the newborn required by law in most states? How would you go about securing the desired information concerning such legislation in the various states of the United States?

6. How does the use of penicillin compare with the use of silver nitrate in the prophylactic treatment of the eyes of the newborn?

7. You are caring for a mother, having her fourth child, who is in very active labor. Suddenly the membranes rupture and she begins to bear down. As you observe the perineum you see the infant's head crowning. Since you are alone with this mother at the time, what will you do?

8. A 21-year-old mother at term, who has attended "natural childbirth" classes for a previous pregnancy, comes to the hospital on her physician's instructions because her membranes have ruptured. She is apologetic because her contractions are only 10 to 12 minutes apart, of mild intensity, lasting about 35 seconds and "not really good enough yet to come to the hospital." On examination, her cervix is found to be 2 cm. dilated and 10 per cent effaced. Discuss the nursing care you would plan for this mother if she were assigned to your care.

Study Questions

UNIT THREE: NORMAL LABOR

Read through the entire question and place your answer in the parentheses.

1. Give the term or the phrase which best fits each of the following statements:
   A. Enlargement of the external os to 10 cm. in diameter (*dilation*)
   B. Maximum shortening of the cervical canal (*effacement*)
   C. A type of drug used in obstetrics which blots out memory of whatever occurs under its influence (*amnesic*)
   D. A condition caused by failure of the uterine muscle to stay contracted after delivery (*uterine atony*)
   E. A surgical incision of the perineum during second-stage labor (*episiotomy*)
   F. Settling of the baby's head into the brim of the pelvis (*lightening*)

2. The character and the frequency of uterine contractions and the location of the discomfort experienced by the mother during labor often provide pertinent information regarding the labor.

Situation No. 1: In the case of a multipara who is having discomfort but is not in real labor, which of these symptoms would most probably serve to identify false labor contractions?

   A. Discomfort may begin as early as 3 or 4 weeks before the onset of true labor.
   B. Discomfort occurs 3 or 4 days before the onset of true labor.
   C. Contractions occur at regular intervals.
   D. Contractions occur at irregular intervals.
   E. Discomfort is confined to the lower abdomen and the groin.
   F. Discomfort is felt in the upper abdomen and the back.

Select the number corresponding to the correct letter or letters.
   1. A only
   2. A and C
   3. A, C and E
   4. All of them (*3*)

Situation No. 2: In the case of a primigravida in the beginning of the first stage of labor, which of the following symptoms would most probably describe her labor contractions?

   A. Contractions occur at regular intervals.
   B. Contractions occur at irregular intervals.
   C. Discomfort is confined to the lower abdomen and the groin.
   D. Discomfort is located in the lower back and the abdomen.
   E. Contractions occur at intervals of from 2 to 3 minutes.
   F. Contractions occur at intervals of from 10 to 15 minutes.

Select the number corresponding to the correct letters.
   1. A and C
   2. A, D and F
   3. B, C and E
   4. All of them (*2*)

Situation No. 3: In the case of a primigravida approaching the end of the first stage of labor, which of the following symptoms would most probably give an accurate description of her labor?
   A. Contractions occur at regular intervals.
   B. Contractions occur at irregular intervals.
   C. Contractions occur at intervals of every 1 to 1½ minutes.
   D. Contractions occur at intervals of from 2 to 3 minutes.
   E. Duration of contractions is from 45 to 60 seconds.
   F. Duration of contractions is from 50 to 70 seconds.
Select the number corresponding to the correct letters.
   1. A, C and E
   2. A, D and F
   3. B, D and E
   4. All of them   (————)

3. Labor is divided into the first, the second and the third stages.
   A. When is the first stage of labor considered to be terminated?
      1. When contractions occur at 10- to 15-minute intervals
      2. When the cervix is completely dilated
      3. When the baby is delivered   (————)
   B. When is the second stage of labor considered to be terminated?
      1. When the cervix is completely dilated
      2. When contractions occur at 2- to 3-minute intervals
      3. When the baby is delivered   (————)
   C. When is the third stage of labor considered to be terminated?
      1. When the baby is delivered
      2. When the placenta is delivered
      3. After the uterus has remained firm for 1 hour   (————)

4. The nurse is caring for a mother during the first stage of labor. Which of the following observations would she report promptly to the physician?
   A. Small amounts of bright blood in the vaginal discharge
   B. Plugs of blood-streaked mucus in the vaginal discharge
   C. Sudden gush of amniotic fluid from the vagina
   D. Mother has a frequent desire to urinate.
   E. Fetal heart rate slows during uterine contractions but returns to its usual rate 10 to 15 seconds following the contractions.
Select the number corresponding to the correct letters.
   1. A and C
   2. A, C and E
   3. B, D and E
   4. All of them   (————)

5. On admission of the mother to the obstetric department, which of the following procedures are usually carried out routinely?
   A. Check mother's temperature, pulse, respirations and blood pressure.
   B. Take the mother to the bathroom and have her void.
   C. Cleanse and shave the vulvar and perineal area.
   D. Listen to the fetal heart sounds.
   E. Prepare the mother for vaginal examination.

Select the number corresponding to the correct letter or letters.
1. A only
2. A and E
3. A, C and D
4. All of them (——3——)

6. Why is an enema frequently given to a mother during the early part of the first stage of labor?
A. To obtain a stool specimen
B. To avoid straining as the mother bears down with contractions
C. To cleanse the lower bowel and/or stimulate labor contractions (——C——)

7. After the cervix is dilated, and particularly if the membranes have ruptured, what facilities would provide the mother with the greatest degree of comfort and safety to expel an enema?
A. Use of toilet facilities in bathroom
B. Remain in bed and use the bedpan
C. Use the bedpan on a chair close to the bed (——B——)

8. Often it is the nurse's responsibility to decide when the mother is ready to be moved from the labor room to the delivery room. Which of the following signs would signify to the nurse that the time of delivery is near?
A. Mother has a desire to defecate.
B. Increase in frequency, duration and intensity of uterine contractions
C. Mother begins to bear down spontaneously with uterine contractions.
D. Bulging of the perineum
E. Increase in amount of blood-stained mucus from the vagina
Select the number corresponding to the correct letter or letters.
1. D only
2. A, C and E
3. B, D and E
4. All of them (——4——)

9. A physician was busy draining mucus from the mouth of the baby immediately after its birth and asked the nurse to let him know as soon as the placenta seemed to be separated. Which of the following would indicate that it was separated?
A. Gradual descent of the uterus farther into the pelvis
B. Protrusion of several more inches of umbilical cord
C. Uterus becomes more firm and rounded
D. A sudden gush of blood from the vagina
E. Large clots of blood slip out of the vagina
Select the number corresponding to the correct letters.
1. A and C
2. B, C and D
3. B, C and E
4. All of them (——2——)

10. As soon as the physician had clamped and cut the umbilical cord, he handed the infant over to the nurse to care for. Which of the following acts would the nurse perform in the immediate care of the infant?

A. Place the infant so that he lies in a head-down position in a heated crib or resuscitator.
B. Wipe the mucus out of the infant's mouth with sterile gauze.
C. Slap the infant's back and soles of the feet sharply to stimulate crying.
D. Gently remove all vernix caseosa and blood in drying the infant's body with the receiving blanket.
E. "Label" infant with required item of identification as soon as he is transferred to the nursery.
Select the number corresponding to the correct letter or letters.
    1. A only
    2. A and C
    3. B, D and E
    4. All of them   (———1———)

11. After the delivery, the infant is cared for by a nurse in the receiving nursery. The nurse who is caring for the mother during the first hour after the delivery of the placenta would include which of the following in her nursing care plan?
A. Keep the mother warm and out of drafts.
B. Express blood clots if they should accumulate in the uterus.
C. Massage the fundus continuously.
D. Administer ergotrate 0.2 mg. intramuscularly.
E. Check the mother's vital signs at frequent intervals.
Select the number corresponding to the correct letter or letters.
    1. B only
    2. A and C
    3. A, B and E
    4. All of them   (———3———)

12. Possibly the most dangerous stage of labor for the mother is the third stage because of the possibility of postpartal hemorrhage and shock.
A. Because there is a certain amount of blood loss, hemorrhage is said to take place when the loss exceeds what amount of blood?
    1. 100 cc.
    2. 300 cc.
    3. 500 cc.   (———3———)
B. The most common cause of postpartal hemorrhage is atony of the uterus. What is the first thing to do as a preventive measure if the uterus appears to be atonic?
    1. Take a firm grasp on the uterus.
    2. Massage the uterus firmly.
    3. Administer an oxytocic drug.   (———2———)

13. The physician told the nurse to watch a mother during labor for evidence of a prolapsed cord which he feared might occur.
A. When would the nurse consider that a prolapsed cord would be most likely to occur?
    1. During the second stage of labor
    2. In breech presentation
    3. If the presenting part was not engaged in the pelvic brim
    4. If the amniotic sac were intact
    5. If the mother were particularly fatigued   (———3———)

B. If the nurse did suspect the cord to be prolapsed, what position should she put the mother in, with the hope of relieving the pressure on the cord?

1. Knee-chest position
2. Fowler's position
3. The Sims' position
4. A prone position   (————)

C. In addition to changing the mother's position to relieve pressure on the cord, what other measures may the nurse employ if she observes the umbilical cord prolapsed out of the vagina?

1. Immediately wash the cord with warm antiseptic solution and replace in vagina.
2. Cover the cord with a wet sponge.
3. Apply a clamp to the exposed cord and cover with a sterile towel.
4. Keep the cord warm and moist by continuous applications of sterile compresses wrung from warm saline solution.   (————)

D. What are the chief objectives of the emergency care given when prolapsed cord occurs?

1. To prevent cold air from prematurely stimulating respiration while the fetus is in the uterus   (————)
2. To prevent drying of the cord while it is still pulsating
3. To stimulate and restore circulation in the cord by vasodilation
4. To prevent or relieve pressure on the cord   (————)

Note: The key to the correct answers to these questions is given on page 533.

UNIT FOUR

Normal Puerperium

ORIENTATION

The study of the reproductive process developed in the previous chapters should serve as a basis for understanding how the generative organs and the various systems of the human body adapt following the delivery. The nurse must have a knowledge of the anatomic and physiologic changes which normally occur in the puerperium, as well as a basic understanding of the psychological and social influences which affect the mother's condition. Although the mother's needs for physical care are relatively simple, exigency for comprehensive nursing care should provide a real challenge to the nurse. Health guidance is an important part of the nursing care during this period, not only for the mother's immediate comfort and well-being, but also to prepare her for returning home more confident in her ability to resume her role as wife and mother. It should be remembered that during the puerperium the mother is not only adjusting from the experience of pregnancy and labor but also, with the coming of the new baby into the family, she must accommodate to a new scheme of living. The foundation for a wholesome mother-child relationship in the expanding family unit is strengthened when real effort is made to meet each mother's individual needs. The continuity of quality medical supervision and nursing care given during the antepartal and intrapartal phases of childbearing must carry over through the puerperium if maternity care is to be really effective.

CHAPTER THIRTEEN

The Physiology of the Puerperium

DEFINITION

The term puerperium (from *puer,* a child; and *parere,* to bring forth) refers to the 6-week period elapsing between the termination of labor and the return of the reproductive tract to its normal condition. This includes both the *progressive changes* in the breasts for lactation and *involution* of the internal reproductive organs. Although the changes brought about by involution are considered to be normal physiologic processes, they border closely between a condition of health and disease, for under no other circumstances does such marked and rapid involution of tissues occur without a departure from a state of health. For this reason, the quality of the mother's care at this time is essential to ensure her immediate as well as her future health.

ANATOMIC CHANGES

Uterus

Involution of the Uterus. Immediately following the delivery of the placenta, the uterus becomes an almost solid mass of tissue, about the size of a grapefruit. Its thick anterior and posterior walls lie in close opposition, so that the center cavity is flattened. The uterus remains about the same size for the first 2 days after delivery but then rapidly decreases in size by an atrophic process called involution. This is effected partly by the contraction of the uterus and partly by autolytic processes in which some of the protein material of the uterine wall is broken down into simpler components which are then absorbed and eventually cast off through the urine.

THE PROCESS OF INVOLUTION. The separation of the placenta and the membranes from the uterine wall takes place in the outer portion of the spongy layer of the decidua, and, therefore, a remnant of this layer remains in the uterus to be cast off in part in the lochia. Within 2 or 3 days after labor, this remaining portion of decidua becomes differentiated into 2 layers, leaving the deeper or unaltered layer attached to the muscular wall from which the new endometrial lining is generated. The layer adjoining the uterine cavity becomes necrotic and is cast off in the lochia. The process is very like the healing of any surface; there is oozing of blood from the small vessels on this surface. The bleeding from the larger vessels is controlled by compression of the retracted uterine muscle fibers. The process of regeneration is rapid, except at the site of former placental attachment, which requires 6 or 7 weeks to heal completely. Elsewhere, the free surface of the endometrium is restored in half that time.

THE PROGRESS OF INVOLUTION. The normal process of involution requires 5 or 6 weeks, and at the end of that time the uterus regains its normal size, although it never returns exactly to its virgin state. One can realize more fully the rapidity of this process by comparing the changes which occur in the weight of this organ. Immediately following the delivery the uterus weighs approximately 2 pounds; at the end of the first week, 1 pound; at the end of the second week, 12 ounces; and by the time involution is complete it should weigh only about 2 ounces. By observing the height of the fundus, which may be felt through the abdominal wall, the nurse is able to appreciate more fully these remarkable changes. Immediately after the birth of the placenta, the uterus sinks into the pelvis, and the fundus is felt midway between the umbilicus and the symphysis, but it soon rises to the level of the umbilicus (5 or 5½ inches above the pubes); and 12 hours later it probably will be found a little higher. Day-by-day careful measurements will show that it is diminishing in size, so that at the end of 10 days or so it cannot be detected by abdominal palpations. The approximate rate of decrease in the height of the fundus is a little over half an inch or one finger breadth a day. Observation of this rate of involution is very important; the physician will want to be informed about any marked delay, especially if accompanied by suppression of the lochia or retention of clots. In measuring the height of the uterus, care should be taken that the observations are made after the bladder is emptied, as a full bladder will raise the height of the fundus.

Apparent indications that involution is not occurring satisfactorily are: the uterus fails to decrease progressively in size, it remains "flabby" and causes the mother much discomfort (see "Subinvolution," Chap. 20, Complications of the Puerperium).

Changes in the Cervix. After the delivery the cervix is a soft, flabby structure but, because it is retracting, by the end of the first week it becomes so narrow that it would be difficult to introduce anything the size of a finger. Unlike the process of involution which is now occurring in the body of the uterus, a very considerable new formation of muscle cells is taking place in the cervix and, simultaneously, any lacerations are healing. Once a mother has delivered a child vaginally, the cervix does not assume its pregravid appearance, but the external os remains open in varying degrees, although the internal os is closed. This is one of the characteristics of the uterus of a multiparous woman.

The Lochia. A knowledge of the healing process by which the lining of the uterus becomes regenerated is a valuable adjunct to the nurse in understanding and interpreting the lochial discharge. At first the discharge consists almost entirely of blood with a small amount of mucus, particles of decidua and cellular debris which escape from the placental site. It should not contain large clots or membrane or be excessive in amount. This discharge lasts about 3 days and is called *lochia rubra*. As the oozing of blood from the healing surface diminishes, the discharge becomes more serous or watery and gradually changes to a pinkish color, the so-called *lochia serosa*. Toward the tenth day the lochia is thinner, greatly decreased in amount and almost colorless, the so-called *lochia alba*. By the end of the third week the discharge usually disappears, though a brownish mucoid discharge may persist a little longer. Lochia possesses a peculiar animal emanation which is quite characteristic and should never, at any time, have an offensive odor.

The quantity of lochia varies with individuals, but, generally speaking, it is more profuse in multiparas. It is to be expected that when a mother is out of bed for the first time there may be a definite increase in the amount of discharge. Nevertheless, the recurrence of fresh bleeding after the discharge has become dark and diminished in amount, or the persistence of bright blood in the lochia or the suppression of the discharge (which may be caused by cold, fright, grief or other emotion) should be reported to the obstetrician. The daily observation of the amount and the character of the lochia is of greatest importance as an index of the progress of healing of the endometrial surface.

The Pelvis

The vaginal walls, the vulva and all other tissues which have become hypertrophied during pregnancy also undergo a process of involution in their return to normal. The *vagina* requires some time to recover from the distention brought about by the delivery. This capacious passage gradually diminishes in size, although rarely returns to its nulliparous condition. The *labia majora* and the *labia minora* become flabby and atrophic as compared with their condition before childbearing. Any abrasions and lacerations of the genital canal caused by the passage of the fetus should heal completely during the puerperium. The *ligaments* which support the uterus, the ovaries and the tubes which have also undergone great tension and stretching are now relaxed and will take considerable time to return almost to their normal size and position. This is one of the reasons why the mother must be given intelligent interpretation of early ambulation.

Abdominal Wall

The abdominal wall recovers partially from the overstretching but remains soft and flabby for some time. The striae, due to the rupture of the elastic fibers of the cutis, usually remain but become less conspicuous because of their silvery appearance. The process of involution in the abdominal structures requires at least 6 weeks. Provided that the abdominal walls have retained their muscle tone, they gradually return to their original condition. However, if these muscles are relaxed because they have lost their tone, there may be a marked separation or *diastasis of the recti muscles,* so that the abdominal organs are not properly supported. Rest, diet, prescribed exercises, good body mechanics and good posture may do much to restore the tonicity of these muscles.

The Breasts

The changes which occurred in the breasts during pregnancy (see Chap. 6) continue much the same for the first 2 days after the infant is born. The breasts secrete a small amount of thin yellowish fluid called *colostrum,* which when taken by the infant acts as a cathartic. The nutritive value of colostrum in comparison with normal mother's milk is low. Colostrum contains more protein material and salts, less fat and has about the same sugar content as human milk. Breast feeding in these first days helps to stimulate lactation and fulfills the infant's need for sucking.

On the third or fourth day after the delivery, the nurse will observe a change in color of the secretion from the nipples, as it becomes bluish-white, the normal color of human milk. At this time the breasts suddenly become larger, firmer and more tender as the lacteal secretion is established, and the mother experiences throbbing pains in the breasts which may extend into the axillae. This congestion, which usually subsides in a day or two, is caused not only by the pressure from the increased amount of milk in the lobes and the ducts but also from increased circulation of blood and lymph in the breast gland, producing a tension on the very sensitive surrounding tissues. Secretion of breast milk is definitely stimulated by the infant's sucking, and without this stimulation the secretion will not continue for more than a few days.

Breast milk varies markedly in its quality and quantity, not only in different individuals, but also in the same individual at various times. This is dependent on several factors, such as the mother's diet, the amount of exercise she gets and her mental and emotional condition (Chaps. 8 and 15). Also, certain drugs not only exert a pronounced influence on the milk flow (e.g., belladonna diminishes it) but also they are excreted in the milk in sufficient quantities to have a marked effect on the infant. The latter is particularly true if the mother is taking large doses of drugs such as salicylates, certain cathartics, iodides, bromides, quinine, atropine, opium, etc.

CLINICAL ASPECTS

Temperature

Slight rises in temperature may occur without apparent cause following the delivery, but, generally speaking, the mother's temperature should remain within normal limits during the puerperium, that is, below 38° C. (100.4° F.) when taken by mouth. Any mother whose temperature exceeds this limit in any two consecutive 24-hour periods of the puerperium (excluding the first 24 hours postpartum) is considered to be febrile.

It was formerly believed that an elevation of temperature naturally occurred with the establishment of lactation on the third or fourth day after the delivery, and the so-called *milk-fever* was considered to be a normal accompaniment of this process. At the present time this is considered to be a fallacy. On rare occasions, a sharp peak of fever for several hours may be caused by extreme vascular and lymphatic engorgement of the breasts, but this does not last longer than 12 hours at the most.

In judging the significance of a rise in temperature, the pulse rate provides a helpful guide, for in a puerperal patient with a slow pulse, a slightly elevated temperature is not likely to signify a complication. Nevertheless, any rise of temperature in the puerperium should excite the suspicion of endometritis (see Chap. 20, Complications of the Puerperium).

Pulse

In the early puerperium a pulse rate which is somewhat slower than at other times is a favorable symptom. The rate usually averages between 60 and 70 but may even become a little slower than this a day or two after the delivery. This is merely a transient phenomenon, so that by the end of the first week or 10 days the pulse returns to its normal rate. On the other hand, a rapid pulse after labor, unless the mother has cardiac disease, may be an indication of shock or hemorrhage.

Blood

Most of the blood and metabolic alterations characteristic of normal pregnancy disappear within the first 2 weeks of the puerperium.

After-pains

Normally, after the delivery of the first child, the uterine muscle tends to remain in a state of tonic contraction and retraction. But if the uterus has been subjected to any marked distention, or if blood clots or tissue have been retained in the cavity, then active contractions occur in an effort to expel them, and these contractions may be painful. In multiparas, a certain amount of the initial tonicity of the uterine muscle has been lost, and these contractions and retractions cannot be sustained. Consequently, the muscle contracts and relaxes at intervals, and these contractions give rise to the sensation of pain, the so-called "after-pains." These after-pains are more noticeable after a pregnancy in which the uterus has been greatly distended, as with multiple births or hydramnios. They are particularly noticeable in the breast-feeding mother, when the infant is put to breast (because sucking stimulates the uterus to contract), and may last for days, although ordinarily they become quite bearable in about 48 hours after delivery. Often after-pains become so sharp that the administration of a sedative is necessary. Any time they are severe enough to disturb the mother's rest and peace of mind, the physician should be notified.

Digestion

Although the mother's appetite may be diminished the first few days after labor, the digestive tract functions normally in the puerperium. Her thirst is considerably increased at this time due to the marked diaphoresis and loss of fluids associated with the puerperium. Moreover, the fact that the mother has probably gone without fluids for some hours in labor undoubtedly increases her thirst.

Loss of Weight

In addition to the 10- or 11-pound loss of weight which results at delivery, there is generally a still further loss of about 5 pounds of body weight during the puerperium due to the marked increase in excretions.

Kidneys

The amount of urine excreted by the kidneys in the puerperium is of particular significance. As previously stated, during pregnancy there is an increased tendency of the body to retain water, so that now the tremendous output of urine represents the body's effort to return its water metabolism to normal. Diuresis regularly occurs between the second and fifth days after delivery, sometimes reaching a daily output of 3,000 cc. After the delivery, in particular, the bladder may distend without any awareness on the part of the mother, especially if she has received any form of analgesia. Therefore, it becomes a major responsibility of the nurse to be alert to signs of a full bladder and thus prevent distention from occurring.

During the first few days after labor there may be a marked increase in the amount of acetone and nitrogen in the urine. The acetone is due to an excessive breakdown of carbohydrate resulting from the increased muscular activity in labor, while, on the other hand, the nitrogen excretion is due to the breakdown of protein material of the uterine wall in the process of involution, as previously mentioned. Occasionally, during the first weeks of the puerperium the urine contains substantial amounts of sugar which has no relationship with diabetes but is due to the presence of lactose, milk sugar, which is absorbed from the mammary glands.

Intestinal Elimination

The mother is nearly always constipated during the first few days of the puerperium. This is due to the relaxed condition of the intestinal and the abdominal muscles, in particular, and to the inability of the abdominal wall to aid in the evacuation of the intestinal contents. In addition, if hemorrhoids are present the mother is often afraid to have a stool because of the discomfort these varicosities cause during elimination.

Skin

It is to be expected that elimination of waste products via the skin is accelerated in the early puerperium, often to such a degree that the mother is drenched with perspiration. These episodes of profuse sweating, which frequently occur in the night, gradually subside and do not require any specific treatment aside from protecting the mother from chilling at such times as they occur.

Menstruation

If the mother does not breast feed her infant, the menstrual flow probably will return within 8 weeks after delivery. Ordinarily, menstruation does not occur so long as the mother is breast feeding, but this is not a certainty. During lactation the first menstrual period may occur as early as the second month but usually occurs about the fourth month following the delivery. It has been known not to reappear until as late as the 18th month. Studies have shown that failure to menstruate during lactation is due to suppression of ovulation, but, since some mothers have been known to become pregnant in the course of breast feeding an infant, we know that this is not always the case.

POSTPARTAL EXAMINATIONS

The condition of the mother is confirmed before she is discharged from the hospital to make sure that her progress has been satisfactory during the early puerperium. In addition to verifying her vital signs and present weight, observations are made to determine the condition of her breasts, the progress of involution and the healing of the perineal wound. A pelvic examination is deferred, since findings made by palpation of the uterus and inspection of the lochia will give satisfactory evidence as to the progress of involution at this time.

Follow-up Examinations

As has been mentioned previously, the reproductive tract should return to its normal condition by the end of the puerperium. In order to investigate the general physical condition of the mother and determine with what normalcy she has completed her maternity experience, she should return to her physician for examination about 6 weeks postpartum. During the visit the weight and the blood pressure are taken, the urine is examined for albumin and a blood count may be done. The condition of the abdominal walls is observed, and the breasts are inspected. If the mother is breast feeding, the condition of the nipples and the degree of lacteal secretion

are a significant part of the observation. A thorough pelvic examination is carried out to investigate the position of the uterus, the healing of perineal wounds, the support of the pelvic floor and whether involution is complete. In addition, this return examination provides an opportunity for the mother and the obstetrician to discuss any other problems relating to this maternity experience. If abnormalities are found, they may be treated at this time and arrangements made for further examinations and treatments as necessary. Regardless, most physicians instruct their patients to return in 6 months for a check-up examination. Many encourage the mothers to return for a check-up again at the end of one year.

SUGGESTED READING

Beck, A. C., and Rosenthal, A.: Obstetrical Practice, ed. 6, Baltimore, Williams & Wilkins, 1955.

Eastman, N. J.: Williams Obstetrics, ed. 11, New York, Appleton, 1956.

Fleming, A. R.: Prophylaxis of postpartum urinary retention, Am. J. Obst. & Gynec. 64:134, 1952.

Gioiosa, R.: Incidence of pregnancy during lactation in 500 cases, Am. J. Obst. & Gynec. 70:162, 1955.

Greenhill, J. P.: Obstetrics, ed. 11, Philadelphia, Saunders, 1955.

Lull, C., and Kimbrough, R.: Clinical Obstetrics, Philadelphia, Lippincott, 1953.

Naish, F. C.: Breast Feeding, ed. 2, London, Lloyd Luke, 1956.

Nickerson, K., et al.: Oxytocin and milk ejection, Am. J. Obst. & Gynec. 67: 1028, 1954.

Udesky, I. C.: Ovulation in lactating women, Am. J. Obst. & Gynec. 59: 843, 1950.

CHAPTER FOURTEEN

Nursing Care During the Puerperium

INTRODUCTION

Changes brought about in the medical management of the puerperium in the last decade have brought about corresponding changes in this phase of nursing care. These changes have redirected the emphasis and given new significance to what heretofore was considered rather routine nursing. The care of the patient during the postpartal period is very important and presents a real challenge to the nurse. The newly delivered mother is a healthy patient who is adjusting physically and emotionally from the experience of pregnancy and labor. In addition, with the arrival of the infant, she must adapt to a new family structure. Her needs for physical care have been greatly modified because of two important developments, namely, the advent of early ambulation following the delivery and the subsequent evolvement of more simplified obstetric nursing procedures. In the hospital the nurse may not necessarily have the responsibility for both the mother and her new baby; nevertheless, the infant must be considered in relation to the mother's care.

REACTION TO DELIVERY

Immediately after labor, the mother experiences a sense of complete fatigue which is comparable to that which would normally follow the exertion of any strenuous muscular activity. At the same time, if she has been awake during the delivery of her infant, she may be so exhilarated by the experience and the feeling of relief which accompanies it that she is not aware of being exhausted. She is interested in seeing and holding her baby and visiting with her husband. Although this first visit of the family together may be rather brief, it is an experience which is particularly gratifying to the parents. Following this, every effort should be made to help the mother to rest, and with little encouragement she usually passes off into a sound natural sleep. The discomforts which may interfere with sleep, such as soreness of the vulva, hemorrhoids, "after-pains," etc., should be mitigated as much as possible.

Many mothers complain of feeling chilled immediately after labor; a few even appear to have a shaking chill. Such chills may be due in part to nervous reaction and exhaustion. There is some disturbance of equilibrium between internal and external temperature caused by excessive perspiration during the muscular exertion of labor. Some authorities believe that the "chill" may be due partly to the sudden release of intra-abdominal pressure which results as the uterus is emptied at delivery. This reaction may be avoided if the mother is made comfortable in a warm bed and given a cup of hot tea, if it is permissible. If her body does begin to quiver, an extra cotton blanket should be placed over her or tucked close around her body for comfort. Many mothers are frightened or disturbed by this, so the nurse must reassure her patient that this is not an unusual occurrence following delivery.

IMMEDIATE CARE

Intelligent interpretation of the condition of the uterus is essential to the mother's safety and welfare. Although she must be observed carefully for bleeding during the first 6 hours after labor, this observation is most important in the first hour after the delivery of the placenta. Considerable information can be gained by palpating the fundus through the abdominal wall to be assured that the uterus remains firm, round and well

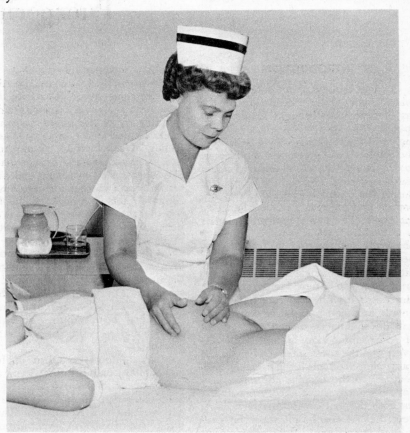

Fig. 180. Nurse palpating fundus of uterus in puerperium. If the uterus is atonic, massage until firm and well-contracted. Then, blood which has collected in the cavity should be expressed with firm but gentle force in the direction of the outlet.

contracted. At the same time it is also important to inspect the perineal pad for obvious signs of bleeding, as well as to take the pulse and the blood pressure. During the first hour these observations should be made at least every 15 minutes, or more often if indicated. In some hospitals it is customary to have a nurse (or a properly prepared nurse's aide) sit at the bedside during this hour, with her hand on the mother's abdomen so that she can feel the fundus constantly. So long as the bleeding is minimal and the uterus remains firm, well-contracted and does not increase in size, it is neither necessary nor desirable to stimulate it. However, if the uterus becomes soft and boggy because of relaxation, the fundus should be massaged immediately until it becomes contracted again. This can be best accomplished if one hand is placed just above the symphysis pubis to act as a guard, as the other hand is cupped around the fundus and rotated gently. It should be remembered that the uterus is a sensitive organ which, under normal circumstances, responds quickly to tactile stimulation. Care must be taken to avoid overmassage, because, in addition to causing the mother considerable pain, this may stimulate premature uterine contractions and thereby cause undue muscle fatigue. Such a condition would further encourage uterine relaxation and hemorrhage. If the uterus is atonic, blood which collects in the cavity should be expressed with firm but gentle force in the direction of the outlet, but only after the fundus has been first massaged (Fig. 180). Failure to see that the uterus is contracted before pushing downward against it could result in inversion of the uterus, an exceedingly serious complication.

During the first hour the mother should be kept clean, dry and comfortable but allowed to rest as much as possible. At the end of this hour it is usually customary to give the mother a partial bath as necessary and take the tempera-ture, in addition to other vital signs, before transferring her to the postpartal division. The nurse must be constantly alert for any changes in the mother's condition, such as her color, character of the pulse, respirations and blood pressure, the status of the fundus and the amount of vaginal bleeding.

DAILY ROUTINE

The daily routine procedures for the postpartal patient vary in different hospitals, but the principles of care are essentially the same. Certain observations should be made and recorded daily. These would include such findings as temperature, pulse and respirations; urinary and intestinal elimination; the physical changes which occur normally in the puerperium. One should note the changes in the breasts, the height of the fundus, the character, the amount and the color of the lochial discharge and the condition of the episiotomy (see Chap. 13). Furthermore, it is equally important for the nurse to be alert to the mother's general comfort and well-being —how she rests and sleeps, her activity, her appetite, and, particularly, because of its vast influence, how she is adjusting to her role as a new mother.

GENERAL CARE

Temperature, Pulse and Respirations

The temperature should be carefully watched during the first 2 weeks of the puerperium, as fever is usually the first symptom of an infectious process. And, as has been stated previously, the pulse rate provides a helpful guide in determining the significance of a rise in temperature. These observations are usually made and recorded every 4 hours for the first few days after delivery, omitting the 2 A.M. observations which would disturb the mother's sleep. Thereafter, they are made every night and morning, so long as the mother is progressing normally. If the temperature rises above 37.8° C. (100° F.) or the pulse rate above 100, the physician should be notified immediately.

Nutrition

Very shortly following the delivery, after having gone without food or fluids for some hours, the mother may express a desire for something to eat. When food is put before her, however, she usually has little appetite. Unless she has received a general anesthetic or is nauseated, there is usually no contraindication to giving her some nourishment. However, it is prudent to give her small amounts of easily digested foods such as milk or tea and toast for this first meal. Thereafter, she may be given a normal diet.

The two factors which the nurse must bear in mind when considering the mother's diet are (1) providing for her general nutrition and (2) providing enough nourishing foods to supply the additional calories and nutrients required during lactation. If these nutritional requirements are provided for, the mother's convalescence will be more rapid, her strength will be recovered more quickly, and the quality and quantity of her milk will be better. She will also be more able to resist infections.

The daily diet of the lactating mother should be like that taken during pregnancy, with the addition of 1,000 calories and amounts of the various nutrients (protein, calcium, iron, vitamin A, thiamine, riboflavin, niacin and ascorbic acid) as recommended by the Food and Nutrition Board of the National Research Council* (see Chap. 8, Antepartal Care). These increased demands in the diet during lactation can be supplied with the addition of a pint of milk, one serving of vegetable and one of citrus fruit, an egg and one large serving of meat. Foods which the mother knows

* Recommended Dietary Allowances, Rev. 1958, Publication 589, National Academy of Sciences, National Research Council, Washington, D. C.

from experience disagree with her should be avoided; but the old belief that certains foods eaten by the mother will cause colic in her infant is now discredited. However, as previously stated in Chapter 13, certain drugs may be excreted in the mother's milk in sufficient quantity to affect the breast-fed infant.

Mothers who are breast feeding their infants usually have good appetites and become hungry between meals. For this reason it is advisable to see that they receive intermediate nourishment in the form of a glass of milk 3 times a day, which also helps to incorporate the additional milk into the diet.

Rest and Sleep

During the puerperium the mother needs an abundance of rest and should be encouraged to relax and sleep whenever possible. This can best be accomplished if she is comfortable and free from worry and other anxiety-producing situations. The need for rest has even more significance for the mother who is breast feeding, because worry and fatigue inhibit her milk supply. With the exception of the husband, visitors should be limited during the first week or so because they can be tiring. A mother who is not getting sufficient rest is usually anxious and worries over minor things which otherwise might cause her little concern. Furthermore, many emotional problems are often precipitated by sleeplessness and fatigue.

Early Ambulation

Although early ambulation of the so-called "normal" mother had its inception out of necessity during World War II, experience with this aspect of management of the puerperium has shown that it possesses certain intrinsic advantages to the mother, and as a result it is almost generally accepted as routine practice today. The mothers seems to get their strength back more quickly and appear to be stronger on the fifth or sixth day than they used to be at the time of discharge under the old regimen. This is proved by multiparas who were kept on bed rest for 7 to 14 days following previous deliveries who state that they feel better and stronger with early ambulation. With this increase in exercise for the newly delivered mother, her circulation is stimulated, and there are fewer complications of thrombophlebitis. Moreover, bladder and bowel function are improved, with the result that bladder complications leading to catheterization are greatly reduced. Abdominal distention and constipation occur less frequently.

The majority of healthy mothers are allowed out of bed in 24 to 48 hours, some as early as 8 hours after delivery. The first time out of bed the mother usually walks a few steps from the bed and sits in a chair for a brief period. On succeeding times up, her activity is increased gradually. The newly delivered mother needs someone to assist her in and out of bed and to go with her when she walks to the bathroom. The nurse should remain close at hand while the mother is in the bathroom so that she can give immediate assistance if the mother becomes weak or faint.

It is important that the nurse explain the purposes of early ambulation to the mother and help her to learn how she can achieve an effective combination of sitting, walking and lying in bed. All too many mothers feel that once they are out of bed they are "on their own" and expected to take care of themselves entirely. Most of them are afraid of being a nuisance and hesitate to ask for help, while others do not realize that help is available. The nurse's attitude is important, for if she acts friendly and interested in the mother, demonstrates a desire to help her and makes her feel comfortable, the mother is more likely to ask for help. New mothers, in particular, are sensitive to the attitudes of those responsible for their care. Many of them are experiencing an enforced dependency for the first time in their adult lives and find this difficult. Others become resentful because they feel that they are being forced toward independence too quickly. It is only as the nurse recognizes each patient as an individual that she is able to gain insight in providing for the mother's total nursing needs.

Although it is customary for mothers to be discharged home on the sixth or seventh day, and in some instances as early as the third or fourth, it should be remembered that early ambulation and the duration of hospital stay are two entirely different matters. Regardless of the day of discharge, mothers should be cautioned to proceed slowly at home during the puerperium, resting a large part of the time. If teaching about "getting back to routine gradually" was begun early in the antepartal period, the mother will be better prepared.

The Bath

As previously mentioned, the mother is prone to have marked diaphoresis in the early puerperium, so that she will find the daily bath refreshing and a source of comfort. The first complete bed bath after delivery should be given by the nurse, even if the mother has already been allowed out of bed for a brief period. This not only conserves a considerable amount of the mother's energy but permits the nurse on the postpartal division, who may be caring for the mother for the first time, to have an opportunity to make certain observations. If the mother is not fatigued, this is an opportune time also to include a considerable amount of health teaching. The nurse will be guided in her teaching by the "readiness" of the mother to learn and should remember that she can absorb only so much information at one time. In addition to answering specific questions asked by the mother, the nurse might include information about breast care, perineal hygiene, elimination, general activity and hospital routines.

After the first bath the mother usually

is able to bathe herself but, nevertheless, should be given help as necessary. Shower baths are frequently permitted after the second or third postpartal day if such facilities are available. The first time or two the mother takes a shower, the nurse, or attendant, should remain with her for safety.

Urinary Elimination

The newly delivered mother does not usually express a desire to void, in part because the bladder capacity is now increased as a result of reduced interabdominal pressure. In addition, if the mother has received analgesia or anesthesia during labor, sensation of a full bladder may be further diminished. The mother should be encouraged to void within the first 6 to 8 hours following the delivery. It is not prudent, however, to adhere to a designated lapse of time to indicate when the mother should empty her bladder, but rather on evidence indicating the degree of bladder distention. It should be kept in mind that there is an increased urinary output during the early puerperium. Moreover, mothers who have received intravenous fluids, or who are having them, are very likely to develop a full bladder. As the bladder fills with urine it gradually protrudes above the symphysis pubis and can be observed bulging in front of the uterus. If the bladder is markedly distended, the uterus may be pushed upward and to the side and may be somewhat relaxed. When a hand is cupped over the fundus to massage it and to bring the uterus back to its midline position, the bladder will protrude still further. When the hand is removed, the uterus will return to its displaced position. Further evidence of bladder distention can be gained by palpation and percussion of the lower abdomen, which will reveal a difference in consistency between the uterus and the bladder. Such observations are of extreme importance and demand immediate attention, first, because a full bladder is considered one of the causes of postpartal

hemorrhage, and, second, because if the bladder is permitted to become distended, urinary retention will follow inevitably.

Some mothers have difficulty in voiding at first. As a result of the labor itself, the tone of the bladder wall may be temporarily impaired or the tissues at the base of the bladder and around the urethra may be edematous. Often the patient's inability to void is due to the fact that she is not accustomed to using the bedpan and would have this same difficulty using one any time. If the mother is allowed early bathroom privileges, urinary elimination may present no problem. On the other hand, some efforts may be needed to excite normal urination. First of all, a positive approach, asking the mother, "Will you try . . ." rather than suggesting, "Do you feel as if you want to . . ." is often helpful to get the mother to void. Also, making her feel at ease by helping her to assume a comfortable position, providing privacy and giving her assurance will help to avoid building up tensions which might further inhibit normal urination.

The nurse should offer the mother a bedpan at intervals of 2 to 3 hours at first and measure the urine at each voiding during the first few days until it has been established that the mother is emptying her bladder completely. A voiding must measure 100 cc. to be considered satisfactory. At the first attempt the mother may void a small amount of urine and obviously not empty her bladder. If the bladder is not distended she may be allowed to wait an hour or so before trying again to empty it, because then she may do so. But if she continues to void in small amounts at frequent intervals, one may suspect that she has a residual urine, and thus these voidings are merely the overflow of a distended bladder. Every effort should be made to encourage the mother to void in sufficient amount so that catheterization will not have to be resorted to, but any time she is unable to do so and there is evidence of bladder distention, she should be catheterized immediately.

Catheterization. Although the procedure for catheterization varies to some degree in different hospitals, the principles involved are essentially the same. Aseptic technic must be maintained throughout in order to avoid introducing bacteria into the bladder or contaminating the birth canal. If the mother is given routine perineal care prior to beginning the catheterization procedure, the potential danger of infection is further reduced.

Because there is a certain amount of soreness of the external genitalia, the nurse should proceed with extreme gentleness. As the labia are separated to expose the vestibule, care should be exercised to prevent pulling on the perineal sutures. Then, as the urinary meatus and surrounding area is cleansed prior to the insertion of the catheter, the nurse should proceed gently, but remember all the while that a certain degree of friction is necessary for proper cleansing of the area. None of the cleansing solution should be permitted to run into the vaginal orifice because of the danger of contaminating the birth canal. Immediately following the cleansing, a dry cotton ball should be placed at the introitus to prevent excretions from the vagina, i.e., blood or lochia, from spreading upward to the urinary meatus from whence it can be carried into the bladder when the catheter is inserted.

Intestinal Elimination

In view of the sluggishness of the bowels in the puerperium, constipation is a problem which can be anticipated unless certain measures are instituted to prevent it. While obstetricians' orders vary, it is common to give a laxative or mild cathartic on the evening of the second day following delivery. If a bowel evacuation has not occurred by the morning of the third day, a soapsuds enema may be prescribed. Where there has been no elimination for several days, especially if the mother has had more

extensive perineal repair done, an oil retention enema followed some hours later by a soapsuds enema sometimes is ordered.

Certain laxatives are excreted in breast milk and therefore affect the infant. The mother who is breast feeding should be advised to follow her physician's prescription if laxatives should need to be used to encourage proper elimination after the mother is discharged from the hospital. In addition, the usual measures employed to encourage good bowel habits, i.e., adequate fluid intake, roughage foods in the diet, establishing a habit time, etc., should be included in the health teaching.

SPECIAL PROCEDURES

Throughout the care of the obstetric patient, emphasis has been directed to the prevention of infection by application of principles of antiseptic and aseptic technics. In view of this, the special procedures employed in the care of the mother during the puerperium should be planned so that individual care technic can be maintained whenever possible. Each mother should have her own equipment for breast care, perineal care, etc., and her equipment should be kept in a designated place separate from her neighbor's. Supplies needed in relation to handling and feeding her infant should be kept on a small tray at the mother's bedside. Individual equipment for perineal care likewise should be kept in a convenient place. This is facilitated in hospitals where the physical plan of the postpartal unit provides a bathroom adjoining each room, in which separate shelves are provided for each mother's equipment and supplies. Such practices are important in the over-all effort to prevent cross contamination.

Breast Care

The care of the breasts during pregnancy has been discussed in Chapter 8, Antepartal Care. Although some aspects differ after the delivery, depending on

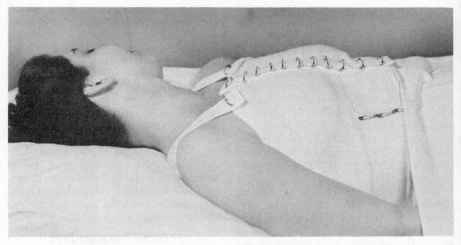

Fig. 181. Breast binder made from straight binder, 10 inches wide. Shoulder straps are attached. (MacDonald House, University Hospitals of Cleveland)

whether or not the mother is breast feeding, the principles of good breast hygiene continue to be of primary importance.

The routine care is directed to maintain cleanliness and adequate breast support necessary for the normal function of the breasts and the comfort of the mother. Precautions should always be exercised to handle the breasts gently, above all to avoid rough rubbing, massage or pressure on these organs. The breasts should be bathed daily with a mild soap and water, with particular attention given to cleansing the nipples first. This can be done most conveniently at the time of the morning bath, but, because the breasts must be protected from all sources of contamination, they should be bathed with a clean washcloth and towel before any other part of the body is washed. To protect them further, they should be covered with a breast towel as soon as they are dried. The nurse has an excellent opportunity for health teaching about postpartal care of the breasts while she is giving the mother her first bath after the delivery.

Some kind of breast support should be worn 24 hours a day after delivery.

Various types of binders or brassières may be used as long as they support the entire breast in the natural position. When a breast is well supported it is not only more comfortable, but also, if pendulous, proper support aids in preventing congestion caused by interference with circulation (Fig. 181). Following the delivery, the breasts are soft, but by the third or fourth postpartal day, as milk replaces colostrum in the breasts, they become heavier, firmer and more tender. The mother may experience throbbing pains in her breasts, which extend back into the axillae. During this time, analgesic medication may be required for pain relief until the congestion subsides in a day or two. Even the mother who is breast feeding experiences temporary discomfort when the breasts become full.

The mother who is breast feeding should wear a binder or brassière not only for support of the breasts but also to ensure further cleanliness. Since the milk secretion is likely to leak from the nipples, they should be directly covered with breast squares, such as sterile 4 x 4 gauze dressings. During the mother's hospital stay she may wear a binder which is convenient for breast feeding (such as the bikini), unless her breasts are pendulous. Heavy breasts require the additional support afforded by the more conventional type breast binder (see Fig. 181). Many mothers prefer to wear a nursing brassière even before the milk comes in. But regardless of which one is used, it should provide uplift support and be well fitted so that it is not too tight and avoids undue pressure on the nipples.

Drying Up the Breasts. The breasts fill with milk initially, whether or not the mother is going to suckle her infant. In the event that she is not going to breast feed, the physician will prescribe orders accordingly. The restriction of fluid intake is believed to lessen the secretion of breast milk, but this should be limited only to such a degree that the mother receives sufficient quantity of fluids to meet normal physiologic requirements of the body. The breasts may become more or less engorged in the course of 24 hours and sometimes so painful that analgesic medication is required. At this time the breasts should not be emptied by pumping or manual expression. Although this gives some temporary relief, it only stimulates further production of breast milk. Furthermore, in the process of engorgement, the vessels within the breast are so compressed that secretory activity is inhibited; thus engorgement subsides, and in a day or two the breasts are soft and painless. On each succeeding day secretion diminishes, and in the course of a week it has practically disappeared.

If a tight breast binder is ordered, it should be applied before the milk "comes in." This binder should fit snugly but not to the extent that it in itself causes discomfort. The mother can assist by supporting her breasts in the normal position while the binder is being applied. And, to encourage uplift support, the binder should be pinned from the bottom up.

The application of ice caps to the breasts may contribute to the mother's comfort when the breasts are full and tender. These should be used on an alternating schedule, i.e., one hour on and one hour off and never used continuously.

Some physicians prescribe various hormones, especially estrogen, to inhibit lactation, although the consensus today is that symptomatic treatment is preferable. One of the disadvantages of prolonged estrogen therapy is that it interferes with regeneration of the endometrium and may cause irregular bleeding. The nurse will observe, for instance, that after the mother has received a course of stilbestrol, the lochial discharge is heavier and contains a greater proportion of bright red blood.

Care of the Nipples. Too much emphasis cannot be placed on "preventive" measures in the care of the nipples to facilitate breast feeding. Cleanliness is a cardinal principle because crustations from dried milk are likely to accumulate and irritate the nipples. Thus, keeping the nipples clean and dry is basic to keeping them in good condition.

Sore nipples are a frequent "complaint" during the mother's early breast-feeding experience, so she should be instructed to report any discomfort in order that corrective measures may be instituted at once. This may result in part from improper methods of breast feeding, even though the nipples are otherwise well cared for (see "Breast Feeding," Chap. 15). They are best treated after each nursing period with the application of a bland cream or ointment, such as lanolin or one of the commercially prepared compounds, e.g., Massé Nipple Cream or Vitamin A and D Ointment. Painting the nipples with tincture of benzoin or alcohol has long been used to toughen tender nipples, but this has a tendency to dry the skin and therefore is less desirable. Many hospitals are now advocating the use of a thermalite (therapeutic) lamp for tender or cracked nipples; the affected breast is exposed for from 20 to 30 minutes twice a day. The mother should be

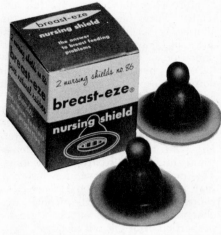

Fig. 182. Nursing shield. In the treatment of sore or cracked nipples this soft, natural rubber shield may be used for their protection during the nursing periods. (The Pyramid Rubber Company, Ravenna, Ohio)

advised that even the exposure of the breast to fresh air for similar periods is beneficial, because this is a measure she may resort to after she returns home.

When a sore nipple is examined it may be found to be fissured (cracked) or to have a small erosion (raw area). The primary treatment for either condition is rest, in order to avoid further irritation and to allow time for healing. In the majority of cases a nipple shield (Fig. 182) may be used for protection so that the infant may continue to nurse. But, if there is any bleeding from the fissure or erosion, all nursing should be discontinued. Under such conditions, manual expression should be instituted to empty the breast, not only to continue to stimulate lactation, but also to relieve engorgement. The nurse should make every effort to recognize the early symptoms of "cracked nipples" so that further problems can be avoided. These raw areas afford an easy portal of entry for pathogenic bacteria to gain access to the

breast and cause mastitis. Abscess of the breast is very painful and often disastrous. Not only does it result in the immediate suspension of breast feeding but it also may prevent the suckling of future babies (see Chap. 20, Complications of the Puerperium).

Expression of Milk. There are some instances when the mother is desirous of breast feeding, but for certain reasons the infant cannot be "put to breast." There are also situations in which the breast-fed infant is not able to empty the breast completely (see "Breast Feeding," Chap. 15). At such times it becomes necessary to utilize artificial means to empty the breasts of milk, otherwise, if this is allowed to persist for several days, lacteal secretion is inhibited and the future milk supply may be jeopardized.

The hands of the person expressing the milk should be washed thoroughly with warm water and soap and dried on a clean towel. Since the daily care of the breasts is designed to maintain cleanliness, the initial cleansing of the nipple for this procedure is the same as that required before putting the infant to breast, i.e., wiping the nipple and the aerola with a sterile water-moistened cotton pledget.

MANUAL EXPRESSION. This can be done by the nurse, but it is preferable to teach the mother how to carry out this procedure while she is in the hospital. In this way she can have guided practice under the supervision of the hospital nurse, so that when she has to do it after she returns home, her confidence and ability will be increased.

A sterile glass or wide-mouthed container should be in readiness before beginning, and if the milk is to be fed to the infant, a sterile bottle and cup also will be needed. It may be desirable first to massage the breast for a few seconds to stimulate the flow of milk, and in such instance it is helpful to lubricate the hands with a drop of mineral oil.

Breast massage should be done with a gliding movement of the hands. The pressure exerted should be firm, even and, above all, gentle. First, place one hand on top of the other above the breast, then as they are drawn apart turn the fingers downward and encircle the breast. As the hands sweep forward toward the areola they should cup the breast, drawing it forward and upward,

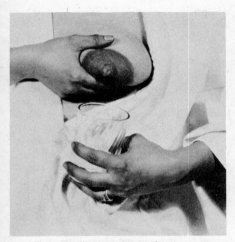

Fig. 183. First position in the expression of breast milk from a large, pendent breast, showing the thumb and fingers properly placed and pressing backward.

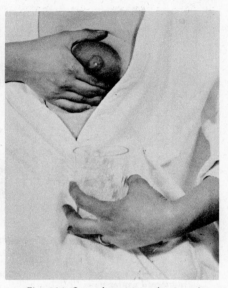

Fig. 184. Second position, showing the thumb and finger pressed deeply into the breast, at the same time compressing the breast well behind the nipple. This deeper pressure is necessary in a round, virginal-shaped breast.

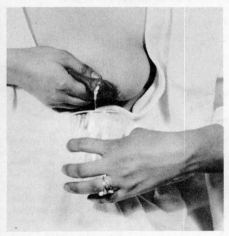

Fig. 185. Second position, showing compression of the breast between the thumb and fingers, well behind the nipple, and the milk coming in a stream. Care is exercised to avoid pinching or bruising the breast tissue.

and glide off without ever touching the areola or the nipple. If the breast is pendulous, care should be taken to allow it to fall gently.

One hand is used to support the breast and express the milk, the other to hold the container which will receive the milk. Although some authorities advocate that the right hand be used to milk the left breast, the decision as to which hand is used should depend on how the mother can accomplish this with the greatest ease. The forefinger is placed below and the thumb above the outer edge of the areola. The forefinger should be kept straight so that pressure can be exerted between the middle of this finger and the ball of the thumb. As they are alternately compressed and released, with the area of the collecting sinuses between them, milk is forced out in a stream (Figs. 183-187). It is of paramount importance here to avoid pinching and possibly bruising the breast tissue. The fingers should not

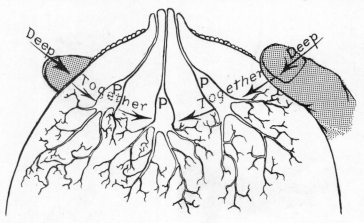

Fig. 186. Illustrating the movements needed to force milk out of the little pockets "P" in which it collects. Place a finger and a thumb on opposite sides of the nipple at "Deep." Press deeply into the breast in the direction of the black arrows. Then compress the breast together in direction of the arrows toward center point "P." This will force the milk out of the ducts in streams. "Deep" and "together" express in two words the motions required. (After U. C. Moore, Nutrition of Mother and Child)

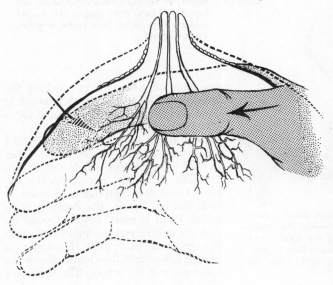

Fig. 187. Diagram showing the method of expressing the milk from the breast, as the mother would view it from above, by compressing the milk pockets between the thumb and forefinger. The 3 unused fingers are used to support the breast. This represents the second or "together" motion. (After U. C. Moore, Nutrition of Mother and Child)

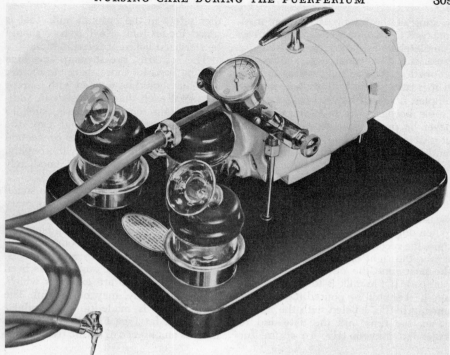

Fig. 188. Electric breast pump. Suction system provides vacuum up to 15" of mercury. Control allows patient to regulate degree of suction to her requirements and comfort. (Gomco Surgical Manufacturing Corp., Buffalo, N. Y.)

slide forward on the areola or the nipple during the milking process. However, they must be moved in clockwise fashion around the areola, each time compressing and releasing the fingers on that area, so that all the collecting sinuses may be emptied.

Many obstetricians advocate this method of emptying the breasts, rather than using the breast pump, because the action more nearly simulates the action of the infant's jaws as it nurses. Furthermore, since no mechanical equipment is required, it is a method which can be readily used when necessary after discharge from the hospital.

ELECTRIC-PUMP EXPRESSION. Several types of electric breast pumps employing the principle of intermittent negative pressure are used in hospitals (Fig. 188). The physician may prescribe their use to empty the breasts of milk, as in some cases to reduce engorgement or to draw out inverted nipples.

The nurse should be familiar with the instructions pertaining to the particular electric pump she is using. If she is teaching the mother how to pump her breasts, it is wise to make sure that she understands how to use it, especially how to control the vacuum.

Low suction will express the milk without discomfort or injury. For whatever purpose the electric breast pump is used, the suction should be increased gradually to prevent irritation to the nipple and needless pain which, in turn, might cause anxiety in the mother and retard the flow of milk. The suction should be intermittent to simulate the sucking of the infant. It takes approximately 5 to 12 minutes to empty a breast completely, depending on the stage of lactation, but pumping should be stopped as soon as milk ceases to flow. If it is used solely to draw out inverted nipples, it should be used only until the nipple becomes erect. A breast should never be pumped longer than 15 minutes at any one time. However, if the mother experiences back or chest pain, an indication that the breast is dry, the pumping should be stopped immediately.

The breast milk obtained should be measured and the amount recorded. When only one breast is pumped at the time, the record should indicate whether it was the right one or the left, so that the next time the other breast can be pumped. If the milk is to be fed to the infant, it should be poured into a sterile nursing bottle, labeled with the infant's name, the time and the date and refrigerated immediately. To ensure fur-

ther safety in the hospital, milk that is saved for an infant in this way should be sterilized before it is fed to him.

The electric breast-pump machine may be used for more than one mother and thus should be washed with soap and detergent each time it is used. In addition, certain removable parts, such as the breast-pump bottle and cap, the breast funnel and the rubber connection tubing, must be washed thoroughly, wrapped and autoclaved immediately after use.

Breast Exercises. Mothers are sometimes concerned about the temporary increase in the size of the breasts during lactation. When breast feeding has been discontinued the breasts soon approximate their previous size and firmness, particularly if needed support has been maintained. There are exercises which, if done regularly, may be helpful. The breast itself is made up of glandular tissue and fat (see Fig. 43), and since there is an absence of elastic tissue, exer-

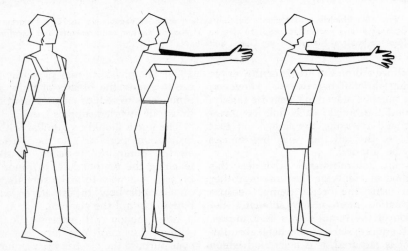

Fig. 189. Breast exercise. After breast feeding has been discontinued the breasts seem to be soft and flabby. These simple exercises may help to restore firmness of tissues because they involve the pectoral muscles which lend secondary support to the breasts. Stand with feet apart, toes turned in slightly, abdomen in and up, buttocks tucked under and head held high. Hold fingertips together, with arms at shoulder level. Press fingers together sharply and firmly. Relax and repeat 10 times.

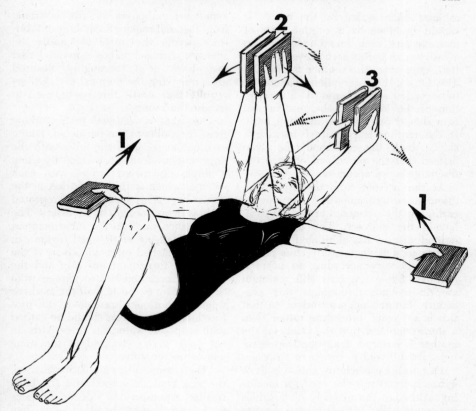

Fig. 190. Breast exercise. Lie flat on back with knees and thighs flexed to place spine firmly on the floor. Abdomen is kept flat. Breathe naturally and do exercises slowly. (1) Holding a small book in each hand, stretch arms out level with shoulders. (2) Raise arms forward from body to bring books together, keeping arms straight. Lower arms to outstretched position. (3) Raise arms forward as in No. 2; then carry them, held straight together, to floor behind head. Return arms to outstretched position. Repeat. Stop all exercises before feeling tired.

cises cannot directly hasten the return of the breasts to their former state. However, exercises which involve the pectoral muscles may be helpful, because these muscles lend secondary support to the breasts (Figs. 189 and 190). These exercises may be started when the mother is no longer breast feeding, should be limited at first and increased only as the mother can tolerate them without fatigue.

Care of the Perineum

Perineal care is a procedure employed to cleanse the vulva, the perineum and the anal region in order to prevent infection, to promote healing of the perineum and to make the mother comfortable. In addition, it provides an opportunity for the nurse to inspect the area and the lochial discharge. Regardless of whether or not an episiotomy has been performed, perineal care should be given at least once a day by the nurse. It should be done as a routine part of morning care, each time the mother uses a bedpan, and after each bowel evacuation, even after the mother is ambulatory. One of the observations that should be recorded each morning is a description of the lochial discharge. Perineal care should precede the morning bath. If the mother is permitted to take a shower bath, this care should be given first so that the nurse can observe the discharge more accurately.

At the present time there is much discussion concerning the best way of caring for the perineum in the days following the delivery. The technic for individual care has simplified this procedure to a large measure, but procedures will vary according to hospital routines. Some hospitals still maintain aseptic technic throughout this procedure, but the majority advocate that this is a "clean" procedure rather than a sterile one and that the safety of the mother is ensured if antiseptic precautions are adhered to conscientiously.

Disposable washcloths, cotton balls or gauze sponges may be used for cleansing. Although the majority of hospitals use cotton balls for this purpose because they are soft, absorbent and economical, the other materials are preferable. When the pubic hair begins to appear, cotton balls tend to catch on the stubble, and particles of cotton remain unless they are picked off. Another variation found is in relation to the cleansing agent, which might be a mild soap or detergent solution, sterile or tap water or an antiseptic solution.

In preparation for the procedure, the nurse should wash her hands thoroughly. After preparing the mother, remove the perineal pad, noting the amount, the odor and the appearance of the lochia and discard the pad in a paper bag. Whether removing the perineal pad or in using the sponges or washcloths in the actual cleansing process, always proceed from the front toward the back to avoid contamination of the vestibule from the anal region. Some hospital routines permit the nurse to handle the sponges with her hands, provided that they have been thoroughly cleansed after removing the perineal pad. Others require that sterile forceps be used to handle the sponges.

The labia is cleansed first, working from the pubis to the perineum, taking care not to separate the labia with the fingers. The cleansing is done by using a single downward stroke with each sponge, which is then discarded in the paper bag. This cleansing is repeated with as many sponges as necessary. The area is then dried in the same manner.

The cleansing of the anal region can be accomplished most effectively if the mother is turned on her side and the buttocks separated before wiping from the perineum to the anus. If the mother's thighs or buttocks are soiled with profuse lochia, these areas should be bathed with soap and water, for these parts do not have to be cleansed in the same manner as the vulva.

When disposable washcloths are used, the first cloth is soaped and the labia washed down on one side to the perineum and then on the other side. Then the anus is washed last and the soaped washcloth discarded. The area is rinsed in the same manner with a second washcloth and dried with a third one. The perineum should be kept clean and dry to promote healing.

The nurse must be mindful of the potential danger of infection if pathogenic organisms ascend the birth canal to the uterus. Care should always be exercised to see that none of the cleansing solution seeps into the vagina because of the possibility of contamination. If the washcloths or moist sponges are used, they should not be dripping wet. If the pitcher douche is used for the purpose of flushing the external genitalia, the solution likewise should not be permitted to enter the vagina.

The clean perineal pad should be

grasped on the outside so that the nurse's fingers do not touch the side which will come in contact with the mother's perineum. Then the pad is applied to the vulva (front to back) and secured to the sanitary belt in front before turning the mother to her side to secure the back tab.

Perineal Self-Care. The first time the mother is allowed up to the bathroom, the nurse should take her and show her where her equipment is kept and how to do perineal self-care. The principles of personal hygiene which were stressed when the nurse gave the mother perineal care in bed should be reviewed again. Instruct the mother to wash her hands carefully before and after carrying out the procedure. Show her how to assemble the necessary equipment, the paper bag, box of small cleansing tissues and wrapped perineal pad, all of which can be placed on a small stool or table adjacent to the toilet. A box of small cleansing tissues is preferable to a roll of tissue for obvious reasons. Have the mother unfasten the perineal pad she is wearing, and instruct her to grasp it by the tabs and remove it from front to back. This perineal pad is placed in the paper bag, which will be disposed of in a step-on can or other covered waste receptacle. After the mother voids, instruct her to cleanse herself from front to back with tissues, using fresh tissues for each stroke and discarding them in the toilet. The mother should again be instructed how to handle the clean perineal pad so that the inner surface is not contaminated by her fingers and to put it on from front to back. It should be fastened immediately to prevent the pad from moving forward. The toilet should be flushed after the mother assumes a standing position to avoid having any of the flushing water spray the perineum.

To ensure further safety, extra precautions should be used if the mother has a bowel evacuation. She should be told that after she has completed self-care she should return to bed so that the nurse may give her routine perineal care.

Perineal Discomfort. Following a spontaneous vaginal delivery, mothers do not usually experience perineal discomfort. It is most likely to be present if an episiotomy has been performed or if lacerations have been repaired, particularly if the perineum is edematous and there is tension on the perineal sutures. Almost all primigravidas experience some degree of discomfort from an episiotomy, depending largely on the extent of the wound and the amount of suturing done. For the most part during the first few days, local treatment in the form of dry heat, analgesic sprays or ointments is all that is necessary to alleviate the discomfort. But if the pain is more severe in the first day or so, such treatment may not be sufficient and analgesic medications may have to be administered by mouth or hypodermic injection. Later on, Sitz baths may be ordered if the discomfort persists.

Exposure of the perineum to heat from the perineal lamp not only provides a considerable measure of comfort to the mother but also supplies a safe amount of heat to promote local healing of the perineal wound. The physician may prescribe such treatment for 20- to 30-minute periods, 2 or 3 times a day. If a lamp such as the one shown in Figure 191 is used, the mother can recline in bed with the lamp between her knees during the treatment, without spreading the thighs too far apart. This lamp is so constructed that the frame can be completely covered with a pillowcase. The excess cover is brought forward over the arch of the frame and tucked securely between it and the shield which is around the bulb. The heat is provided by an ordinary 25-watt light bulb. When the mother has assumed the dorsal recumbent position, the lamp can be easily slipped between her legs and placed about 10 to 12 inches from the perineum. After the perineum is exposed, the bulb should be adjusted so that the

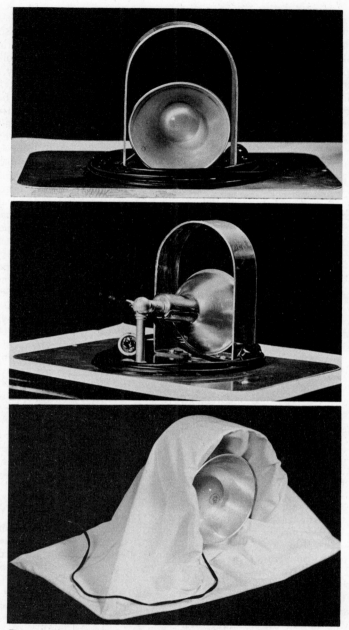

Fig. 191. Three views of a lamp designed for "light treatment" of the perineum. This lamp is simple in design and inexpensive. It is equipped with a bracket which acts as a "cradle" over which the bedclothes may be supported. When in use, the frame is completely covered with a pillow-case. The heat provided by such a lamp gives great comfort to patients when perineal stitches are painful. (University Hospitals of Cleveland)

light shines directly on it. The mother can be completely covered during the treatment, because the arch of the lamp frame acts as a cradle to support the top bedclothes.

Mothers who have discomfort from perineal sutures will usually find it uncomfortable to sit for the first few days. Many of them will be observed sitting in a rigid position, bearing their weight on one side of the buttocks or the other, with obvious discomfort to the back as well as the perineum. Therefore, it is important to teach the mother how to sit comfortably with her body erect. In the sitting position, the perineum is suspended at the lowermost level of the ischial tuberosities which bear the weight of the body. Thus, in order to achieve a greater measure of comfort, the mother must bring her buttocks together to relieve pressure and tension on the perineum, in the same manner described in the exercise for contraction and relaxation of pelvic floor muscles (see p. 177). After assuming a sitting position, the mother should be instructed to raise her hips very slightly from the chair, only enough to permit her to squeeze her buttocks together and contract the muscles of the pelvic floor, and hold them this way momentarily until after she has let her full weight down again. This exercise will also prove to be helpful to the mother when she is reclining in bed.

Abdominal Binder

At the present time there is general agreement that an abdominal binder is unnecessary. It was formerly routine practice to apply one to the newly delivered mother because it was thought that it aided involution and helped to restore the mother's figure. Actually, a binder is of no value for such purposes and, because it inhibits the movements of the abdominal wall, may actually retard the soft, flabby structures in regaining tone. However, the physician may advise the use of a binder if the mother's abdomen is unusually flabby or pendulous, particularly if the mother believes that she would feel more comfortable with some support. If the mother is ambulatory, the straight abdominal binder may be preferable to the scultetus binder because it is more likely to stay in place when the mother moves about. It must be remembered that the binder is applied from the waist down to avoid pushing the uterus upward.

HEALTH GUIDANCE

A considerable amount of health supervision throughout the mother's pregnancy is devoted to anticipatory guidance, not only to provide for her immediate care, but also to help her plan and prepare for the time when she takes her new infant home from the hospital. A good foundation to facilitate this transition has been laid in this way, but it may lose some of its effectiveness unless certain aspects are reinforced in the immediate puerperium.

Each mother's understanding and ability will vary, depending largely on her background and previous experiences. Undoubtedly, the primipara who has not been accustomed to infants will have much to learn about the care and handling of her new baby. On the other hand, the multipara may feel uncertain about the response of an older child to the new baby and thus require guidance in understanding and dealing with sibling rivalry. Many mothers need to know more about their own care, others how to facilitate certain adjustments within the home or the family group. If the mother knows what she can expect and what to do, she usually can handle simple problems which might otherwise cause fear or apprehension.

Proper care for the mother during the puerperium emphasizes the need for rest, nourishing food and protection from worry. Parents, as a rule, seem to be under the impression that once the delivery is over normalcy is restored and

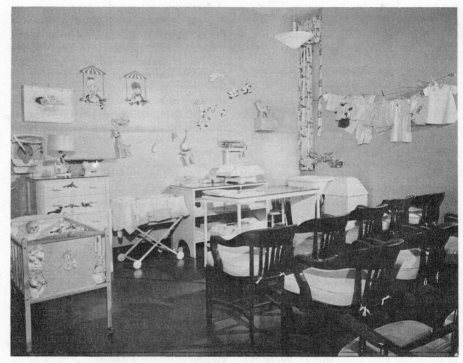

Fig. 192. Sloane Babies Alumni Classroom. Well-cushioned chairs add to the mother's comfort during postpartal classes. (Sloane Hospital for Women, Medical Center, New York)

they can resume their usual activities immediately. However, it is agreed that it may be weeks before the generative organs have returned to normal size and position, and the emotional and endocrine adjustments may be even more delayed. The mother should be cautioned to proceed slowly in the postpartal period at home. The general feeling of well-being and the excitement of having the baby all too often provide such a stimulus that the mother has a tendency to overdo. If it is at all possible, the major responsibilities of housekeeping should be taken over by a "helper," so that the mother can take it easy and devote herself primarily to caring for her new infant and spending more time with the immediate family. This is the

time when family relationships can be strengthened if the mother is not overwhelmed with apprehension and fatigue.

By the time the mother leaves the hospital she should understand about the daily care of her baby, what to expect of him and any other important details related to his care. Parents should know how and where to contact the physician if any medical problems arise before the next scheduled visit. In addition, if they have been given information about the services of the public health nursing agency in their community, and how they may use these services, much of the normal anxiety related to the new baby's care may be alleviated. Husbands who have accompanied their wives to parents' classes are usually much more

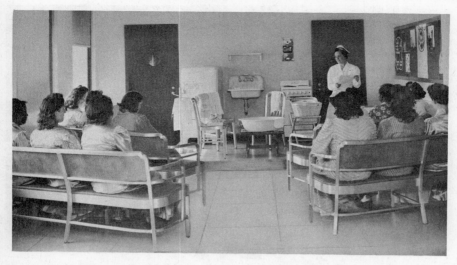

Fig. 193. A special room for mothers' classes, equipped with all the essentials, kitchenette, stove, sink and refrigerator, as well as demonstration equipment for the care of the baby. This room is used for antepartal classes as well as for demonstrations to mothers before discharge. Teaching of this kind is a routine part of the nursing care in almost all hospitals. (Margaret Hague Maternity Hospital, Jersey City, N. J.)

conscious of, and prepared for, this period. Often they plan their time to be at home to help assume some of the responsibilities. It is not so much physical help that is needed as it is the satisfactions gained by the mutual "sharing" engendered by the partnership.

Postpartal Blues

Sometime during the puerperium the mother may quite suddenly experience a "let-down" feeling for no reason which she can explain. She may become irritable and tearful and may even lose her appetite and find it difficult to sleep. These are usually normal manifestations of "postpartal blues"; they are very temporary and may occur while the mother is in the hospital or after her discharge home. The nurse can help the mother most effectively if she is able to recognize and interpret the mother's behavior and, in turn, is kind and understanding with her about the problem. It is true

that the mother appears to recover with amazing rapidity after the delivery, but this may help to obscure the fact that her entire being is still going through a period of transition. She is more vulnerable to stress at this time, and problems which she might otherwise be able to handle with relative ease may stimulate emotionally charged situations as she faces the responsibility for the protection and the care of her new baby, family and home. At the same time, the mother's own need for affection and attention may bring about feelings of jealousy when the major attention more often than not is directed to the infant.

Mothers' Classes

Many hospitals now provide regularly scheduled mothers' classes (Figs. 192 and 193), in which certain procedures relating to the care of the infant at home are demonstrated and discussed by a member of the nursing staff. These

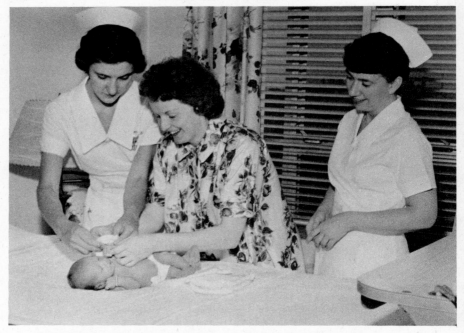

Fig. 194. Individual teaching in the hospital. A new mother has opportunity for learning to care for her baby with the help and guidance of the nursing staff. (MacDonald House, University Hospitals of Cleveland)

classes are particularly valuable because the new mother is usually most receptive and ready for such guidance when her new baby is here. When the mother is permitted to leave her room she should be encouraged to attend the infant-bath and formula-preparation classes in the mothers' classroom. Even mothers who are breast feeding benefit from the formula-preparation class because they learn about the care of nursing bottles used for orange juice or water and how to prepare a supplementary feeding. Some hospitals have special classes for mothers who are breast feeding. Such classes have the advantage of encouraging the mothers to share their experiences and problems related to feeding their infants, under the guidance of a nurse. More recently, some hospitals have included a pediatrician's class for all mothers, in which the physician discusses the newborn infant—its appearance, behavior, growth, development and, in general, the care of the normal newborn infant.

Individual Teaching

Regardless of the fact that a mother may attend all the group classes offered in the maternity hospital, each mother should be given individual help to learn how to handle and care for her infant while she is in the hospital, particularly if this is her first baby. Many new mothers are timid at first because they do not know what to expect of their infants, or they are afraid of what they will do to them because of their own feelings of inadequacy. A mother who has had no previous experience with infants will need some guided practice in changing diapers, dressing her baby and handling the infant in general (Fig. 194). Rooming-in units provide an environment in which the mother can have such an experience over an extended period of time. However, even in situations where the infants are kept in a central nursery, the nurse should plan to spend some time with the mother, in addition to the regular feeding periods,

to help her learn to care for her baby. If hospital staffing permits the time, it may be desirable for some mothers to bathe their own infants at the bedside, under the nurse's guidance, before leaving the hospital. There is no reason why such practices should violate the "clean nursery technic" if they have been properly planned. A rooming-in experience is undoubtedly beneficial for both mother

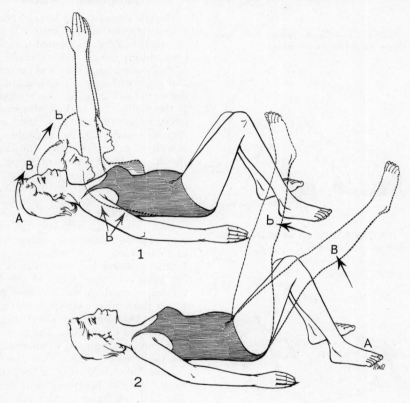

Fig. 195. Postpartal exercises. To prevent low back strain with these calisthenics the knees and the hips should be flexed to place the pelvis firmly on the floor. Double leg raising exercises and "sit-ups" are not advised because these exercises place considerable strain on the back muscles and may injure them. (1) Lie on the back with knees and hips flexed. Bring the head forward to flex the chin on the chest, and at the same time contract the abdominal muscles. In time, gradually increase this action to lift the shoulders and upper back from the floor, but avoid efforts to bring the body to an erect position. (2) Lie on the back with knees and hips flexed. Raise one leg at a time by bringing it up to straighten the knee. Increase the action gradually so that eventually each leg is brought to a vertical position.

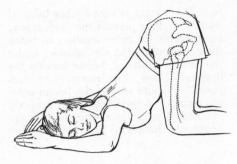

CORRECT — Chest resting on bed, thighs perpendicular to surface.

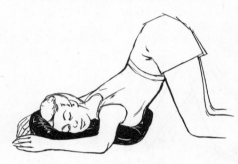

INCORRECT—Chest on pillow, thighs slant away from body.

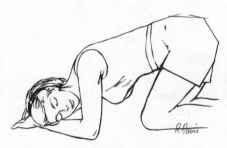

INCORRECT—Resting on elbows, thighs slant inward toward body.

Fig. 196. Knee-chest position may be advised by the physician if the uterus has not returned to its almost normal position.

and baby. But when this is not possible because of hospital facilities or policies, a daily extended visiting period can be extremely helpful. In this way the mother and the baby can become better acquainted in the security of the maternity division, where experienced personnel are near at hand to answer the mother's questions and offer advice.

Postpartal Exercises

Certain exercises are advantageous to the mother during the postpartal period to strengthen the abdominal muscles, to promote involution and a general sense of well-being. Such exercises are *advised and regulated by the physician,* according to the individual mother's condition. If the mother has had an abnormal delivery or any extensive perineal repair, exercises may not be advisable. Any exercises prescribed for the mother should not be strenuous or tiring when used in moderation. They should be practiced slowly and rhythmically, only a few times at first and gradually increased from day to day.

Soon after the delivery the mother may assume relaxation position on her abdomen for 20 to 30 minutes at a time. In this position her arms should be at her sides with the palms of the hands turned upward. A small pillow placed under the mother's waistline will greatly increase her comfort by alleviating pressure against her breasts. The Sims' position may also be used to encourage relaxation (see Fig. 112). Exercises which can be done while lying in bed, such as diaphragmatic breathing and contraction and relaxation of the pelvic floor muscles, are usually suggested for the early postpartal period (see Chap. 8). The patient may be advised to include more exercises later on when she is at home. It is preferable to do exercises on a firm surface, such as the floor. A good exercise for the abdominal muscles is shown in Figure 195, top. From a reclining position on the back, with knees flexed, bring the head forward to flex the chin on the chest and, at the same time, contract the abdominal muscles. As this exercise is practiced from day to day, the action can gradually be increased to lift the shoulders and upper back from the floor, but no attempt should be made to bring the body to an erect position. Some persons find it more helpful to lift the shoulders if the arms are extended above the head, as if reaching toward the ceiling. Another exercise is to lie on the back with the knees and hips flexed and feet flat on the floor (Fig. 195, bottom). Raise one leg at a time by bringing it up to straighten the knee. The legs can be raised gradually, so that eventually each leg is brought to a vertical position. In order to prevent low-back strain when such calisthenics are done, the hips and the knees should be flexed to place the pelvis firmly on the floor. It is advisable to avoid double leg raising and "sit-ups" because these exercises place considerable strain on the back muscles and may injure them.

The knee-chest position may be advised by some physicians to encourage the uterus to return to its normal position, particularly if the organ is retroverted. When employed, the physician usually instructs the patient to start this exercise about the third postpartal week, beginning with 2-minute periods each morning and evening and gradually increasing the time to 5 minutes twice daily. Patients should never be put in the knee-chest position *without specific orders from the physician.* Because of the anatomic relationship of the bladder to the uterus, the patient should empty her bladder first. The advantage to be gained from this exercise depends on the position of the pelvis. In order to attain the correct attitude of the pelvis, the patient's thighs should remain erect (perpendicular to the floor) while her back is carefully positioned so that it does not sag (Fig. 196). Care must be taken to see that the external genitalia are not drawn open to allow air to enter the vagina. The danger of an air embolism occurring in such situations has been reported.*

Discharge Instructions

Before the mother is discharged from the hospital, the physician will give her instructions about her care and the rate at which it is prudent for her to resume normal activities in the following weeks at home. She is told to avoid any heavy work and to get as much rest as possible during the next 3 weeks. Her schedule should be planned to include morning and afternoon rest periods and adequate sleep at night. Stair climbing should be limited until the second week at home. If the mother is advised to take exercises to strengthen abdominal and perineal muscles, the physician will specify when such calisthenics may be started and the frequency with which they are to be done. The hair may be washed at any time, and tub baths or showers are permissible. The mother is usually advised not to have intercourse or take a vaginal douche until after the "6-week checkup." Instructions concerning eating habits and regulation of the bowels are discussed.

If the medical care of the infant is being supervised by a pediatrician, he may give the mother going-home instructions concerning her baby, otherwise this is taken care of by the obstetrician. The mother should be given specific information about feeding, skin care, clothing, sleep, bowel habits, behavior and the early growth and development of her infant.

Many hospitals provide printed going-home instructions for maternity patients. When these are used it is important to

* Redfield, R. L., and Bodine, H. R.: Air embolism following knee-chest position, J.A.M.A. 113:671, 1939.

make sure that the mother understands them before she leaves the hospital.

The maternity programs of most public health agencies include home visits by the nurse. When a referral has not been made by the hospital nurse, the mother should be informed that such services are available in the community and how to secure them should she need help with the care of the baby.

The importance of follow-up care for both mother and baby should be stressed. The mother is instructed that it is essential for her to keep the appointment for her "6-week check-up." The infant should be checked in 4 weeks and regularly thereafter by a private physician or in one of the well-baby clinics sponsored by the department of health.

SUGGESTED READING

Bookmiller, M., and Bowen, G.: Textbook of Obstetrics and Obstetric Nursing, ed. 3, Philadelphia, Saunders, 1958.

Brodsky, J. D., and Greenstein, C.: Air embolism associated with pregnancy and the puerperium, Illinois M. J. 112:5, 1957.

Caplan, G.: The mental hygiene role of the nurse in maternal and child care, Nursing Outlook 2:14, 1954.

Corbin, H.: Meeting the needs of mothers and babies, Am. J. Nursing 57:54, 1957.

Davis, M. E., and Scheckler, C. E.: DeLee's Obstetrics for Nurses, ed. 16, Philadelphia, Saunders, 1957.

DeClue, J. F.: Early ambulation in a postpartum unit, Am. J. Nursing 54: 295, 1954.

Hanfrect, F.: A procedure to reduce perineal discomfort in the puerperium, Am. J. Obst. & Gynec. 70:205, 1955.

Herbut, H. R.: Clean perineal care, Am. J. Nursing 56:1124, 1956.

Lesser, M. S., and Keane, V. R.: Nurse-Patient Relationships in a Hospital Maternity Service, St. Louis, Mosby, 1956.

McClure, M. H.: When she chooses breast feeding, Am. J. Nursing 57: 1002, 1957.

Mercer, M. E.: The growth and development of parents, Bull. Maternal Welfare 5:15, 1958.

Millsap, J. G.: Teaching is a part of nursing, Am. J. Nursing 53:54, 1953.

Naish, F. C.: Breast Feeding, ed. 2, London, Lloyd Luke, 1956.

Newton, M., and Newton, N.: Postpartum engorgement of the breast, Am. J. Obst. & Gynec. 61:664, 1951.

Newton, N.: Nipple pain and nipple damage; problems in management of breast feeding, J. Pediat. 41:411, 1952.

Van Blarcom, C. C.: Obstetrical Nursing, ed. 4, Rev. by Erna Siegel, New York, Macmillan, 1957.

Wiedenbach, E.: Family-Centered Maternity Care, New York, Putnam, 1958.

——: Safeguard mother's breasts, Am. J. Nursing 51:544, 1951.

CONFERENCE MATERIAL

1. The patient's husband is severely injured the day after her infant is born. What provision can be made by the hospital to keep the patient informed about conditions at home and the care of her three other children?

2. What instructions should be given to the primipara and her husband concerning her care following delivery and discharge from the hospital? How can the public health nurse participate most effectively in this family's care?

3. What line of reasoning would you use to convince parents of the importance of breast feeding? What are the responsibilities of the physicians and nurses in this respect?

4. Why is the postpartal examination important? What is the nurse's role in relation to the examination?

5. A mother tells the nurse that she wants to breast feed her baby for 6 to 8 months because she knows she cannot become pregnant so long as she is nursing. How can the nurse reply?

6. What are the pros and the cons of early ambulation for the maternity patient?

7. How can the nurse help a nursing

mother so that she can make her limited food budget provide well-balanced meals for the family? The family consists of the mother, the father (employed as a factory worker) and two small children.

8. A young mother is concerned that her 2-year-old child will be jealous of the new baby. How can this problem be handled?

9. What health teaching would you consider necessary to include as you give a bath to a primipara the first morning after delivery? A multipara?

Study Questions

UNIT FOUR: NORMAL PUERPERIUM

Read through the entire question and place your answer in the parentheses.

1. Soon after the mother was normally delivered, she complained of feeling chilly. The nurse observed that she was having a chill. In addition to reporting this to the physician, which of the following measures would the nurse carry out?
   A. Provide external warmth to the mother with blankets.
   B. Give a heart stimulant.
   C. Prepare to give oxygen.
   D. Give a hot drink.
   E. Place the mother in shock position.
   Select the number corresponding to the correct letter or letters.
   1. A only
   2. A and C
   3. A and D
   4. B and E

                                                                   (———3———)

2. If a mother making satisfactory progress has a pulse rate of 90 immediately before delivery, what average rate or rates would be considered to be favorable soon after delivery?
   A.   60
   B.   70
   C.   80
   D.   90
   E. 100
   Select the number corresponding to the correct letter or letters.
   1. C only
   2. A, B and C
   3. C, D and E
   4. All of them

                                                                   (———2———)

3. The appearance of the lochial discharge normally changes during the process of involution. In the space provided after the descriptive phrase in Column 2, place the letter of the period of time in Column 1 that corresponds to it.

Column 1	Column 2	
A. First day	1. Clotted blood with strings of membrane	(———G———)
B. From 1 to 2 days		
C. From 4 to 7 days	2. Brownish color; thin, scanty	(———D———)
D. From 8 to 14 days		

E. Third week
F. Seventh week
G. Not at all

3. Blood mixed with small
amounts of mucus (——B——)
4. Pinkish color; moderate
amount (——C——)
(——E——)
5. Yellow, creamish color
6. Dark-brown with occa-
sional bright-red (——G——)
7. Characteristic stale odor (——D——)
8. Characteristic foul odor (——C——)

4. A good understanding of the physiologic changes taking place in the mother during the puerperium is a basis for good nursing. Which of the following processes are believed to accomplish involution of the uterus?
A. The contraction of stretched muscle fibers
B. The elimination of endometrium along with blood and serous discharge
C. The casting off of a portion of the spongy layer of the decidua
D. The generation of new endometrial lining from the layer of decidua attached to the muscular wall
E. The formation of new endometrium
Select the number corresponding to the correct letters.
1. A, B and D
2. A, C and D
3. C and E
4. All of them

(——4——)

5. The nurse should be able to evaluate the observations she makes of her patient's condition. Which of the following changes in the height of the fundus would you consider to be indicative of normal progress of involution?
A. Twelve hours after delivery—1 cm. above umbilicus
B. Second day after delivery—6 in. above pubis
C. Fourth day after delivery—3 in. above pubis
D. Eighth day after delivery—2 in. above pubis
E. Tenth day after delivery—1 in. above pubis
Select the number corresponding to the correct letter or letters.
1. A only
2. A and C
3. B, D and E
4. All of them

(——2——)

6. Which of the following seem to be the advantages gained from early ambulation after delivery?
A. Improved bowel and bladder function
B. Mothers seem to regain their strength more readily
C. Minimizes the chances of hemorrhage
D. Hastens involution of the uterus
E. Eliminates incidence of thrombophlebitis
Select the number corresponding to the correct letters.
1. A and B
2. A, C and D
3. B, C and E
4. All of them

(——1——)

7. Although the procedures for perineal care vary from hospital to hospital, in what respects do they all agree?
   A. Requiring the nurse to carry out surgical aseptic technic
   B. Endeavoring to protect the patient against infection from external sources
   C. Using forceps to handle sponges in cleansing vulva
   D. Requiring that each sponge be used for one stroke only
   E. Requiring that perineal pads be sterile when applied
   Select the number corresponding to the correct letters.
   1. A and E
   2. A, B and C
   3. B, D and E
   4. All of them

(—————)

8. To keep the nipples in good condition for breast feeding, which of the following should be included in their daily care?
   A. Keep the nipples clean and dry.
   B. Wash with bland soap and warm water once a day.
   C. Wash with mild antiseptic solution prior to each feeding period.
   D. Cover the nipples and areola with clean plastic breast squares to prevent contamination.
   E. If nipple is sore, discontinue breast feeding until tenderness subsides.
   Select the number corresponding to the correct letters.
   1. A and B
   2. A, C and D
   3. B, D and E
   4. All of them

(—————)

Note: The key to the correct answers to these questions is given on page 533.

The Normal Newborn

ORIENTATION

One of the stimulating phases of the obstetric experience is the opportunity to observe and to care for the "brand-new" baby. Before birth the baby is protected physically from jars and injury by the amniotic fluid and has been in an environment where the temperature was most suited to his growth and development. His birth may be anticipated by the mother with the greatest of joy, or his arrival may be looked forward to with agony or an almost indifference. What effect this reception may have on the baby is not known. The birth process is bound to necessitate prompt and extensive adjustment for the baby. It might be a painful experience for both the baby and the mother. The readjustment which has to be made may be the most drastic and dramatic that he ever will be called upon to make. What fears or inhibitions may be carried over from this experience is a conjecture. At birth, the baby's brain is more than one fourth its adult size, and his nervous system is in an impressionable state. The care of this new baby, which for the student nurse extends through the delivery and the baby's hospital stay, should be one of real consideration. It is very often during this time that much is determined in the way of habits for the new baby. It should be remembered that during these first days the nurse is introducing the baby to a new way of life and laying some of the foundations, thereby shaping his behavior. Beginning habits are very significant. Needless to say, the most careful and thoughtful attention on the part of the nurse should be given to aid this new baby to make these adjustments.

Today, approximately 95 per cent of the infants born annually in the larger cities of the United States are born in hospitals—about 4 million babies born each year—and because their welfare is of major concern, stringent measures for their protection in the hospital must be adhered to.

Although the general care of newborn infants has been greatly simplified in recent years, the importance of quality newborn care must not be minimized. There has been a gradual decline in the neonatal mortality rate since 1935; nevertheless, it is still high (Figs. 3 and 4). In 1957, 37.8 per cent of infant deaths occurred within the first day of life, 63 per cent within the first week.

Most hospitals have established policies which require nurses and physicians to have a physical examination, including a chest roentgenogram, before assigning them to the maternity service and at regular intervals thereafter. Infection is a potential hazard to the infants, and personnel with infections of any nature, regardless of how minor, should not be permitted in the nursery or allowed to care for maternity patients.

The Committee on the Fetus and Newborn of the American Academy of

Pediatrics has prepared a helpful manual.* "The purpose of this manual is to define optimum standards for those procedures which will safeguard the physical well-being of the newly born infant and foster wholesome and normal relationships between him and his environment."

* Committee on the Fetus and Newborn, American Academy of Pediatrics: Standards and Recommendations for Hospital Care of Newborn Infants (Rev.), Evanston, Ill., The Academy, 1957.

CHAPTER FIFTEEN

Care of the Newborn Infant

INTRODUCTION

The 10 most important months of a baby's life are the nine months before he is born and the first month after birth. During pregnancy, the baby has been protected and nourished by the mother, but at birth the baby becomes an "independent" individual and undergoes the most profound physiologic changes that are encountered at any period of life. Certain of these alterations are immediate and others are delayed, but they are all permanent and therefore significant.

It is necessary to use the utmost care in handling the baby, keeping him warm and protecting him from exposure and injury. The first 4 weeks of life is the *neonatal period*. From the standpoint of maternity care, the infant is considered through this period.

Initial Care

In the delivery room the initial care has been given to the infant's eyes and the cord, and appropriate identification has been added. The baby should be

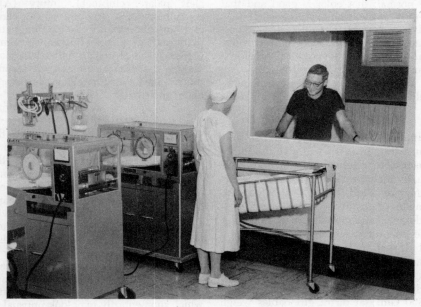

Fig. 197. A father sees his new baby immediately after delivery through the viewing window of the receiving nursery. (MacDonald House, The University Hospitals of Cleveland, Cleveland, Ohio)

329

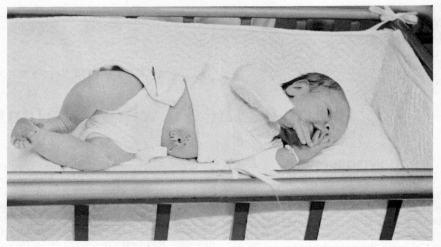

Fig. 198. A healthy newborn infant 4 hours after birth. *Note:* The umbilical cord has been clamped with a Hesseltine clamp (see Fig. 166). (MacDonald House, The University Hospitals of Cleveland, Cleveland, Ohio)

watched to see that he is kept warm (a most important detail), that respirations are normal, that color is good and that there is no bleeding from the cord.

It is customary in many maternity hospitals today to provide a "receiving" nursery on the labor and delivery division so that closer supervision and care for the infant may be assured immediately following the delivery (Fig. 197).

PHYSICAL EXAMINATION

Immediately, or within the next few hours, the physician will give the infant a complete physical examination. This usually includes: head (fontanels, overriding of skull bones), eyes, mouth (palate, gums, tongue), heart, lungs, abdomen, extremities, genitalia and anus. The measurements of the infant are noted, such as the circumference of the head and the shoulders, and weight and length. The average full-term boy baby weighs from 7 to 7½ pounds (about 3,300 Gm.) at birth; girl babies weigh a little less. The average length of a full-term infant at birth is about 20 inches (51 cm.).

The physician will scrutinize the infant carefully for any deformity (e.g., cleft palate, clubfoot), injury (e.g., cephalhematoma, fracture of the clavicle) or abnormality (e.g., tonguetie, phimosis). If a malformation or injury is found, the physician will advise concerning the infant's care and will assume the responsibility for telling the parents about their baby.

General Appearance

The nurse should be familiar with the characteristics of the normal newborn so that she can distinguish them from the abnormal. For example, certain symptoms which might be cause for concern in an older child, e.g., rapid rate and rhythm of respirations, when observed in a newborn infant may merely represent normal neonatal physiology. Also, it is well for the nurse to take a look at him from the standpoint of how he appears to his mother. The healthy newborn infant has many characteristics which momentarily may look unusual to her. The nurse should be ready to talk with the mother about her baby and to answer her questions.

The newborn infant usually lies with his arms and legs flexed, or tending to imitate the position he has been accustomed to in utero. When the infant is awake he sucks, yawns, sneezes, blinks and stretches. His movements for the most part are purposeless. For the first day or two he sleeps most of the time, but even while he is relaxed and quiet he occasionally may exhibit some coarse, jerky movements. During the first few weeks of life he may lie with his head turned to one side and the arm and leg on that side extended, while the other arm and leg are drawn up (tonic neck reflex). If he is awakened suddenly or startled by jarring or a loud noise, he will thrust his arms out in an "embracing motion" (Moro reflex).

The infant's head is large, comprising about one quarter of his size, and with cephalic presentations may initially appear to be asymmetrical because of the molding of the skull bones during labor. The suture lines between the skull bones and the anterior and the posterior fontanels can be palpated easily (Fig. 70). When the nurse's hand is passed over the fontanels, the areas should feel soft but neither bulged nor depressed. The anterior fontanel, the diamond-shaped and larger of the two, may feel smaller for the first several days when there is marked overriding of the skull bones. Occasionally the scalp is covered with a thick growth of hair which sheds for the most part before the permanent hair appears.

The face is small and round, and the lower jaw appears to recede. The eyes are closed much of the time but will open spontaneously if the infant's head is lifted (a valuable point to remember when one wants to inspect the eyes). The movements of the eyes are not coordinated and they cannot focus, although they react to bright lights and large objects passed directly in front of them. Many new mothers become exceedingly anxious when they observe strabismus or nystagmus in their infants, thus they should be reassured that this lack of co-ordination is normal during the first few months of life. The lips are sensitive to touch, and any stimulation of this nature usually elicits the sucking reflex. Moreover, the rooting reflex is well developed, so that when the cheek is stroked on one side the infant will turn his head in that direction. In conjunction with sucking, a labial tubercle may be present on the center of the upper lip, as well as the sucking pads (fat) in the cheeks. At this time the tongue does not extend far beyond the margin of the gums because the frenum is normally short. A mother's concern that her baby is tonguetied is usually unwarranted.

The infant's neck is short. His chest is round and slightly smaller in circumference than his head. The breasts may be engorged initially and may even secrete "witch's milk." This condition, like menstruation, a vaginal tag or enlarged labia in girl babies, is due to a hormonal factor and without interference will disappear spontaneously. In boy babies the scrotum appears to be relatively large, and the prepuce is long and adherent to the glans penis (this separates in several months). The abdomen is round and protruding due to the relative size of the abdominal organs and weak muscular structures. The respiratory movements are largely diaphragmatic, and breathing is rapid, shallow and irregular.

The infant's skin appears to be thin and delicate and is often dry and peeling. The baby's color may be pink, reddish or pale, becoming very ruddy when he cries. Initially, the hands and the feet are quite blue, but this cyanosis of the extremities soon disappears, often within a few hours. Vernix caseosa, a white cheesy material which has been a protection to the infant's skin while floating in amniotic fluid in the uterus, may be apparent, particularly in the creases of the body. Also, on the body there may be large areas of fine downy hair called lanugo. Milia may be present on the nose and the forehead, and small flat hemangiomas may be apparent on the

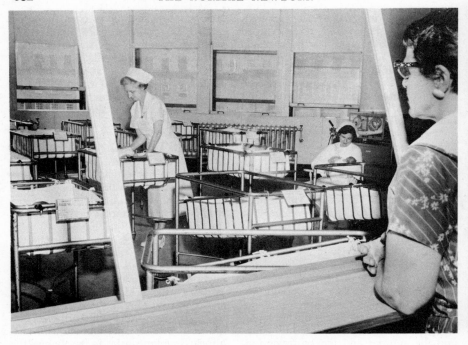

Fig. 199. The layout of the nursery provides for adequate space between cribs to decrease chances of cross-infection. Each infant is given individual care in his own crib. *Note:* The crib in the foreground is tilted to keep the newborn infant in Trendelenburg position for the first 12 hours after delivery. (MacDonald House, The University Hospitals of Cleveland, Cleveland, Ohio)

nape of the neck, the eyelids or over the bridge of the nose. These so-called "stork bites," clusters of small capillaries, usually disappear spontaneously during infancy.

In nonwhite infants, dark bluish areas are usually apparent on the buttocks or the lower back. These "mongolian spots" have no relationship to mongolism and will disappear spontaneously during late infancy. A pilonidal "dimple" resulting from an irregular fold of skin sometimes is seen in the mid-line over the sacrococcygeal area.

NURSERIES

Regular Nursery. The regular newborn nursery on the postpartal division is designed for the care of a variable number of healthy newborn infants

(Fig. 199). Some of the protection provided for the infants is accomplished by careful control of the physical facilities, requiring all personnel to wash their hands thoroughly and put on clean gowns before entering the nursery, limiting the number of individuals who may enter the nursery and requiring strict adherence to nursery aseptic technic on the part of all nursery personnel. Although the nurse "scrubs," i.e., washes her hands and arms to the elbows and scrubs her fingernails thoroughly before entering the nursery, she must wash her hands carefully before and after handling each baby.

The regular nursery is a so-called "clean" nursery. But it must be understood that there is a difference in nursery technic between what is considered to

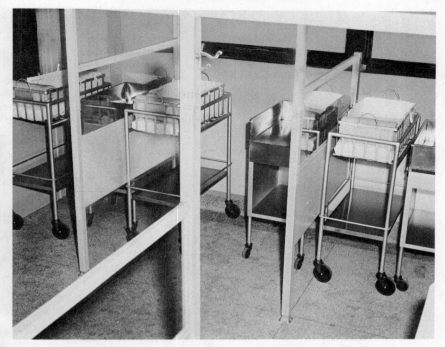

Fig. 200. Observation nursery with cubicles which provide complete isolation for each infant. Each unit is complete, containing all the equipment necessary for the care of the baby. (Margaret Hague Maternity Hospital, Jersey City, N. J.)

be "nursery clean" and what is considered to be "baby clean," i.e., what is clean for an individual baby. There should be no common equipment, such as a common bath table, used in providing care for the babies. There should be provisions in the nursery so that individual technic can be followed. Each infant should have his own crib and general supplies so that he can be given such care as his daily inspection bath, or be diapered or dressed in his own bed. Some cribs are constructed with a built-in cabinet for the infant's own supplies (clean diapers, shirts and linens) and a drawer to hold the containers for cotton balls, safety pins, thermometer, etc. When such cribs are not available, improvised units for the infant's crib should be obtained so that individual-care technic can be carried out.

If there is any evidence of a question-able infection at the time of delivery, if the infant is born on the way to the hospital, or if the infant is suspected of having an infection of the eyes, the skin, the mouth or the gastro-intestinal tract, the infant should not be admitted to the central nursery.

Observation Nursery. Maternity hospitals should have an observation nursery where infants suspected of developing an infectious condition may be kept until the presence or absence of infection is determined (Fig. 200). When a definite diagnosis of infection is made, the infant must be transferred immediately to an isolation nursery away from the maternity division.

Aside from the fact that infants in the "suspect" nursery must be segregated apart from others, and naturally require closer supervision and care because of suspected infection, their nursing care

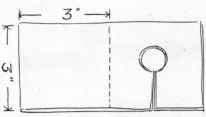

Fig. 201. Method of making the cord dressing.

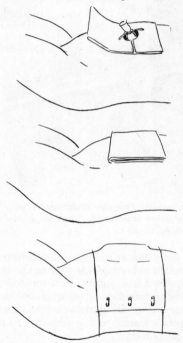

Fig. 202. Application of the cord dressing.

otherwise should be like that given a healthy newborn infant.

DAILY CARE
Eyes

In the daily care of the baby, no special treatment is given the baby's eyes unless there is a discharge. Any redness, swelling or discharge should be reported

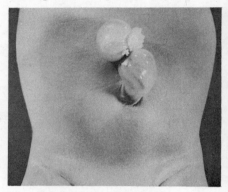

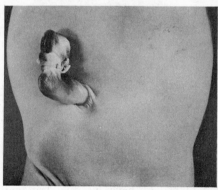

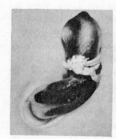
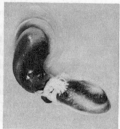
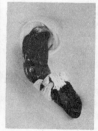
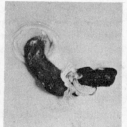

Fig. 203. The umbilical cord drying.

and recorded on the chart. There may be some reaction from the medication used for prophylaxis against ophthalmia neonatorum, but the physician will prescribe treatment if necessary.

Cord

Babies do not receive a tub bath until the cord has separated and the umbilicus has healed. The cord dressing is considered to be unnecessary in most hospitals, but, nevertheless, it is still used in some institutions (Figs. 201-202). When a cord dressing is used it is replaced when it becomes soiled. The condition of the cord and the umbilicus should be inspected and noted daily.

No attempt should be made to dislodge the cord before it separates completely. If there is a red inflamed area around the stump or any discharge with an odor, this condition should be recorded and brought to the physician's attention immediately. The cord usually becomes detached from the body between the fifth and eighth days after birth, but its detachment may be delayed until the twelfth or fourteenth day without causing any concern (Fig. 203). When the cord drops off, the umbilicus is depressed somewhat and usually free from any evidence of inflammation. No further treatment is necessary, except to keep the part clean and dry. When inflammation is present the physician will give specific orders for care.

Genitals

Adherent Foreskin. In a male infant, adhesions between the prepuce and the glans penis are very common. The foreskin may be extended beyond the glans. Reduction to a very small opening is spoken of as a "phimosis." A curdy secretion, called "smegma," may form in considerable amount and collect under the prepuce behind the glans. Also, small amounts of urine may be retained. Any of these conditions favor irritation and, if found, should be reported to the obstetrician. He may perform the delicate operations of separating the adhesions, stretching the prepuce or circumcising the baby (see Chap. 21).

The manipulation following dilation and retraction is difficult, at first, and should be done gently. The foreskin must be replaced immediately; if not, edema may result, rendering the replacing difficult.

Care Following Circumcision. When the newborn infant is circumcised, the main principles of postoperative care are to keep the wound clean and to observe it closely for bleeding. For the first 24 hours, the area is covered with a sterile gauze dressing to which a liberal amount of sterile petrolatum has been added.

Mothers are naturally anxious about their babies at this time, so, as soon as it is feasible after the circumcision has been done, the nurse should take the baby to his mother for a brief visit.

The infant's diaper should be applied so that only one layer of the material covers the penis. This lessens the danger of masking any bleeding which might occur. When changing the infant's diaper the nurse should hold his ankles with one hand so that he cannot kick against the operative area. Unless the physician orders otherwise, the circumcision dressing can be removed postoperatively when the infant voids for the first time. Cleansing must be done gently but can be accomplished as necessary with cotton balls moistened with warm tap water. A fresh sterile petrolatum dressing is usually applied to the penis each time the diaper is changed for the first day. The penis must be observed closely for bleeding, and during the first 12 hours should be inspected every hour. It is advisable to place the infant's crib where he can be watched conveniently. Moreover, in order to keep all the nursing personnel alerted, some signal, such as a red tag, can be attached to the identification card on the crib. If bleeding occurs, usually it can be controlled with gentle pressure. Some physicians leave a p.r.n. order for local application of Adrenalin 1:1,000 solution to the bleed-

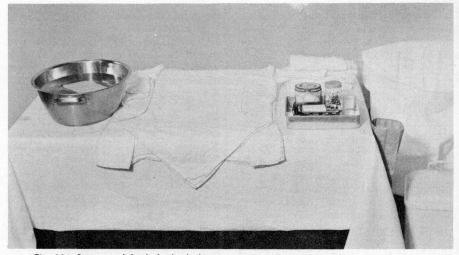

Fig. 204. Setup used for baby bath demonstration in the mothers' classroom. Note paper bag for discarded cotton balls, pillowcase for a laundry hamper and step-on can for diaper pail. (MacDonald House, The University Hospitals of Cleveland, Cleveland, Ohio)

ing point, but if bleeding persists the physician should be notified immediately.

Because circumcision is usually done on the 5th or 6th day, many times on the day preceding discharge, the nurse should make certain that the mother knows how to care for her newly circumcised infant.

Care of Girl Babies. Similar adhesions are sometimes found about the clitoris in female infants and, when observed, should be reported to the obstetrician. The smegma which may accumulate between the folds of the labia should be gently and carefully cleansed with moistened cotton balls, using the front-to-back direction and a clean cotton ball for each stroke. Occasionally a slight bloody discharge may come from the vagina. It may be due to injury or it may be apparently menstrual in character. If menstrual, it rarely reappears, and cleanliness is the only treatment necessary.

Weight

The baby should be weighed on the birth date and every day or every other day thereafter. If the infant remains in the hospital longer than 5 days, he should be weighed at intervals prescribed by the medical staff. His weight should be recorded accurately. The first few days after birth he usually loses weight because of the minimal amount of nutrients he takes in and probably because the digestive apparatus is barely learning to function. About the time the meconium begins to disappear from his stools, the weight commences to increase and, in normal cases, does so regularly until about the tenth day of life, when it may equal the birth weight. Then he should begin to gain from 4 to 6 ounces per week during the first 5 months. After this time, the gain is from 2 to 4 ounces weekly. At 6 months of age, the baby should be double his birth weight, and triple it when a year old. This is one way to note the baby's condition and progress, and when the baby is not gaining, that fact should be reported to the physician. Besides gaining regularly in weight and strength, the baby should be happy and good-natured when awake but inclined to sleep a good part of the time between nursings.

Pulse and Temperature

The clinical record of a normal baby should show a variation in pulse of from 110 to 150. Only experience can teach a nurse to count an infant's pulse rate accurately. Touching his wrist will generally startle him and noticeably accelerate the heart beat. It can always be felt at the temporal artery to best advantage, particularly during sleep. The rectal temperature may normally vary a whole degree, from 98° to 99° F. A premature baby may have a temperature below this. He will stabilize his temperature within 24 to 72 hours somewhere between 96° and 98° F., depending on his weight—the smaller the baby, the lower the temperature will be.

Cries

After the baby is born and has cried lustily, he becomes quiet and usually sleeps. After the eyes, the cord and the skin have received the necessary care, he is dressed and placed in a warm crib and does not usually cry unless he is wet, hungry or ill. A nurse soon will learn to distinguish an infant's condition and needs from the character of his cry, which may be described as follows. A loud, insistent cry with drawing up and kicking of the legs denotes colicky pain; a fretful cry, if due to indigestion, will be accompanied by green stools and passing of gas; a whining cry is noticeable when the baby is ill, premature or very frail; a fretful, hungry cry, with fingers in the mouth, is easily recognized; and there is a peculiar, shrill, sharp-sounding cry which suggests injury. A nurse should make every effort to recognize any deviation from the usual manner in which a baby announces his normal requirements.

Care of the Skin

The skin is thin, delicate, extremely tender and very easily irritated. Since the skin is a protective covering, breaks in its surface may initiate troublesome infection, hence skin disturbances constitute an actual threat to the baby's well-being.

The new baby does not perspire, usually, until after the first month, and he does not react to cold by having "goose flesh." In warm weather, or if the baby is dressed too warmly, he may develop prickly heat, a closely grouped pin-head-size rash of papules and vesicles, on the face, the neck and wherever skin surfaces touch. Fewer clothes and some control over the room temperature will help to relieve the discomfort.

In the majority of hospitals today, elaborate procedures for bathing the infant have been discarded. The skin is cleansed with sterile cotton and warm water. Oil or water baths as such should not be given during the hospital stay. Blood should be removed from the skin after the delivery, but no attempt should be made to remove the vernix caseosa unless it is stained with blood or meconium. The vernix caseosa serves to protect the skin and soon disappears spontaneously. During the first days of life a daily inspection bath is given, and at this time the infant can be "spot cleansed" with moistened cotton balls, as mentioned above. The use of soap, oil and baby powder is discouraged by many pediatricians because of the sensitivity of the newborn's skin. The nurse should pay particular attention to cleansing (and drying) the scalp and all creases at the neck, behind the ears, under the arms, the palms of the hands and between the fingers and the toes, under the knees, the soles of the feet, and in the groins, the buttocks and the genitals. The cord tie should be left in place until the cord drops off; the clamp is removed on the morning of the second day, provided that the umbilical stump has dried sufficiently. The nurse should observe whether the skin is clear, pink, cyanotic, blotchy or jaundiced and if there is dryness present.

It is not unusual, despite good nursing care, for the infant's buttocks to become reddened and sore. Since this "diaper rash" is due primarily to the irritating effect of urine and feces on the delicate skin, the most important prophylaxis lies in keeping the diaper area clean and dry. When the slightest evidence of irritation is apparent on the skin, immediate treatment should be instituted. Mineral oil may be prescribed for cleansing the buttocks. Sometimes the application of a bland protective ointment, such as vitamin A and D ointment, is used. Buttocks pastes are not advised, partly because they are much more adhesive than ointments and thus create cleansing problems. A simple treatment which is often effective is merely to expose the infant's reddened buttocks to air and light several times a day, using care to keep the infant covered otherwise. Warm daylight may be all that is necessary, although the use of a "lamp" treatment is more effective and at the same time provides a measure of warmth. An ordinary gooseneck lamp with a screened bulb (no stronger than 40 watt) can be placed on a table so that it is a foot or more away from the infant's exposed buttocks. The light may be used for 30 minutes at a time. Because the skin is already irritated, the nurse should exercise care not to burn it further by using too strong a bulb or placing the light too close.

Sleeping

After the profound experience of being born, the baby will need rest and sleep with as little handling as possible. If he is well and comfortable, he should sleep much of the time and wake and cry when he is hungry or uncomfortable. His clothes should be light in weight, warm but not too warm and free from wrinkles and bunches. His position should be changed often, from side to side. Criterion for placing a baby on his abdomen is his physical ability to raise his head.

Elimination

Intestinal. During fetal life the content of the intestines is made up of brownish-green tarlike material called "meconium." It is composed of epithelial and epidermal cells and lanugo hair that probably were swallowed with the amniotic fluid. The dark greenish-brown color of the meconium is due to the bile pigment. During fetal life and for the first few hours after birth the intestinal contents are sterile. Apparently there is no peristalsis until after birth, because normally there is no discoloration of the amniotic fluid. For the first 2 or 3 days the stools are meconium. After this, the color gradually changes to a soft yellow of a smooth pasty consistency with a characteristic odor if the infant is formula-fed. Stools of breast-fed infants tend to be golden yellow and of mushy consistency. Most newborns pass the first stool within 12 hours of birth—nearly all have a stool in 24 hours. If an infant has not passed a stool by this time, intestinal obstruction must be considered as a possible reason for the delay and the baby observed closely. The number of daily stools on about the fifth day of life is usually 4 to 6. As the infant grows, this number decreases to 1 or 2 each day. The type of stool may be influenced by the mother's diet. However, there may be slight variations from the normal, which may have little significance if the baby appears to be comfortable and sleeps and nurses well. If the baby's stools have a watery consistency, are of a green color and contain mucus or gas, the condition may be evidence of some digestive or intestinal irritation and should be reported to the physician. The number, color and consistency of stools should be recorded daily on the baby's record.

Urinary. Urinary activity of the fetus is evidenced by the presence of urine in the amniotic fluid. The baby usually voids during delivery or immediately after birth, but the function may be suppressed for several hours. However, if the baby does not void within 24 hours,

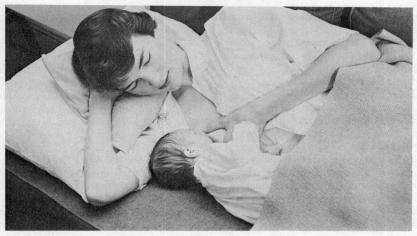

Fig. 205. Both the mother and the baby should be comfortable during the nursing period. The mother should hold the breast so that it does not interfere with the baby's breathing. When he cannot breathe freely, he becomes irritated and may refuse to nurse altogether.

the condition should be reported to the physician, as retention of the urine may be due to an imperforate meatus. After the first 2 or 3 days, the baby voids from 10 to 15 times a day. When the urine is concentrated, red or rusty stains on the wet diaper may be due to uric-acid crystals in the urine.

Infant Feeding

Breast Feeding

The adoption early in pregnancy of measures that will prepare the mammary glands for the function of supplying milk, and the very meticulous follow-up care necessary during the early postpartal period, have much to do with the mother's ability to furnish milk sufficient in quality and quantity. The best food for a baby is that designed for it by nature—breast milk. Nursing and the complete emptying stimulate the breasts to produce sufficient milk from day to day. Usually the milk from one breast will be enough for a feeding for a very young baby; therefore, alternate breasts should be used for each nursing. As the baby grows older, it may be necessary to put him to both breasts at every feed-

ing. This may be done at any time when the milk of one breast alone does not seem to be sufficient to satisfy the baby.

Routines vary, but usually the infant is put to breast 24 hours following delivery and every 4 hours thereafter. For the first two days the nursing periods are limited to 5 minutes. Thereafter they are increased to 20 minutes at each feeding. This allows the nipples (which can easily become sore) to become accustomed gradually to this manipulation.

When the nursing period arrives, the breasts, under normal conditions, should be firm and tense but never painful, and at this time a very slight pressure should be enough to cause the milk to flow. Many mothers need help with this new experience of nursing, and many babies must be taught to nurse. Therefore, the nurse has a definite responsibility in relation to breast feeding.

Advantages of Breast Milk. Breast milk is to be preferred to any modified milk, which at best is only a substitute. The advantages are:

Exactly the correct composition for babies

Emotional satisfaction, which is very

important in establishing mother-child relationships

Convenient and economical

Constantly available, no preparation necessary

Even temperature

Free from bacteria

Lowered incidence of allergy

Earlier involutionary processes in the mother after the termination of pregnancy.

Self-regulatory Feedings. Self-demand, as it is popularly referred to, is being used more and more frequently as an increasing number of hospitals are adopting the rooming-in plan. Demand feeding is the idea of putting a baby on a feeding schedule that seems to fit his individual needs, instead of the previous practice of putting all babies on one rigid feeding schedule of every 4 hours. On this feeding regimen the hours are flexible. Basically, the infant is allowed to regulate his own schedule within limits. Because infants cry for numerous reasons, food being only one of them, the mother must be familiar with the "hunger cry" and be able to differentiate it from other demands. The majority of infants set up a fairly stable eating pattern after the first few weeks of life. Even on an ad lib schedule, the infant should nurse only for short periods at a time during the first 2 days to prevent

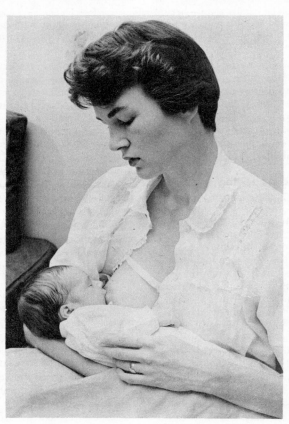

Fig. 206. Babies nurse better if the mother is relaxed and both the mother and the baby are comfortable.

sore nipples. The baby is usually put to the breast 24 hours following delivery. At first the breast secretes colostrum, which is characterized by a yellowish color. It contains more protein material but less fat than breast milk, while its sugar content is about the same. It is important to the baby because of its cathartic properties. Some authorities state that babies who nurse this colostrum have less initial weight loss.

Position During Nursing. If the baby is to nurse satisfactorily, he must be held properly by the mother; while some mothers seem to know how to support a baby at the breast, many are awkward, and definite instructions are helpful. First of all, both the mother and the baby must be comfortable and in such a position that the baby can grasp the nipple and areola without any effort —not just the nipple (Figs. 205 and 206). If the mother is lying down, she should be on her side with her arm raised and her head comfortably supported. The baby should lie on his side, flat on the bed, or supported by pillows. When the mother is sitting up to nurse the baby, she should use a comfortable chair with a stool to support her feet, and, if necessary, a pillow may be used to support her arm or may be placed under the baby. The mother should guard against feeding the baby either too rapidly or too slowly, or allowing his position to interfere with his breathing (i.e., nose mashed against the breast).

Effects of Menstruation and Pregnancy. Changes may occur in the mother's milk during menstruation. Formerly it was thought best to omit breast feeding if the menstruation returned during lactation. As long as the baby is satisfied, there is no contraindication to breast feeding during this time. Should the mother become pregnant during this period, she should discontinue breast feeding her baby immediately, for she cannot properly nourish herself, the baby and the fetus in utero. This is too much of a demand on any individual,

no matter how healthy she may seem to be.

Composition of Human Milk. Breast milk, as it leaves the mother's breast, is a sterile fluid. It should have an alkaline or possibly a neutral reaction, but never an acid reaction. Colostrum cells should be absent after the twelfth day, and the fat globules should be small, numerous and of uniform size.

Milk is a natural emulsion and consists of about 10 per cent of solids and 90 per cent of water. The solid substances are fat, sugar, proteins and salts. The fat of milk is the cream, the sugar is the kind known as "lactose," or "milk-sugar," and the protein makes up the bulk of the curd.

COMPARISON IN COMPOSITION OF HUMAN AND COW'S MILK

	Human	Cow's
Protein	1.15%	3.5%
Fat	3.5–4.0%	3.5–4.0%
Carbohydrate	7.0%	4.0–5.0%
Salts	0.2%	0.75%

Artificial Feeding

Today, more infants in American hospitals are artificially fed than breast fed. In artificial feeding it is necessary to modify the milk to approximate as nearly as possible the chemical and physical characteristics of human milk. When human and cow's milk are compared, the differences in protein and carbohydrate content explain the reason why cow's milk is diluted (e.g., one part milk to two parts water) and carbohydrate may be added for a newborn infant's formula. The carbohydrate may be in the form of granulated sugar, corn syrup or a commercially prepared carbohydrate modifier. The physician will always prescribe the formula for the infant and give specific directions for its use.

Various formulas are used today: diluted pasteurized milk with added carbohydrate, diluted evaporated milk with or without carbohydrate added, fresh skimmed milk, powdered skimmed milk

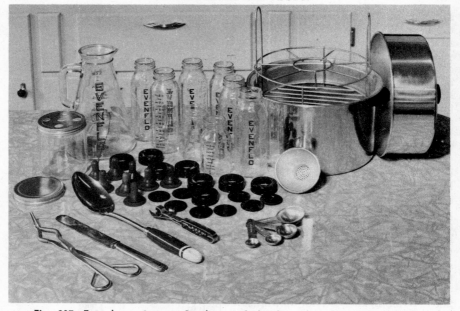

Fig. 207. Formula equipment. Sterilizer with bottle rack and tight-fitting lid; six 8-ounce nursers (for formula) and two 4-ounce nursers (for water and orange juice) complete with nipples, caps and sealing disks; quart-size formula pitcher with clearly marked graduations; nipple jar with perforated (for sterilizing) and solid lids; long-handled tongs; table knife; long-handled mixing spoon; can opener; set of measuring spoons and a funnel-strainer. (Pyramid Rubber Company, Ravenna, Ohio)

or one of the brands of prepared-milk preparations. Of these, the most widely used for formula is diluted evaporated milk with added carbohydrate. Evaporated milk has several advantages: it is safe (sterile in the unopened can), it is convenient to store, the cost relatively low, and the formula is simple to prepare. The following is an example of a formula that is often used to make the quantity necessary for a full day's supply, i.e., six 3-ounce feedings:

12 ounces water (2 parts)
6 ounces evaporated milk (1 part)
2 tablespoons corn sirup

The schedule for feeding is regulated, basically, in the same way for both breast-fed or formula-fed infants (Fig. 211).

If mothers receive the proper instructions they usually have no problems in preparing the infant's formula at home.

Formula may be sterilized by either the terminal or the aseptic method, but since the terminal method is so much safer and easier to do, this is almost always advised. Even though the mothers may attend a formula-demonstration class while they are in the hospital, they should be informed that public health nurses in the community agencies give instructions in preparing formula, if necessary, when they make a home visit.

Directions for Making Formula. The hands should be washed before assembling the equipment. All equipment used for the preparation of the formula should be kept separate (Fig. 207). If bottled milk is used, the outside of the bottle should be washed with soap and cool water as soon as received, and the bottle should be placed in the refrigerator. If canned milk is used, the top of the can should be washed with soap and

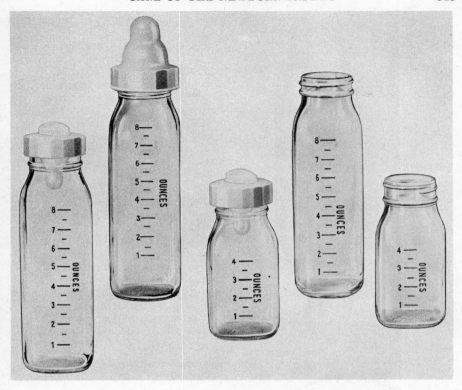

Fig. 208. A modern "nurser" for formula feeding is a complete unit consisting of a wide-mouthed bottle, nipple and screw-top all-in-one. It is safe and convenient because the cap seals the nipple and formula against contamination until used. During the feeding the collar can be screwed tighter or looser to regulate the rate of flow of the formula. (Davol Rubber Company, Providence, R. I.)

water, using friction, and then thoroughly rinsed. Hot water should be poured over the top just before it is opened. All equipment should be washed thoroughly in warm soapy water and rinsed well so that no milk film remains to hold bacteria.

Bottles and Nipples. The 8-ounce bottle is a good size to use and should be graduated in ounces and half ounces so that it will be possible at all times to know exactly how much food the baby has taken. A sufficient number of bottles and nipples should be sterilized to supply the feedings for the 24-hour period. It is always safer to have one or two extra bottles and nipples in reserve in case of breakage (Fig. 208).

The shape of the bottle should be such that every part of the inner surface can be reached with a brush to facilitate cleaning.

The holes in the nipple are usually small, but they may be made the required size by heating a fine sewing needle with its eye fixed in a cork used as a handle. The point is held in the flame until red hot, then accurately plunged into one of the three holes and withdrawn quickly. It needs practice before holes of proper size can be made. Some nipples have crucial incisions in-

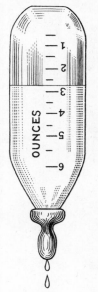

stead of punctured holes to prevent them from clogging.

The test of proper hole size is made by holding the bottle, filled with milk and with the nipple attached, upside down. The milk should escape drop by drop, and if it runs in a stream, the hole is too large (Fig. 209). The objection to the large hole is that the baby nurses too rapidly, which causes indigestion, colic and other disorders. If the stream is very rapid, the baby may have difficulty in swallowing.

PREPARATION OF EQUIPMENT. The equipment may vary with the type of formula prescribed and the method of sterilization used.

ASEPTIC METHOD. Wash all equipment in hot soapy water and rinse thoroughly in clear hot water. Place the following articles in the sterilizer half-full of cool water: quart-size graduate, measuring cup, measuring spoon, tablespoon, bottles, funnel, nipple protector, can opener (if canned milk is used) and

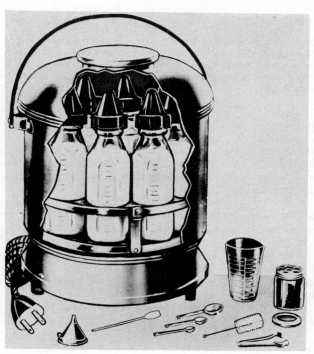

Fig. 210. Electric model of "Baby-All" formula and sterilizer outfit which may be used for regular or terminal sterilization. A nonelectric model is also obtainable. (Sanit-All Products Corporation)

forceps (place in sterilizer last to be removed first). Bring water to a boil, and boil vigorously for 10 minutes.

In the aseptic method the bottles, the nipples and the equipment used in making the formula are sterilized before the formula is prepared. The formula is then made according to directions. A specific amount of the formula is put into each bottle. The bottles are then nippled, capped and refrigerated.

Terminal Sterilization. In this method the formula is prepared under a clean but not aseptic technic. The bottles, the nipples and the nipple protectors are washed thoroughly but are not sterilized. The formula is prepared and poured into the bottles, and the nipples and the protectors are applied loosely. They are then placed in the sterilizer, covered with a tight-fitting lid and sterilized by having water boil rapidly in bottom of sterilizer for 25 minutes. In this method, formula, bottles, nipples and protectors are all sterilized in one operation. Before the formula is refrigerated the screw collar should be made secure. The majority of hospitals

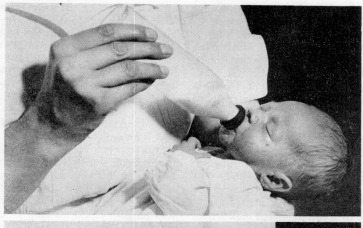

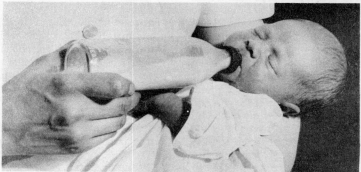

Fig. 211. (*Top*) The right way to hold a bottle. The baby's head should be turned slightly to one side, and the bottle held so that the baby will grasp the nipple squarely. To prevent the baby from swallowing air, the neck of the bottle should be filled with milk at all times. (*Bottom*) The wrong way to hold a bottle. If the bottle is held flat, air enters the nipple, and the baby may suffer as a result of swallowing air.

use the autoclaving method, but in the home the above procedure is used. In each method the formula must remain sterile and the nipple untouched and sterile until it reaches the baby's mouth (Fig. 211).

There is a variety of bottles and nipples on the market, many of them sold as "units" (bottle, nipple and nipple protector) (see Fig. 208).

Milk. Milk is usually graded by letter or special names to designate the conditions of production and processing demanded by United States Public Health Service standards. Standards vary somewhat in the various states for milk fat content and bacteria count allowed.

CERTIFIED MILK. Certified milk is produced under conditions which must conform to standards set by the American Association of Medical Milk Commissioners. Certified milk is very expensive and available mostly in the eastern part of the country.

VITAMIN D MILK. Vitamin D milk is produced by adding a concentrate "by the approved method to 400 units per quart," as stated in the Milk Ordinance, Code of the U.S.P.H.S., 1953. The addition of the concentrate must be specified on the label.

SKIMMED MILK. Skimmed milk is milk from which the cream (fat) has been removed. Sometimes it is ordered for babies who have simple diarrhea, but it should be used only when prescribed by the physician.

PASTEURIZED MILK. Pasteurized milk is milk which has been heated to a temperature of not less than 143° F. and kept at that heat for half an hour and cooled promptly. A "short-time" method of pasteurization is to heat the milk to not less than 160° F. and maintain this temperature for 30 seconds. This is sometimes done at home in a double boiler. Pasteurized milk is not boiled, since it is heated to a temperature of 143° or 160° F. only. Pasteurized milk offers excellent protection, for it destroys the common disease organisms in addition to most of the spoilage organisms which are responsible for souring, bad flavors, etc.

STERILIZED MILK. Sterilized milk means milk that is boiled for at least 10 minutes, during which few, if any, bacteria survive. It should be stirred constantly while boiling so that there will be no loss of the proteins which otherwise may stick to the sides of the pan. The nutritive value is reduced somewhat, especially through the effect of heat on vitamin C, and orange or tomato juice and cod-liver oil always should be added to the diet, replacing this loss.

THREE-MINUTE BOILED MILK. This shorter time of boiling produces less change in the milk than the boiling for 10 minutes, but it is still considered wise to add orange or tomato juice and cod-liver oil to the baby's diet. Boiling does not change the fats or the solids of milk. The protein goes through certain changes, but not enough to prevent the milk from providing the nourishment which its protein should furnish.

EVAPORATED MILK. Evaporated milk is cow's milk which has been evaporated so that it is twice as concentrated as whole milk. It is safe because the milk is sterilized in the cans in which it is sold and remains sterile as long as the cans are unopened.

HOMOGENIZED MILK. Homogenized milk is merely regular milk which, just before pasteurization, has been forced through a tiny opening under tremendous pressure. This breaks up the butter fat globules into much smaller ones and distributes them permanently throughout the milk. As a result, cream will not rise on homogenized milk, and so the last drop of it as rich and nourishing as the first.

POWDERED MILK. Powdered milk is milk from which all the fluids have been removed. It consists of about 10 per cent solids that are found in milk, for the 90 per cent of water is eliminated by the drying process. Powdered milk is obtainable in various forms: powdered whole milk, partially skimmed milk, modified milk, protein milk, lactic-acid milk and other special preparations. These are very simple to use when traveling, for all that is necessary is to add the specified amount of boiled water. The physician should be consulted before powdered milk is given to the baby.

Hunger. If the baby is not getting enough food, he will wake before his regular nursing time and be obviously hungry. He will cry and fret, refuse water with apparent disgust and, when nursing is permitted, seize the nipple ravenously and nurse with great vigor.

He may continue to nurse long after the breast is empty, in his effort to secure enough food; and he will cry in a fretful way when an attempt is made to remove him from the breast. Between nursings, he will suck his fingers or any article which may come in contact with his lips. In such cases, the breast, when examined just before nursing, will contain very little milk, and, when manual expression is attempted, it may be impossible to express any milk from the nipple.

Occasionally, a baby appears to be hungry between feedings when in reality he is only thirsty. He may be given a small amount of tepid boiled water to satisfy his thirst (but this must not be done immediately before or after a feeding).

Bubbling. After 5 minutes or so, or in the middle and at the end of each feeding, the infant should be held in an upright position or against the nurse's (or mother's) shoulder, while she gently pats his back to aid him in bringing up any air he may have swallowed (Fig. 212). Because the new infant's gastro-intestinal tract is labile, milk may be eructated with gas bubbles. Care should be taken to ensure adequate "bubbling" before the infant is placed back into the crib, thus preventing milk regurgitation.

Regurgitation. Regurgitation, which is merely an overflow and occurs immediately after nursing, should not be confused with vomiting, which may

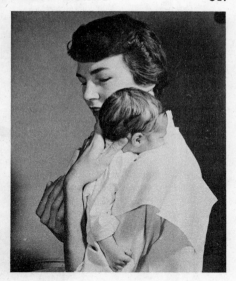

Fig. 212. "Bubbling" the baby. While in the hospital the mother should be taught to "bubble" her baby. Holding the baby upright against the shoulder during and immediately after nursing, gently pat his back to bring up air. Cuddly babies are sometimes difficult to put in this position.

occur at any time and is accompanied by other symptoms. This regurgitation is the means of relieving the distended stomach and indicates that the baby has either taken too much food or has taken it too rapidly.

Weaning

When, for any reason, it is necessary to wean the baby while the breasts are still secreting milk, it will be necessary to "dry up" the breasts. In general, the breasts should be emptied as completely as possible and a snug breast binder applied. The milk should disappear in a few days, but if the breasts become engorged, the physician should be consulted immediately. He may order ice caps to be applied to the breasts or he may give stilbestrol or both.

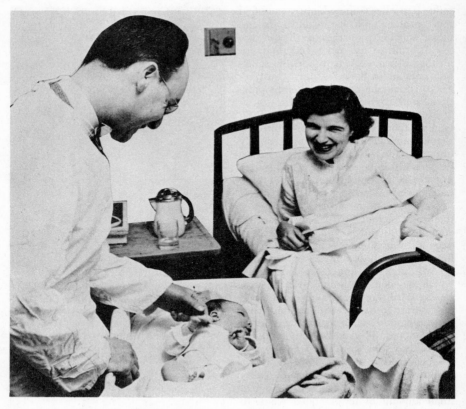

Fig. 213. Rooming-in makes it possible for the father to handle and become acquainted with the new baby. (French Hospital, New York; photo by Three Lions, Inc.)

Rooming-In

"Rooming-in" is the name given to the present plan of having the new infant share his mother's hospital unit so that they may be cared for together as mother and baby (Figs. 213-215). Although this plan for maternity care seems to have gained more widespread interest in this country in recent years, it is not really new, for it was practiced by mothers far back in history. However, the rooming-in program today in the modern maternity hospital must be regarded as a new departure from the old idea. Certainly, attitudes in maternal and infant care have changed, in part because of increased insight into the needs of the mother, her baby and the family as a unit. Rooming-in plays an important part in the family-centered approach to maternity care, for it not only provides an environment which fosters a wholesome, natural mother-child relationship from the very beginning, but it also affords unlimited opportunities for the parents to learn about the care of their baby.

To have a rooming-in program function successfully requires administrative planning and sound preparation of the entire hospital staff and the parents who use it. Generally, it demands a differ-

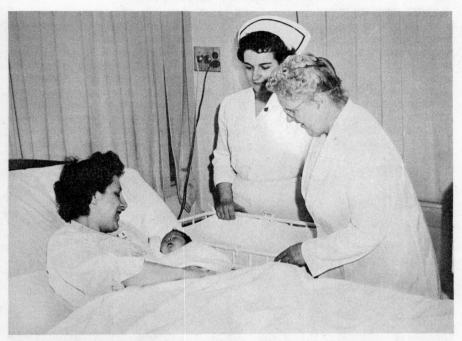

Fig. 214. Rooming-in. Pediatrician and nurse offer advice and consultation. This is a learning experience for the parents. (Grace-New Haven Community Hospital.)

ent architectural arrangement. Adequate space must be allowed for the mother's unit to accommodate the regular equipment needed for her, as well as that needed for the infant's care. Different physical plans for rooming-in arrangements have been developed, some units to accommodate one mother, others for as many as 4 of them. Each rooming-in unit should have an adjoining nursery and its own "workroom." Where it has not been feasible to make major changes in the physical plan of a maternity hospital to provide for continuous rooming-in, some hospitals have adopted a modified rooming-in program, providing extended time for the mother and her baby to be together during the day but otherwise utilizing the general nursery.

The newborn infant must be protected from sources of infection regardless of where he is cared for. The same basic principles for asepsis employed in the nursery must be followed in infant care in the rooming-in unit. Some years ago Dr. Edith Jackson said that it was possible to provide "the essential psychological satisfactions" which the mother and baby derive from a rooming-in experience "without losing the hard-won safeguards to physical health."* This has been demonstrated, for epidemic infections, such as diarrhea and skin infections, which sometimes occur in large hospital nurseries have not been observed in rooming-in programs.

Individual mothers must be taken into consideration as to whether or not they should have rooming-in. Some mothers

* Jackson, E. B.: Should mother and baby room together?, Am. J. Nursing 46:17, 1946.

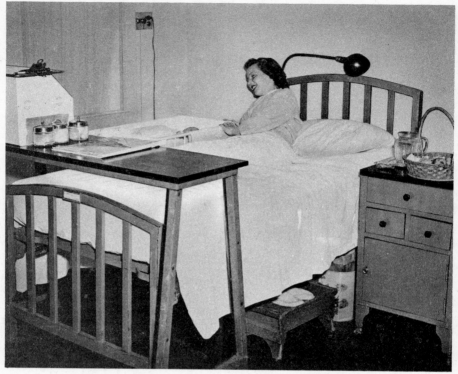

Fig. 215. A cubicle in the rooming-in unit of the Grace-New Haven
Community Hospital. (Photos by John J. Curran)

will want to have their babies with them most of the time so that they can get to know them and learn to care for them under the guidance of the nurses and the physicians. Other mothers may not want rooming-in, particularly multiparas, because they feel that this is an opportunity for rest and freedom from responsibility. Many mothers feel that they would enjoy rooming-in but hesitate because they do not feel sufficiently able to assume the care or the responsibility for the baby at this time. These mothers need help, of course, to understand that the nurse is there to help them, and they do not have to take over any more of the infant's care than they feel able or want to do.

Nurses with understanding and inter-est often can anticipate the mother's needs and desires and can be of invaluable help to her. Much of the practical care of the new baby must be learned by the new mother during her brief hospital stay to supplement the theoretical knowledge she has gained during the antepartal period. At this time the mother usually needs close supervision and guidance from the nurse in order that she may develop confidence in her own ability to handle and care for her baby. The father, also, may share in some of these experiences and learn much about his baby and his baby's care. With this kind of preparation, parents of first babies in particular do not feel so helpless when they return home. These shared experiences undoubtedly contribute toward an excellent foundation for stable and secure family relationships.

SUGGESTED READING

Adams, Margaret: Appraisal of a newborn infant, Am. J. Nursing 55:1336, 1955.

Berner, H. M.: New techniques in individual infant care, Hospital Management 77:42, 1954.

Boak, Walter E.: Medical and hospital care during pregnancy and early infancy, Pediatrics 22:538, 1958.

Bolby, John: Maternal Care and Mental Health, Geneva, World Health Organization, 1952.

Breast, bottle or both for your baby?, Parents Magazine 31:36, 130-133, 1956.

Clifford, S. H., and Davison, W. C.: The origin of obstetric nurseries, J. Pediat. 44:205, 1954.

Eastman, Nicholson J.: William's Obstetrics, ed. 11, New York, Appleton, 1956.

Grayson, R., and Cranch, G.: Care of the foreskin, Am. J. Nursing 56:75, 1956.

Gyorgy, Paul: Trends and advances in infant nutrition, Nursing Outlook 6:516, 1958.

Hurlock, Elizabeth: Child Development, ed. 3, New York, McGraw-Hill, 1956.

Jackson, Edith: New trends in maternity care, Am. J. Nursing 55:584, 1955.

Jackson, R.: Feeding healthy infants, Am. J. Nursing 55:1076, 1955.

Jeans, P. C., Wright, F. H., and Blake,

F. G.: Essentials of Pediatrics, ed. 6, Philadelphia, Lippincott, 1958.

Larsen, E.: Terminal rooming-in, Am. J. Nursing 56:1442, 1956.

McClure, Muriel H.: When she chooses breast feeding, Am. J. Nursing 57:1002, 1957.

McKerlie, E., and Einarson, L.: The psychological impact of and on the new arrival, Canad. Nurse 50:262, 1954.

Meyer, Herman F.: Infant feeding practices in hospital maternity nurseries, Pediatrics 21:288, 1958.

Naish, F. Charlotte: Breast Feeding, London, Lloyd-Luke, 1956.

Paterson, Donald, and McCreary, John Ferguson: Pediatrics, Philadelphia, Lippincott, 1956.

Smith, Christine S.: Demand feeding in the newborn nursery, Nursing Outlook 6:514, 1958.

Smith, Clement A.: Human milk technology, J. Pediat. 20:616, 1942. (Also available in reprint form.)

——: The Physiology of the Newborn Infant, ed. 3, Springfield, Ill., Thomas, 1959.

Stott, K. B.: Rooming-in is not a passing fad, Hospitals 29:80, 1955.

Volinsky, Thomas J.: Care of the newborn, Nursing World 131:24, 1957.

Wiedenbach, Ernestine: Family Centered Maternity Nursing, New York, Putnam, 1959.

Zabriskie, Louise: Mother and Baby Care in Pictures, ed. 4, Philadelphia, Lippincott, 1953.

CHAPTER SIXTEEN

Care of the Premature Infant

DEFINITION

A premature infant is arbitrarily defined as any infant, of single or multiple birth, born prematurely, at term or even past term, with a birth weight of 2,500 Gm. (5½ lbs.) or less. Such an infant is usually less than 48 cm. (19 in.) in length and usually has been born prior to the thirty-sixth week of gestation. Nonwhites, because they generally have smaller infants than whites, have a higher percentage of premature infants. Infants over this empirical weight, even though apparently born at full term, occasionally may be diagnosed by a physician as "premature" on the basis of other considerations, such as faulty maintenance of body temperature, particular feeding difficulties or certain physical characteristics. This may apply particularly to infants born to diabetic or prediabetic mothers. Although the upper limit of weight has been established, the lower never has been accepted by any authoritative group, and the level at which a dividing line is drawn between abortions and premature infants remains a matter of personal or local preference. The lower limit will depend on the definition of abortion, but the 1,000 Gm. figure is the one most frequently used. If the baby is from 6 to 8 weeks or more premature, the diagnosis is comparatively easy because of his weight, length and physical characteristics. The closer to full term the greater the chances for survival.

CAUSES OF PREMATURITY

Since more than half of the neonatal deaths in the United States are due to prematurity and since these rates have remained constant for many years, the emphasis on preventive care must be stressed. If the money expended on premature care were applied to preventive care, it would be interesting to prognosticate the results. However, the causes of prematurity present a challenging problem. Multiple pregnancy is the most common single cause of prematurity. Other causes are chronic hypertension, toxemia, infectious diseases (such as syphilis), acute abdominal conditions resulting in surgical interference, cardiac and diabetic diseases and thyroid disturbances.

Pregnancy itself also has its contributing causes—malformation in the embryologic development, erythroblastosis fetalis dependent on the Rh factor and faulty nutrition of the fetus. Abnormalities of placental structure resulting in the rupture of the membranes, placenta previa, abruptio placenta and hydramnios may cause prematurity. Then too, there is a fairly large group of premature births due to undiagnosed causes. From analysis of the causes, prematurity is very definitely an obstetric problem, because it occurs during pregnancy and terminates in a premature delivery.

CAUSES OF PREMATURE DEATHS

The main cause of the death of these infants is usually due to abnormal pulmonary ventilation. Faulty resuscitation method is one factor. Other causes are those conditions such as pneumonia, without hyaline-membranes, malformations, cerebral hemorrhage, atelectasis, anoxia and trauma. The blood vessels of the premature baby lack the supporting wall structure and, therefore, are very easily damaged.

Prevention of Prematurity

Edith L. Potter, M.D., of Chicago, says:

The ideal solution to the problem of prematurity is through the mother; more important than saving the life of a premature infant is the prevention of a premature birth. In many instances there is no recognizable cause of premature labor, although in a study of mortality made at the Chicago Lying-In Hospital, the common causes were toxemia, placenta praevia and premature separation of the placenta. Prevention of these conditions would aid materially in decreasing the number of premature births.*

Other authorities state that poor or inadequate diet and lack of rest are predisposing causes of prematurity.

DESCRIPTION AT BIRTH

As there are many degrees of prematurity, so also are there various stages of anatomic and physiologic development. Many of the symptoms described below may vary in infants of approximately the same fetal age, depending on the cause of prematurity and the physical condition of the mother and the infant. At birth the premature baby lacks the subcutaneous fat which is deposited during the last two months of intra-uterine

* Engle: Pregnancy Wastage, Springfield, Ill., Thomas, 1953.

development. This gives the skin a transparent appearance with the blood vessels easily seen through the skin, which is often of a deep red color, sometimes with a cyanotic hue. Also, these premature babies are prone to develop icteric skin changes. Lanugo is usually abundant all over the skin surface but disappears within a few weeks.

The external ears and the nose are very soft, due to the underdeveloped cartilage. The ears lie very close to the head. The skull is round, in contrast with the long anteroposterior skull diameter of the full-term infant. The fontanels are large, and the sutures prominent. The finger- and toenails may be immature, often not reaching the ends of the fingers and the toes.

The infant may be puny and small or he may approximate full-term weight, yet the internal organs may be imperfectly developed, and these babies appear to be reluctant to assume the responsibility to live. The respirations are shallow and irregular, due to the lack of lung expansion and proper gaseous exchange. There are often periods of apnea. Due to the irregular respirations and the poorly developed function of swallowing, there is danger of aspiration of milk or vomitus, causing cyanosis and predisposing to pulmonary infections. The premature baby regurgitates his food readily because the stomach is tubular in form and the sphincters are poorly developed. The urine is usually scanty.

The walls of the blood vessels are weak, and the tendency to hemorrhage is great. Since the central nervous system is not fully developed, the premature infant is sluggish, must be wakened to be fed, and the muscular movements are feeble. The temperature is usually subnormal and fluctuating, due to the underdeveloped heat-regulating center. The cry is monotonous, whining, "kittenlike" and effortless, showing a lack of energy. All these symptoms are evidenced in varying degrees, according to the stage of prematurity.

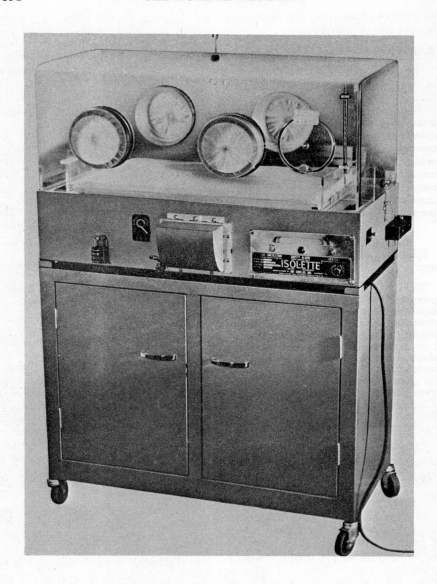

Fig. 216. The Isolette incubator. (Air-Shields Inc., Hatboro, Pa.)

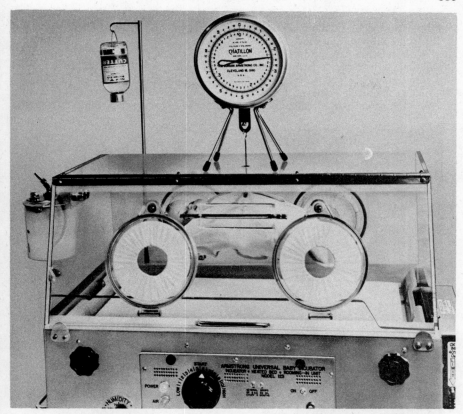

Fig. 217. The Armstrong Universal baby incubator. (The Gordon Armstrong Company, Inc., Cleveland, Ohio)

IMMEDIATE CARE

The care given the premature baby at birth may differ from that given to the full-term baby, depending on his condition. For the very small and feeble premature baby, the urgency of providing immediate warmth, humidity and oxygen as indicated may precede the care of the eyes and completion of the care of the cord. Whenever possible, it is advisable to wait until the cord pulsation weakens before clamping it, so that the baby will benefit from the placental blood. The cord should be clamped or tied with special care because of the softness of the tissues, leaving space for a second ligature close to the body when the linen cord tie is used. The cord should be inspected at frequent intervals for bleeding, because prematurity is a predisposing cause of secondary hemorrhage. Since premature babies are also more susceptible to infections, asepsis is imperative. The head and the shoulders should be level or slightly elevated but not in a head-down position.

As soon as the head emerges, the eyes should be wiped gently with moist sterile gauze. The instillation of prophylactic drops may have to be deferred until the condition of the baby warrants this treatment.

Because of the baby's underdeveloped and delicate structures, the resuscitation of the premature infant must be managed with extreme care and gentleness. Often the method of resuscitation will determine the baby's chances to live. The mucus should be removed from the nose and the throat with great care. Any injury to the delicate tissues is an avenue to trauma and infection which may lead to pneumonia.

Since the maintenance of body heat is so essential, a baby should be wrapped in a warmed blanket, and a heated bed or incubator (Figs. 216 and 217) should be ready to receive him. When the

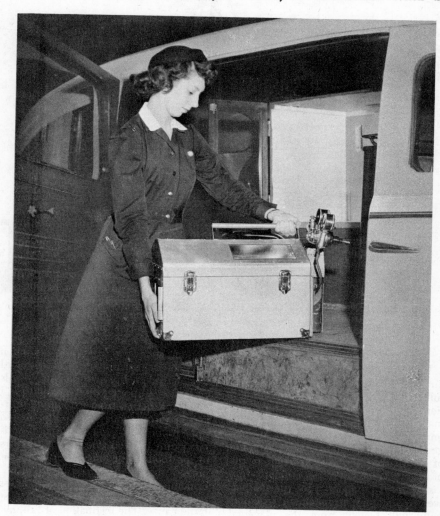

Fig. 218. Nurse of the New York City Department of Health placing the portable premature incubator into the Department's Premature Transport Service Ambulance. (City of New York, Department of Health; photo by George Doherty)

baby's condition permits, his temperature and weight should be recorded. The infant should be turned gently from side to side periodically and occasionally stimulated to cry (though handled as little as possible).

NURSING CARE

Management

Because of the nationwide interest in reducing deaths among premature infants, there have developed special premature nurseries and special premature referral centers in municipalities and other major health jurisdictions. Space is usually allotted in the hospital separate from the nursery for the full-term babies. Some centers concentrate on the care of the smaller babies. Generally, provision

is made for the safe transport to and from the hospital (Figs. 218 and 219). As discharge time approaches, plans are made for the follow-up care in the home. In these programs the premature infants spend the initial period in an incubator. During this time skilled medical and nursing care is aimed at maintaining adequate oxygenation, stabilizing the body temperature, safeguarding the baby against infection, supplying proper nutrition and feeding, maintaining a fluid and electrolyte balance and recognizing early abnormalities and infections.

Some hospitals have special premature nurseries which are air-conditioned in respect to temperature (85° to 90° F.), ventilation and humidity (50 to 65%) control. This may not be necessary where infants are "housed" in modern incuba-

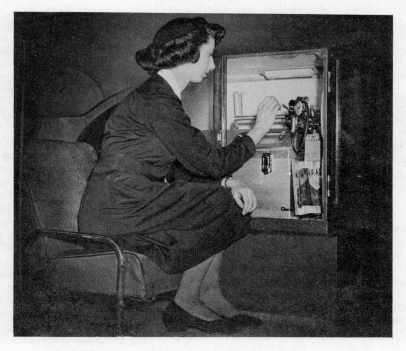

Fig. 219. Nurse regulating oxygen in portable incubator in the heated compartment of the Premature Transport Service Ambulance of the New York City Department of Health. (City of New York, Department of Health; photo by George Doherty)

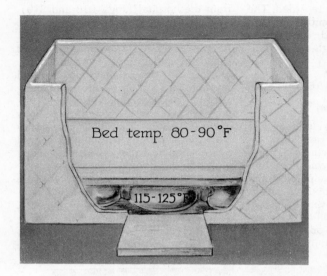

Fig. 220. Homemade, heated bed made from small canned goods box. The platform is 4 inches above the floor. The box is padded inside and outside with quilting. Three quarters of the bed is covered with a blanket. (Lundeen and Kunstadter: Care of the Premature Infant, Philadelphia, Lippincott)

Bed temp. 80-90°F

115-125°F

tors. From a recent study by Silverman and his colleagues, is reported the following:

Survival rates of premature infants are higher in those kept at an incubator temperature of 89° F. during the first five days of life than those maintained at 84° F.*

In an emergency situation, for example when the infant is born prematurely at home in an outlying, rural area, some means to protect the premature must be devised until an incubator can be brought from the local health agency. An incubator can be improvised from a box or a cardboard carton (Fig. 220). Such a specially prepared bed may be heated by electricity from a wire-screened 25- or 40-watt light bulb or, if electricity is not available, by the use of hot-water bottles, or heated bricks or sandbags.

A large majority of premature infants must receive oxygen initially because of

* Silverman, W. A., Fertig, J. W., and Berger, A. P.: Pediatrics 22:876, 1958.

respiratory difficulties or cyanosis. Nevertheless, this should not be used routinely and, except in an emergency, should always be prescribed by the physician. Oxygen therapy is often a life-saving measure for the premature infant, but it must be used judiciously. The oxygen requirements for these infants vary, and, thus, it should be administered at the lowest concentration compatible with life. As a temporary measure, after necessary suctioning, the newborn may be given oxygen by mask or funnel placed over the infant's nose and mouth. The flow of oxygen should be set at a maximum of 3 liters when this method is used. When the premature infant is in an incubator, the lowest oxygen concentration to relieve the respiratory symptoms should be employed, if possible *not* over 40 per cent. Occasionally, higher concentrations are necessary, but in any case, oxygen therapy should be discontinued as soon as the infant can get along without it. One of the inherent dangers is the development of retrolental fibroplasia (see Chap. 21). Evidence has shown that there is a relationship between the use of relatively high concentrations of oxygen and the occurrence of retrolental fibroplasia.

The modern air-conditioned incubator is a miniature room in which the infant can live and be cared for under ideal atmospheric conditions, i.e., desirable levels of heat, humidity and oxygen. The very immature infant may require a completely air-conditioned environment, receiving heat, humidity and oxygen in the incubator, while an infant who is more mature may need only heat, and sometimes humidity. Many kinds of incubators are currently used, but the principle is the same, the difference being in the special construction details developed by various manufacturers.

The new incubators have controls on the outside of the unit to regulate atmospheric conditions accurately and to adjust the bed proper from the horizontal to the tilted positions (i.e., Trendelenburg and reverse-Trendelenburg positions). Special oxygen inlets provide either 40 per cent maximum concentration or high oxygen concentration in case it may be needed. Regardless of this, at regular intervals the nurse should check and record the oxygen concentration of the incubator with a reliable oximeter, i.e., an oxygen analyzer, placed at the level of the infant's nose. The incubator can be ventilated with fresh air from the room through a large, replaceable air filter or through an outside air attachment when oxygen therapy is no longer

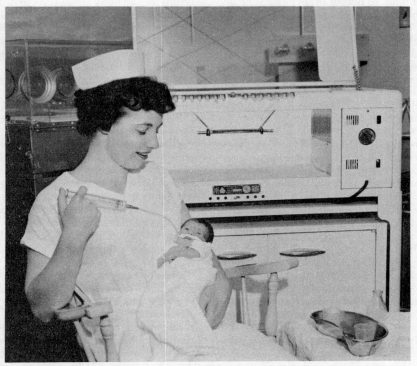

Fig. 221. Gavage feeding. When the premature infant does not require oxygen, the nurse can take him out of the incubator and hold him as she feeds him. (Babies and Childrens Hospital, The University Hospitals of Cleveland, Cleveland, Ohio)

required for the infant. Humidity can be controlled, and, by means of a nebulizer, supersaturated atmosphere can be created. Constant temperatures within the incubator can be regulated and maintained with a double-thermoswitch-controlled, sealed heating unit. Other features which are none the less important to the nurse are that these incubators are so designed that the infant can be observed from all sides through transparent windows. Moreover, hand holes with air-tight doors and self-adjusting "sleeves" permit the nurses and the physicians to care for the infant without disturbing the atmospheric conditions. The incubators are made of stainless steel and plastic and constructed for easy removal of all essential parts, without tools, to permit proper cleansing and sterilizing.

Some persons have the impression that once the baby is placed in a good incubator no further special precautions need be taken. This is a mistaken idea. Premature or underdeveloped infants require the most solicitous care in every way; merely to keep them in a proper atmosphere will avail nothing unless the other details of their care are executed carefully. The maintenance of asepsis in every detail is essential for these inadequately fortified babies. It is also urgent that doctors, nurses or anyone caring for a delicate premature baby should avoid contact with any possible source of infection which might be transferred to the baby.

Rest is a most important factor, and the baby must be shielded from excitement and disturbing influences. Light should be curtailed, and loud or sudden noises should be avoided. As long as the infant requires high humidity or oxygen therapy routine care is given in the premature bed, such as administering nourishment, altering his position, cleansing his skin and changing his linen as necessary. The skin is extremely delicate and tender; and if diapers are used they should be changed as soon as they become wet or soiled. Sometimes only a small pad is placed under the baby. The skin does not require bathing or oiling if care is taken so body folds do not become irritated and the diaper area kept clean and dry. If an incubator is not available, he is dressed in a jacket of cotton and gauze or flannel. The weight and the temperature of the baby are both matters of importance and are carried out according to the hospital routine.

Feeding

When planning the feeding schedule for the premature infant, it is important to establish a food tolerance since the intestinal tract (as well as other organs) is underdeveloped. The caloric needs of the premature baby are estimated according to the body weight. At first, the feeding should be in small amounts and increased gradually to the amount that will produce a consistent gain, since vomiting, distention and diarrhea may be due to overfeeding.

According to some authorities the general plan involves an initial period of rest, followed by small amounts of water at frequent intervals; gradual replacement of water feedings by milk feedings; gradual increase in amounts of milk and water at each feeding until caloric and fluid requirements are met. Some physicians advise adding a 5 per cent glucose solution to the drinking water.

In some areas of the country breast milk is considered to be the feeding of choice for premature infants. In other sections, however, modified formulas are preferred.

Prematures who weigh 3 pounds or less may be fed every 2 or 3 hours. Infants who weigh over 3½ pounds may be placed on a 4-hour feeding schedule. In addition to the feedings, premature diets usually include vitamin and iron preparations. These additions are introduced when the feeding and schedule are fairly well established and the infant is able to tolerate them. The stomach of the premature baby needs rest between feedings as much as that of the full-term baby; therefore, the interval should be regulated accordingly. The schedule should be as near that of a normal infant as is compatible with his progress.

When a very small and weak infant is on a 3-hour feeding schedule, gavage feeding is usually indicated. It is common practice today to introduce a polyethylene retention catheter to the stomach rather than the gavage catheter at frequent intervals. The end to be introduced must be rounded and smooth (using very fine sandpaper, and immersing the tip in melted wax). The distance between the bridge of the infant's nose and the estimated area of the stomach should be measured and marked on the catheter. The tubing is then introduced into the lower end of the esophagus (by the physician) and may be left in place from 3 to 7 days. Before each feeding the nurse inserts a No. –20 needle into the distal end of the tubing to act as an adapter for the Luer syringe which holds the milk. No air should precede the milk. The milk should be introduced very slowly and at the correct temperature, while the infant is supported in a semi-reclining position. If the infant requires oxygen he must be fed in the incubator. After the feeding the infant may need to be placed in the incubator with his head and shoulders slightly elevated. When the infant is able to suck, gavage feeding may be discontinued in favor of a bottle with a small soft nipple.

Currently, in premature care a medicine-dropper feeding is usually not used. When a medicine-dropper feeding is indicated for some specific reason, the glass tip should be protected by a small piece of rubber tubing which extends at least one quarter of an inch beyond the glass tip. When the infant is unable to suck, the swallowing reflex is also extremely weak. If a medicine dropper is to be used to feed such an infant, the procedure should be managed only by the most skilled practitioner.

Precautions

Since the life of the premature baby may depend on his nursing care, the nurse should realize the seriousness of this responsibility during this period of her nursing experience and make every effort to increase her knowledge and develop her skill.

Often the first hours of the premature baby's life determine the outcome. He needs warmth, meticulous care, gentle handling, precise and careful feeding and protection from infection. It must always be remembered that the word "premature" means that this baby has arrived before he had the opportunity to develop completely and, if he is to live, this intricate development has to be completed against odds almost unsurmountable—under conditions sometimes difficult even for the normal full-term baby. It is important that home conditions be investigated by the visiting nurse or social worker before the baby is discharged from the hospital.

GROWTH AND DEVELOPMENT

Growth and development of the premature baby is primarily dependent on the degree of prematurity at the time of birth. Much will depend on the ability of the infant to meet the conditions attendant at birth and to adjust to the changes in his new environment. Those infants who react well to prompt treatment and care make their adjustment by the end of the first year, but there are others who may require several years to match the normal child at that age.

The nurse is often asked if a premature baby will ever develop as well and become as strong and sturdy as one born at term. While the premature baby is slower in regaining his birth weight, by the end of the first year his weight should approximate that of the normal baby. Evidences of progress in his development are temperature stability, the increased vigor of his cry, stronger muscular activity, evidence of appetite and hunger, more normal periods of sleep, changes in the appearance and the character of his skin due to the addition of the subcutaneous fat, the development of reflexes and general signs of health. Parents of prematurely born infants invariably need special guidance and support to help them develop confidence in their ability to care for their baby, particularly in anticipation of taking him home from the hospital. The nurse has a real responsibility to help them so that they are adequately prepared for the baby's homecoming.

SUGGESTED READING

Baumgartner, Leona: Nation-wide plan for réduction of premature mortality, J.A.M.A. 146:893, 1951.

Clifford, S. H.: The problem of prematurity, J. Pediat. 47:13, 1955.

Committee on the Fetus and Newborn, American Academy of Pediatrics: Standards and Recommendations for Hospital Care of Newborn Infants (Rev.), Evanston, Ill., The Academy, 1957.

Crosse, Victoria M.: Premature Infants, New York, Hoeber, 1955.

Dancis, Joseph: The possibilities of total elimination of retrolental fibroplasia by oxygen restriction, Pediatrics 17: 247, 1956.

Dancis, Joseph, and Spitz, Rose: Your Premature Baby (Children's Bureau Folder No. 40), Washington, D. C., U. S. Dept. of Health, Education and Welfare, 1954.

DiMaggio, G., and Gelina, Marguerite: Parents learn about their premature babies, The Child 17:106, 1953.

Dunham, E. C.: Premature Infants, ed. 2, New York, Hoeber, 1955.

Folsome, Clair E., et al.: Maternal factors in prematurity, Am. J. Obst. & Gynec. 72:62, 1956.

Greene, D. M., and Zetzsche, L.: Premies are human beings too!, Pub. Health Nursing 44:253, 1952.

Jeans, P. C., Wright, F. H., and Blake, F. G.: Essentials of Pediatrics, ed. 6, Philadelphia, Lippincott, 1958.

Losty, Margaret A., Orlofsky, Irene, and Wallace, Helen M.: A transport service for premature babies, Am. J. Nursing 50:10, 1950.

Lundeen, E. C., and Kunstadter, R. H.: Care of the Premature Infant, Philadelphia, Lippincott, 1958.

Parke, Priscilla C.: Naso-gastric tube feeding for premature infants, Am. J. Nursing 51:517, 1951.

Prugh, Dane G.: Emotional problems of the premature infants' parents, Nursing Outlook 1:461, 1953.

Silverman, William A., and Blanc, William A.: The effect of humidity on survival of newly born premature infants, Pediatrics 20:477, 1957.

Taylor, E. Stewart: The prevention of deaths from prematurity, Pub. Health Nursing 42:280, 1950.

Wallace, Helen M., Losty, Margaret A., and Wishik, Samuel M.: Prematurity as a public health problem. Am. J. Pub. Health 40:41, 1950.

Weidman Olt, Esther, and Lubehenco, Lula: The premature infant's reaction to illness, Am. J. Nursing 57:1431, 1957.

Weintraub, David and Tabankin, Alvin: Relationship of retrolental fibroplasia to oxygen concentration, J. Pediat. 49:75, 1956.

CONFERENCE MATERIAL

1. What is the responsibility of the hospital and the nurse in preparing the mother to care for her baby after they leave the hospital?

2. What advice and help could you give the mother to help her to adjust the new baby in the home and to prevent (or deal with) sibling rivalry when there is a 2-year-old brother who is accustomed to having the undivided love and attention of his parents?

3. Compare the physiologic development of the premature infant with that of the normal full-term infant.

4. What are some other means which could be employed to supply external heat for the premature infant who requires it when a mechanical incubator is not available?

5. What information can you give parents about the "well-baby clinic" in your community?

Read through the entire question and place your answer in the parentheses.

1. The neonatal period constitutes one of the most important periods of life because of the profound physiologic changes which occur. Which of the following statements concerning these alterations are correct?
   A. Certain of these physiologic changes are immediate, some are delayed.
   B. All of these physiologic changes are immediate.
   C. All of these physiologic changes are permanent.
   D. Certain of these physiologic changes are temporary.
   Select the number corresponding to the correct letters.
   1. A and C
   2. A and D
   3. B and C
   4. B and D

(——1——)

2. Which of the following reasons best explain why the maternity hospital should adopt the "rooming-in" plan for the mother and her newborn?
   A. All mothers need the experience gained thereby.
   B. Selected mothers and babies may profit where the plan could be adopted.
   C. All mothers want this type of service.
   D. Most infants cry too much in a "central" nursery.
   E. All infants need this added attention.
   Select the number corresponding to the correct letter or letters.
   1. A only
   2. B only
   3. A, C and D
   4. B, C and E

(——2——)

3. What type of initial bath is usually given the newborn infant?
   A. Tub bath
   B. Spray bath
   C. Oil bath
   D. Cleansing only as necessary with warm water and sterile cotton
   E. Sponge bath with mild, unscented soap and warm water

(——D——)

4. What is the reason for selecting this method of skin care in the above question?
   A. The infant's skin must be washed thoroughly to prevent irritation.
   B. It stimulates the circulation.
   C. Special oils provide nourishment to the tissues.
   D. It is the best means of applying external heat.
   E. It lessens the danger of infection.

(——E——)

5. What is the usual procedure for the daily care of the genitals of the male infant who is not in need of circumcision?

A. Wash externally with soap and water, otherwise let alone.
B. Retract and cleanse under the foreskin with cotton ball moistened with warm water.
C. Retract and cleanse under the foreskin with alcohol.
D. After cleansing, apply sterile petrolatum under the foreskin.
E. Stretch the prepuce and lubricate with mineral oil.

(——B——)

6. What is the principle underlying the concept of demand feedings for the newborn infant?
A. Maintaining a regular 4-hour schedule to establish eating habits
B. Feeding the infant every 2 to 3 hours to stimulate digestion
C. Fitting individual feedings to individual needs
D. Permissive feeding schedule causes less conflict with the mother's household activities.
E. More frequent feedings assure an adequate nutritional intake.

(——C——)

7. The young mother asks how she will know when her baby is hungry. Which of the following responses would be most appropriate for the nurse to reply?
A. "All crying indicates hunger."
B. "Feed the baby whenever he is awake."
C. "He will cry, fret and suck on anything in contact with his lips."
D. "Offer him water first; if he refuses the water, then feed him."

(——C——)

8. What is the established birth weight below which the infant is considered to need special premature care, regardless of whether or not he is born prematurely according to dates?
A. 4 pounds
B. 4½ pounds
C. 5 pounds
D. 5½ pounds
E. 6 pounds

(——D——)

9. The appearance of a healthy newborn infant's stools will normally change during the neonatal period. Which of the following types of stools, in sequence of appearance, would the nurse observe in the healthy infant?
A. Dark, tarlike
B. Clay-colored, soft
C. Mottled greenish-brown, soft
D. Smooth, yellow
E. Green, curdy
Select the number corresponding to the correct letters.
1. A and D
2. A, C and D
3. B, C and E
4. All of them

(——2——)

10. How does the composition of mother's milk compare with cow's milk?

A. Human milk contains more protein.
B. Human milk contains less protein.
C. Human milk contains more carbohydrate.
D. Human milk contains larger fat globules.
E. Human milk contains less iron.
Select the number corresponding to the correct letters.
   1. A and C
   2. A, C and E
   3. B, C and D
   4. B, D and E

(———)

11. Which of the following features are characteristic of the premature infant and distinguish him from the full-term infant?
A. The infant is usually puny and weighs less than 2,000 Gm.
B. The infant's head is proportionately large, his skull is round or ovoid in shape, and his facial features are small and angular.
C. The skin is soft, transparent and may be covered with lanugo.
D. These infants whimper and cry rather constantly, although the cry is weak.
E. The body temperature is unstable and thus responds rather readily to changes in the temperature of the environment.
Select the number corresponding to the correct letters.
   1. A and B
   2. B, C and D
   3. B, C and E
   4. All of them

(———)

12. When the mother learned that her premature infant was receiving gavage feedings she asked the nurse why this was being done. Which of the following reasons may be correct for the nurse to reply?
A. "This method of feeding your baby was indicated because he became exhausted when he tried to swallow."
B. "Feeding your baby this way prevents him from vomiting and thus eliminates the danger of his aspirating formula into his lungs."
C. "Feeding your baby this way conserves his strength and permits him to receive food into his stomach when sucking or swallowing may be difficult."
D. "He can be given his formula quickly this way and so he does not have to be handled as much."
E. "A tiny baby's resistance to infection is poor, so gavage feeding is really a protective measure against such infections as thrush, which he might acquire if he were bottle fed."
•Select the number corresponding to the correct letter or letters.
   1. A only
   2. C only
   3. B, C and D
   4. B, D and E

(———)

13. When caring for premature infants, which of the following precautions should be taken against retrolental fibroplasia?
A. The administration of oxygen should be discontinued as soon as feasible.

B. The concentration of oxygen in the incubator housing the infant should be tested periodically and kept at less than 40 per cent.
C. Daily determinations of the serum bilirubin level should be done when there is any indication of proliferation of the retinal capillaries.
D. High humidity should be maintained in the incubator constantly.
E. The infant's eyes should be protected from bright lights.
Select the number corresponding to the correct letters.
1. A and B
2. A, C and D
3. B, D and E
4. All of them

(————)

14. How can the public health nurse assist the family in the care and the supervision of the premature infant?
A. Visit the home before the infant leaves the hospital to evaluate the home situation and give anticipatory guidance to the parents as necessary.
B. Help the family to understand that the infant is still premature and must have the same kind of skillful, protective care in a sheltered environment similar to that in the hospital premature nursery.
C. Make daily visits to the home to bathe the infant, prepare the formula and, in general, give suggestions and guidance to the mother about her infant's care.
D. Visit the home again after the infant is discharged from the hospital to give the family guidance and assistance as necessary.
E. Help the family to understand that this infant requires a great amount of undisturbed rest and thus should not be held or cuddled as much as the full-term infant.
Select the number corresponding to the correct letters.
1. A and D
2. A, C and E
3. B, C and E
4. All of them

(————)

15. The premature infant has difficulty in regulating his body temperature because heat regulation is one of the least developed functions of his body. Which of the following conditions are responsible for this?
A. The surface area of the premature infant is relatively smaller than that of a normal full-term infant in proportion to body size.
B. Lack of subcutaneous fat which would furnish a measure of insulation
C. Limited ability to produce body proteins
D. Poor reflex control of skin capillaries
E. Frequent episodes of diaphoresis causing loss of body heat
Select the number corresponding to the correct letters.
1. A and C
2. B and D
3. B, C and E
4. All of them

(————)

Note: The key to the correct answers to these questions is given on page 533.

Operative Procedures in Obstetrics

Episiotomy and Repair of Lacerations
Forceps
Version
Cesarean Section
Destructive Operations
Induction of Labor

CHAPTER SEVENTEEN

Operative Obstetrics

Although the nurse will rarely be called upon to perform obstetric operations, she will be a much more intelligent and understanding assistant to the obstetrician if she knows why the more common operations are done and how they are carried out. The only operative procedure of major importance which the nurse may be obliged to perform in emergencies is breech extraction. This will be discussed on page 436 in connection with the management of breech delivery.

EPISIOTOMY AND REPAIR OF LACERATIONS

Except for clamping and cutting the umbilical cord, episiotomy is the most common operative procedure performed in obstetrics. In view of the fact that this incision of the perineum, made to facilitate delivery, is employed almost routinely in primigravidas, the procedure has been discussed in the section on the conduct of normal labor (see Chap. 12).

Lacerations of the perineum and the vagina which occur in the process of delivery (see Fig. 175) have also been covered earlier in the text because some tears are unavoidable even in the most skilled hands. The suturing of spontaneous perineal lacerations is similar to that employed for the repair of an episiotomy incision but may be more difficult be-cause such tears are often irregular in shape with ragged, bruised edges.

FORCEPS

The common types of obstetric forceps are illustrated in Figures 222-225. The instrument, it will be seen, consists of two steel parts which cross each other like a pair of scissors and lock at the intersection. The lock may be of a sliding type, as in the first three types shown, or a screw type, as in the Tarnier instrument. Each part consists of a handle, a lock, a shank and a blade; the blade is the curved portion designed for application to the sides of the baby's head. The blades of most forceps (the Tucker McLane is an exception) have a large opening or window (fenestrum) in them to give a better grip on the baby's head, and usually they have two curves: a cephalic curve, which conforms to the shape of the baby's head, and a pelvic curve, to follow the curve of the birth canal. Axis-traction forceps, such as the Tarnier, are used less frequently today than formerly; this instrument has a mechanism attached below which permits the pulling to be done more directly in the axis of the birth canal.

The two blades of the forceps are designated as right and left. The left blade is the one which is introduced into the vagina on the patient's left side; the right blade goes into the right side. In

369

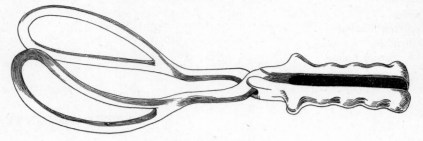

Fig. 222. Simpson forceps.

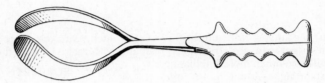

Fig. 223. Tucker McLane forceps.

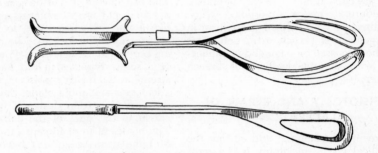

Fig. 224. Kielland forceps. (A) Front view; (B) side view.

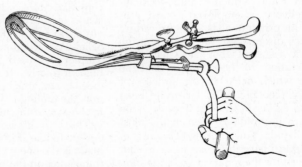

Fig. 225. Tarnier axis-traction forceps.

the majority of hospitals today, the nurse does not scrub for delivery but assists the obstetrician as a "circulating" nurse in the delivery room. However, if the nurse is ever expected to scrub and assist the obstetrician, she should articulate and disarticulate the forceps a few times and make sure that she knows which blade is which. Otherwise, this may prove to be rather confusing.

It may become necessary to deliver the baby by forceps because of reasons related to the mother's welfare (maternal indications), or because of conditions associated with the baby's condition (fetal indications). Among the more common maternal indications are: inability of the mother to effect delivery after 2 hours or so of complete dilatation of the cervix, maternal exhaustion, heart disease, toxemia of pregnancy and threatened rupture of the uterus. The chief fetal indication for forceps delivery is fetal distress, as shown by a slow, irregular fetal heart. Many obstetricians, however, deem it desirable to deliver almost all primigravidas with forceps in the belief that the operation spares the mother many minutes of exhausting bearing-down efforts and relieves pressure on the baby's head. This is usually referred to as "elective forceps."

Forceps operations never are attempted unless the cervix is completely dilated. In the vast majority of cases today, the procedure is carried out at a time when the baby's head is on the perineal floor (visible or almost so) and, as a rule, internal rotation has occurred so that the baby's head lies in a direct antero-posterior position. This is called "low forceps," sometimes "outlet forceps." When the head is higher in the pelvis, with its lowermost point near the level of the ischial spines, the operation is called "mid-forceps." If the head has not yet engaged, the procedure is known as "high forceps." High-forceps delivery is an exceedingly difficult and dangerous operation for both mother and baby and is rarely done. The obstetrician will in-

form the nurse of the type of instrument he wishes to use. Autoclaving is the usual type of sterilization employed, so several pairs of the generally approved forceps, each encased in suitable wrappings, are autoclaved and kept in the delivery room for immediate use. If the latter procedure is not done, most obstetricians will request that a pair of forceps be sterilized with the other instruments prepared for delivery in case they should be necessary in an emergency. The other instruments needed for a forceps delivery are the same as those required for a spontaneous delivery, plus those necessary for repair work (see Chap. 12).

Complete anesthesia is necessary, but in low-forceps deliveries it may be light, and in many institutions this type of operation is performed successfully under local infiltration anesthesia. The patient is placed in the lithotomy position and prepared and draped in the usual fashion. The obstetrician will first catheterize the patient. After checking the exact position of the baby's head by vaginal examination, he will introduce two or more fingers of his right hand into the left side of the vagina; these fingers will guide the left blade into place and at the same time protect the maternal soft parts (vagina, cervix) from injury. Taking the left blade of the forceps in his left hand, he introduces it into the left side of the vagina, gently insinuating it between the baby's head and the fingers of his right hand (Fig. 226). The same procedure is carried out on the right side, and then the blades are articulated. Traction is not continuous but intermittent (Fig. 227); and between traction, the obstetrician will partially disarticulate the blades in order to release pressure on the baby's head. Episiotomy is almost routine nowadays in these cases.

VERSION

Version consists of turning the baby in the uterus from an undesirable into a desirable position. There are three types of version: external, internal and Braxton-Hicks.

External Version. This is an operation designed to change a breech presentation into a vertex presentation by external manipulation of the fetus through the abdominal and the uterine walls. It is attempted in the hope of averting the difficulties of a subsequent breech delivery. Obstetricians find the procedure most successful when done about a month before full term; it often fails, however, either because it proves to be impossible to turn the fetus around or because the fetus returns to its original position within a few hours. Some obstetricians disapprove of it altogether.

Internal Version. Sometimes called internal podalic version, this is an operation designed to change whatever presentation may exist into a breech presen-

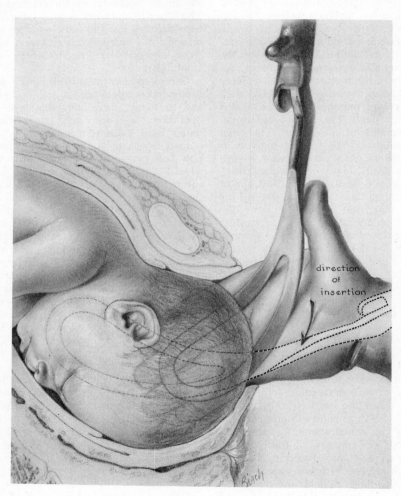

direction of insertion

Fig. 226. Insertion of forceps blade.

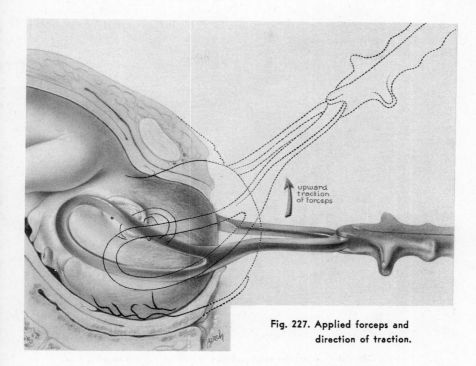

Fig. 227. Applied forceps and direction of traction.

upward
traction
of forceps

tation (see Fig. 228). With cervical dilatation complete, the whole hand of the operator is introduced high into the uterus, one or both feet are grasped and pulled downward in the direction of the birth canal. With his external hand the obstetrician may expedite the turning by pushing the head upward. The version usually is followed by breech extraction (p. 433). Internal version finds its greatest usefulness in cases of multiple pregnancy in which the birth of the second twin is retarded.

Braxton-Hicks Version. In this procedure, two fingers are introduced into a partially dilated cervix and, after manipulating the fetus to effect turning, one leg is drawn through the cervix. The operation is not designed to bring about immediate delivery and never is followed at once by extraction. Its purposes are either to compress the lower uterine

segment with the infant's buttock (see placenta previa, p. 413), or, more rarely, to stretch the cervix with the infant's thigh so that labor may be initiated. It is rarely used in modern obstetrics.

CESAREAN SECTION

Cesarean section is the removal of the infant from the uterus through an incision made in the abdominal wall and the uterus. The main indications for cesarean section fall into 5 groups: (1) disproportion between the size of the fetus and that of the bony birth canal, that is, contracted pelvis (p. 440), tumor blocking birth canal, etc.; (2) certain cases in which the patient has had a previous cesarean section, the operation being done because of fear that the uterine scar will rupture in labor; (3) certain cases of very severe toxemia of pregnancy, but rarely in eclampsia; (4)

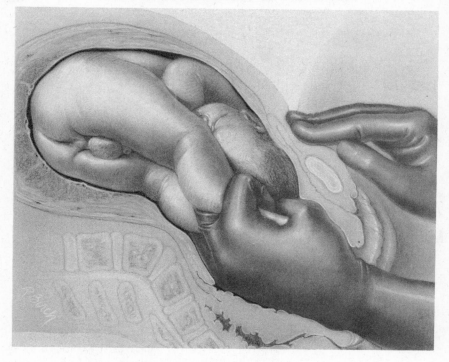

Fig. 228. Internal podalic version. Elbow length gloves are usually worn for this operation.

certain cases of placenta previa and premature separation of the normally implanted placenta; (5) miscellaneous complications.

There are 4 main types of cesarean section.

Classic Cesarean Section. The incision is made directly into the wall of the body of the uterus; the baby and the placenta are extracted, and the incision is closed by three layers of catgut sutures (Figs. 229 and 230). As a rule, classic cesarean section is employed only in those cases in which the operation is done prior to the onset of labor. At this time, the uterine contents are sterile, but after 6 or more hours of labor, particularly if the membranes have been ruptured, bacteria ascend from the vagina into the uterus and are potential sources of infection. When done after the patient has been in labor many hours, this type of operation is considered to be dangerous because of the ease with which infectious material, during the puerperium, may escape directly through the uterine wound into the peritoneal cavity. When any type of cesarean section is done prior to the onset of labor, as the result of a prearranged plan, it is known as "elective" cesarean section. (As with "elective low forceps," the obstetrician is not forced to perform the operation but elects to do it as the best procedure for mother and baby.)

Low Cervical Cesarean Section. (Synonyms: 2-flap cesarean section; laparotrachelotomy.) The initial incision (the abdomen having been opened) is made transversely across the uterine

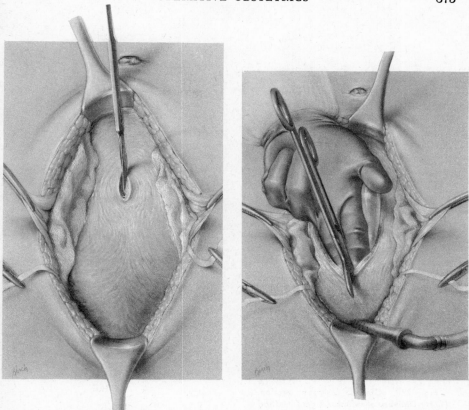

Fig. 229. Classic cesarean section. (*Left*) Uterus packed off with warm, moist gauze pads. Start of incision with knife. (*Right*) Continuation of incision with bandage scissors.

peritoneum where it is attached loosely just above the bladder. Two flaps of peritoneum are thus created. The lower flap and the bladder are now dissected off the uterus, and the uterine muscle is incised either longitudinally or transversely. The baby is ordinarily delivered head first, usually with forceps. After the placenta has been extracted and the uterine incision sutured, the lower flap is imbricated over the upper (Figs. 231 and 232). This two-flap arrangement seals off the uterine incision and is believed to prevent the egress of infectious lochia into the peritoneal cavity. When low cervical cesarean was first intro-

duced in this country, by Dr. Alfred C. Beck of Brooklyn, N. Y., about 1919, the operation was employed chiefly on patients who had been in labor for a number of hours, and it is undoubtedly safer than the classic procedure in such cases. But it has other advantages, and many obstetricians today prefer it in elective cases as well.

Extraperitoneal Cesarean Section. There are two extraperitoneal operations, one devised by Dr. W. Latsko, formerly of Vienna, Austria, and the other by Dr. E. G. Waters, of Jersey City, N. J. By appropriate dissection of the tissues around the bladder, access to the lower

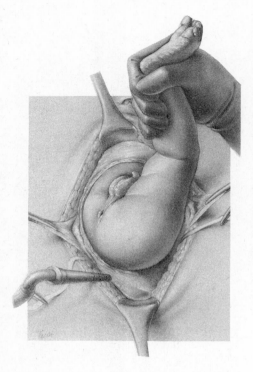

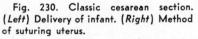

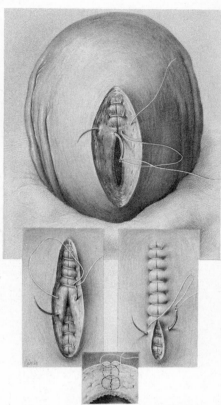

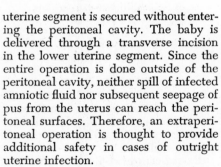

Fig. 230. Classic cesarean section. (*Left*) Delivery of infant. (*Right*) Method of suturing uterus.

uterine segment is secured without entering the peritoneal cavity. The baby is delivered through a transverse incision in the lower uterine segment. Since the entire operation is done outside of the peritoneal cavity, neither spill of infected amniotic fluid nor subsequent seepage of pus from the uterus can reach the peritoneal surfaces. Therefore, an extraperitoneal operation is thought to provide additional safety in cases of outright uterine infection.

Cesarean Section—Hysterectomy. (Synonyms: radical cesarean section; Porro operation.) This operation comprises cesarean section (usually classic) followed by removal of the uterus. It is a procedure which also gives protection against infection, since it removes the infected organ. Obviously, it is most undesirable in younger women, and obstetricians avoid it whenever possible. However, it may be necessary in certain cases of premature separation of the placenta and in patients with multiple fibroid tumors of the uterus. (See "Moral Considerations," p. 403.)

Preparations for cesarean sections are similar to those for any other abdominal operation, except that in these cases it includes preparations for the care of the infant. When the operation is an elective procedure, the patient is admitted 24 hours or more prior to surgery, so there is ample time for physical examination, routine laboratory studies, typing and

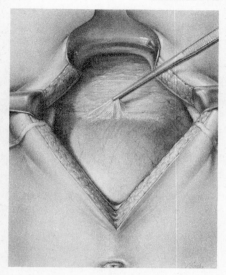

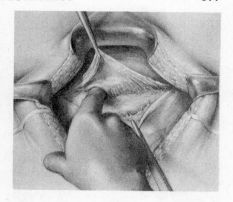

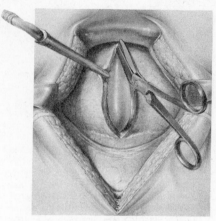

Fig. 231. Low cervical cesarean section. (*Left*) High Trendelenburg position, bladder empty, with catheter in place. The peritoneum over lower portion of uterus is picked up with tissue forceps to determine how far up it is loosely attached to uterus. A transverse incision of the peritoneum, slightly concave downward, is to be made about 1 inch below the point where the peritoneum is firmly attached to the uterus.

(*Right, top*) The lower edge of the incised peritoneum is picked up by the tissue forceps and gently stripped off the underlying uterine segment by finger dissection.

(*Right, bottom*) The upper flap of loose peritoneum has been stripped from the underlying muscle by finger dissection and is held back by a retractor. A small incision with a scalpel is made at the upper end of the lower uterine segment and carried downward with bandage scissors.

cross-matching blood and other customary procedures. However, if there is an emergency or labor has started, then such preparations must be made with expediency. In any event, the usual hospital procedure should be followed.

Nursing Care. When the patient is admitted for an elective cesarean section, nursing care which is routine for any waiting mother, e.g., checking fetal heart tones and being alert to prodromal signs of labor, is employed. A short time before the operation the skin should be shaved to remove all hair from the abdomen and the vulva. The abdomen is shaved first, beginning at the level of the xiphoid cartilage and extending out to the far sides and down to the pubic area. Then the vulvar region is shaved. A retention catheter is inserted to ensure that the bladder remains empty during the operation, and it is unclamped during

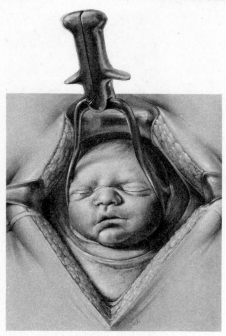

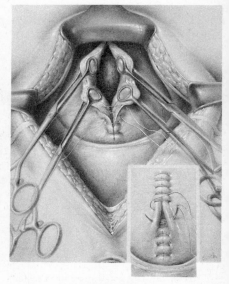

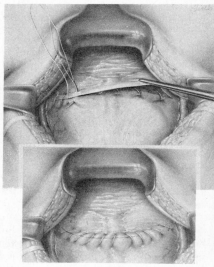

Fig. 232. Low cervical cesarean section. (*Left, top*) Extraction of baby with forceps. Pitocin (1 cc.) intramuscularly is usually given as soon as the head is delivered. (*Right, top*) After delivery of baby and placenta, edges of the lower segment incision are grasped with ring forceps and sutured. (*Right, bottom*) After upper peritoneal flap is pulled down over the uterine wound and sutured, the lower flap is pulled upward and sutured with running suture.

this procedure. The preoperative medication usually ordered is atropine. The use of narcotic drugs prior to delivery is avoided because of their depressant effect on the infant, but these medications should be readily available. Oxytocic drugs, i.e., Pitocin and ergonovine, should be ready in the operating room so that they can be administered promptly upon the verbal order of the obstetrician when the infant is born.

In addition to the preparation of the operating room for the surgical procedure, preparations for the care of the infant must ·be accomplished. There must be a warm crib and equipment for the resuscitation of the infant. An infant resuscitator, such as the Kreiselman shown in Figure 263, is an efficient mechanical device because it is equipped with heat, suction, oxygen (open mask and positive-pressure) and an adjustable frame to permit the proper positioning of the infant. Furthermore, such a resuscitator provides a convenient place to give initial care to the newborn. A competent person should be present at cesarean section to give the infant initial care and to resuscitate it, if necessary. This person may be a nurse, but in many hospitals today it is customary to have a pediatrician present so that he may "take over" the care of the infant as soon as it is born and thus free the obstetrician to devote all of his attention to the mother.

The obstetrician will direct the treatment of the mother, but usually postoperative care is the same as that following abdominal surgery. It is well to remember that the patient who has had a cesarean section has had both an abdominal operation and a delivery. The patient must be watched for hemorrhage, both from the abdominal incision and the vagina, so the abdominal dressings and the perineal pad must be inspected frequently. If the abdominal dressings are bulky it is impossible to palpate the fundus to see if the uterus is well contracted, but if the dressings are not massive, and do not extend above the level of the umbilicus, the nurse may feel the consistency of the fundus without difficulty. She should employ extreme gentleness if this is done in order not to traumatize the uterus, and remember that the uterus must not be massaged in the process. Oxytocics may be ordered to keep the uterus contracted and to control bleeding. The vital signs should be checked regularly until they have stabilized, and if there is any indication of shock or hemorrhage it should be reported promptly. Although there may be no visible signs of external hemorrhage, one would suspect internal hemorrhage if the pulse rate becomes accelerated, the respirations increase in rate or the blood pressure falls, bearing in mind, of course, that the drop in blood pressure

could be due to the effects of some types of anesthetic drugs.

If the retention catheter is to remain in place until the following morning, it should be attached to "constant drainage" and should be watched to see that it drains freely. Intravenous fluids are usually administered during the first 24 hours, although small amounts of fluids may be given by mouth after nausea has subsided. A record of the mother's intake and elimination is kept for the first several days or until the need is no longer indicated.

Sedative drugs should be used to keep the mother comfortable and encourage her to rest. Her position in bed during the early postoperative hours may be dictated by the type of anesthesia that she received, but, nevertheless, she should be encouraged to turn from side to side every hour. Deep breathing and coughing should also be encouraged at this time to promote good ventilation. Today most mothers delivered by cesarean section are allowed early ambulation 12 to 48 hours following operation. It is felt that this contributes considerably to maintaining good bladder and intestinal function.

The patient's husband should be permitted to have a short visit with his wife as soon as it is feasible. The mother will be anxious to see her infant, too, and it should be brought to her as soon as she is able to see it. The nurse should remain with the mother while she has her infant with her.

An effort should be made to encourage breast feeding, both because of the advantage to the infant and because the maternal processes need this stimulation. If the mother progresses satisfactorily, there should be no reason why the infant should not be put to breast after 24 hours and regularly thereafter.

The general care of the mother will be similar to that given any postoperative or postpartal patient. Daily breast care and perineal care are carried out per routine. The mother may have "after-pains," engorgement of the breasts and emotional reactions which often accompany a normal delivery.

DESTRUCTIVE OPERATIONS

Destructive operations (designed for the most part to reduce the size of the baby's head and thus expedite delivery) are rarely done in modern obstetrics and are *never* performed on a living child. Even in large maternity hospitals several years may pass without a single destructive operation. This salutary state of affairs is attributable in part to the widespread extension of prenatal care, in part to better management of women in labor and in part to the recent development of cesarean section which makes it reasonably safe to effect abdominal delivery even in neglected cases. In the event that a destructive operation is necessary, the obstetrician will choose the necessary instruments.

INDUCTION OF LABOR

By the induction of labor is meant the artificial bringing on of labor after the period of viability. This may be attempted by medication, by instrumental means or by a combination of both methods. Toxemia of pregnancy is the most frequent reason for the procedure, since in this disorder continuation of pregnancy is often fraught with considerable danger to both mother and infant. Labor is also induced occasionally in patients who have gone beyond their calculated date of confinement and whose babies are large.

Medicinal Induction. Since it is believed that the intestinal peristalsis produced by a cathartic is somehow transferred to the uterus, with the consequent initiation of uterine contractions, castor oil has long been employed to induce labor. It is given in the amount of 1 ounce and followed by the administration of a hot soapsuds enema as soon as the castor oil has acted. While this is a harmless procedure, it usually fails and

is employed less frequently today than it was formerly.

A much more efficient method for the induction of labor is the administration of *Pitocin*. The properties of this oxytocic agent and its use in the third stage of labor have already been discussed on page 269. For inducing labor, Pitocin may be used in one of two ways: intramuscularly or intravenously.

Since Pitocin has dangerous potentialities when administered to a pregnant woman, the dosage used is always extremely small. The physician will specify the dosage to be employed and will make the injection himself. For the intramuscular administration of Pitocin, the dose is usually ½ to 3 minims (⅛ to 2 International Units). Because of the very small amount of solution to be given, the physician will want, as a rule, a tuberculin syringe for the injection and a small quantity of sterile intravenous saline solution for dilution of the Pitocin.

For the intravenous administration of Pitocin, the physician will usually ask for a flask containing 500 cc. of 5% glucose into which he will add the quantity of Pitocin which he wishes to use. The intravenous equipment is set up as usual so that the number of drops flowing per minute can be closely observed in the observation tube. This is extremely important, and the physician will specify the precise number of drops per minute which he wishes employed.

As already mentioned, the administration of Pitocin to a gravida carries certain hazards, and it is obligatory for her safety and that of the baby that a physician or a nurse be in constant bedside attendance to make certain that the number of drops flowing per minute does not change and to watch for certain untoward effects that may ensue. This is usually the responsibility of the physician, but occasionally it may fall to the nurse. If so, she must check the rate of flow of the Pitocin solution at frequent intervals to make certain that it remains constant. Whether Pitocin is administered intramuscularly or intravenously, the duration and the intensity of each uterine contraction must be watched closely and recorded, because any contraction lasting over 2 minutes indicates that the quantity of solution is too great and the rate of flow should either be decreased or tentatively discontinued altogether. Furthermore, the fetal heart rate should be counted after each contraction and recorded. It will be recalled that the fetal heart tones should return to their normal rate and rhythm within 15 seconds or so after the termination of a contraction, and any persistence of fetal bradycardia is another indication for discontinuation of the Pitocin drip. In the event that the nurse should be left alone with the patient while the intravenous-drip Pitocin technic is being employed, and she observes any abnormalities in the uterine contractions or the fetal heart tones, she should turn off the solution *immediately* and report her findings to the physician.

The advantages of intravenous Pitocin over its intramuscular injection are severalfold. In the first place, it assures a uniform, although infinitesimal, concentration of the agent in the blood stream which can be maintained at the same concentration over long periods, whereas with intramuscular Pitocin there must necessarily be fluctuations in the blood and tissue concentration of Pitocin depending on varying rates of absorption from time to time. Another advantage is that the Pitocin drip may be discontinued immediately in the event that untoward effects should be observed—an obvious safety factor.

Artificial Rupture of the Membranes. This is today the most common method of inducing labor. It is accomplished after placing the patient in the lithotomy position and carrying out antiseptic preparation of the vulva. The first two fingers of one hand are inserted into the cervix until the membranes are encountered. The cervix is stretched gently, and the membranes are stripped from the region of the internal os. A long hook, similar to one blade of a disarticulated vulsellum tenaculum, is inserted into the vagina, and the membranes are simply hooked and torn by the tip of the sharp instrument. As much fluid as possible is allowed to drain. Provided that the patient is near term, with other conditions favorable, artificial rupture of the membranes will almost always initiate labor within a few hours.

So far as the nurse is concerned, these obstetric operations do not differ greatly from any other surgical procedures. The direction of these operations is entirely the responsibility of the physician, and the nurse's share consists of these 3 responsibilities: (1) having everything in readiness beforehand, (2) giving reassuring advice to the patient and her family and (3) making sure that no opportunity is lost in rendering all possible assistance to the doctor.

SUGGESTED READING

Bishop, Edward H.: Dangers attending elective induction of labor, J.A.M.A. **166**:1953, 1958.

Bookmiller, Mae, and Bowen, George: Textbook of Obstetrics and Obstetric Nursing, ed. 3, Philadelphia, Saunders, 1958.

Brierton, John F.: Rupture of the pregnant uterus, Am. J. Obst. & Gynec. **59**:113, 1950.

Broomes, E. L. C.: Full term abdominal pregnancy with the delivery of a living child, J.A.M.A. **145**:399, 1951.

Cosgrove, Robert A.: Management of pregnancy and delivery following cesarean section, J.A.M.A. **145**:884, 1951.

Danforth, D. N.: A method of forceps rotation in persistent occiput posterior, Am. J. Obst. & Gynec. **65**:120, 1953.

Davis, M. E., and Scheckler, C. E.: DeLee's Obstetrics for Nurses, ed. 16, Philadelphia, Saunders 1957.

Douglas, R. Gordon, and Landesman, Robert: Recent trends in cesarean section, Am. J. Obst. & Gynec. **59**:96, 1950.

Eastman, Nicholson J.: Williams Obstetrics, ed. 11, New York, Appleton, 1956.

Fish, Stewart: The Barton forceps, Am. J. Obst. & Gynec. **66**:1290, 1953.

——: The Tucker McLane forceps: a history, Am. J. Obst. & Gynec. **65**: 1042, 1953.

Lull, Clifford, and Kimbrough, Robert (eds.): Clinical Obstetrics, Philadelphia, Lippincott, 1953.

Moon, R. E., and Wall, D. D.: Midforceps delivery, Am. J. Obst. & Gynec. **72**:954, 1956.

Randall, J. H.: Newer trends in cesarean section, J. Iowa M. Soc. **45**:173, 1955.

Swann, R. O.: Induction of labor by stripping membranes, Obst. & Gynec. **11**:74, 1958.

Van Blarcom, Carolyn C.: Obstetrical Nursing, ed. 4 (rev. by Erna Siegel), New York, Macmillan, 1957.

Weinberg, Arthur: Midforceps operations, J.A.M.A. **146**:1465, 1951.

CONFERENCE MATERIAL

1. A mother, para ii, is admitted to the hospital at 42 weeks' gestation for induction of labor. Her membranes have been artificially ruptured and intravenous Pitocin has been started. Discuss the nursing care of this mother from this time until she is in active labor.

2. What specific nursing care would you give to a mother who sustained a third-degree perineal laceration as the result of a precipitous labor?

3. A 38-year-old gravida v had an uneventful pregnancy until the last trimester when she developed preeclampsia. Now, at term, she is admitted to the hospital because of suspected abruptio placenta and, after consultation, is to have an emergency cesarean section. Discuss the nursing care of this mother from the time of admission until she is taken to the operating room for surgery.

4. A primigravida, who has 3-year-old adopted twins, is delivered by low cervical cesarean section because of pelvic injuries received in an auto accident 6 years earlier. Discuss the nursing care of this mother following cesarean section.

Study Questions

UNIT SIX: OPERATIVE PROCEDURES IN OBSTETRICS

Read through the entire question and place your answer in the parentheses.

1. Which of the following structures are involved when an episiotomy is performed?
   A. The vaginal mucosa.
   B. The levator ani muscle.
   C. The glans clitoris.
   D. The cardinal ligament.
   E. The fourchet.
   Select the number corresponding to the correct letter or letters.
   1. A only
   2. A and B
   3. A, B and E
   4. All of them

(———)

2. Obstetric forceps are frequently used to facilitate delivery. In which of the following conditions would it be indicated to deliver the infant by forceps?
   A. The cervix fails to dilate completely.
   B. The mother has heart disease.
   C. The mother has a contracted pelvis.
   D. Prolapse of the umbilical cord.
   E. Passage of meconium-stained amniotic fluid in vertex presentation.
   Select the number corresponding to the correct letters.
   1. A and B
   2. B, D and E
   3. C and E
   4. All of them

(———)

3. Which of the following principles should be observed in the use of intravenous Pitocin to stimulate labor?
   A. The condition of the fetus must be satisfactory.
   B. It should be used only in cases of secondary uterine inertia.
   C. It should not be given to a multipara who has had 4 or more full-term pregnancies.
   D. It should be used in cases of borderline pelvis.
   E. A responsible person should be in constant attendance while the mother is receiving intravenous Pitocin.
   Select the number corresponding to the correct letters.
   1. A and B
   2. A, C and E
   3. B, D and E
   4. All of them

(———)

4. What specific treatment should be included in the care given a mother who has had a repair of a second-degree laceration of the perineum?
A. Daily routine perineal care.
B. Soft diet until the fifth postpartal day.
C. Omit enemas until the fifth postpartal day.
D. Limit activities in regard to early ambulation.
E. Encourage the mother not to sit erect until wound has healed.
Select the number corresponding to the correct letter or letters.
    1. A only
    2. A, D and E
    3. B, C and D
    4. All of them

(————)

5. After a cesarean section, which of the following symptoms might indicate that the patient is having excessive bleeding?
A. Accelerated pulse and respirations and drop in blood pressure.
B. Pain and tenderness in operative area.
C. Abdominal distention.
D. Sanguineous drainage from the abdominal wound and the vagina.
E. Apprehension and restlessness.
Select the number corresponding to the correct letters.
    1. A and B
    2. A, C and D
    3. A, D and E
    4. All of them

(————)

6. In caring for a mother who has been delivered by cesarean section, which of the following are usually employed to keep the uterus contracted and control bleeding?
A. Oxytocic drugs.
B. Gentle massage of the fundus if it becomes relaxed.
C. Icebag to the operative area.
D. Pressure dressings and tight abdominal binder.
E. Keep the patient flat in bed for the first 6 hours postoperatively.
Select the number corresponding to the correct letter or letters.
    1. A only
    2. A, C and D
    3. B, C and E
    4. All of them

(————)

Note: The key to the correct answers to these questions is given on page 533.

UNIT SEVEN

Abnormalities of Obstetrics

CHAPTER EIGHTEEN

Complications of Pregnancy

Regardless of the fact that from a biologic point of view pregnancy and labor should be considered to be a normal process of the female reproductive system, the borderline between health and illness is less distinctly marked during this time because of the numerous physiologic changes which occur in the mother's body during pregnancy. The importance of early and continued medical supervision during pregnancy is paramount for the health of the mother and her infant, for such preventive care enables detection of warning signals of potential pathologic conditions, so that serious problems may be averted or controlled by prompt treatment (see Chap. 8).

There are certain common complaints which most expectant mothers experience to some degree, the so-called minor discomforts of pregnancy, which are not serious in themselves but, nevertheless, detract from the mother's feeling of comfort and well-being. Since these discomforts are usually related to normal physiologic changes occurring within the mother's body and are not in themselves pathologic, they have been included in the chapter on antepartal care (see Chap. 8). However, minor discomforts, if neglected, may lead to a major complication. There are certain complications of pregnancy which very seriously jeopardize the health of both mother and infant. The more common of these major disturbances are discussed in five groups:

1. Hyperemesis gravidarum
2. Toxemias
3. Hemorrhagic complications
4. Blood groups and the Rh factor
5. Coincidental diseases and pregnancy

HYPEREMESIS GRAVIDARUM

A mild degree of nausea and vomiting, "morning sickness," is the most common complaint of women in the first trimester of pregnancy. This manifestation is considered in the realm of a minor discomfort rather than a complication, and it usually responds to measures discussed in Chapter 8. It is uncommon today for this mild form of nausea and vomiting to progress to such serious extent that it produces systemic effects, i.e., marked loss of weight and acetonuria; but when it becomes thus exaggerated, the condition is known as hyperemesis gravidarum, sometimes called "pernicious vomiting." Because even the gravest case of hyperemesis starts originally as a simple form of nausea, all cases of nausea and vomiting should be treated with proper understanding and judgment and none should be regarded casually. When simple remedies do not prove to be effective, and symptoms of hyperemesis appear to be imminent, the patient should be hospitalized for more intensive treatment. At the present time, less than 1 pregnant woman in 300 has to be admitted to the hospital because of this complication of pregnancy, and, indeed, the grave cases of hyperemesis gravidarum are becoming rare. The recovery of those who are admitted to the hospital is usually rapid.

Cause. It is currently recognized that during pregnancy there are certain organic processes which are basic to all cases of vomiting, regardless of whether the symptoms are mild or severe. The endocrine and metabolic changes of normal gestation, fragments of chorionic villi entering the maternal circulation and the diminished motility of the stomach might well give rise to clinical symptoms.

It has long been thought that hyperemesis gravidarum is in large measure a *neurosis*. The term "neurosis," it will be recalled, is employed very loosely to designate a large array of conditions in which symptoms occur without demonstrable pathologic explanation, the symptoms being due, it is thought, to a functional disturbance of the patient's psyche. Some psychiatrists estimate that 40 per cent of patients who visit physicians belong in this neurotic class. As many examples show (quite apart from pregnancy), nausea is often psychic in origin. For instance, a repellent sight, an obnoxious odor or the mere recollection of such a sight or odor may give rise to nausea and even vomiting. Our general use of the adjective "nauseating" to depict a repulsive object is further acknowledgment that an upset mind may produce an upset stomach.

In all life's encounters there are probably few experiences which are at first more upsetting, mentally and emotionally, than the realization by a young woman that she is pregnant. At the onset, there are several weeks of anxious uncertainty before she can be sure of the diagnosis. Then, numerous adjustments must be made and plans changed. Emotionally, the implications of pregnancy extend far back into the past when she first met her husband, while its future ramifications are endless. The responsibilities entailed are plain enough,

also, and seem, on first thought, perhaps more than can be assumed. These and a thousand other thoughts crowd themselves into the mind; and in women who cannot adjust themselves to all these new circumstances, it is understandable that the groundwork for a neurosis is laid. Beyond question, there is a large neurotic element in most cases of hyperemesis, a factor which looms large in the treatment of the condition.

The neurotic factor, on the other hand, is not the whole cause of hyperemesis, nor in all probability even the basic cause. As has been stated previously, in every case an important, underlying organic process is also at work—either the dissemination of toxins into the maternal blood stream or some maladjustment of the metabolism to the changes wrought by the growing fetus. It is this toxic or organic element which is doubtless the fundamental cause of the disease. To what extent the patient reacts to this underlying process by vomiting seems to be determined in large measure by neurotic factors, that is, by her psychic and emotional stability and by the mental stress and strain which pregnancy has imposed.

Clinical Picture. The clinical picture of the patient suffering from pernicious vomiting varies in relation to the severity and the duration of the condition. In any event, the condition begins with a typical picture of "morning sickness." The patient experiences a feeling of nausea on arising in the morning, she may even be unable to retain her breakfast, but she recovers in a few hours and has no further episodes until the next morning. With the majority of these patients this pattern persists for a few weeks and then suddenly ceases.

A small number of patients who have "morning sickness" develop persistent vomiting which lasts for 4 to 8 weeks or longer. These patients vomit several times a day and may be unable to retain any liquid or solid foods, with the result that marked symptoms of dehydration and starvation occur. *Dehydration* is pronounced, as evidenced by a diminished output of urine and a dryness of the skin. In some instances slight jaundice may develop. Further results of dehydration may be observed in the patient's vital signs. The pulse is usually accelerated, often to 130 or over, and a low-grade fever may be present. The temperature seldom rises above 101° F. (38.4° C.), but it may persist despite therapy to combat dehydration.

Starvation, which is regularly present, manifests itself in a number of ways. Weight loss may vary from 5 pounds to as much as 20 or 30 pounds. This is tantamount to saying that the digestion and the absorption of carbohydrates and other nutrients has been so inadequate that the body has been forced to burn its reserve stores of fat in order to maintain body heat and energy. When fat is burned without carbohydrates present, the process of combustion does not go on to completion. Consequently, certain incompletely burned products of fat metabolism make their appearance in the blood and in the urine. The presence of acetone and diacetic acid in the urine in hyperemesis is common. In severe cases considerable changes associated with starvation and dehydration become evident in the blood chemistry. There is a definite increase in the nonprotein nitrogen, uric acid and urea, a moderate decrease in the chlorides and little alteration in the carbon dioxide combining power. Then, too, vitamin starvation is regularly present, and in extreme cases, when marked vitamin B deficiency exists, polyneuritis occasionally develops and disturbances of the peripheral nerves result.

The severe type of vomiting may occur in either acute or chronic form. With prompt, persistent and intelligent therapy, the prognosis of hyperemesis is excellent.

Treatment and Nursing Care. The principles underlying the treatment of hyperemesis gravidarum are as follows:

(1) combat the dehydration by liberal administration of parenteral fluids; (2) combat the starvation by administration of glucose intravenously and thiamine chloride subcutaneously and, if necessary, by feeding a high-caloric, high-vitamin fluid diet through a nasal tube; (3) combat the neurosis by psychotherapy, sedatives and isolation.

Although it may be necessary on occasion to treat cases of hyperemesis in the home, hospitalization is urgently desirable, because isolation from relatives, change of atmosphere and better facilities for intravenous medication confer unusual benefits in this condition. During the first 24 hours in the hospital, it is customary to withhold all food and fluids by mouth in order to give the gastro-intestinal tract as complete a rest as possible. Glucose solution, usually in 10 per cent concentration, is administered intravenously and, in addition, normal saline solutions subcutaneously or intravenously. The total fluid intake should approximate or exceed 3,000 cc. in the 24 hours. The nurse must keep a careful record of the exact quantity of fluids given, the amount of urine excreted and the quantity of the vomitus. Sedation is accomplished either by Luminal Sodium hypodermically in dosage of 1 or 2 grains (0.06 to 0.12 Gm.) every 4 hours, or by the rectal instillation of some barbiturate drug such as Sodium Amytal, 3 grains (0.2 Gm.) every 6 hours. Thiamine hydrochloride, 50 mg. daily hypodermically, supplies the most urgent vitamin needs during the first 24 hours. All visitors are excluded during this period, including husband and relatives.

After such a regimen for 24 hours, dry toast, crackers or cereal are given by mouth in small quantities every 2 or 3 hours. Fluids are given on alternate hours in small amounts (not over 100 cc. at a time); hot tea and ginger ale usually are tolerated better than plain water. If no vomiting occurs, the amounts and the variety of the food are increased gradually until the patient is on a regular soft, high-vitamin diet. The intravenous administration of fluids may have to be continued for several days, depending on the oral intake.

The success of the treatment will depend in large measure on the tact, the understanding and the attitude of the nurse. While optimism must be the keynote of the nurse's approach to the patient, this must be coupled with a plainly avowed determination to conquer the complication. The patient must be led gradually to understand that, in the treatment of vomiting, the nurse knows no such word as "failure." Not a few of these patients are in psychological conflict because of family, financial or social difficulties, and many are averse to the whole idea of pregnancy. If one can only get to the root of these difficulties in a tactful, sympathetic way, and help the patient to become reconciled to becoming a mother, a great deal will have been accomplished.

The nurse must exercise great care in preparing and serving trays for patients suffering from hyperemesis. The portions should be extremely small and attractively arranged. Cold liquids such as ginger ale or lemonade must be ice-cold; and hot foods, such as soups, cocoa and tea, must be steaming hot, since lukewarm liquids may be nauseating. It is best not to discuss food with the patient, even when serving the tray, but simply assume that she will enjoy it and talk about other matters. At all times keep the emesis basin out of view, since the sight of it may start vomiting. Likewise, the smell of food may be nauseating; accordingly, the patient's room should be kept well-aired and should be as far from the kitchen as possible.

If vomiting continues despite these measures, as it rarely does, the physician may institute nasal feeding. A small rubber tube (Levin tube) is inserted by the physician through a nostril and on down into the stomach. The tube is strapped to the patient's cheek, connected with an overhanging bottle and left in place. By this means, large amounts of vitamin-rich liquid foods may be administered. The secret of success with nasal feeding lies in very slow but constant introduction of food into the stomach. The apparatus should be so arranged that the number of drops per minute passing through the tube can be counted. This should not exceed 50 per minute. Even this slow rate, it may be noted, yields about 200 cc. per hour.

Even the most severe cases of hyperemesis usually will respond favorably to the treatment described if patience and persistence are exercised; but, in extremely rare instances, the patient may continue to vomit despite all efforts, and such grave signs may develop that the physician is forced to the conclusion that further continuation of pregnancy will be at the cost of the woman's life. The following signs are grave omens and, especially when several are present, may call for therapeutic abortion if it has been decided that the mother is to be removed from danger: (1) jaundice; (2) delirium; (3) steadily rising pulse rate to levels of 130 or above; (4) fever of 101° F. (38.4° C.) or above which persists despite liberal fluid intake; and (5) hemorrhages in the retina, as observed by the physician during ophthalmoscopic examination. (See "Moral Considerations," p. 403.)

TOXEMIAS OF PREGNANCY

"The toxemias of pregnancy are disorders encountered during gestation, or early in the puerperium, which are characterized by one or more of the following signs: hypertension, edema, albuminuria, and in severe cases, convulsions and coma."[*] Despite decades of intensive research, the cause of toxemia is still unknown. The name itself would give rise to the supposition that these conditions are due to circulating toxins

[*] Definition established by The American Committee on Maternal Welfare, April 1, 1952.

in the blood, derived presumably from the products of conception; but this is probably not correct. Whether toxemia represents an exaggeration of the various physical changes which normally accompany pregnancy or whether it depends on some entirely new deviation from the normal course of pregnancy is still one of the most important unsolved problems in the whole field of human reproduction.

The toxemias of pregnancy are a very common complication of gestation, being seen in 6 or 7 per cent of all gravidae. They rank among the three major complications (hemorrhage, puerperal infections and the toxemias of pregnancy) responsible for the vast majority of maternal deaths and account for some 1,000 maternal deaths in the U.S. each year. As a cause of fetal death they are even more important. It can be estimated conservatively that at least 30,000 stillbirths and neonatal deaths each year in this country are the result of toxemias of pregnancy. The great majority of these deaths are due to prematurity of the infant.

The huge toll of maternal and infant lives taken by the toxemias of pregnancy is in large measure preventable. Proper antepartal supervision, particularly the early detection of signs and symptoms of oncoming toxemia and appropriate treatment, will arrest many cases and so ameliorate others that the outcome for baby and mother is usually satisfactory. The nurse is often the first to encounter the early signs and symptoms, not only in the hospital out-patient department, but also on home visits, and it is of utmost importance that she be constantly on the lookout for them so that treatment may be instituted at the earliest possible moment.

Classification. The toxemias of pregnancy have heretofore been classified in many forms. In 1952, The American Committee on Maternal Welfare revised their classification as follows:

1. Acute Toxemia of Pregnancy

A. Preeclampsia
   1. Mild
   2. Severe
B. Eclampsia
2. Chronic Hypertensive (Vascular) Disease with Pregnancy
A. Chronic hypertensive vascular disease without superimposed acute toxemia
   1. Those cases in which hypertension was definitely known to exist before the onset of pregnancy
   2. Cases of early hypertension before the twenty-fourth week
B. Chronic hypertensive vascular disease with superimposed acute toxemia
3. Unclassified Toxemias

Acute toxemia of pregnancy is divided into two stages: *preeclampsia* (the nonconvulsive stage) and *eclampsia* (the convulsive stage). The condition is classified as *preeclampsia* when, after the 24th week of pregnancy, a gravida who previously has been normal in the following respects develops sudden elevation of blood pressure, albuminuria or edema (either one or more of the symptoms). Certain criteria have been established to divide preeclampsia into two groups: "preeclampsia mild" and "preeclampsia severe," depending on the symptoms. In *preeclampsia mild,* the systolic blood pressure is found to be 140 mm. Hg. or more, or is elevated 30 mm. or more above the usual level; the diastolic pressure will be 90 mm. Hg. or more, or is elevated 15 mm. or more above the usual level. Abnormal blood pressures must be observed on two occasions or more at least 6 hours apart, because a single reading may be misleading. The albumin in the urine is small in amount but must be of sufficient degree on 2 or more successive days. Persistent edema involving the hands and the face is present. The condition is classified as *preeclampsia severe* if any one of the following signs or symptoms is present:

(1) a systolic blood pressure of 160 mm. Hg. or more, or a diastolic pressure of 110 mm. or more; (2) marked albuminuria; (3) oliguria; (4) cerebral or visual disturbances; (5) pulmonary edema or cyanosis. Once the preeclamptic patient has a convulsion, she passes into the stage called *eclampsia*.

Chronic hypertensive vascular disease, sometimes called essential hypertension, is a disease which is not peculiar to pregnancy. When pregnancy aggravates the already existing hypertension so that the gravida with this chronic process develops an acute elevation of blood pressure and a significant degree of albuminuria, the condition is called *chronic hypertensive vascular disease with superimposed acute toxemia.* This disease is seen in all stages of gestation but is prone to occur between the 24th and 30th weeks. Furthermore, the symptoms may increase in severity to the stage of eclampsia.

Preeclampsia

As has been stated in the previous classification of the toxemias of pregnancy, preeclampsia is characterized by a sudden elevation in blood pressure, albuminuria and edema in a gravida who previously has been normal in these respects. It is the forerunner or prodromal stage of eclampsia; in other words, unless the preeclamptic process is checked by treatment or by delivery, it is more or less likely that eclampsia (convulsions and coma) will ensue. Characteristically, preeclampsia is a disease of the last 2 or 3 months of pregnancy, and is particularly prone to occur in young primigravidae. The underlying disease processes of preeclampsia and eclampsia are probably identical, the chief difference being that the latter goes on to convulsions and coma, while the former does not.

The earliest warning signal of preeclampsia is sudden development of hypertension. Accordingly, the importance of frequent and regular blood pressure estimations during pregnancy cannot be emphasized too strongly. The absolute blood pressure reading is probably of less significance than the relationship it bears to previous determinations and to the age of the patient. For example, a rise from 110/70 to 135/85 in a young woman is a more urgent danger signal than a rise from 135/85 to 150/90 in a patient of 35.

The next most constant sign of preeclampsia is sudden, excessive weight gain. If cases of preeclampsia are studied from the viewpoint of fluid intake and output, it is at once apparent that these sudden gains in weight are due entirely to an accumulation of water in the tissues. Such weight gains, in other words, represent latent edema and almost always precede the visible face and finger edema which is so characteristic of the advanced stages of the disease. From what has been said, it is apparent that a pair of scales is essential equipment for good antepartal care. Weight gain of 1 pound a week or so may be regarded as being normal. Sudden gains of more than 2 pounds a week should be viewed with suspicion; gains of more than 3 pounds, with alarm. Weight increases of the latter magnitude call for more frequent blood pressure determinations, and if these latter are also abnormal, hospitalization with intensive treatment is indicated. In investigating suspected edema, it is well to ask the patient if her wedding ring is becoming tight, since finger and facial edema is a more valuable sign of preeclampsia than is swelling of the ankles. In the facies of a patient with outspoken preeclampsia, the eyelids are swollen, and, associated with the edema, marked coarseness of the features develops (Fig. 233).

The sudden appearance of *albumin in the urine,* with or without other findings, always should be regarded as a sign of preeclampsia. Usually it develops later than the hypertension and the gain in weight and for this very reason must be regarded as being of serious omen

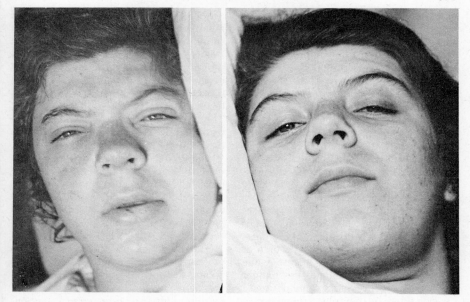

Fig. 233. (*Left*) Facies in preeclampsia. Note edema of eyelids and facial skin and general coarsening of features. (*Right*) Same patient 10 days after delivery.

when superimposed on these other two findings.

But the very essence of preeclampsia is the lightninglike fulminance with which it strikes. Although the above physical signs of preeclampsia usually give the physician ample time to institute preventive treatment, it sometimes happens that these derangements develop between visits to the office or the clinic, even though they be only a week apart. For this reason it is imperative that all expectant mothers be informed, both verbally and by some form of printed slip or booklet, in regard to certain danger signals which they themselves may recognize. Insofar as the toxemias of pregnancy are concerned, the following symptoms demand immediate report to the doctor: (1) severe, continuous headache; (2) swelling of the face or the fingers; (3) dimness or blurring of vision; (4) persistent vomit-

ing; (5) decrease in the amount of urine excreted; and (6) epigastric pain (a late symptom).

It should be emphasized that these three early and important signs of preeclampsia, namely, hypertension, weight gain and albuminuria, are changes of which the patient is usually unaware. All three may be present in substantial degree, and yet she may feel quite well. Only by regular and careful antepartal examination can these warning signs be detected. By the time the preeclamptic patient has developed symptoms and signs which she herself can detect (such as headache, blurred vision, puffiness of the eyelids and the fingers), she is usually in an advanced stage of the disease and much valuable time has been lost. Headache is rarely observed in the milder cases but is encountered with increasing frequency as the most severe grades are met. In general, patients who actually develop eclampsia often have a severe headache as a forerunner of the first convulsion. The visual disturbances range from a slight blurring of vision to various degrees of temporary blindness. Although convulsions are less likely to occur in cases of mild preeclampsia, the possibility cannot be entirely eliminated. Patients with severe preeclampsia should always be considered as being on the verge of having a convulsion.

Treatment. Prophylaxis is most 'important in the prevention and the control of preeclampsia. Since in its early stages preeclampsia rarely gives rise to signs or symptoms which the patient herself will notice, the early detection of this disease demands meticulous antepartal supervision. Rapid weight gain or an upward trend in blood pressure, while still in the "normal" range, are danger signals. Every pregnant woman should be examined by her obstetrician every week during the last month of pregnancy and every 2 weeks during the 2 previous months. The most promising prophylaxis of the disease lies in reduction of salt intake and curtailing weight gain in all pregnant women. Finger edema is a frequent forerunner of preeclampsia, which may precede the hypertension by several weeks, and is a valuable warning sign.

When the patient's symptoms are mild, i.e., minor elevation of blood pressure and minimal or no signs of edema and proteinuria present, treatment may be instituted at home in the hope that symptoms will abate. During this period the patient should be examined by the physician at least twice a week, and she should be given a strict regimen to follow, as well as careful instructions in regard to symptoms to report promptly. The patient's activities should be restricted, and she should understand that bed rest during the greater part of the day is most desirable. Sedative drugs, such as phenobarbital, may be prescribed to encourage rest and relaxation, the dosage being dependent on the severity

of the condition. Of major importance is a salt-poor diet. Therefore, the patient should be instructed so that she understands which foods have appreciable sodium content and therefore must be excluded from her diet, in addition to the fact that no salt may be added to her food in the kitchen or at the table. The diet should be well balanced but restricted in caloric content if the patient's weight gain indicates the need. It should contain ample protein, particularly lean meat, eggs and a quart of milk daily. Fluid intake should be maintained at 2,500 cc. daily; in hot weather 3,000 cc. Carbonated beverages should be avoided because of their sodium content.

The restriction of salt in the diet of the preeclamptic patient is directed at reducing the edema. Even in normal, nonpregnant persons an increased intake of sodium chloride causes water retention. Pregnant women, particularly gravidae suffering from preeclampsia, show a marked tendency to retain sodium, and there is reason to believe that this tendency of the tissues to retain sodium is closely correlated with their tendency to hold water. To superimpose still more salt in the diet on this already existing sodium and water retention is obviously unwise.

By means of the above measures it is often possible to relieve the signs and symptoms of preeclampsia so that the patient proceeds to term satisfactorily. In the event that the patient's condition does not respond promptly to ambulatory treatment, she should be hospitalized without delay. A systematic method of study should be instituted upon admission to the hospital. A general physical examination and history should be obtained promptly, followed by constant vigilance for the development of such symptoms as headache, visual disturbances and edema of the fingers and the eyelids. Body weight should be obtained on admission and every other morning thereafter. Blood pressure readings should be taken every 4 hours except between midnight and morning, unless the midnight blood pressure has risen. Daily fluid intake and output records should be kept, and urine specimens sent to the laboratory daily for analysis for albumin and casts. Retinal examination is always included as part of the admission physical examination and is done every 2 to 3 days thereafter, depending on the findings. Blood chemical determinations are also included.

Once the patient is admitted to the hospital, complete bed rest is essential. Even in milder cases, minimal doses of sedative drugs are helpful. Phenobarbital, 32 mg. (½ grain), may be given 4 times a day, or twice this dosage in cases of moderate severity. The dietary regimen previously described should be adhered to, or it may be indicated to restrict the sodium chloride to less than 3 Gm. daily. In such cases it may become necessary to substitute one of the commercial sodium-free milk powders in place of regular milk, since a quart of milk itself contains about 1.25 Gm. of sodium chloride. In many instances diuretics may be used routinely. Magnesium sulfate (epsom salts), 15 Gm., or citrate of magnesia, 200 cc., may be used every second or third day, although these merely increase water loss from the bowel, not sodium excretion. Ammonium chloride, 4 Gm. daily for 3 days, is frequently used. This may never be given for more than 3 days consecutively because of the acidosis which it tends to produce when used for longer periods. Two other diuretic drugs sometimes employed in the toxemias are Diamox and Diuril. The usual dose of Diamox is 250 mg. daily, but since, like ammonium chloride, it produces a mild acidosis, it is ordinarily administered for not more than 5 days at a stretch. Diuril increases the elimination of both sodium and water from the body without causing acidosis and is occasionally employed to relieve edema in normal pregnancy as well as in the toxemias. The dose is 0.5 to 1.0 Gm. daily.

When severe preeclampsia exists, immediate and intensive medicinal therapy is imperative. Sedation is of major importance to forestall convulsions. The dosage of the drugs should be regulated so that they produce drowsiness and sleep from which the patient can be easily awakened. Morphine sulfate, 16 mg. (¼ grain) may be given hypodermically, followed by either paraldehyde per rectum or one of the barbiturates. If paraldehyde is employed, the dose should be about 10 to 15 cc., depending on the weight of the patient, and administered in 30 cc. of olive oil. Magnesium sulfate administered intramuscularly is another drug frequently chosen because it protects the patient with toxemia against convulsions during labor. In addition to its action as a vasodilator and diuretic, it has a sedative effect, because when given intramuscularly it acts as a central nervous system depressant. Recently the new tranquilizing drugs and hypotensive drugs have been used effectively.

Despite all efforts, the condition may persist to a marked degree, and in that event induction of labor may become necessary for the welfare of mother and infant. In occasional instances when the preeclampsia is severe and fulminating, and conditions for induction of labor are not favorable, cesarean section may be the procedure of choice.

The signs and symptoms of preeclampsia usually abate rapidly after delivery, but the danger of convulsions does not pass until 48 hours have elapsed postpartum. Therefore, continuation of sedation throughout this interval is indicated. In the majority of cases the elevated blood pressure as well as the other derangements have returned to normal within 10 days or 2 weeks. In about 30 per cent of cases, however, the hypertension shows a tendency either to persist indefinitely or to recur in subsequent pregnancies. For this reason the prolonged follow-up of these patients is highly important.

Nursing Care. The nurse's responsibility in the detection and care of cases of preeclampsia is manifold. Since this complication of pregnancy is seen more commonly in certain localities and among particular groups of women, and may occur antepartally, intrapartally or postpartally, it is important for the nurse to observe all maternity patients closely for the first indication of early symptoms, as well as to be quick to recognize and report any evidence pointing to an aggravation of the process. The early symptoms and the manifestations related to more severe preeclampsia, such as persistent headache, blurred vision, spots or flashes of light before the eyes, epigastric pain, vomiting, torpor or muscular twitchings, are all vastly important. Data collected in relation to these symptoms, in addition to an accurate record of weight gain, fluid intake and elimination, diet and attitudes and behavior, when it is accurately recorded, can assist the physician in evaluating the symptoms and planning his course of therapy.

In setting the therapeutic atmosphere, the nurse should see that the environment is as comfortable and pleasant as possible. The patient should be in a single room, free from the stimuli of noise, strong lights and the presence of unnecessary equipment which might frighten her. To the best of her ability, the nurse must protect the patient from needless traffic into the room; otherwise, the coming and going of personnel to the bedside may be so constant that it could interfere with the efficacy of the treatment being carried out. Every effort should be exerted to relieve the patient's anxiety, which sometimes is brought about by apprehension regarding her illness or may be due to concern for the welfare of her family at home.

Regardless of the severity of the toxemia, certain responsibilities are carried out by the nurse. Medications ordered must be administered promptly, the prescribed diet should be supervised, a careful record of intake and elimination kept, blood pressure readings and basal weights taken, specimens collected and labeled accurately, and observations of slight symptoms or change in condition should be reported immediately, both verbally and on the patient's record. Since rest is a major consideration in the care of this patient, the nurse should plan a schedule of activities so that the patient is disturbed as little as possible. Medications, treatments and nursing procedures should be administered at the same time as far as the physician's orders will permit, but always with the thought in mind that only as much as will not overtire the patient should be planned for any one time. When any treatment is ordered, the procedure is best carried out after sedation has been administered. Before heavy sedation is initiated, any removable dentures or eyeglasses should be removed and stored in a secure place. If the patient is not in labor, the nurse must be alert to watch for signs of labor, particularly after sedation has been given. Any time intravenous fluids are administered, if the physician has not specified the rate at which the fluid is to flow, it should be given slowly.

The nurse should see that the equipment necessary for the safe and efficient care of the patient is immediately available and in good working order. A padded mouth gag should always be ready for use at the bedside to prevent the patient from biting her tongue in the event that a convulsion develops. Trays for catheterization equipment and for the administration of special medications constitute part of the necessary equipment. Since water retention plays such a large role in the disease, and urinary output is likely to be diminished, an indwelling bladder catheter may be ordered to ensure accuracy in obtaining output from the kidneys. Since the urinary output must be watched carefully, it is imperative to see that the retention catheter is draining properly at all times. In severe cases suction apparatus should be readily available for aspirating mucus, as well as equipment for the administration of oxygen, should symptoms such as cyanosis or depressed respirations indicate the need.

Eclampsia

Clinical Picture. As indicated, the development of eclampsia is almost always preceded by the signs and symptoms of preeclampsia. A preeclamptic patient, who may have been conversing with you a moment before, is seen to roll her eyes to one side and stare fixedly into space. Immediately, twitching of the facial muscles ensues. This is the *stage of invasion* of the convulsion and lasts only a few seconds.

The whole body then becomes rigid in a generalized muscular contraction; the face is distorted, the eyes protrude, the arms are flexed, the hands are clenched, and the legs are inverted. Since all the muscles of the body are now in a state of tonic contraction, this phase may be regarded as the *stage of contraction;* it lasts 15 or 20 seconds.

Suddenly the jaws begin to open and close violently, and forthwith the eyelids also. The other facial muscles and then all the muscles of the body alternately contract and relax in rapid succession. So forceful are the muscular movements that the patient may throw herself out of bed, and almost invariably, unless protected, the tongue is bitten by the violent jaw action. Foam, often blood-tinged, exudes from the mouth; the face is congested and purple, and the eyes are bloodshot. Few pictures which the nurse is called upon to witness are so horrible. This phase in which the muscles alternately contract and relax is called the *stage of convulsion;* it may last a minute or so. Gradually the muscular movements become milder and farther apart, and finally the patient lies motionless.

Throughout the seizure the diaphragm has been fixed with respiration halted. Still no breathing occurs. For a few seconds the woman appears to be dying from respiratory arrest, but just when this outcome seems almost inevitable, she takes a long, deep, stertorous inhalation, and breathing is resumed. Then coma ensues. The patient will remember nothing whatsoever of the convulsion or, in all probability, events immediately before and afterward.

The coma may last from a few minutes to several hours, and the patient may then become conscious; or the coma may be succeeded by another convulsion. The convulsions may recur during coma, or they may recur only after an interval of consciousness, or they may never recur at all. In the average case, from 5 to 10 convulsions occur at longer or shorter intervals, but as many as 20 are not uncommon. Convulsions may start before the onset of labor (antepartum), during labor (intrapartum) or any time within the first 48 hours after delivery (postpartum). About a fifth of the cases develop postpartum.

Upon physical examination, the findings of eclampsia are similar to those in preeclampsia, but exaggerated. Thus, the systolic blood pressure usually ranges around 180 mm. Hg. and sometimes exceeds 200 mm. Hg. Albuminuria is frequently extreme, from 10 to 20 Gm. per liter. Edema may be marked but sometimes is absent. Oliguria, or suppression of urinary excretion, is common and may amount to complete anuria. Fever is present in about half the cases.

In favorable cases, the convulsions cease, the coma lessens, and urinary output increases. However, it sometimes requires a day or two for clear consciousness to be regained. During this period eclamptic patients are often in an obstreperous, resistant mood and may be exceedingly difficult to manage. A few develop actual psychoses. In unfavorable cases the coma deepens, urinary excretion diminishes, the pulse becomes more rapid, the temperature rises, and edema of the lungs develops. The last is a serious symptom and usually is interpreted as a sign of cardiovascular failure. Edema of the lungs is readily recognizable by the noisy, gurgling respiration and by the large quantity of frothy mucus which exudes from the mouth and the nose. Toward the end, convulsions cease altogether, and the final picture is one of vascular collapse, with falling blood pressure and overwhelming edema of the lungs.

Like preeclampsia, eclampsia is a disease of young primigravidae, the majority of cases occurring in first pregnancies. It is more likely to occur as full term approaches and is rarely seen prior to the last 3 months. Eclampsia is particularly prone to develop in twin gestations, the likelihood being about four times that in single pregnancies.

Prognosis. Eclampsia is one of the gravest complications of pregnancy; the maternal mortality ranges, in different localities and in different hospitals, from 10 to 20 per cent of such cases. The outlook for the baby is particularly grave, the fetal mortality being about 50 per cent. Although it is difficult in a given case to forecast the outcome, the following are unfavorable signs: prolonged coma; a sustained pulse rate over 120; temperature over 103° F.; more than 10 convulsions (but patients with 200 have been known to recover); 10 or more Gm. of albumin per liter in the urine; systolic blood pressure of more than 200; edema of lungs. If none of these signs is present, the outlook for recovery is good; if two or more are present, the prognosis is serious. .

Even though the patient survives, she may not escape unscathed from the attack but sometimes continues to have high blood pressure indefinitely. This statement applies both to preeclampsia and eclampsia. Indeed, about 10 per cent of all preeclamptic and 5 per cent of all eclamptic patients are left with chronic, permanent hypertension. It is of even more importance to note that a still larger percentage of these women (about 50% of preeclamptics and 30% of eclamptics) again develop hypertensive toxemia in any subsequent pregnancies. This is known as "recurrent" or "repeat"

toxemia. These facts make it plain that careful, prolonged follow-up of these mothers who have suffered from preeclampsia or eclampsia is imperative. Moreover, the prognosis for future pregnancies must be guarded, although, as the figures indicate, such patients stand at least an even chance of going through subsequent pregnancies satisfactorily.

Principles of Treatment. Since the cause of eclampsia is not known, there can be no "specific" therapy, and treatment must necessarily be empirical. By "empirical" treatment is meant the utilization of those therapeutic measures which have yielded the best results in other cases. It is thus based on experience. Since the experience of different doctors and different hospitals varies considerably, the type of therapy employed from clinic to clinic differs somewhat in respect to the drugs used and in other details. However, the general principles followed are almost identical everywhere. For the nurse to memorize some particular regimen of therapy, as given in this textbook or as used in this or that hospital, will serve little purpose in her later career and conduces to an undesirable rigidity of attitude. However, she should grasp thoroughly the general principles involved. These are enumerated as follows.

1. PREVENTION. Let it be emphasized again that eclampsia is largely (but not entirely) a preventable disease. Vigilant antepartal care and the early detection and treatment of preeclampsia will do more to reduce deaths from eclampsia than the most intensive treatment after convulsions have once started.

2. CONSERVATIVE TREATMENT. Since eclampsia never occurs in nonpregnant women nor in men, it is reasonable to believe that it must be due in some way to the pregnant condition. By the same token it might be concluded that the best way to treat eclampsia would be to terminate the pregnancy at once, that is, empty the uterus. This was the therapy employed in the early years of the cen-

tury and is known as the "radical treatment" of eclampsia; either the cervix was forcibly dilated and the baby extracted, or cesarean section was employed. The results were disastrous. A quarter to a third of the mothers died, often on the operating table from shock.

Dissatisfied with the poor results yielded by the radical treatment of eclampsia, about 1910, physicians began treating the convulsions with sedative drugs, ignored the pregnancy and allowed labor to start whenever it would. The most famous method of therapy of this sort is the Stroganoff regimen, based on sedation by means of morphine and chloral hydrate. The results were dramatic: the maternal mortality fell to 10 per cent, and the fetal mortality was no worse than before. Other physicians tried other sedative drugs and other means of combating the convulsions, but as long as they refrained from interfering with the pregnancy, the results were as good as Stroganoff's, that is, only 1 woman in 10 was lost. This program, whereby the eclamptic convulsions are treated by sedation or otherwise, the pregnancy ignored, and labor allowed to start when it will, is known as the "conservative treatment" of eclampsia. This is the policy generally followed today, because, in the majority of cases, it gives the best results.

Although the conservative treatment has shown itself to be the program of choice in most cases, hard-and-fast rules in eclampsia are unwise. Now and then cases occur in which cesarean section may be the best therapy.

3. SEDATION. The purpose of administering sedative drugs is to depress the activity of the brain cells and thereby stop convulsions. The drugs most commonly employed are described below.

Morphine. Because of its quick action and readiness of administration, morphine is usually the first drug which the eclamptic patient receives. Thus, it is often given at the patient's home to allay convulsions during transport to the hospital, or in the admission room of a hospital pending the institution of other types of medication. When given as a single initial dose, the amount ordered by the physician is likely to be large, from one quarter to one half a grain (0.016 to 0.032 Gm.), depending on the size of the patient. Morphine may also be administered during the subsequent course of the treatment, but the modern tendency is to rely on other drugs for the main sedative program.

Paraldehyde. Although pungent in odor and somewhat difficult to administer, paraldehyde is being used more and more in eclampsia. In this condition it is almost always given per rectum, diluted with an equal amount of olive oil, and in dosages which may range from 20 to 35 cc. of the pure paraldehyde, according to the severity of the disease and the size of the patient. Usually it is repeated from time to time, in somewhat smaller doses perhaps, in order to maintain a fairly deep narcosis.

Magnesium Sulfate. Magnesium sulfate is not only a central nervous system sedative (employed in tetanus) but it is believed to cause a dilatation of the peripheral blood vessels and thus lower the blood pressure. For these reasons this drug is frequently used both in the treatment of preeclampsia and eclampsia. It may be given either intravenously or intramuscularly. When administered intravenously, it is sometimes given in amounts of 20 cc. of a 10 per cent solution, sometimes in a 2-cc. injection of a 50 per cent solution.

The intramuscular use of magnesium sulfate is more widely employed perhaps than the intravenous technic. Here the dosage varies considerably from institution to institution but may be given in amounts as large as 10 Gm. intramuscularly in a 50 per cent solution as an initial dose, followed by 5 Gm. every 6 hours. A 1 per cent concentration of procaine is frequently introduced in the injected solution to minimize discomfort following the injection. The initial dose is divided, 5 to 10 cc. being given into each buttock. In order to avoid tissue irritation as much as possible, the needle is moved about while injecting the solution in order to obtain wider dispersion. After withdrawal of the needle the area is massaged with a dry warm pack, which is then taped over the injection site. These injections are always made by the physician.

Barbiturates. The more commonly employed of these are Luminal Sodium (0.3 Gm. subcutaneously) and Amytal Sodium (0.3 to 0.6 Gm. intravenously). The drugs produce sleep, muscular relaxation and lowering of the blood pressure.

Chloral Hydrate. As already mentioned, chloral hydrate in conjunction with morphine forms the basis of the Stroganoff treatment.

4. PROTECTION OF PATIENT FROM SELF-INJURY. The eclamptic patient must never be left alone for a second. When in the throes of a convulsion, she may crash her head against a bedpost or throw herself onto the floor; or she may bite her tongue violently. To prevent the latter injury, some device should be kept within easy reach which can be inserted between the jaws at the very onset of a convulsion. A piece of very heavy rubber tubing, a rolled towel or a padded clothespin is often employed (Fig. 234). The nurse must take care in inserting it not to injure the patient (lips, gums, teeth) and not to allow her own finger to be bitten.

Eclamptic patients must never be given fluids by mouth unless thoroughly conscious. Failure to adhere to this rule may result in aspiration of the fluid and consequent pneumonia.

5. PROTECTION OF PATIENT FROM EXTRANEOUS STIMULI. A loud noise, a bright light, a jarring of the bed, a draft —indeed, the slightest irritation—may be enough to precipitate a convulsion.

6. PROMOTION OF DIURESIS. When an eclamptic patient begins to excrete substantial quantities of urine, the outlook is encouraging. Accordingly, efforts are generally made to stimulate renal activity. This is most often done by the intravenous administration of hypertonic glucose solutions, usually about a 20 per

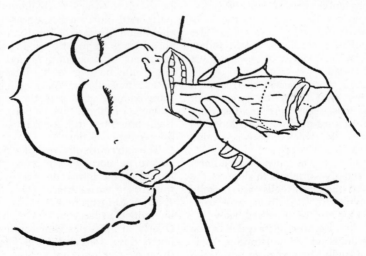

Fig. 234. Improvised mouth gag inserted between jaws of eclamptic patient to prevent tongue injury. (Putnam, Tracy J.: Convulsive Seizures, Philadelphia, Lippincott)

cent solution in amounts ranging from 200 to 500 cc.

7. OTHER THERAPEUTIC PROCEDURES. Although the above principles of treatment may be regarded as more or less standard, the nurse will encounter many experienced obstetricians who secure good results with other procedures. Thus, in many hospitals various hypotensive drugs, such as Veratrone and Apresoline, are favored. These agents produce relaxation of the arterioles throughout the body and by thus reducing peripheral resistance to blood flow lower the blood pressure, often dramatically. They are frequently employed in combination with other drugs.

Nurse's Responsibilities in Eclampsia. The nurse's responsibilities in the management of a case of eclampsia are serious. Some of them have already been mentioned in the discussion of treatment. Although eclampsia is regarded usually as the climax to a mounting preeclamptic toxemia which has been present, the nurse must remember that it is occasionally observed as a fulminating case in an apparently normal woman who may develop severe symptoms in the span of 24 hours. In the event that eclampsia occurs, the best quality of nursing care is necessary. The attack may come on at any time, even when the patient is sleeping. During the seizure it is necessary to protect the patient from self-injury. Never leave the patient for an instant unless someone is actually at the bedside to relieve you. Gentle restraint should be used to guide the patient's movements whenever necessary to prevent her from throwing herself against the head of the bed or out of it. Canvas sides, as well as pads at the head and the foot of the bed, are helpful. The padded mouth gag should be inserted between the upper and lower teeth at the onset of a convulsion to prevent the tongue from being bitten. Regardless of the fact that the nurse is exceedingly "busy" with the patient when a seizure occurs, she should make careful and complete observations of the duration and the character of each convulsion, the depth and the duration of coma, the quality and the rate of pulse and respirations and the degree of cyanosis. A careful record should be kept so that this information can be used by the physician in treating the patient. During the coma which follows, care must be taken to see that the patient does not aspirate. It is understood, of course, that one never gives an eclamptic patient fluids by mouth unless it is certain that she is fully conscious. The position of the patient in bed should be such that it promotes drainage of secretions and the maintenance of a clear airway. It may be necessary to raise the foot of the bed of the comatose patient a few inches to promote drainage of secretions from the respiratory passage. When this measure must be resorted to, it is particularly important to watch for signs of pulmonary edema, which would be aggravated by this position. The head of the bed may need to be elevated to relieve dyspnea. Even though the patient should be disturbed as little as possible, her position should be changed at hourly intervals.

The patient should be protected from extraneous stimuli. Light in the room should be eliminated except for a small lamp, so shaded that none of the light falls on the patient. Although the room should be darkened, the light should be sufficient to permit observations of changes in condition, such as cyanosis or twitchings. A flashlight, directed well away from the patient's face, may be used during catheterization and rectal instillations and during the physician's examinations. Sudden noises, such as the slamming of a door or the clatter of a tray as it is placed on a table, and jarring of the bed must be avoided because they are often sufficient stimuli to send the patient into convulsions. Only absolutely necessary conversation should be carried on in the room, and this should be in the lowest tones possible.

The fetal heart tones should be checked as often as time will permit. Also, the nurse must watch for signs of labor. In eclampsia this may proceed with few external signs, and occasionally such a patient gives birth beneath the sheets before anyone knows that the process is under way. Be suspicious when the patient grunts or groans or moves about at regular intervals, every 5 minutes or so. If this occurs, feel the consistency of the uterus, watch for "show" and bulging and report your observations to the physician. Convulsions which occur during labor may speed up this process, and more rapid preparation for delivery should be made. During the delivery, the same atmosphere of quiet should be maintained, and glaring lights kept away from the patient's face.

Throughout the care of the eclamptic patient a careful account of fluid intake and output should be recorded, along with all the other observations and pertinent data. And, since further complications of pregnancy may occur in eclampsia, the patient should be observed for signs and symptoms of cerebral hemorrhage, abruptio placentae, pulmonary edema and cardiac failure.

Chronic Hypertensive Vascular Disease

Preeclampsia and eclampsia have been discussed in some detail because the nurse's role in the management of these conditions is extremely important.

As the name indicates, this disease is a chronic disorder of the vascular system associated with high blood pressure. In other words, these patients have a tendency to have hypertension, whether pregnant or not. Not infrequently the kidneys are also affected, with the result that albuminuria may be present as well as diminution in the excretory power of the kidneys. The age of these patients is usually in the thirties; most of them are multiparae with a number of children. The course of pregnancy in these chronic

hypertensive women is often troublesome, the blood pressure showing a tendency to reach higher and higher levels as the last 3 months of pregnancy are reached. In general, the outlook for the baby is poor. The fetus often dies in utero. Following delivery, there may be a slight recession in the blood pressure, but it usually remains at a figure only slightly below that observed during pregnancy. Each subsequent pregnancy adds its increment to the hypertension, and, as a rule, the exacerbation in blood pressure occurs earlier and earlier in each succeeding pregnancy.

Aside from the high blood pressure, the signs and symptoms of hypertensive vascular disease may be surprisingly few. Headache is rather common, but even this complaint may be absent. The doctor's examination of the retina very often shows a narrowing of the arterioles, indicative of the fact that there is a generalized sclerosis of the small arterioles throughout the body.

In patients with chronic hypertensive vascular disease, we cannot prevent the occurrence of hypertension since it was already present when conception took place. These patients already had the sclerosed, inelastic arterioles mentioned above, and it is understandable that the 50 per cent increase in minute output of the heart which pregnancy imposes (p. 123) will place a severe burden on such a vascular system. In the face of this chronic process and this burden imposed by pregnancy, very little can be done in such cases to relieve the hypertension. The physician will have a plan which he will discuss with the expectant parents. Hence, the problem is largely one of preventive medicine, in the sense that pregnancies either should be avoided altogether or limited.

Decision as to the best way of managing a case of hypertensive vascular disease will be made by the physician after taking into consideration a number of circumstances, such as the severity of the hypertensive process, the number of children in the family, the duration of the pregnancy when first seen, etc. If the process is mild, the pregnancy may be allowed to continue with the patient under close observation for signs of impending trouble. On the other hand, if the process is very severe, the mother's life may be at stake. In most cases in this group, the doctor may wish to prevent further pregnancies and may recommend either ligation of the fallopian tubes or the use of some method of contraception.

Moral Considerations. The nurse should remember that such recommendations are not always acceptable to the patient, particularly if this involves ethical problems related to her religious beliefs. In such instances it is well to encourage the patient to discuss the problem with her priest or minister, as well as with her husband and her physician. Some pertinent references have been included in the suggested readings at the end of the chapter.

HEMORRHAGIC COMPLICATIONS

The causes of bleeding in pregnancy are usually considered in relation to the stage of gestation in which they are most likely to cause complications. Frequent causes of bleeding during the first half of pregnancy are abortion, ectopic pregnancy and hydatidiform mole. Although hydatidiform mole is a less common cause (occurs once in about 2,000 pregnancies), it is nevertheless important because uterine bleeding is its outstanding symptom. The two most common causes of hemorrhage in the latter half of pregnancy are placenta previa and abruptio placentae.

Abortion

Definitions. Abortion is the termination of pregnancy at any time before the fetus has attained a stage of viability, that is, before it is capable of extra-uterine existence.

It is customary to use the weight of the fetus as an important criterion in abortion. Infants weighing 1,000 Gm. (2 lbs. 3 oz.) or less at birth possess little chance for survival, while those above this weight have a substantial chance of living. Thus, many authorities regard a pregnancy which terminates when the fetus weighs 1,000 Gm. (about 28 weeks of gestation) or less as an abortion. On the other hand, a small percentage of infants weighing 1,000 Gm. or less do survive. Modern advances in the management and care of premature infants have made it possible for smaller and smaller infants to survive, so fetuses weighing only 800 to 900 Gm. (1 lb., 13 oz. to 2 lbs.) may live. For this reason many authorities now maintain that fetal weight of 1,000 Gm. or less but more than 400 Gm. is classified as immature, and that fetal weight of 400 Gm. (about 20 weeks of gestation) or less constitutes an abortion. It is obvious, therefore, that how the termination of pregnancy is classified in different hospitals will depend wholly on the interpretation to which they subscribe. In summary, the following definitions are generally used. The termination of pregnancy at any time when the fetus weighs 400 Gm. or less is defined as an *abortion*. Infants weighing between 401 and 1,000 Gm. are called *immature*.

A premature infant is one born after the stage of viability has been reached but before it has the same chance for survival as a full-term infant. By general consensus, an infant which weighs 2,500 Gm. or less at birth is termed *premature;* one which weighs 2,501 Gm. (5½ lbs.) or more is regarded as *full term*.

It is well to remember that premature labor does not refer to abortion. *Premature labor* is the termination of pregnancy after the fetus is viable but before it has attained full term. Although the cause of many premature labors cannot be explained, the condition can be brought on by maternal diseases, such as chronic hypertensive vascular disease, abruptio placentae, placenta previa, untreated syphilis or a mechanical defect in the cervix.

As a measure to bring about greater uniformity in the interpretation of the terms "abortion," "miscarriage" and "viability," the World Health Organization, in 1950, introduced certain new definitions which, in effect, would substitute the term "early fetal death" for "abortion" and would tabulate all live births and fetal deaths in 4 groups, according to length of gestation.

Terminology of Abortion. The term abortion includes many varieties of termination of pregnancy prior to viability but may be subdivided into 2 main groups, namely, spontaneous and induced. *Spontaneous abortion* is one in which, through natural causes, the process starts of its own accord. *Induced*

abortion is one which is artificially induced, and may be in the form of either a therapeutic abortion or a criminal abortion. The laity, however, is inclined to associate the word "abortion" with instances in which criminal interference with pregnancy has been perpetrated, and to them, therefore, the term often carries a definite stigma. They employ the word "miscarriage" to designate spontaneous abortion, and the nurse will do well, in discussing the matter with patients or relatives to use that term.

In medical parlance the word "miscarriage" is rarely employed.

THREATENED ABORTION. An abortion is regarded as threatened if a patient in early pregnancy has vaginal bleeding or spotting; this may or may not be associated with mild cramps. The cervix is

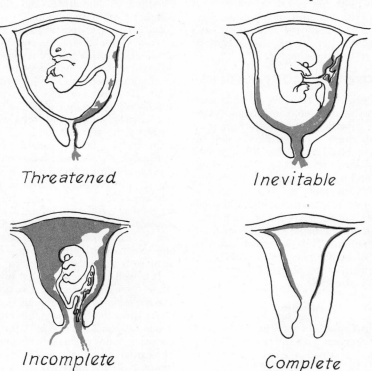

Threatened *Inevitable*

Incomplete *Complete*

Fig. 235. Stages of abortion. (Cooke, Willard R.: Essentials of Gynecology, Philadelphia, Lippincott)

closed. The process has presumably started but may abate under suitable treatment (Fig. 235).

INEVITABLE ABORTION. Inevitable abortion is so called because the process has gone so far that termination of the pregnancy cannot be prevented. Bleeding is copious, and the pains are more severe. The membranes may or may not have ruptured, and the cervical canal is dilating.

INCOMPLETE ABORTION. An incomplete abortion is one in which part of the product of conception has been passed, but part (usually the placenta) is retained in the uterus. Bleeding persists until the retained secundines of the uterus have been passed.

COMPLETE ABORTION. Complete abortion is the expulsion of the entire product of conception.

MISSED ABORTION. In a missed abortion the fetus dies in the uterus, but, instead of being expelled, it is retained indefinitely. The term is generally restricted to cases in which 2 months or more elapse between fetal death and expulsion. During this period the fetus undergoes marked degenerative changes. Of these, maceration, or a general softening, is the most common. Occasionally it dries up into a leatherlike structure (mummification) and very rarely it becomes converted into stony material (lithopedion formation). Symptoms, except for amenorrhea, are usually lacking, but occasionally such patients complain of malaise, headache and anorexia. Hypofibrinogenemia, a hemorrhagic complication, may result (see p. 416).

HABITUAL ABORTION. By this term is meant a condition in which spontaneous abortion occurs in successive pregnancies (3 or more). This is a most distressing condition, some women having 6 or 8 spontaneous abortions.

THERAPEUTIC ABORTION. Therapeutic abortion is the instrumental termination of pregnancy by a physician because of some grave maternal disease which would make continuation of the pregnancy extremely hazardous to the mother. As a rule, one or more physicians are called into consultation to make certain that the procedure is absolutely necessary. Modern methods of antepartal care are making the necessity for therapeutic abortion relatively rare. The nurse must recall, moreover, that ethical principles of the Roman Catholic Church forbid the procedure, and that it may not be performed in hospitals of that faith.

CRIMINAL ABORTION. Criminal abortion is the termination of pregnancy without medical and legal justification. Since these operations always are performed surreptitiously, accurate figures concerning their frequency are difficult to secure, but the very minimum estimate is 100,000 annually in the United States, while some authorities put the figure at over half a million a year. This means that each year in this country between 100,000 and 500,000 potential lives are destroyed simply for "convenience," a frightful wastage of human life and a sorry reflection on our civilization. Quite apart from this destruction of fetal life, criminal abortion is one of the most common causes of maternal death. No reputable physician will induce an abortion without medical justification. Consequently, these clandestine operations usually are performed by hands which are not only unskilled but unclean. Fatal infections are common. Of those who survive many are left invalids, others permanently sterile. Most cases of so-called "infected abortion" are of this origin.

Every year huge quantities of castor oil, quinine and other "powerful" drugs are bought for the express purpose of interrupting early pregnancy. As a rule, these concoctions merely produce nausea and vomiting, while pregnancy is not interrupted. However, certain of the patent medicines used for this purpose contain ingredients which act with such violence that hemorrhages into the bowel and the kidneys sometimes ensue, with results that may be exceedingly grave. The reputation of these drugs rests on the circumstance that the menstrual interval in the same woman often varies widely; a woman who has been accustomed to menstrute every 28 days may occasionally experience a 35-day cycle without apparent cause or detriment to health. If, in such a long cycle, when she thinks herself 5 or 6 days "overdue," she takes one of these medicines and starts menstruating the next day, naturally the drug is acclaimed as the benefactor. It is obvious that the same end would have been attained had she done nothing. At the present writing there is no drug known to the medical profession which will produce abortion in the human being, whether given by mouth or hypodermically.

Clinical Picture. About 75 per cent of all spontaneous abortions occur during the second and the third months of pregnancy, that is, before the twelfth week. The condition is very common; it is estimated that about 1 pregnancy in every 10 terminates in spontaneous abortion. Almost invariably the first symptom is bleeding due to the separation of the fertilized ovum from its uterine attachment. The bleeding is often slight at the beginning and may persist for days before uterine cramps occur; or, the bleeding may be followed at once by cramps. Occasionally the bleeding is torrential in nature, leaving the patient in shock. The uterine contractions bring about softening and dilatation of the cervix and expel the products of conception either completely or incompletely.

Causes. What causes all these spontaneous abortions—so tragic and shattering to so many women? If the evidence is reviewed with some perspective and with full fairness to all concerned, it is the inevitable conclusion that most of these abortions, far from being tragedies, are blessings in disguise, for they are Nature's beneficent way of extinguishing embryos which are imperfect. Indeed, careful microscopic study of the material passed in these cases shows that the commonest cause of spontaneous abor-

tion is an inherent defect in the product of conception. This defect may express itself in an abnormal embryo, in an abnormal *trophoblast* (p. 75) or in both abnormalities. In early abortions, 80 per cent are associated with some defect of the embryo or trophoblast which is either incompatible with life or would result in a grossly deformed child. The incidence of abnormalities passed after the second month is somewhat lower, but not less than 50 per cent. Whether the germ plasm of the spermatozoon or the ovum is at fault in these cases it is usually difficult, if not impossible, to say. Abortions of this sort are obviously unpreventable and, although bitterly disappointing to the parents, serve a useful purpose.

Spontaneous abortions may be due to causes other than defects in the product of conception. Severe acute infections, such as pneumonia, pyelitis and typhoid fever, often lead to abortion. Heart failure is another etiologic factor. Occasionally, abnormalities of the generative tract, such as a congenitally short cervix, produce the accident. Retroposition of the uterus rarely causes abortion, as was formerly believed. Many women tend to explain miscarriage on the grounds of injury of one type or another, or excessive activity. Different women exhibit the greatest variation in this respect. In

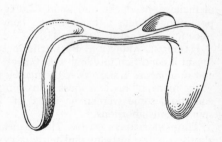

Fig. 236. Sims speculum for inserting into the vaginal canal so as to expose the cervix to view.

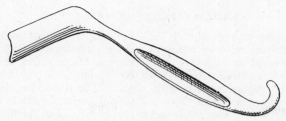

Fig. 237. Schroeder vaginal retractor for drawing back the
vulvar or vaginal walls during an operation.

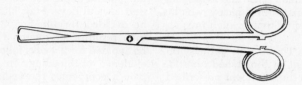

Fig. 238. Bullet forceps used in grasping
the lips of the cervix.

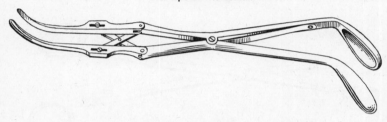

Fig. 239. Modified Goodell-Ellinger dilator used for enlarging the
canal of the cervix.

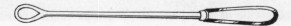

Fig. 240. Uterine sound.

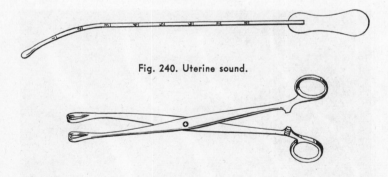

Fig. 241. Placental forceps with heart-shaped jaws.

Fig. 242. Sims sharp curette, a scraper or spoonlike instrument
for removing matter from the walls of the uterus.

some the pregnancy may go blithely on despite falls from second-story windows and automobile accidents so severe as to fracture the pelvis. In others a trivial fall or merely overfatigue seems to contribute at least to abortion. Since there is no way of telling who is susceptible and who is not, it would seem prudent for every expectant mother to follow the dictates of common sense and avoid long automobile trips, lifting heavy weights and any form of activity which involves jolting.

Treatment. The severity of the symptoms manifested in threatened abortion will determine the treatment prescribed. If the patient is having only a slight vaginal bleeding or even spotting, without pain, she should be advised to stay in bed, eat a light well-balanced diet, avoid straining at bowel evacuation and the use of cathartics. If she appears to be apprehensive, a mild sedative may be given. She should be further advised to save all perineal pads, as well as all tissue and clots passed, for the physician's inspection. If the bleeding disappears within 48 hours, she may get out of bed but should limit her activities for the next several days. Stair climbing should be avoided for the first 24 hours and then resumed gradually. Coitus should be avoided for 2 weeks following the last evidence of bleeding. In cases where pain accompanies the vaginal bleeding, the prognosis for saving the pregnancy is poor. Usually bleeding is observed first, and then, in a few hours, sometimes

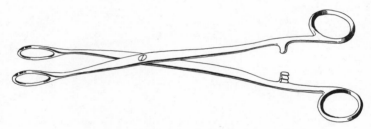

Fig. 243. Sponge holder.

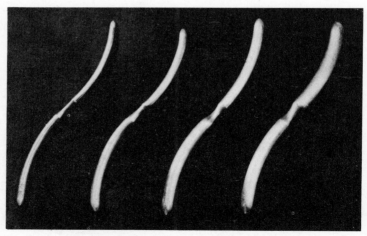

Fig. 244. Hegar dilators, of graduated diameters from 5 to 12 mm. Larger sizes are also used.

days later, uterine contractions ensue. This is treated by absolute bed rest, narcotic drugs (paregoric, morphine, etc.) and some preparations of progesterone (see Chap. 3). When the pain and the bleeding increase, the patient should be hospitalized, if this has not already been done. If the abortion is incomplete, ordinarily efforts are made to aid the uterus in emptying its contents. Pituitary extract may be administered, but if this is ineffectual, surgical removal of the retained products of conception should be done promptly, provided that the patient is afebrile and no other evidence of infection exists. Active bleeding may make this urgently necessary. Many times the tissue lies loose in the cervical canal and can be simply lifted out with ovum forceps, otherwise curettage of the uterine cavity must be done. The instruments commonly used in completing an incomplete abortion are shown in Figs. 236 to 244. If evidence of infection is present (fever, foul discharge or suspicious history of criminal abortion), the physician may prefer to withhold any invasion of the uterine cavity, lest it disseminate bacteria into the venous sinuses of the uterus and thence into the general circulation. Although the use of antibiotics has greatly reduced this hazard, it has not eliminated it entirely. On the other hand, bleeding and certain other circumstances may make removal of the uterine contents desirable despite the presence of infection. Complete abortion requires exactly the same care as that given during the postpartal period. As already indicated, habitual abortion may be helped by endocrine therapy as well as by meticulous attention to general hygiene, rest, vitamin requirements, etc.

Nurse's Responsibilities in Abortion Cases. Bleeding in the first half of pregnancy, no matter how slight, always must be considered as threatened abortion. The patient must be put to bed and the physician notified. An episode of this nature is indeed distressing to the expectant mother, many times alarming.

The nurse should bear in mind that while the emotional support she gives her patient is important, she must never try to reassure her that "everything will be all right," because in fact the patient may lose this pregnancy. Perineal pads and all tissue and blood clots passed by the patient should be saved. The physician will wish to examine these to determine the amount of bleeding and, when tissue has been passed, to examine the products of conception to ascertain, among other facts, whether or not the abortion is complete. If bleeding is so copious as to be alarming, elevate the foot of the bed (shock position) while awaiting the physician's arrival. If surgical completion of the abortion is to be carried out, the same aseptic regimen is carried out as for delivery.

All cases of criminal abortion must be regarded as potentially infected, and strict antiseptic precautions must be carried out to prevent spread of infection to others. In regard to criminal abortion, the nurse can have only one attitude, to regard it as the murder of a potential human being and also as a procedure which kills thousands of mothers each year. In caring for a woman who has had a criminal abortion recently, or one whose history is suspicious, the nurse may find it difficult to handle her own feelings so that she does not reflect a judgmental attitude. It is helpful to remember that it is not within the province of the nurse to pass moral judgments as she gives nursing care. In such situations the nurse should direct her concern to the gravity of the patient's illness. Occasionally circumstances make it possible for the nurse to be of definite educational help on the question of criminal abortion, both to her patients and to the public.

Ectopic Pregnancy

An ectopic pregnancy is any gestation located outside the uterine cavity. The majority of ectopic pregnancies are tubal gestations. Other types, which

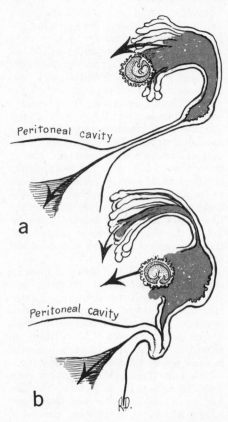

Peritoneal cavity

a

Peritoneal cavity

b

Fig. 245. (a) Tubal abortion, showing passage of the products of conception, together with much blood, out the fimbriated end of the tube. (b) Rupture of tubal pregnancy into peritoneal cavity. There is an outpouring of blood into the abdomen from vessels at the site of the rupture.

This condition is known as "ectopic pregnancy" (literally, a pregnancy which is out of place), or as "tubal pregnancy" or "extra-uterine pregnancy." Since the wall of the tube is not sufficiently elastic to allow the fertilized ovum to grow and develop there, rupture of the tubal wall is the inevitable result. Rupture most frequently occurs into the tubal lumen with the passage of the products of conception, together with much blood, out the fimbriated end of the tube and into the peritoneal cavity—so-called "tubal abortion." Or, rupture may occur through the peritoneal surface of the tube directly into the peritoneal cavity; and, again, there is an outpouring of blood into the abdomen from vessels at the site of rupture (Fig. 245). In either case, rupture usually occurs within the first twelve weeks.

Occasionally an ectopic pregnancy may develop in that portion of the tube which passes through the uterine wall, a type known as "interstitial pregnancy." In very, very rare instances, the product of conception, after rupturing through the tubal wall, may implant itself on the peritoneum and develop to full term in the peritoneal cavity. This extraordinary occurrence is known as "abdominal pregnancy." Surprisingly enough, quite a few living infants have been delivered in such cases by means of abdominal incision.

Ectopic pregnancy may be due to any condition which narrows the tube or brings about some constriction within it. Under such circumstances, the tubal lumen is large enough to allow spermatozoa to ascend the tube but not big enough to permit the downward passage of the fertilized ovum. Among the conditions which may produce such a narrowing of the fallopian tube are: previous inflammatory processes involving the tubal mucosa and producing partial agglutination of opposing surfaces, such as gonorrheal salpingitis; previous inflammatory processes of the external peri-

make up about 5 per cent of all ectopic pregnancies, are: interstitial (in the interstitial portion of the tube), cornual (in a rudimentary horn of a uterus), cervical, abdominal and ovarian gestations.

About once in every 300 pregnancies the fertilized ovum, instead of traversing the length of the fallopian tube to reach the uterine cavity, becomes implanted within the wall of the fallopian tube.

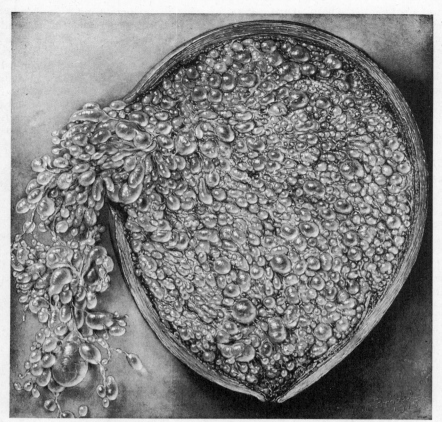

Fig. 246. Hydatidiform mole ×½. (Eastman, N. J.: Williams Obstetrics, New York, Appleton-Century)

toneal surfaces of the tube causing kinking, such as puerperal and postabortal infections; and developmental defects resulting in a general narrowing of the tubes.

In cases of ectopic gestation the woman exhibits the usual early symptoms of pregnancy and, as a rule, regards herself as being normally pregnant. After missing one or two periods, however, she suddenly experiences pain which is knifelike in nature and often of extreme severity in one of the lower quadrants. This is usually associated with very slight vaginal bleeding, commonly referred to as "spotting." Depending on the amount of blood which has escaped into the peritoneal cavity, she may or may not undergo a fainting attack and show symptoms of shock.

Ectopic pregnancy is a grave complication of pregnancy and is an important cause of maternal death. Moreover, if a woman has had one ectopic pregnancy and subsequently becomes pregnant, she is more likely than the average woman to have another such accident.

The treatment of ectopic pregnancy is removal of the tube,* supplemented by blood transfusion. While transporting

* See "Moral Considerations," p. 403.

such a patient to the hospital or awaiting operation, the nurse can be of immeasurable assistance in combating the shock which is frequently present. Elevation of the foot of the bed and maintenance of body heat by means of hot-water bottles and blankets may help to save the patient's life.

Hydatidiform Mole

Hydatidiform mole is a benign neoplasm of the chorion in which the chorionic villi degenerate and become transparent vesicles containing clear, viscid fluid. The vesicles have a "grapelike" appearance and are arranged in clusters involving all or part of the decidual lining of the uterus (Fig. 246). Although there is usually no embryo present, occasionally there may be a fetus* and only part of the placenta involved. Hydatidiform mole is rather an uncommon con-

* See "Moral Considerations," p. 403.

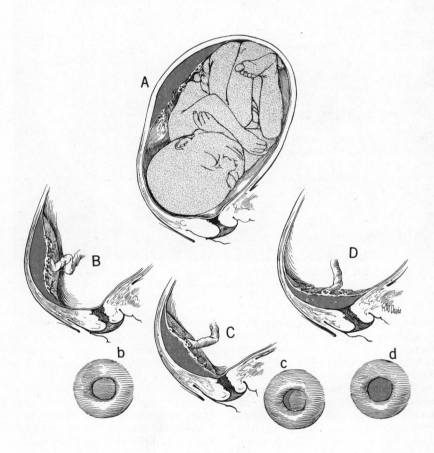

Plate 8. The 3 types of placenta previa, showing position of the placenta in relation to the internal os (B, C and D) contrasted with normal placental insertion (A). Below (b, c and d), on vaginal examination the placenta can be felt during effacement and dilatation of the cervix in low implantation, partial and complete placenta previa.

dition, occurring about once in every 2,000 pregnancies. The pregnancy appears to be normal at first. Then bleeding, a usual symptom varying from spotting to that of a profuse degree, occurs, so that one might suspect threatened abortion. If the patient does not abort, the uterus enlarges rapidly, and profuse hemorrhage may occur, at which time these vesicles may be evident in the vaginal discharge. Vomiting in rather severe form may appear early. Severe preeclampsia, a complication which does not usually occur until the later months of pregnancy, may appear early in the second trimester. The treatment consists in emptying the uterus by dilating the cervix and carefully extracting the uterine contents. There is always great danger of injury to the uterine wall, which is weakened and of spongy consistency due to the growth of the mole. Some physicians advise hysterectomy. The follow-up care is very important because, although this is a benign process, extremely malignant chorioncarcinoma (formerly called chorionepithelioma) sometimes further complicates the picture.

Placenta Previa

While abortion is the most frequent cause of bleeding early in pregnancy, the most common cause during the later months is placenta previa. In this condition the placenta is attached to the lower uterine segment (instead of high up in the uterus as usual) and either wholly or in part covers the region of the cervix. There are three types, differentiated according to the degree to which the condition is present (Plate 8):

1. *Total placenta previa,* in which the placenta completely covers the internal os.

2. *Partial placenta previa,* in which the placenta partially covers the internal os.

3. *Low implantation of placenta,* in which the placenta encroaches upon the region of internal os, so that it can be palpated by the physician on digital exploration about the cervix, but does not extend beyond the margin of the internal os.

Painless vaginal bleeding during the second half of pregnancy is the main symptom of placenta previa. The bleeding usually occurs after the seventh month. It may begin as mere "spotting" and increase or it may start with profuse hemorrhages. The patient may awaken in the middle of the night to find herself in a pool of blood. The bleeding is caused by separation of the placenta as the result of changes which take place in the lower uterine segment during the later months. This separation opens up the underlying blood sinuses of the uterus from which the bleeding occurs.

Fortunately, placenta previa is not a very common condition, occurring about once in every 200 deliveries. It occurs much more frequently in multiparae than in primigravidae. Placenta previa always must be regarded as a grave complication of pregnancy. Until recent years it showed a maternal mortality of approximately 10 per cent. Modern methods of management, plus the more liberal use of blood transfusion, have reduced this figure considerably. The outlook for the baby is always dubious, not only because the placental separation interferes with the infant's oxygen supply, but also because many of these babies are very premature when delivery must necessarily take place.

Treatment. There are two main forms of treatment: (1) pressure therapy exerted *per vaginum* and (2) cesarean section. The principle underlying the first of these is to compress the bleeding sinuses by exerting pressure on them and the overlying placenta. Depending on the nature of the case, the physician may choose to do this in one of several ways: (1) rupture of the membranes, which allows the head to gravitate downward and exert a certain amount of pressure on the placenta and the lower uterine segment; (2) application of Willett's forceps to the scalp with traction (Fig. 247); (3) Braxton Hicks' version, by which the fetus is turned and a leg brought down so that a thigh and a buttock of the fetus compress the lower segment. In addition to checking hemorrhage by pressure effects, these measures serve to dilate the cervix and to hasten the moment when delivery can be effected. The other main form of treatment, cesarean section, has been used more and more in recent years, particularly in the severe forms of the complication, such as complete and partial placenta previa. As in other hemorrhagic complications of pregnancy, blood transfusion plays an important—often a lifesaving—role in the management of these cases.

Bleeding, shock and infection are the main dangers. Before the arrival of the physician, the nurse should keep a solicitous eye on the amount of bleeding and the pulse rate and watch for signs of oncoming shock (pallor, increased pulse rate, cold extremities, etc.). Should the bleeding be profuse, elevation of the foot of the bed and application of external heat may forestall shock. If the diagnosis is not clear, the nurse may be asked to watch the patient for amount of bleeding. Under such circumstances, the patient should be instructed to report feeling the escape of fluid from the vulva. The nurse, in turn, should inspect the pad or bed frequently for hemorrhage.

One of the important facts about placenta previa to keep in mind is that a vaginal or rectal examination may precipitate severe hemorrhage. Therefore,

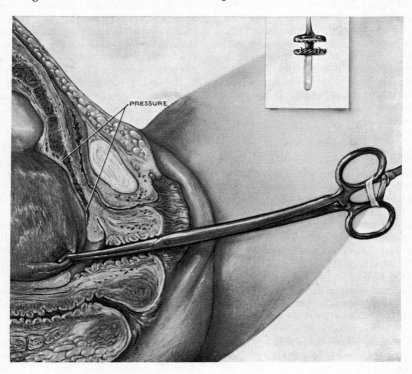

Fig. 247. Willett's forceps in place, showing one method of exerting pressure of baby's head on placenta and the lower uterine segment in placenta previa. Insert shows front view of forceps' tip.

any patient who bleeds to any extent greater than "show" during the last half of pregnancy should never have a digital examination, either rectal or vaginal, at home. She should be sent to the hospital promptly, where everything is available for the immediate carrying out of any procedure which may be necessary for treatment. In the hospital, digital examination is performed only in the operating room, and then only after complete preparations are in readiness for carrying out abdominal and vaginal surgery as well as blood transfusion. This is usually referred to as the "double setup" (i.e., a setup for both vaginal and abdominal delivery).

Patients with placenta previa may later develop puerperal infection. This is understandable when one recalls that the open venous sinuses, low down about the cervix, are particularly accessible to infection and toxic conditions due to any bacteria which might have been introduced into the vagina. Hemorrhage, moreover, lowers the patient's resistance to infection. It is essential, therefore, that meticulous attention be given to antiseptic and aseptic precautions in the handling of these cases.

Abruptio Placentae

Abruptio placentae (meaning that the placenta is torn from its bed) is a complication of the last half of pregnancy, in which a normally located placenta undergoes separation from its uterine attachment. The condition is frequently referred to as "premature separation of the normally implanted placenta"; other synonymous terms such as "accidental hemorrhage" (meaning that it takes place unexpectedly) and "ablatio placentae" (ablatio means a carrying away) are sometimes used. Bleeding may be apparent, in which case it is called *external hemorrhage;* or bleeding may be concealed, in which case it is called *concealed hemorrhage.* In other words, if a separation occurs at the margin, the blood is apt to lift the membranes and

trickle down to the cervical os and thus escape externally. If the placenta begins to separate centrally, a huge amount of blood may be stored behind the placenta before any of it becomes evident (Fig. 248). Although the precise cause of the condition is not known, it is frequently encountered in association with cases of toxemia of pregnancy.

Premature separation of the normally implanted placenta is characterized not only by bleeding beneath the placenta but also by pain. The pain is produced by the accumulation of blood behind the placenta, with subsequent distention of the uterus. The uterus also enlarges in size as the result of the accumulated blood and becomes distinctly tender and exceedingly firm. Because of the almost woody hardness of the uterine walls, fetal parts may be difficult to determine. Shock is often out of proportion to blood loss, as manifested by a rapid pulse,

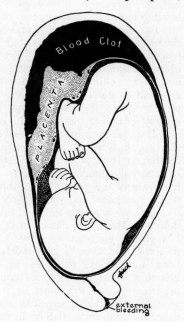

Fig. 248. Abruptio placentae with large blood clot between placenta and uterine wall.

dyspnea, yawning, restlessness, pallor, syncope and cold, clammy perspiration.

Clear-cut examples of this complication occur much less frequently than placenta previa and are uncommon. Treatment consists either in cesarean section or in rupturing the membranes, but whatever course is indicated, the immense gravity of the situation demands the organized teamwork of physicians, nurses and laboratory technicians. Transcending all else in importance is therapy of shock, which is almost invariably present. Where blood loss has been substantial, it should be replaced before proceeding with abdominal delivery. In less severe cases, artificial rupture of membranes, when instituted promptly, may initiate labor, and vaginal delivery may be accomplished before the extent of detachment increases and the bleeding becomes more extensive. In more severe cases, a further complication may be encountered because of extravasation of blood into the uterine musculature and beneath the uterine peritoneum, so-called *"utero-placental apoplexy"* or *"Couvelaire uterus."* Here the uterus remains flaccid, and, after either vaginal delivery or cesarean section, bleeding may be so profuse as to indicate prompt hysterectomy. Another hemorrhagic complication which may follow in severe cases of abruptio is due to a deficiency in the fibrinogen level of the blood, so-called hypofibrinogenemia. The nurse should be aware of the possibility of this additional complication, particularly when the patient continues to bleed following delivery. The usual measures to stimulate uterine contractions prove to be of no avail, and even if hysterectomy has been performed, evidence of steady bleeding from the vagina continues. Needless to say, this must be reported promptly so that corrective measures may be begun immediately, in this case to restore the fibrinogen level of the blood. This could be accomplished eventually by blood transfusions but would require such a massive volume of blood that it would not be feasible in severe cases, whereas the administration of fibrinogen injected intravenously can promptly restore the deficiency. Hemorrhage and/or trauma in labor must always be considered as predisposing factors to puerperal infection, so the nurse must guard against infection and be alert for any symptoms. In many cases antibiotic therapy may be used as a prophylactic measure. Although abruptio placentae constitutes one of the gravest accidents which can befall a pregnant woman, the maternal mortality rate has been markedly reduced as a result of more intelligent management. The out-come for the infant depends to a great extent on the severity of the process. In the milder cases the infant may be born alive, but it is often born prematurely; in severe cases almost all infants die.

Mistaken Diagnosis of Hemorrhage

A false alarm concerning hemorrhage is sometimes due to a normal "show" at the beginning of labor. It simply means that dilatation of the cervix has begun, causing slight bleeding. No treatment is required. However, the nurse should reassure the patient and watch to determine whether or not the bleeding which is present is more than the normal show.

BLOOD GROUPS AND THE RH FACTOR

An important complicating factor in childbearing may exist when the pregnant woman is Rh negative, because this condition may contribute to a chain of events which exerts a harmful effect on the fetus. There are other circumstances, however, which must be present before this condition can affect the unborn child. When the mother is Rh negative, blood group differences between the fetus and the mother may arise: (1) if the Rh negative woman has had one or more transfusions of Rh positive blood, (2) if the male parent of the fetus is Rh positive, and (3) if the developing fetus is Rh positive. In a small percentage of pregnancies *erythroblastosis fetalis,* a hemolytic disease of the fetus and the newborn, develops (see Chap. 21). The nurse must have some knowledge of certain basic facts regarding blood groups in order to understand this phenomenon.

Blood Groups

Following the discovery in 1900-1901 that certain antigens exist in human red blood cells, it became possible to divide all human blood into 4 main types or groups, now called A, B, AB and O, on the basis of the antigen or antigens within the erythrocytes. It was observed that the red blood cells of certain individuals became clumped (agglutinated) or dissolved (hemolyzed) when transfused into certain other individuals, thus preventing any advantage from the transfusion and, moreover, causing injurious or toxic effects due to the reaction of incompatible substances. In general,* an O person's blood may be given with safety to any one of the other 3 types (in the case of A-B-O genes, A and B are dominant over O). Therefore, O individuals are often called "universal donors." However, an O individual is least able to receive blood from the other 3 types; if transfusion is necessary, he should be given O blood. Any person of the other 3 blood types may be transfused with O type blood, but he is preferably transfused with blood of his own type, that is, A with A type, B with B type and AB with AB type. Thousands of tests show that about 40 per cent of our population are O type and about 40 per cent are A type.

These blood groups are not related to racial differences. All 4 types have been reported in all known nationalities, though they differ in proportions. In the United States the average for the white race is roughly 45 per cent O and 40 per cent A, but in the American Indians

* Important exceptions in O and other persons are concerned with the Rh situation, discussed later in this section.

about 75 per cent are of O type and 25 per cent the A type.

It was once thought that blood from one member of a family would be compatible with that of any other member, but blood types may differ greatly within a given family. It is possible for a child born to an O and an AB parent to have O, A, B or AB blood. If the child had O blood it might receive transfusions from the O parent but not from his AB parent. However, his O blood might be transfused with safety to either his O or his AB parent.

The Rh Factor

Even carefully matched blood, e.g., A to A, or universal O to one of the other 3 types, has not always been free from undesirable effects. It is now known that there are several other antigens within erythrocytes, in addition to the 4 (A, B, AB and O) which resulted in the division of human blood into 4 major types. The most important of the recently discovered antigens is the Rh substance or factor. Its name is derived from the first two letters of the scientific term for the rhesus monkey, which always has the factor present in its blood. A person's Rh type depends on the presence or absence of the Rh antigen within the red blood cells. The Rh factor is an hereditary characteristic, transmitted according to the principles set forth in Mendel's law. About 85 per cent of our white population and slightly more of our Negro population are Rh positive. Therefore, such persons are said to be Rh positive (Rh+); persons lacking the Rh factor are called Rh negative (Rh—).*

When the blood of an Rh-positive person is introduced, through blood transfusion or otherwise, into the blood stream of an Rh-negative individual, the latter develops antibodies against the Rh factor present in the blood administered. Antibodies are substances which the body manufactures as a protective mech-

* Only about 7 per cent of Negroes and about 1 per cent of Chinese are Rh negative.

anism to counteract the effect of various kinds of new materials which may be introduced into the blood and the tissues. For instance, when bacteria gain access to the blood stream, antibodies against that particular kind of bacteria are usually developed and, sooner or later, destroy the bacteria. Accordingly, antibodies may be regarded as a sort of defensive army which the blood and the tissues muster against foreign invading forces. It is these antibodies which cure most infectious diseases, from the common cold to typhoid fever. Moreover, they often remain present in the blood and the tissues long after the disease has been combated successfully, making the person immune to that particular type of infection; in other words, should the same bacterium or material which incited the original manufacture of the antibodies be again introduced into the body, these defensive substances now stand ready to attack and destroy it.

Rh and Transfusions. As stated above, when an Rh-negative person is given a blood transfusion from an Rh-positive donor, antibodies are developed by the recipient against the Rh substance present in the administered blood. But, as is true when bacteria invade the body, these antibodies against the Rh factor do not form instantaneously but only after a period of time. Consequently, with the first transfusion, nothing out of the ordinary occurs. However, should this Rh-negative recipient receive at some later date another transfusion from an Rh-positive donor, antibodies probably will have been developed and these will immediately attack the Rh factor. Since the Rh substance is an integral part of the red blood cells, this conflict causes a violent reaction in the blood stream with the destruction of many red cells. As the broken-down products of these fragmented red cells are disseminated throughout the body, they exert a poisonous effect, and, as a result, the recipient of the blood transfusion suffers a reaction usually manifested by a chill

and fever but sometimes by more grave symptoms. In World War II, when many Rh-negative soldiers had to be given repeated blood transfusions, this Rh problem was a serious one. It was met by using Rh-negative donors for transfusions of Rh-negative persons—in other words, by administering blood without any Rh factor in it to cause the trouble described above. Nowadays physicians and surgeons everywhere are careful to determine the Rh status of any prospective recipient of a blood transfusion; if it is negative, blood from an Rh-negative donor is employed.

The greatest danger lies in giving Rh-positive blood (male or female) to an Rh-negative woman. This Rh blood difference has caused more cases of erythroblastosis fetalis than the mating of an Rh-positive father and an Rh-negative mother. Although the results from transfusions with incompatible Rh blood may not be manifested at the time, it may show up years later during childbirth in erythroblastotic infants.

Rh Differences in Mates. Since at least six sevenths of all persons, male or female, are Rh positive, Rh incompatibility is not as frequent as one might at first suppose. Even when an Rh-positive male parent mates with an Rh-negative female, there may be no erythroblastosis in the offspring, for the father may be *heterozygous* for Rh (has both Rh-positive and Rh-negative genes), and no difficulty occurs if the fetus has Rh-negative inheritance from both parents. The danger is much greater when the father is *homozygous* (has all Rh-positive genes), for the fetus will inherit the Rh-positive factor against which the mother produces antibodies which (as in the transfusion of incompatible Rh-positive blood to Rh-negative mothers) may lead to the destruction of the Rh-positive blood cells of the fetus. The danger to the fetus is increased with the ability of the mother's antibodies to pass through the placenta (Fig. 249).

In Rh differences in mates, as well as

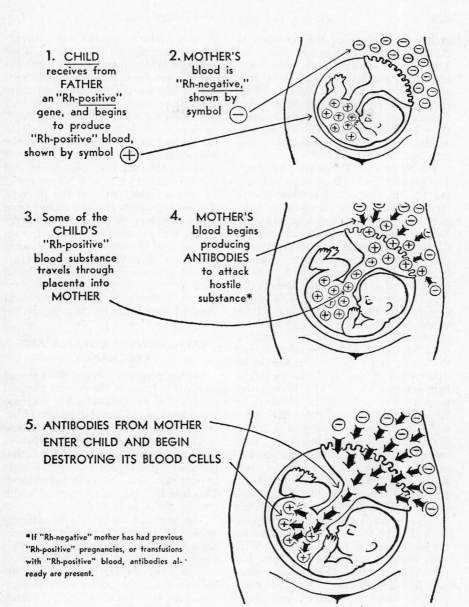

1. CHILD receives from FATHER an "Rh-positive" gene, and begins to produce "Rh-positive" blood, shown by symbol ⊕

2. MOTHER'S blood is "Rh-negative," shown by symbol ⊖

3. Some of the CHILD'S "Rh-positive" blood substance travels through placenta into MOTHER

4. MOTHER'S blood begins producing ANTIBODIES to attack hostile substance*

5. ANTIBODIES FROM MOTHER ENTER CHILD AND BEGIN DESTROYING ITS BLOOD CELLS

*If "Rh-negative" mother has had previous "Rh-positive" pregnancies, or transfusions with "Rh-positive" blood, antibodies already are present.

Fig. 249. Effect of the Rh factor. (Scheinfeld, Amran: The New You and Heredity, Philadelphia, Lippincott)

in blood transfusions, the reactions of the Rh-negative mother are slow, and 1 or even 2 normal births may occur before the mother has an infant with erythroblastosis. Once it occurs, all later pregnancies are risky, and future pregnancies may be contraindicated because there is a substantial chance for the condition to recur in subsequent pregnancies.

Rh-Negative Pregnant Women. The present fund of knowledge concerning the Rh factor and erythroblastosis fetalis makes certain routines in antepartal management and care essential. Every pregnant woman should have her Rh type determined early in pregnancy. If the mother is Rh negative, it should be ascertained if she has had previous blood transfusions, and the father's Rh type should be determined. If he also is found to be Rh negative, there will be no danger of hemolytic disease affecting this fetus, or subsequent ones, because the offspring will be Rh negative. In case the father is Rh positive, it should be determined if he is homozygous or heterozygous for Rh. The Rh-negative mother's blood should be checked by laboratory tests several times during the first two trimesters of pregnancy to see if her antibody titer is increasing, indicating harmful reactions against Rh-positive factors. Only after the 34th week of gestation is it necessary to do this every two weeks. At the present time, the Coombs test is the one most frequently employed because it is considered to be the most sensitive test for the detection of Rh antibodies. With such checks, mating between an Rh-positive man and an Rh-negative woman may be perfectly safe, unless earlier Rh-positive blood transfusions complicate the situation. Even then, some degree of control is possible.

The nurse should bear in mind that when an Rh-negative woman's husband is Rh positive, this mother is often apprehensive about the outcome of her pregnancy. These patients must not be given any false hopes, but it is relatively safe to assume that when there is no serologic evidence to indicate sensitization, the prospects for normal childbearing for her are no different from those of an Rh-positive mother. However, this is not the case if the mother is sensitized, for then the outlook depends entirely on the severity of the manifestation in the individual.

As already indicated, certain cases of erythroblastosis fetalis may be prevented by proper investigation of the Rh type of women patients and any donors from whom they receive blood. During pregnancy, if the mother's antibody titer increases markedly, there is an additional problem in that the infant may be delivered prematurely by either induced labor or cesarean section. In such instances, a supply of Rh-negative blood should be available for treating the infant, if born alive.

COINCIDENTAL DISEASES AND PREGNANCY

During pregnancy every effort should be made to improve the general physical condition of the mother and to decrease any attendant strain and depletion of her energy due to illness. When chronic conditions, such as cardiac disturbances or kidney disease, are present, the pathologic condition should be checked early in pregnancy and preferably beforehand. This is really a part of the general health control of the individual.

The pregnant woman is quite naturally subject to diseases, both medical conditions and those requiring surgical intervention, which affect the nonpregnant woman. Any disease which affects the individual's health adds inevitable complications in pregnancy. The pregnancy may be jeopardized by the disease; or the disease process may be aggravated by the pregnancy, and at this time a latent condition may even become active.

One cannot group the adverse effects of coincidental complications of pregnancy wholly into these two specific categories, for one or the other, or both, may occur. A number of diseases in which either one of these effects, or both, may be seen includes rheumatic heart disease, diabetes mellitus, chronic hypertensive vascular disease, pyelonephritis, pneumonia and untreated syphilis. In addition to these mentioned, other general physiologic disturbances and infectious diseases and their relations to pregnancy are discussed briefly on the following pages.

General Physiologic Disturbances

Anemia. During pregnancy the blood volume is increased (p. 123). Because of this hydremia, hemoglobin estimations in gestation are likely to be lower than ordinarily considered normal. This is not a true anemia, since the total amount of hemoglobin in the body remains the same, and sometimes the condition is referred to as the "pseudo-anemia of pregnancy." Hemoglobin standards which have been established for nonpregnant women, i.e., 12 to 15 Gm. per 100 cc. of blood, are applicable for normal pregnant women also. The diagnosis of true anemia is made when the hemoglobin falls below 12 Gm., or the hematocrit below 35 per cent.

The hemoglobin levels of pregnant women fall as the result of a number of factors. Most of these cases represent a true anemia due to iron deficiency. The need of the fetus and the growing uterus for iron, inadequate iron intake in the diet and a low hemoglobin level at the start of pregnancy combine to bring about this anemic state. It is encountered more commonly in Negro women than in white women.

The symptoms are few, but some of these patients complain of becoming tired easily; many are pale; and in a few the pulse rate is fast. Because of the rather frequent occurrence of anemia in pregnancy, hemoglobin determinations are a routine part of antepartal care. The treatment consists of an iron-rich diet (emphasis on liver, meat, eggs, spinach, etc.) supplemented by the administration of some iron compound such as ferrous sulfate. In patients with anemia who do not tolerate orally ingested iron well, as shown by gastrointestinal disturbances, or in whom rapid effects are desired, injections of intramuscular iron in the form of Imferon are most helpful.

Cardiac Complications. Rheumatic heart disease is a serious complication of pregnancy. Heart lesions, especially those of the mitral valve, may be greatly aggravated by pregnancy. Constant medical supervision of the pregnant woman with any degree of cardiac involvement, however mild, is imperative, for, fortunately, much can now be done to aid cardiac patients. If the patient has placed herself under medical care at the beginning of gestation, and if the physician has made a proper and thorough examination of all her organs at that time, he will be in a position to administer promptly such treatment as may be necessary. In this day of heart specialists, the specialist and the obstetrician must work hand in hand; and each, in his own province, is of the greatest help to the other. It is also absolutely essential to have close co-operation between the patient and the physician. In this situation the nurse may play an important part—by helping the patient to understand and to observe with care the primary principles of antepartal care.

The treatment of heart disease in pregnancy is governed to a large measure by the functional capacity of the heart. Rest probably will accomplish more than any other single measure, and the amount of rest needed will naturally vary with each individual, some patients having to be kept at rest a great part of the time. Strenuous activity and undue excitement must be avoided during pregnancy. The great majority, however, may safely indulge in moderate activity, and all should be in the fresh air as much as possible. Upper respiratory infections play great havoc in patients with heart disease and they may even precipitate heart failure; accordingly, the nurse should advise all such patients to take special precautions against catching cold—that is, they should avoid large gatherings and people known to have sore throats, colds, etc. All of these safeguards will be advised by the physician, but the nurse may aid greatly in helping the patient to carry out his instructions.

Although heart failure usually occurs suddenly, the onset may be gradual. The nurse should be alert to particular signs and symptoms which may be warning signals and report her observations to the physician promptly. Such symptoms include sudden limitation in the patient's ability to carry on her usual household activities, increased dyspnea on exertion, tachycardia, coughing or attacks of smothering with the cough. It is well to remember that serious cardiac lesions complicating pregnancy may predispose to premature labor or may be responsible for premature death. In the past many cardiac patients have had their pregnancies terminated by therapeutic abortion, but today many a mild heart case is carried to a happy completion by providing thorough medical supervision and nursing care during pregnancy and labor. However, these successes should not lead us to forget that, if not adequately cared for, even mild cardiac disorders as well as the severe types result in definite invalidism or even death.

Diabetes. The diabetic woman who becomes pregnant requires meticulous supervision, and the nurse can be of much help in such cases by stressing the extreme importance of rigid adherence to the prescribed diet and regular visits to the physician. The younger the patient when diabetes manifests itself, the more severe the disease is likely to be. A patient who co-operates and in whom the diabetes has been and is easily controlled is more likely to have a suc-cessful pregnancy than one who is difficult to control. During pregnancy the patient should be observed carefully, with special reference to control of diet to maintain good nutritional status and prevent undue weight gain. She should have salt restricted from the beginning. Careful checking of the diabetes is essential at frequent intervals. The patient should be under the care of an internist who is thoroughly competent in the management of diabetes, as well as under the care of a qualified obstetrician. Diabetic patients are more apt to have complications. They are inclined to produce large babies and to suffer from toxemias of pregnancy. The last trimester is the most trying time, and during this stage the patient should be watched for early signs of toxemia. Patients with this disease should be acquainted with the fact that they may have diabetic children.

Urinary Tract Infection. Inflammation of the ureter and the pelvis of the kidney is not uncommon during pregnancy. It seldom occurs earlier than the fourth month, and occasionally an acute attack of great severity occurs in the puerperium, in which case care will be required to distinguish it from puerperal infection. It is due to several causes, each of which may aggravate the condition: improper intestinal elimination, an increase of colon bacilli, pressure from the gravid uterus upon the ureter at the pelvic brim, leading to retention of urine above the line of pressure, and certain displacements of the bladder due to pregnancy itself. The symptoms may be gradual and slight, or quite acute in their onset, with chills and high temperature, 103° or 104° F. (39.4° or 40° C.). The patient often complains of frequency of urination, pain in the kidney region and malaise. In the acute form the patient is seized suddenly with acute abdominal pain, sometimes attended with chills or shivering; after a few hours the abdomen may become distended, and vomiting may occur. The pain, diffused at first, usually localizes in the right side. It is necessary for the nurse to secure definite instructions from the physician concerning the treatment; but rest, forced fluids and a bland, non-irritating diet (chiefly milk) may be advised in the interim. Heat over the kidneys will relieve pain.

DRUGS. The main aim of treatment in urinary tract infection is to rid the urine and the urinary tract of bacteria. During recent years the treatment of infections of the urinary tract has been revolutionized by the introduction of the sulfonamide group of drugs. The fluid intake is maintained between 2,500 and 3,000 cc. daily. The physician will follow the results of treatment not only by means of the temperature chart but also by thorough and repeated examinations of the urine. These examinations will entail both a microscopic study of the number of pus cells present and a survey of the bacteria yielded on culture. Accordingly, the nurse will be asked to secure frequent catheterized urine specimens. Follow-up of these cases is highly important and must be carried out not only during the remainder of pregnancy but also for several months after delivery, until it is certain that the urine is sterile and x-ray studies of the kidney reveal a normal state.

Ptyalism. While this is one of the rarer complications of pregnancy, it is one which is most annoying to the patient and very stubborn in resisting treatment. It is due entirely to altered innervation, or changes in nerve control, and is characterized by an enormously increased secretion of the salivary glands. Women at times have been known to discharge as much as 2 quarts of saliva daily from this cause. This complication, if it occurs at all, usually appears in the early months of pregnancy and lasts a considerable time, but, fortunately, it is inclined to cease spontaneously. It is seen in highly nervous women of low vitality and is likely to cause great mental depression and interfere with nutrition.

The treatment consists in building up the general health and the administration of such medication as may be prescribed by the physician. The use of astringent mouthwashes often contributes to the patient's comfort. Any treatment may seem to be inadequate, and the condition is most disagreeable.

Infectious Diseases

Certain infectious diseases have no proved specific ill effect on the mother or the baby, but, if possible, any communicable disease should be avoided during pregnancy, for even mild diseases add strain at this particular time.

With infectious diseases two types of effects may occur: (1) on the mother and (2) on the fetus. The diseases which often have serious effects on the infant are discussed in Chapter 21. Among those directly affecting the mother are the following.

The Common Cold. The susceptibility to acute upper respiratory infections is apparently greater during pregnancy. Therefore, the pregnant woman should make every effort to avoid contacts with these infections. When she does acquire a cold, prompt medical attention is usually desirable, because the common cold often precedes more serious conditions affecting the upper respiratory tract. Prescribed medication should be used in preference to the various antihistamine drugs obtainable without a prescription. Rest in bed helps the individual and aids in checking the spread of the disease.

Pneumonia. Pneumonia, which often follows the common cold, may frequently lead to complications of pregnancy. The pneumonia organisms, especially streptococci, may also infect the uterus, causing puerperal infections. Prompt use of penicillin and other antibiotics is most helpful. Since antibiotics have been employed, the occurrence of abortion and premature labor is less common.

Influenza. Serious complications may

follow influenza, especially in the pneumonic type in which pregnancy is sometimes interrupted. Sulfa drugs and such antibiotics as penicillin are usually given to help forestall pneumonia, but they do not control the influenza virus.

Measles. Ill effects are not commonly noted in pregnancy, but pregnant mothers who contract measles are said to be more likely to have premature labors. No other definite effects are reported, although eruptions have been noted on infants at birth.

German Measles. Rubella, or German measles, is caused by a virus—distinct from the virus of measles (rubeola). German measles produces most serious effects on the mother's unborn infant if it occurs in the first trimester of pregnancy. These infants are often afflicted with congenital malformations such as cataracts, deafness, heart lesions and mental defects (see Chap. 21). There are no antiserums against German measles, although globulin is considered by some to be a wise precaution for pregnant mothers.

Typhoid Fever. Typhoid fever, which is now relatively rare in this country, may cause serious complications in pregnancy, resulting in abortion, prematurity and infant mortality. Immunization is not contraindicated during pregnancy, and antityphoid vaccine should be administered when necessary.

Brucellosis (Undulant Fever, Malta Fever). These debilitating diseases in humans are contracted mainly from unpasteurized milk. In this country today, conditions for the production and the processing of milk are set by U.S. Public Health Service standards. When these diseases are seen, the bacteria have been found in the human placenta, but abortion in humans is very infrequently traced to this organism, although brucella bacteria do cause abortion in cattle. Good results have been attained with Aureomycin and also with combined streptomycin-sulfadiazine.

Scarlet Fever. There seems to be greater susceptibility to scarlet fever during the puerperium. The cause is a streptococcus, so the risk of developing puerperal fever is clear. Antibiotics are effective in treating the disease, but sometimes abortion is caused by scarlet fever contracted during early pregnancy, due to the mother's high fever.

Erysipelas. This disease, usually caused by streptococci, may be very serious at any time, but in pregnant women there is the danger of developing puerperal fever. Care must be taken to avoid transferring streptococci from any local lesion to the genital area. Strict isolation is essential. Appropriate drugs (penicillin, sulfa drugs, etc.) should be used if necessary. The streptococci may pass through the placenta and cause the death of the fetus.

Smallpox. Cases of abortion and prematurity increase with the severity of the attack, especially with the hemorrhagic type. As in measles, smallpox may be transmitted through the placenta, for eruptions may be present in live births.

Malaria. In more severe cases of malaria the incidence of abortion and premature labor is increased. Prompt therapy is of utmost importance. Malaria organisms have been found in the blood of the cord and the fetus; they are frequently found in the placenta, although no ill effects have been noted on the infants. Quinine or the newer related drugs, such as Atabrine, should be administered to women with malaria history to prevent recrudescence during pregnancy and the puerperium. The decrease in malaria reported (1951) by the Communicable Disease Center of the U. S. Public Health Service makes malaria much less important as a complication of pregnancy.

Tuberculosis. The average case of tuberculosis in itself has only a slight effect on the course of pregnancy, since it rarely predisposes to abortion, premature labor or even stillbirth. (Fortunately, the disease is seldom acquired congenitally, although a small number of authentic cases have been reported in which, in addition to a tuberculous condition of the placenta, tubercle bacilli were found in the cord blood, together with tuberculous lesions in the baby.) Medical opinions differ, but the consensus is that pregnancy does not exert an adverse effect on tuberculosis. Some authorities think that this disease becomes aggravated by pregnancy and that only an arrested case should consider becoming pregnant. Pregnancy is undertaken with some risk, for while a tuberculous lesion may remain latent for an indefinite time, provided that the natural resistance is not overtaxed, it must be noted that pregnancy is one of the factors often responsible for overtaxing the resistance sufficiently to convert a latent, inactive lesion into an active one. Proper hygiene, nutrition and excellent surroundings so as to conserve health in every possible way will do much to prevent activity in a latent focus. Other authorities deny that the tuberculosis is necessarily aggravated by pregnancy, basing this belief on statistics of large series of tuberculous patients who have progressed satisfactorily in pregnancy.

The symptoms of tuberculosis in pregnancy do not differ materially from those that accompany the disease in other conditions. During the early months of gestation, the characteristic anemia and general malnutrition of tuberculosis are usually pronounced, but in the latter months there is often considerable improvement. Too often, however, this is followed by a rapid decline after delivery.

Treatment will depend on the type of involvement as well as on the particular stage of pregnancy. Prophylactic treatment is most important, since it offers most chance of success. The patient must be given every medical and hygienic advantage, wholesome food (milk is of very great value), fresh air and sunshine and absolute rest. Any cough or rapid loss of weight should be reported. It is rarely indicated for the physician to interrupt the pregnancy. When a tuberculous patient reaches term, the labor is made as easy as possible to conserve her strength. Under no circumstances should a tuberculous woman be allowed to nurse her baby, for the baby's sake as well as for her own. Months of careful follow-up treatment will be necessary. The patient should not consider becoming pregnant again until a sufficient time has elapsed to establish a reasonable certainty that her disease has been arrested.

It is in the group in which tuberculosis is unsuspected that tragedies occur, many of which could be avoided. Therefore, a complete medical history always should be taken. Exposure to tuberculosis in the family, a history of hemoptysis, pleurisy, or fistula in ano, and a cough or loss of weight over a period of time suggest strongly the presence of possible tuberculosis. These danger signals are of the utmost value, and if heeded will often enable the physician to recognize tuberculosis symptoms developing during pregnancy which he might otherwise attribute to the pregnancy itself.

Examinations of the chest (roentgenographic) and the sputum (microscopic) should be done routinely in suspected cases. The newer antibiotics (streptomycin, hydrostreptomycin, neomycin) should be available if need is indicated. There may be undue alarm due to confusion of tuberculosis with the milder disease, histoplasmosis, unless expert testing (skin and sputum) facilities are available.

Poliomyelitis. Poliomyelitis generally does not complicate pregnancy or delivery, except in the very unusual cases where respiratory paralysis develops; in these rare cases cesarean section has given satisfactory results. Fortunately, the fetus rarely contracts the disease. Of about 80 cases reported during pregnancy, less than one fifth occurred in the first trimester. A milder form of infection of poliomyelitis is attributed to a different virus, the Coxsackie virus, which has less paralysis but is often unrecognized.

Gonorrhea. This disease should be studied by the nurse with the other infectious diseases; but, because of the consequences of gonorrheal infection to the mother at the time of labor and during the puerperium, as well as the risk of permanent injury to the baby's eyes at the time of birth, this disease is of special concern to the obstetric nurse.

The disease is due to a micro-organism, known commonly as the gonococcus organism (*Micrococcus gonorrhoeae* or *Neisseria gonorrhoeae*). It may affect any mucous membrane, e.g., that of the eye, but usually attacks the mucosa of the genital tract, particularly the opening of the bladder and the crypts around the cervix, causing a catarrhal discharge of pus. It is called a venereal disease simply because the usual mode of transfer of this infection is by sexual intercourse. The infection often extends into the uterus and the tubes, causing a very serious localized peritonitis, and may cause sterility by a mechanical blocking of the tubes. Gonorrhea is not commonly considered to be a fatal disease, in the sense that a high proportion of the cases terminate in death, but in the list of diseases causing chronic ill health, especially in the female sex, gonorrhea is most important.

Gonorrhea does not greatly modify the course of pregnancy, and its existence is often unsuspected by the patient. The vaginal discharge may increase, as it normally does during pregnancy, and, with the local congestion of the venous system, the patient may have some irritation in the vulvar region. Pregnancy may act as a barrier to the ascent of the gonococcus, and thus the fetus may be protected during development. The patient may abort, but more commonly she carries the baby to full term and delivers normally. However, after delivery, conditions are quite different. Even when a patient has had a normal labor, the cervix is dilated, and the minute tears

and abrasions offer many avenues for the spread of the infection, and the lochial discharge makes an ideal culture medium for the bacteria. This condition may lead to the development of a form of puerperal fever.

It is now routine practice to obtain a specimen of vaginal secretions for culture on the first antepartal visit. In the female, the diagnosis of gonorrhea is confirmed by culturing the organisms from fresh vaginal secretions.* If the culture is positive, penicillin is given promptly, for it yields dramatic results in treatment of this disease. Cure may be effected by a single intramuscular injection of suitable dosage of penicillin in at least 90 per cent of the cases. In chronic cases 1 or 2 repeated doses may be necessary.

Gonorrhea is not hereditary, but, if a woman is infected at the time of her confinement, the organism may get into the baby's eyes and cause blindness. This infection of the eyes is called ophthalmia neonatorum. The prophylactic treatment of the baby's eyes at this time never should be neglected (see Chap. 12).

Syphilis. Formerly, syphilis was one of the most important complications of pregnancy and prior to the advent of efficient antepartal supervision was responsible for a high percentage of fetal deaths. Today serologic tests for syphilis are a routine part of antepartal care. The study of infant mortality rates shows that as a result of syphilis infants may be stillborn, die in the early months of life or, if they live, are infected. Like gonorrhea, this venereal disease is best studied with the other infectious diseases, but because of its definite relation to the life and the health of mothers and babies, a few facts are mentioned here.

DEFINITION. Syphilis may be defined as an infectious systemic disease which runs a prolonged course and, during this course, may, at one time or another, attack nearly every part of the body. Many

* U.S. Public Health Service Publication No. 573, 1958.

women do not know that they or their children are infected; therefore, they seek no advice. In many patients, even with no history of infection or any manifestations of the disease, the first intimation of the existence of syphilis is a positive Wassermann (or other blood test) reaction or the birth of a premature or macerated fetus. Although macerated fetuses may be produced in consequence of other diseases and accidents during pregnancy, the suspicion of syphilis may arise in instances when the mother's S.T.S. is not known. Unlike the effects of gonorrhea, syphilis does not cause sterility.

SYPHILIS AND PREGNANCY*

Causal Organism. Syphilis is a specific infectious disease caused by a spirochete, *Spirochaeta pallida* or *Treponema pallidum,* discovered by Schaudinn and Hoffmann in 1905.

Types of Syphilis. Syphilis in any individual may be acquired or congenital. The acquired form is usually transmitted by sexual intercourse; however, other forms of personal contact may transmit the infection, such as kissing, an examination of the patient by a contaminated physician and the nursing of the newborn by an infected person.

Congenital syphilis is a term applied to syphilis transmitted to the child before birth. An infected mother may transmit syphilis to the fetus through the placenta. Such transfer may occur from mothers whether they were syphilitic at the time of conception or whether they acquired syphilis during early pregnancy.

In this discussion of syphilis and pregnancy, we may focus our attention on three points: (1) the detection of syphilis in the pregnant mother; (2) the treatment of such infected mothers; and (3) the prompt detection of syphilis in the baby after birth.

Diagnosis of Syphilis in Pregnant Mothers: Clinical Symptoms. In syphilis there is usually a primary lesion or hard

* By William T. Daily, M.D., Department of Obstetrics and Gynecology, The Long Island College Hospital, Brooklyn, N. Y.

chancre located where there was a defect in the surface epithelium, allowing the entrance of the spirochete. In women, the initial lesion of syphilis is less easily observed than in men, and, unless seen on the vulva, is usually unnoticed. In a large proportion of recently infected women, no evidence of a scar of a chancre of the genitals may be seen. The secondary manifestations, likewise, are often unnoticed. The skin eruptions are mild and disappear rather rapidly. On the other hand, the presence of condylomata lata may cause the patient to consult her physician.

Previous Pregnancy History. The history of previous pregnancies is most significant in indicating syphilis in the mother. In a series of pregnant syphilitic women studied, a large proportion of pregnancies failed to go to term, ending in a miscarriage, in a premature, a full-term stillbirth, or in the birth of a syphilitic infant. Abortion in the first trimester of pregnancy is noted but slightly more frequently than in ordinary pregnancy; on the other hand, interruption of pregnancy during the fifth, sixth or seventh month is common.

Blood Tests. Blood tests constitute a third method of detecting syphilis. The importance of blood tests is evident when we realize that syphilis complicating pregnancy in a primigravida is seldom recognized until the damage is done, unless the practice of making routine serologic tests is followed. The advantage of this third method of detecting syphilis is shown by the fact that out of 144 pregnant women thus shown to have syphilis, only 6 gave evidence of a primary lesion, and the history and physical examination were suggestive of syphilis in but 34 patients in the series. Without the blood tests, over 100 of these mothers would have failed to receive the necessary treatment.

The tests devised by Wassermann, Kahn, Kline, Mazzini and the U. S. Public Health Service test V.D.R.L. are the ones now most frequently used in this country. If the blood test is found to be positive or questionable, the test is repeated to make sure that any possible laboratory error is eliminated. Should a test be strongly positive, treatment is inaugurated, even though there were no other indications of syphilis (lesions, pregnancy history). Treatment is also given to all patients with a definite pregnancy history indicating syphilis, even though the blood test may be but mildly positive or negative.

Several types of tests are used to determine the condition of the infant.

1. The cord blood test should be made on every suspicious or treated case. However, this test is not wholly reliable; but a positive cord blood test indicates the need for close follow-up and frequent examinations.

2. The placenta may furnish suspicion, if not evidence, of pathologic changes. The normal placenta at full term weighs about 500 Gm. Normally, the relative weight of the baby to placenta is about 6:1. The placenta of syphilitic infection is larger, heavier and paler than normal. Since a premature placenta is relatively heavier than a placenta at term, and because many syphilitic babies are born prematurely, this may account for the too common opinion regarding the great size and weight of a syphilitic placenta. Histologically, the chorionic villi are greatly enlarged; they show diminished branching and they are more club-shaped. On cross section, the vessels are seen to be diminished in number and stenosed or obliterated by endoarteritic changes. The stroma is more granular, and the stroma cells lose their normal stellate appearance. The villi, due to their greater size or thickness, approach each other, reducing the intervillous spaces. Syphilis of the placenta is not a common lesion, and many hesitate to make a positive diagnosis unless the spirochete is seen in microscopic darkfield examination.

3. The umbilical cord vein, in an area near the placenta, may be scraped and studied for spirochetes under a darkfield examination.

4. An x-ray examination of the long bones, especially the lower and upper ends of the femur, upper fibula and tibia, and the upper humerus and lower radius, is most valuable in determining the syphilitic condition of the infant. The usual lesion is an epiphysitis.

5. Blood tests may also be used. The newborn baby of a treated mother should be referred to a pediatrician familiar with the treatment of syphilis in the newborn about the sixth week after birth, for repeated serologic and x-ray examinations.

Conclusion. Syphilis of the newborn is preventable, and, if a child is delivered with the infection or succumbs to its virulence, either before delivery or neonatally, two and only two persons are largely responsible: first, the mother for her failure to be examined early in her pregnancy, and, secondly, the physician (or clinic) whom she consults, if he neglects to take routine serologic tests and which, if positive, he fails to treat intensively.

TREATMENT OF SYPHILITIC MOTHERS. The present-day treatment of syphilis in pregnancy consists in the intensive administration of penicillin as soon as the disease is recognized. The earlier in pregnancy therapy is started, the better are the results. The course of treatment consists of the administration of approximately 6 million units of penicillin, given over a period of 10 days. It is well established that this dosage is several times that necessary to protect the baby from syphilis, and it is believed to be enough to cure the mother also; but it is quite possible that further experience will result in a still higher dosage in order to make certain of permanent maternal cure. The intensive treatment schedule has posed a difficult problem for these patients, but it has been met in many cities by special treatment centers.

Penicillin, with rare exceptions, has been free from serious toxic effects. The frequent injection schedules formerly used have now been replaced by schedules permitting 1, 2 or 3 injections a week for from 1 to 2 weeks. This relatively short treatment period with its freedom from severe toxic reactions has a great advantage over the previously accepted 1 to 2 years of arsenical and bismuth therapy. However, for patients who do not tolerate penicillin, massive arsenotherapy is the treatment of choice. Penicillin also possesses the ability of being filtered through the placenta and consequently can act as a very potent agent in the treatment of congenital syphilis in utero. Unfortunately, failures do occur as the result of relapse or reinfection, and this accounts for most of the rare instances of congenital syphilis resulting from treated mothers.

INCOMPETENT CERVICAL OS

Recently, a mechanical defect in the cervix, incompetent cervical os, has gained recognition as a cause of late habitual abortion or premature labor. When repeated termination of pregnancy in the second trimester is due to an anatomic factor such as this, surgical treatment may make fetal salvage possible. One of the various treatments used to prevent relaxation and dilatation of the cervix when it is incompetent to carry on a "good" pregnancy is the modified Shirodkar technic.* In this, the vaginal mucous membrane is elevated and a narrow strip of some material such as Mersilene is carried around the internal os of the cervix and tied. Then the vaginal mucosa is restored to its original position and sutured.

The patient is kept in bed for the first several days postoperatively, often in Trendelenburg position initially, to prevent undue pressure on the cervix. The patient should be watched closely for signs of bleeding or labor. Demerol and Phenergan may be prescribed routinely for the first day, not necessarily for pain, but to keep the uterus quiet. Actually, these patients experience relatively little discomfort and usually feel quite well in a day or so. At the time of discharge, about the 5th postoperative day, the physician generally advises certain restrictions about coitus and the patient's daily activities. He frequently recommends at least one rest period in the horizontal position during the day. By and large, the expectant mother may resume a "normal" life during the rest of her pregnancy.

* Durfee, R. B.: Surgical treatment of the incompetent cervix during pregnancy, Obst. & Gynec. 12:91, 1958.

The nonabsorbable band is left in place until the patient is ready for labor. Then she may be delivered either by elective cesarean section or vaginal delivery. If the latter is the choice, the band must be cut and removed. Definitive cervical repair is done at a later date.

SUGGESTED READING

Abramson, Julius, and Tenny, Benjamin: Cardiac disease in pregnancy, New England J. Med. 253:279, 1955.

Alter, N. M., and Cosgrove, S. A.: Hydatidiform mole: practical considerations, Obst. & Gynec. 5:755, 1955.

Bartholomew, R. A., et al.: The mechanisms of bleeding during pregnancy, Am. J. Obst. & Gynec. 66:1042, 1953.

Black, Marion E., and Miller, Max: Management of diabetes and pregnancy, Clin. Obst. & Gynec. 1:229, 1958.

Bookmiller, Mae, and Bowen, George: Textbook of Obstetrics and Obstetric Nursing, ed. 3, Philadelphia, Saunders, 1958.

Bunim, Joseph J., and Appel, S. Baer: Pregnancy and rheumatic heart disease, J.A.M.A. 142:90, 1950.

Burt, K. L., Donnelly, J. F., and Fleming, S. P.: Acute toxemia of pregnancy associated with organic heart disease, Am. J. Obst. & Gynec. 68:528, 1954.

Bysshe, Stanley M.: Premature separation of the normally implanted placenta, Am. J. Obst. & Gynec. 62:38, 1951.

Cherny, W. B., Carter, F. B., Thomas, W. L., and Peete, C. H., Jr.: Hypotensive drugs in pregnancy toxemia, Obst. & Gynec. 9:505, 1957.

Cosgrove, S. A.: Therapeutic abortion, J. Michigan M. Soc. 55:795, 1956.

Curtis, Arthur C., et al.: Penicillin treatment of syphilis, J.A.M.A. 145:1223, 1951.

de Alvarez, Russell: Toxemias of pregnancy, Am. J. Nursing 54:1486, 1954.

Eastman, Nicholson J.: Williams Obstetrics, ed. 11, New York, Appleton, 1956.

Fox, Max J., and Belfus, Frank H.: Poliomyelitis in pregnancy, Am. J. Obst. & Gynec. 59:1134, 1950.

Giblin, Elizabeth, and Osmond, Thelma: Nursing care in toxemias of pregnancy, Am. J. Nursing 54:1488, 1954.

Groasmun, Ruth: Nursing care of the pregnant diabetic, Am. J. Nursing 58:102, 1958.

Horowitz, W.: Management of the pregnant patient with cardiac disease, New England J. Med. 252:511, 1955.

Lund, Curtis J.: Studies on the iron deficiency anemia of pregnancy, Am. J. Obst. & Gynec. 62:947, 1951.

McElin, Thomas W., Faber, John E., Randall, Lawrence M.: True toxemia of pregnancy occurring before the third trimester, Am. J. Obst. & Gynec. 61:379, 1951.

Oxorn, Harry: Rubella and pregnancy, Am. J. Obst. & Gynec. 77:628, 1959.

Pearse, Harry A., and Ott, Harold A.: Hospital control of sterilization and therapeutic abortion, Am. J. Obst. & Gynec. 60:285, 1950.

Pearse, Warren H.: ABO blood groups in obstetrics, Am. J. Obst. & Gynec. 74:538, 1957.

Pritchard, Jack A.: Anemia in obstetrics and gynecology: an evaluation of therapy with parenteral iron, Am. J. Obst. & Gynec. 77:74, 1959.

Rauh, Louise W.: Rubella and pregnancy, Ohio M. J. 51:875, 1955.

Reid, Duncan E., et al.: Maternal afibrinogenemia associated with long-standing intrauterine fetal death, Am. J. Obst. & Gynec. 66:500, 1953.

Rolf, Bruce B.: The obstetrician's responsibility to the Rh-negative patient, Am. J. Obst. & Gynec. 61:139, 1951.

Rosenbach, L. M., and Gangemi, C. R.: Tuberculosis and pregnancy, J.A.M.A. 161:1035, 1956.

Rouse, George P.: Pregnancy and diabetes, Am. J. Nursing 58:100, 1958.

Russell, K. P., et al.: Acute renal failure as obstetric complication, J.A.M.A. 157:15, 1955.

Schaefer, George: Clinical management of the pregnant woman with tuberculosis, New York J. Med. 55:1189, 1955.

Semmens, James P.: Placenta previa: the role of conservative management in a controlled study, Am. J. Obst. & Gynec. 77:63, 1959.

Smith, Kaighn: Cesarean section in the treatment of placenta previa, Am. J. Obst. & Gynec. 77:55, 1959.

Tietze, Christopher, Guttmacher, Alan F., and Rubin, Samuel: Unintentional abortion, J.A.M.A. 142:1348, 1950.

Tolstoi, E., et al.: Management of the pregnant diabetic, J.A.M.A. 153:998, 1953.

U. S. Public Health Service, Washington, D. C.: An Outline of Venereal Disease Management (Pub. No. 573), 1958.

——: Prenatal Health Examination Legislation: Analysis and Compilation of State Laws (Pub. No. 369), 1954.

Van Blarcom, Carolyn C.: Obstetrical Nursing (rev. by E. Ziegel), ed. 4, New York, Macmillan, 1957.

Weil, R. J., and Stewart, L. C.: The problem of spontaneous abortion: psychosomatic and interpersonal aspects of habitual abortion, Am. J. Obst. & Gynec. 73:322, 1957.

Wesselfoeft, Conrad: Acute infectious diseases in pregnancy, Ann. Int. Med. 42:555, 1955.

World Health Organization, Geneva: Venereal Diseases: A Survey of Existing Legislation, 1956.

Zuspan, F. P., et al.: Abdominal pregnancy, Am. J. Obst. & Gynec. 74:259, 1957.

LEGAL AND ETHICAL CONSIDERATIONS

Ethical and Religious Directives for Catholic Hospitals, ed. 2, St. Louis, Catholic Hospital Association, 1959.

Holman, Edwin: Medicolegal aspects of sterilization, artificial insemination and abortion, J.A.M.A. 156:1309, 1954.

Kelly, Gerald: Medico-Moral Problems, St. Louis, Catholic Hospital Association, 1958.

McFadden, Charles J., Medical Ethics, ed. 4, Philadelphia, Davis, 1956.

Rosen, H.: Therapeutic Abortion: Medical, Psychiatric, Legal, Anthropological, and Religious Considerations, New York, Julian Press, 1954.

Stevens, Dom Gregory: Principles of Ethics, ed. 5, Philadelphia, Lippincott, 1959.

CHAPTER NINETEEN

Complications of Labor

MECHANICAL DYSTOCIA

Occasionally the nurse will see cases in which hours and hours of labor pass without progress and in which even a day or two may transpire without the birth of the infant. In such instances, obviously there is something wrong with the mechanics or "machinery" of labor. In other words, these are cases of dystocia (difficult labor) in which the mechanics of the process are at fault—cases of mechanical dystocia. But what precisely *is* wrong?

Reduced to its simplest constituents, the process of labor resolves itself into the propulsion by certain *forces* of an irregular object (the infant or *passenger*) through the birth canal (the *passage*). There are only three factors involved in labor therefore—the forces, the passenger and the passage. When, despite many hours of labor, the infant fails to come, one of these three factors or some combination of them must be at fault.

Let us make this clear by a homely example. If a person were trying to force his foot into a boot and was unable to do so, what could be the causes of his failure? First, he might not be pushing hard enough. (Forces at fault.) Second, he might not be holding his foot in the correct position; the foot cannot be jammed in any way but must be flexed sharply so that the smallest diameters present themselves. (Faulty position.) Third, the boot may be too small or (what amounts to the same thing) the foot may be too big. (Disproportion between size of foot and boot.)

Likewise, when Nature tries to propel an infant through the birth canal and fails to do so, there can be only three causes of the failure—the same three. The forces are inadequate (uterine inertia); or the position of the infant is at fault; or there is disproportion between the size of the infant and that of the birth canal.

Uterine Inertia

In some cases, from the very beginning of labor, the contractions are weak, irregular, brief in duration and ineffectual. Even after 12 or 15 hours the contractions are still 8 or 10 minutes apart, last only 20 or 30 seconds and are of weak intensity. This matter of the intensity of labor contractions is something with which the nurse must familiarize herself in order that she may report intelligently about such cases. At the height of an excellent uterine contraction it is impossible to indent the uterine wall with one's finger tips. With a fairly good contraction it may be possible to cause some slight indentation, but if the uterine wall can be indented easily at the height of a contraction, it is a poor one. In evaluating the intensity of a labor contraction, reliance should be placed on this tactile examination and not on the amount of complaining done by the patient about her pain.

431

Primary Uterine Inertia. When contractions are poor from the very onset of labor, the condition is known as primary uterine inertia. The cause is unknown. The essence of the treatment is to give the patient more time, a program which calls for much patience and waiting on the part of everyone concerned. The nurse can be very helpful in encouraging the patient and in keeping up her morale during the long hours. Fluids should be offered to the patient frequently, and unless delivery seems to be imminent, liquid diet should be given at frequent intervals in order to maintain strength. Hot soapsuds enemas probably will be ordered from time to time in the hope of stimulating more effectual uterine contractions. In certain cases (in some it may be dangerous) the physician may ask that the patient be allowed to walk about, in the belief that this may favor descent of the head, which in turn will exert greater pressure on the lower uterine segment and thereby stimulate stronger contractions. In very stubborn cases some physicians may order extremely minute doses of Pitocin intramuscularly (½ to 1 minim). However, unless used with the utmost caution and in very small doses, the employment of Pitocin in labor is fraught with dangerous possibilities—tetanic contraction of the uterus with asphyxiation of the fetus and even rupture of the uterus. Because it affords better control of dosage, the intravenous administration of Pitocin by the continuous drip technic, as described on page 380, is being used extensively in the treatment of uterine inertia.

Secondary Uterine Inertia. In another group of cases, the contractions are excellent for the first 10 or 15 hours of labor, then become gradually weaker, irregular and far apart. There is often an associated quickening of the pulse rate. This condition is called secondary uterine inertia because it is secondary to (that is, caused by) exhaustion. The treatment is rest and fluids. This is usually accomplished by giving a hypodermic of morphine plus the administration of from 500 to 700 cc. of glucose solution (usually 10%) intravenously. The morphine, as a rule, stops the contractions altogether for a few hours and gives the patient a much-needed sleep. Upon awakening, the contractions are likely to return to their original vigor, and the remainder of labor progresses without difficulty.

In such patients who have been in labor for more than 24 hours, whether from uterine inertia or other causes, bacteria are likely to ascend into the uterus and give rise to infection. This is known as *intrapartal infection* and is a serious complication. It is signalized by a rise in temperature, often in association with a chill. Because of this danger, it is customary to take temperatures every 2 hours in patients whose labors have lasted more than 24 hours. Even an elevation of half a degree should be reported at once to the physician. Intrapartal infection is much more likely to occur if the membranes have been ruptured for a long time. Treatment is usually in the form of antibiotics.

Abnormal Fetal Positions

Persistent Occiput Posterior Positions. As stated on page 20 and illustrated in Figures 13 and 14, the fetal head usually enters the pelvic inlet transversely and therefore must traverse an arc of 90° in the process of internal rotation to the direct occiput anterior position. In about a quarter of all labors, however, the head enters the pelvis with the occiput directed diagonally posterior, that is, in either the R.O.P. or L.O.P. position. Under these circumstances, the head must rotate through an arc of 135° in the process of internal rotation.

With good contractions, adequate flexion and a baby of average size, the great majority of these cases of occiput posterior position undergo spontaneous rotation through the 135° arc just as soon as the head reaches the pelvic floor.

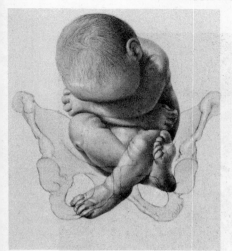

Fig. 250. Footling breech.

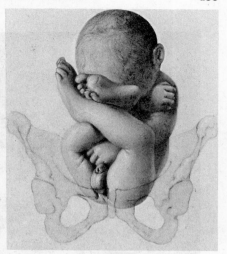

Fig. 251. Frank breech.

This is a normal mechanism of labor. In a small minority of cases, however, perhaps 5 or 10 per cent, these favorable circumstances do not exist, and rotation may be incomplete or may not take place at all. If rotation is incomplete, the head becomes arrested in the transverse position, a condition known as *transverse arrest*. If anterior rotation does not take place at all, the occiput usually rotates to the direct occiput posterior position, a condition known as *persistent occiput posterior*. Both transverse arrest and persistent occiput posterior position represent deviations from the normal mechanisms of labor and often require operative delivery.

Breech Presentations. These are presentations in which the breech instead of the vertex presents at the pelvic brim. They occur in about 3 per cent of all term deliveries. In breech cases, the infant often passes meconium from its rectum during the course of labor; and if, after the membranes are ruptured and the liquor amnii has escaped, the nurse finds a black, tar-colored discharge coming from the patient's vagina, she may very properly suppose that the case is one of breech presentation.

Breech presentations are classified as follows:

1. *Complete,* when the feet and the legs are flexed on the thighs, and the thighs are flexed on the abdomen, so that the buttocks and the feet present (see Fig. 75).

2. *Footling,* when one or both feet present through the cervix (Fig. 250).

3. *Frank,* when the legs are extended and lie against the abdomen and the chest, with the feet meeting the shoulders, and the buttocks present (Fig. 251).

With strong contractions, particularly in multiparae, breech cases may be delivered spontaneously, or at least with very little aid by the attendant. The breech is pushed through the vulva as the result of the mother's bearing-down efforts and rises upward in front of the symphysis pubis. With the emergence of the trunk, the legs descend, the attendant simply receiving them and steadying the breech. With further bearing-down efforts, the shoulders are expelled; then, as the attendant holds up the body, the head is extruded with the face directed back at the perineum (Fig. 252, A to F).

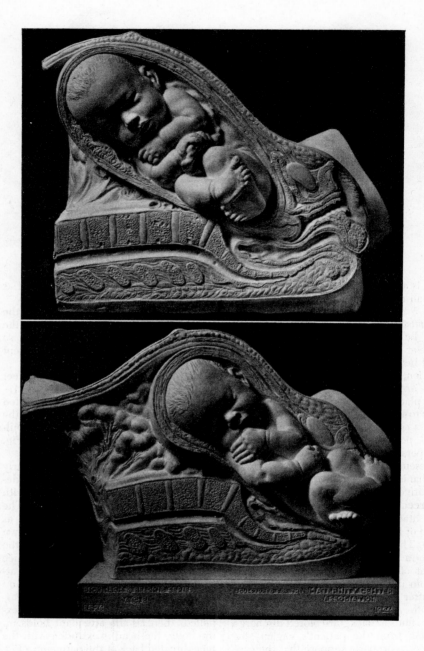

Fig. 252. (A and B) Delivery in footling breech presentation. (From the Dickinson-Belskie Breech Delivery Series, sculptured for the Maternity Center Association, New York)

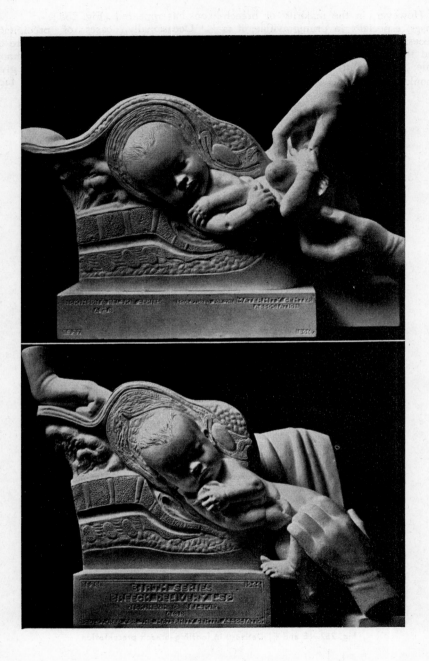

Fig. 252. (C and D) Delivery in footling breech presentation.

Occasionally, cases of precipitate
breech delivery may fall to the care of
the nurse. These cases are uncommon
and, when they do occur, seldom give
rise to difficulty because the very fact

However, in the majority of breech
cases, especially in primigravidae, it is
necessary for the physician to give more
aid than is indicated above, and, as a
rule, this amounts to extraction of the
shoulders and the head after the umbili-

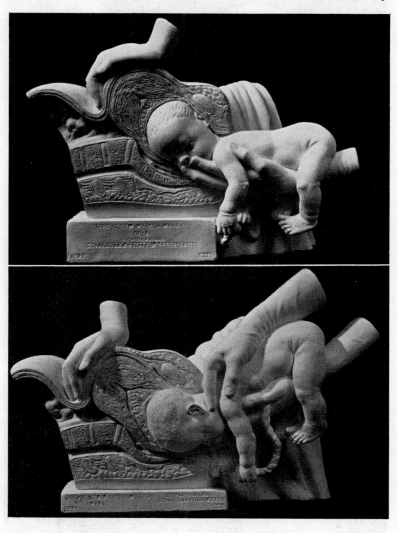

Fig. 252. (E and F) Delivery in footling breech presentation.

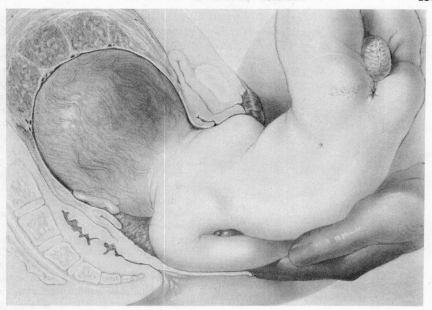

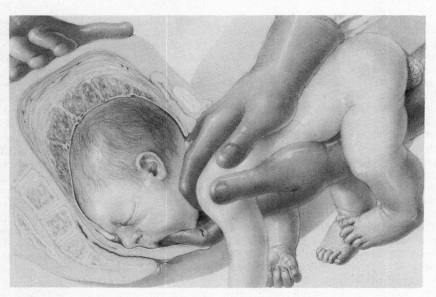

Fig. 253. (*Top*) Extraction of posterior shoulder in breech delivery. (*Bottom*) Extraction of head in breech delivery (Mauriceau maneuver).

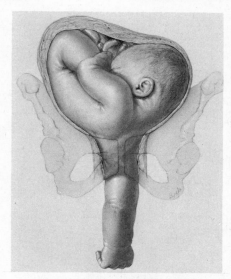

Fig. 254. Shoulder presentation with
prolapse of arm.

that they are precipitate presupposes a
small infant, excellent expulsive forces
and a capacious birth canal. As the
breech emerges, it is received and is
steadied with a sterile towel and sterile
hands, and the mother is urged to bear
down strongly. This will usually effect
delivery of the shoulders in cases of this
sort, but if it does not, the arm which is
the more posterior is drawn out of the
vagina by passing the first and the
middle fingers over the infant's shoulder, down the arm to the elbow, and
then drawing the forearm and the hand
across the face and the chest and out.
The other arm is delivered in the same
way; and then, to favor the birth of the
head, the body of the baby is raised upward in a vertical position. If there is
any great delay, the nurse may pass her
two fingers into the baby's mouth, with
the trunk resting on the palm of the
same hand and the legs straddling her
forearm. Then, with the other hand, upward and outward traction is made on

the shoulders, while firm downward
pressure is made by an assistant on the
lower abdominal wall.

The great danger in breech delivery
is to the baby as the result of the trauma
which it may sustain in delivery. In footling presentations, prolapse of the umbilical cord (see p. 445) is common.
Even in the most skilled hands, and considering only full-term infants, about 1
breech infant in 15 succumbs as the
result of delivery. The danger to the
mother is not appreciably greater than
in vertex deliveries, but lacerations of
the birth canal are more frequent.

**Shoulder, Face and Brow Presen-
tations.** In shoulder presentations, the
infant lies crosswise in the uterus instead
of longitudinally (see Fig. 77). This
complication occurs about once in every
200 cases and is seen most often in multiparae. Not infrequently an arm prolapses into the vagina, making the problem of delivery even more difficult (Fig.
254). The physician usually will turn
the infant in these cases, bringing a foot
or both feet into the vagina, an operation
known as "version" (p. 372). Shoulder
presentation is a serious complication,
occasionally causes rupture of the uterus
(p. 444) and carries a much greater risk
to the infant than either vertex or breech
presentations.

Face presentations are also seen about
once in every 200 cases. They usually
terminate spontaneously, the face coming through the vulva with the chin anterior. As edema of the scalp is common
in vertex presentations (caput succedaneum), so in face presentations the
presenting part, the face, becomes
greatly swollen and purplish. This disappears within a few days. Brow presentations are even more rare and are
much more difficult to deliver because
the largest diameter of the fetal head,
the occipitomental, presents. They frequently convert themselves into face or
occipital presentations; or the physician
may convert them or perform version.

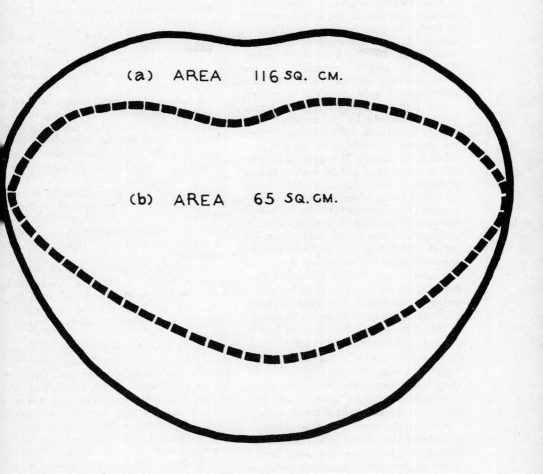

(a) AREA 116 SQ. CM.

(b) AREA 65 SQ. CM.

Fig. 255. Areas (actual size) of normal pelvic inlet (a) and contracted inlet (b). The extreme degree of pelvic contraction shown in (b) occurred in a 26-year-old Negro woman who had had severe rickets in infancy. This might have been prevented by giving cod-liver oil in infancy and childhood. (J. H. H. 283193)

Disproportion

Contracted Pelvis. Disproportion between the size of the infant and that of the birth canal (commonly spoken of simply as "disproportion") is caused most frequently by contracted pelvis. The pelvis may be contracted at the inlet, the midpelvis or the outlet. Inlet contraction is most often due to *rickets,* a fact indicating how much good may be accomplished by the prevention of rickets in infants and children through the routine administration of cod-liver oil or some vitamin D preparation (Fig. 255). Contracted pelvis due to rickets is much more common in the Negro race than in the white. In midpelvic contraction, the distance between the ischial spines is diminished; it is often found in conjunction with outlet contraction. In outlet contraction, the angle formed by the pubic rami is narrow, and the ischial tuberosities are close together; it thus resembles a male pelvis in so far as the outlet is concerned. This type of pelvic contraction occurs with equal frequency in the white and the Negro races, but its cause is not known. It is not only likely to hinder the egress of the infant at the outlet but also may be responsible for deep lacerations, since the narrow pubic rami tend to push the infant's head posteriorly in the direction of the rectum.

One of the main functions of antepartal care is to detect pelvic contraction during pregnancy so that—long before labor begins—some intelligent decision can be reached about how best to deliver the infant. Of course, in such a case as shown in Figure 255, cesarean section is obligatory. But all gradations of contracted pelvis are encountered, and, depending on the size of the infant and other factors, many patients with moderate degrees of the condition can be delivered vaginally without difficulty. In doubtful cases, the physician may give the patient a "trial labor," that is, 6 or 12 hours of labor to ascertain whether or not, with adequate contractions, the head will pass through the pelvis.

Oversize Baby. Excessive size of the infant is not commonly a cause of serious dystocia unless the fetus weighs over 4,500 Gm. (10 pounds). About one infant in a hundred will fall in this class. The trauma associated with the passage of such huge infants through the birth canal causes a decided increase in fetal mortality; this has been estimated as 15 per cent (almost 1 in 6), in contrast with the usual death rate for normal-size infants of 4 per cent. Uterine inertia is frequent in labors with excessive-size infants, and, at the time of delivery, the shoulders may give great difficulty. Even though these infants are born alive, they often do poorly in the first few days because of cerebral hemorrhage and must be watched closely for signs of that condition (see Chap. 21).

One of the common causes of excessive-size infants is diabetes. Large infants are also more commonly seen in older multiparae and after prolonged pregnancies; the majority of such infants are boys.

Despite tales to the contrary, tremendously large infants—weighing over 13 pounds—are extremely rare and almost all are born dead. In 50,000 deliveries at the Johns Hopkins Hospital, there have been only two such cases. Both these infants were boys: the smaller, who weighed 13 pounds, 7 ounces, was the ninth child of a 34-year-old negress; and the larger, 14 pounds, 4 ounces, was the seventh child of a white woman aged 44. The largest infant born at the New York Lying-In Hospital in 100,000 cases weighed 15 pounds. While there may be rare exceptions, most stories that one hears of infants weighing over 15 pounds at birth are the result of either gross exaggeration or incorrect scales.

Hydrocephalus. Hydrocephalus, or an excessive accumulation of cerebrospinal fluid in the ventricles of the brain with consequent enlargement of the cranium, is encountered in 1 fetus in

2,000, approximately, and accounts for some 12 per cent of all malformations at birth. Associated defects are common, spina bifida being present in about one third of the cases. Varying degrees of cranial enlargement are produced, and not infrequently the circumference of the head exceeds 50 cm., sometimes reaching 80 cm. The amount of fluid present is usually between 500 and 1,500 cc., but as much as 5 liters has been reported. Since the distended cranium is too large to fit into the pelvic inlet, breech presentations are exceedingly common, being observed in about one third of such cases. Whatever the presentation, gross disproportion between the size of the head and that of the pelvis is the rule, and serious dystocia the usual consequence. This is a tragic and serious complication of labor, and the obstetrician will find it necessary, as a rule, to puncture the cranial vault and aspirate as much of the cerebrospinal fluid as may be necessary to permit delivery. This does not injure the child.

HEMORRHAGIC COMPLICATIONS
Postpartal Hemorrhage

It has been said of the three stages of labor that the first stage is the most difficult for the physician and the nurse (because of the patience required during the long hours of waiting); that the second is the most difficult for the infant (because of the trauma and asphyxia it may undergo in passing through the birth canal); while for the mother the third stage is the most dangerous because of the likelihood of postpartal hemorrhage and shock.

Definition and Incidence. The average blood loss postpartum is about 300 cc. The term "postpartal hemorrhage," as ordinarily used, does not refer to bleeding of this magnitude, but only to excessive blood loss; and, by rather general consensus, when postpartal bleeding reaches 500 cc. or more, it is designated as "postpartal hemorrhage."

Bleeding of this degree occurs in every 20 or 30 cases despite the most skilled care. Hemorrhages of 1,000 cc. and over are encountered once in about every 75 cases, while blood losses of even 1,500 and 2,000 cc. are encountered now and then. In other words, postpartal hemorrhage is a fairly common complication of labor. Moreover, it is one with which the nurse must be intimately familiar, because she will be expected to assume an important role in the prevention and treatment of the condition.

The Three Causes. In order of frequency, the three causes of postpartal hemorrhage are:

1. Uterine atony
2. Lacerations of the perineum, the vagina and the cervix
3. Retained placental fragments

Uterine atony is by far the most common cause. Again let us recall that the uterus contains huge blood vessels within the interstices of its muscle fibers and that those at the placental site are open and gaping. It is essential that the muscle fibers contract down tightly on these arteries and veins, if bleeding is to be controlled. They must *stay* contracted down, for only a few seconds' relaxation will give rise to sudden, profuse hemorrhage. They must stay *tightly* contracted down, because continuous, slight relaxation gives rise to continuous oozing of blood, one of the most treacherous forms of postpartal hemorrhage.

Lacerations of the perineum, the vagina and the cervix are naturally more common after operative delivery. Tears of the cervix are particularly likely to cause serious hemorrhage. Bright red arterial bleeding in the presence of a hard, firmly contracted uterus (no uterine atony) suggests hemorrhage from a cervical laceration. The physician will establish the diagnosis by actual inspection of the cervix (retractors are necessary) and, after locating the source of bleeding, will repair the laceration.

Retained Placental Fragments. Small, partially separated fragments of placenta may cause postpartal hemorrhage by interfering with proper uterine contraction. Careful inspection of the placenta to determine whether a piece is missing will rule out or confirm the diagnosis; the treatment, obviously, is to remove the placental fragment. This is an uncommon cause of postpartal hemorrhage, but occasionally the nurse will encounter cases in which profuse bleeding occurs suddenly a week or more after delivery. These late hemorrhages are usually designated by the term "puerperal hemorrhage." They are almost always caused by a retained placental fragment.

Predisposing Factors. There are certain factors which predispose to postpartal hemorrhage so that, to a certain extent, it may be anticipated in advance. Among these, one of the most important is the size of the infant. With a 9-pound infant, the chances of postpartal hemorrhage are 5 times as great as they are with a 5-pound infant. Excessive bleeding is twice as common in twin pregnancy. Hydramnios (excessive amount of amniotic fluid) is another predisposing factor. Other conditions in which postpartal hemorrhage is extremely frequent are premature separation of the placenta and placenta previa. Finally, operative delivery, particularly if a prolonged general anesthetic has been given, greatly increases the likelihood of this complication.

Clinical Picture. Excessive bleeding may occur prior to the birth of the placenta, but it is seen more commonly thereafter. Although it is occasionally torrential in character, the most common type is a continuous trickle—minute by minute. These small constant trickles are not alarming in appearance, consequently no one may become alarmed and no one may do anything. This is what makes this type of hemorrhage so treacherous. This fact has been emphasized particularly by Doctor Beecham, of Philadelphia, in his survey of 52 deaths from postpartal hemorrhage which occurred in that city. The average

interval between delivery and death in this series was 5 hours and 20 minutes. Only 6 patients, 11.5 per cent, died within 2 hours of delivery, and none in less than 1½ hours. In other words, there would have been ample time for intensive treatment in any of these cases, had the attendant known how much blood was being lost.

Treatment. The first and most important thing to do is to grasp the uterus and massage it vigorously. This must be continued until the uterus assumes a woody hardness; if the slightest relaxation occurs, the massage must be re-instituted. In many cases, the uterus stays contracted most of the time but occasionally relaxes; it is therefore obligatory to keep a hand on the fundus constantly for a full hour after bleeding has subsided. Even then the danger is not over, since relaxation sometimes occurs 2 or more hours after delivery; in these cases, the uterus may balloon with blood, with very little escaping externally. Accordingly, the size and the consistency of the uterus should be checked frequently until several hours have elapsed. The nurse must make absolutely certain that she is actually massaging the uterus. Frequently, these big, boggy, relaxed uteri are difficult to outline through the abdominal wall, and it may be necessary to push the hand well posteriorly to the region of the sacral promontory to reach it. The very fact that the uterus is hard to identify usually means that it is relaxed. If the nurse is not sure that she is feeling the uterus, she should inform the physician at once.

If the bleeding occurs prior to delivery of the placenta, the physician may find it necessary to extract the placenta manually. (Change of gloves as well as gown may be called·for). Oxytocics will invariably be requested—ergonovine or pituitary extract intramuscularly, or both. One or another of these may be given by the physician intravenously. If these measures fail to stop the bleeding, the physician probably will either pack the uterus or carry out bimanual compression of the organ (Figs. 256 and 257). The latter provides the most efficient means of massaging the uterus as well as compression. Packing may be done either manually or by means of the Holmes packer; this instrument prevents contamination of the gauze by vaginal bacteria. If shock threatens, the Trendelenburg position should be employed, external heat applied, and preparations for blood tranfusion made.

In the handling of a case of postpartal hemorrhage, the nurse may be taxed to her utmost. The physician in charge may have to search for and suture a cervical laceration or start a blood transfusion or even resuscitate the infant; another physician may be needed to give the anesthesia. To the nurse, or nurses, will usually fall the important tasks of massaging the uterus, giving oxytocics, helping with the transfusion and keeping an eye on the infant. The nurse must be prepared to act quickly and efficiently if the lives of these bleeding mothers are to be saved.

If postpartal hemorrhage should occur

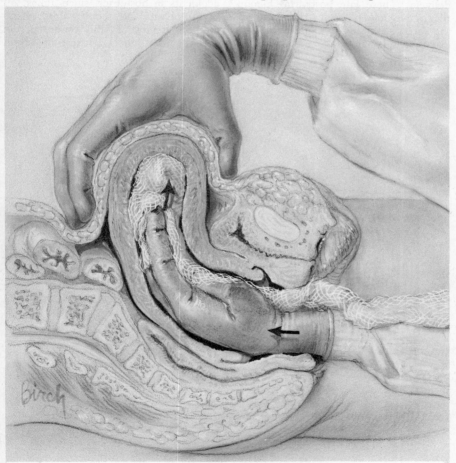

Fig. 256. Uterus tamponed by the manual method.

after the physician has left, the nurse should grasp the uterus at once, press out as much blood as possible and begin vigorous massage, sending word, of course, to the physician. If massage fails to stop the bleeding, the physician usually will not object if the nurse gives the patient an intramuscular injection of ergonovine or Pitocin. If possible, this arrangement should be understood beforehand.

Late Postpartal Hemorrhage. Occasionally postpartal hemorrhage may occur later than the first day following delivery. These late postpartal hemorrhages may take place any time between the second and twenty-eighth day, are usually sudden in onset and may be so massive as to produce shock; they are due almost always to retained placental fragments. Late postpartal hemorrhage is fortunately uncommon, occurring perhaps once in a thousand cases. The physician probably will carry out instrumental dilatation of the cervix, followed by removal of the placental fragments either with a curet or ovum forceps.

Rupture of Uterus

Rupture of the uterus is fortunately a rare complication, but when it does occur it constitutes one of the gravest accidents in obstetrics, since almost all of the infants and about a third of the mothers are lost. In this condition, the uterus simply bursts, because the strain

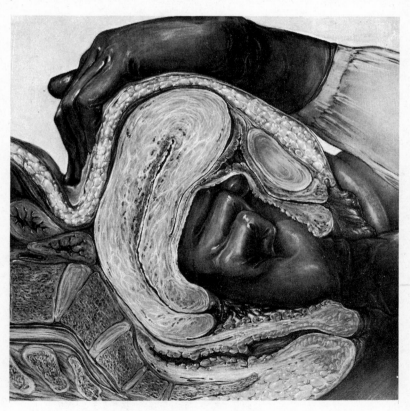

Fig. 257. Bimanual compression of uterus in treatment of postpartal hemorrhage.

placed upon its musculature is more than it can withstand. It may occur in pregnancy but is more frequent in labor. In modern obstetrics, the most common cause is rupture of the scar of a previous cesarean section. Accordingly, when observing labor in a patient who has had a previous cesarean section, the possibility of this accident always should be borne in mind. Other causes are disproportion, traumatic delivery, such as version and extraction, and the injudicious use of Pitocin in labor. In a patient who is having strong labor contractions, a sudden tremendously severe, lancinating pain followed by complete cessation of regular contractions suggests rupture of the uterus; due to the outpouring of blood into the abdominal cavity, signs of shock are a frequent but not invariable accompaniment. As soon as the diagnosis of rupture of the uterus is made, rapid preparations for an abdominal operation should be made, since hysterectomy is the usual treatment.

AMNIOTIC FLUID EMBOLISM

At any time after the membranes have ruptured there is a possibility that amniotic fluid may enter the gaping venous sinuses of the placental site as well as the veins in the cervix, be drawn into the general circulation and in this way reach the pulmonary capillaries. Since the amniotic fluid invariably contains small particles of matter, such as vernix caseosa, lanugo and sometimes meconium, multiple tiny emboli may reach the lungs in this manner and cause occlusion of the pulmonary capillaries. This complication, amniotic fluid embolism, is almost invariably fatal and, as a rule, causes the death of the mother within an hour or two. Fortunately, this tragic condition is rare, occurring only once in many thousand labors.

The clinical characteristics of the condition are sudden dyspnea, cyanosis, pulmonary edema, profound shock and uterine relaxation with postpartal hemorrhage. A highly important feature of amniotic fluid embolism is a diminution in the fibrinogen content of the blood, or hypofibrinogenemia. The mechanism is similar to, if not identical with, that which occurs in abruptio placentae and missed abortion, as described on pages 405 and 416.

The treatment consists of oxygen therapy, blood transfusion and the intravenous administration of fibrinogen, but, as indicated, this is usually futile.

ACCIDENTAL COMPLICATIONS

Lacerations of Perineum

Lacerations have already been referred to as a cause of postpartal hemorrhage. In addition, perineal tears may do great damage in destroying the integrity of the perineum and in weakening the supports of the uterus, the bladder and the rectum. Unless these lacerations are repaired properly, the resultant weakness, as the years go by, may cause prolapse of the uterus (called by the laity "falling of the womb"), cystocele (a pouching downward of the bladder) or rectocele (a pouching forward of the rectum). These conditions, which originate from perineal lacerations at childbirth, give rise to many discomforts and often necessitate operative treatment.

Because lacerations of the birth canal sometimes occur during the process of normal delivery, and are sometimes unavoidable even in the most skilled hands, this subject has already been discussed in Chapter 12.

Prolapse of Umbilical Cord

In the course of labor, the cord prolapses in front of the presenting part about once in every 400 cases. It is a grave complication for the fetus, since the cord is then compressed between the head and the bony pelvis, and the fetal circulation is shut off (Fig. 258). The accident is usually due to premature rupture of the membranes when the head, the breech or the shoulder is

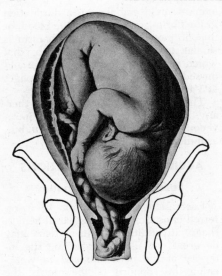

Fig. 258. Prolapse of the umbilical cord (Bumm). As the head comes down, the compression of the cord between the fetal skull and the pelvic brim will shut off its circulation completely.

not sufficiently down in the pelvis to prevent the cord from being washed past it in the sudden gush of amniotic fluid. After the membranes rupture, the cord comes down, and it may be either a concealed or an apparent prolapse. In the latter instance, the diagnosis is made when the cord is seen; but when the cord is not visible, the correct diagnosis will not be made unless the patient is examined and the cord is felt, or examination of the fetal heart reveals distress due to pressure on the cord. This is why it *must* be a routine practice to listen to the fetal heart sounds immediately after the membranes rupture.

If the nurse is alone with the patient, she should send immediately for the physician and then attempt to relieve the pressure on the cord by elevating the patient's hips, thus allowing the head to gravitate away from the pelvis. This takes place in either the "knee-chest

position" (see Fig. 196) or the Trendelenburg position. In the home, the latter is arranged by slipping the back of a straight-backed chair, covered with a flat pillow, under the buttocks and the shoulders, with the knees down over the rungs of the chair. In putting the patient in such positions, her hips must be kept raised above the level of her shoulders. If the patient is unable to remain in either of these positions very long, she may be put in the elevated Sims' position, that is, on her side with the hips elevated by pillows in order to raise the hips higher than the thorax. Any change in position must be carried out slowly!

If the physician is expected to arrive on the scene within the next 15 minutes, this is all that the nurse should do. If he can be reached by telephone in this period, instructions about further therapy should be sought. If no medical advice can be obtained at the end of 15 minutes and the umbilical cord is protruding from the vagina, the nurse should protect the exposed cord with sterile wet saline dressings, if they are available. In handling the cord, great care must be exercised not to compress it. The nurse should *never* attempt to replace a prolapsed cord into the vagina.

Inversion of Uterus

Inversion of the uterus is a rare and highly fatal accident of labor in which, after the birth of the infant, the uterus turns inside out. Shock is profound, in many cases causing the death of the mother. This rare complication is mentioned here only to stress the two common causes: (1) pulling on the umbilical cord and (2) trying to express the placenta when the uterus is relaxed. In the former case, the traction on the attached placenta simply pulls the uterus inside out, while in the latter the hand pushes the relaxed muscular sac inside out. The umbilical cord never should be pulled on, and the uterus never should be pushed upon unless it is firmly contracted.

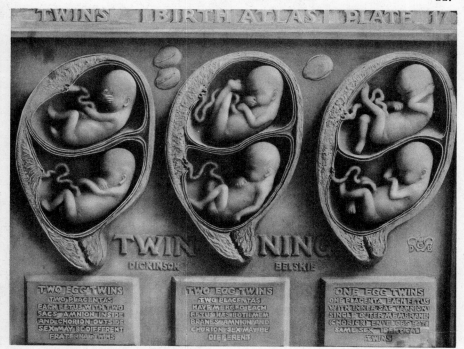

Fig. 259. One-egg and two-egg twins. (Dickinson-Belskie Series, *Birth Atlas* published by Maternity Center Association, New York)

MULTIPLE PREGNANCY

When two or more embryos develop in the uterus at the same time, the condition is known as multiple pregnancy. Twins occur once in 92 births, approximately; triplets once in 9,400 births; and quadruplets once in 620,000. Over 30 cases of quintuplets have been recorded, but with two notable exceptions, none of these infants has survived more than a few weeks. The familiar one, of course, is the Dionne quintuplets, and the fact that all 5 of these little girls lived is one of the miracles of modern times. Heredity plays an important causative role in twin pregnancy, and if there are twins in the family of either the expectant mother or her husband, the likelihood of twins is greater.

Twins may be of two kinds: identical and nonidentical. Identical twins *are* identical because they come from a single egg; hence they are called "single-ovum twins." Fertilization takes place in the usual way, by a single spermatozoon, but then, very early in the ovum's development, it divides into 2 identical parts instead of continuing as a single individual. Such twins are always of the same sex and, as we have implied, show close physical and mental resemblances. Nonidentical twins come from the fertilization of two ova by two spermatozoa and are therefore known as "double-ovum twins" (Fig. 259). Such twins, according to chance, may be of the same sex or of opposite sexes; and the likelihood of their resembling each other is no greater than that of any brother and sister.

Single-ovum twins have 1 placenta

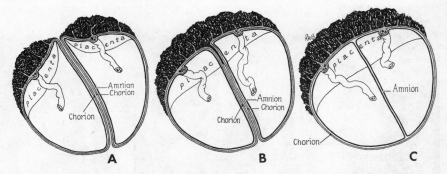

Fig. 260. Single- and double-ovum twin differences. A and B, double-ovum twins; there are two chorions; in B the two placentas have fused. C, single-ovum twins; there is only one chorion and one placenta.

and 1 chorion, but there are normally 2 amnions and 2 umbilical cords (Fig. 260). In double-ovum twins, each fetus has its own chorion, amnion, cord and placenta, but the placentas may be partially fused. These double-ovum twins are much the more common of the two types, making up about 85 per cent of all twins.

In the majority of instances (but not all) it is possible for the physician to make a diagnosis of twins by abdominal examination during the last few months; in doubtful cases, a roentgenogram may be necessary to settle the question.

Twins are likely to be born about 2 weeks before the calculated date of delivery. Even though pregnancy goes to full term, twins are usually smaller than single infants by nearly one pound; however, the outlook for such infants, provided that the pregnancy continues into the last month, is almost as good as that for single infants.

The patient with a multiple pregnancy faces greater discomforts and greater hazards than does a woman with a single pregnancy. The latter weeks of a twin pregnancy are likely to be associated with heaviness of the lower abdomen, back pains and swelling of the feet and the ankles. Moreover, there are two serious complications which such patients are particularly prone to develop:

toxemia and postpartal hemorrhage. Eclampsia is four times more common in twin pregnancy. Therefore, the antepartal course of these patients should be followed with especial care for signs of beginning toxemia. Postpartal hemorrhage is twice as common in twin pregnancy. Mechanical difficulties in labor are less frequent than might be expected. Uterine inertia, however, is encountered rather often. Not infrequently, the physician has to rupture the membranes of the second twin and occasionally deliver it by version and extraction.

SUGGESTED READING

Bookmiller, Mae, and Bowen, George: Textbook of Obstetrics and Obstetric Nursing, ed. 3, Philadelphia, Saunders, 1958.

Bradley, Chester D.: Retained placenta, Am. J. Obst. & Gynec. 59:141, 1950.

Brandeberry, Keith R., and Kistner, Robert W.: Prolapse of the umbilical cord, Am. J. Obst. & Gynec. 61:356, 1951.

Cole, J. T.: Method of treating massive obstetric hemorrhage, J.A.M.A. 135: 142, 1947.

Davis, M. E., and Scheckler, C. E.: DeLee's Obstetrics for Nurses, ed. 16, Philadelphia, Saunders, 1957.

Eastman, Nicholson J.: Williams Obstetrics, ed. 11, New York, Appleton, 1956.

Gordon, C. A.: Hemorrhage as the most

frequent cause of maternal death. An analysis of the puerperal deaths in Brooklyn, 1944, Am. J. Surg. **70**:277, 1945.

Greenhill, J. P.: Obstetrics, ed. 11, Philadelphia, Saunders, 1955.

Gusberg, S. B.: Prolapse of the umbilical cord, Am. J. Obst. & Gynec. **52**:826, 1946.

Guttmacher, A. F.: An analysis of 521 cases of twin pregnancy: (1) differences in single and double ovum twinning, Am. J. Obst. & Gynec. **34**:76, 1937.

——: An analysis of 473 cases of twin pregnancy: (2) hazards of pregnancy itself, Am. J. Obst. & Gynec. **38**:277, 1939.

Macklin, Madge T.: The use of monozygous and dizygous twins in the study of human heredity, Am. J. Obst. & Gynec. **59**:359, 1950.

Moore, W. T., and Steptoe, P. P., Jr.: The experience of the Johns Hopkins Hospital with breech presentation, South. M. J. **36**:295, 1943.

Potter, Edith L.: Fundamentals of Human Reproduction, New York, McGraw-Hill, 1948.

Van Blarcom, Carolyn C.: Obstetrical Nursing (rev. by E. Ziegel), ed. 4, New York, Macmillan, 1957.

CHAPTER TWENTY

Complications of the Puerperium

PUERPERAL INFECTION

When inflammatory processes develop in the birth canal postpartally, as the result of bacterial invasion of these highly vulnerable areas, the condition is known as "puerperal infection." It is really a postpartal wound infection of the birth canal, usually of the endometrium. As is true of other wound infections, the condition often remains localized but may extend along various pathways to produce diverse clinical pictures. Febrile reactions of more or less severity are the rule, and the outcome varies according to the portal of entry, the type, the number and the virulence of the invading organisms, the reaction of the tissues and the general resistance of the patient.

Puerperal infection is one of the most common causes of death in childbearing. Frequently used (but less satisfactory) synonyms are puerperal fever, puerperal sepsis, puerperal septicemia and childbed fever.

Causative Factors

The vast majority of puerperal infections are caused by the streptococcus, but most of the well-known pathogenic bacteria—such as the staphylococcus, the colon bacillus and the Welch bacillus—may be responsible for the disease.

What are the sources of these bacteria? The late Dr. John Osborne Polak,

of Brooklyn, N. Y., used to teach that there are "eleven causes" of puerperal infection—the 10 fingers and the nasopharynx. He meant by this that the attendants themselves are most likely to carry infection to the parturient uterus. The physician may inadvertently do so in two ways. In the first place, gloved and sterile though his hands may be during the vaginal examinations or the operative manipulations, he may carry bacteria already in the vagina upward into the uterus. Secondly, his hands and the instruments he uses may become contaminated by virulent streptococci as the result of droplet infection, dispersed by himself or some of the attendants, and in this manner he may be responsible for introducing bacteria into the birth canal. Even in modern obstetrics, the latter is a very common mode of infection, and unless the utmost vigilance is used in masking all attendants in the delivery room (both nose and mouth) and in excluding therefrom all persons suffering or recovering from an upper respiratory infection, it is a constant source of danger.

Although a less common means of transfer today than a few decades ago, careless physicians and nurses have been known to carry bacteria to the parturient from countless extraneous contacts—from other cases of puerperal infection, from suppurative postoperative wounds, from cases of sloughing carcinoma, from patients with scarlet fever, from infants with impetigo neonatorum, from umbilical infections of the newborn and, finally, from the autopsy table. The physician himself may have the infection on his own person, such as an infected hangnail or felon. Not too many years ago, a Baltimore midwife with an ulcer on her finger gave a patient a fatal case of puerperal infection.

Coitus late in pregnancy is more common than ordinarily believed and may introduce extraneous organisms to the birth canal or carry upward bacteria already present on the vulva or in the lower vagina. Tub baths, particularly in multiparae with gaping vulvae, may permit the bath water to gain access to the vagina and thus introduce surface bacteria from the whole body.

During the second stage of labor, the chances of fecal matter being transferred to the vagina are great, another constant source of danger.

Following completion of the third stage of labor, the site of previous placental attachment is a raw, elevated area, deep red in color and about 4 cm. in diameter. Its surface is nodular, due to the presence of numerous gaping veins, many of which are occluded by clots. These form excellent culture media for bacteria. Furthermore, at this time, the condition of the entire endometrium is peculiarly favorable to bacterial invasion, since it is less than 2 mm. thick, is infiltrated with blood and presents numerous small wounds. Since the cervix rarely escapes some degree of laceration in labor, it is another ready site for bacterial invasion. Vulvar, vaginal and perineal wounds offer still other possible portals of entry.

Puerperal infection is much more likely to occur if the mother has had a traumatic labor or a postpartal hemorrhage. Therefore, hemorrhage and trauma must be regarded as important predisposing causes of this infection. Other causes in this respect are pro-longed labor, retention of placental tissue and pre-existing physiologic conditions which lower the mother's general resistance to disease.

Prevention of Infection

The prevention of infection throughout the maternity cycle has been emphasized in foregoing sections as an important factor in the maintenance of health and the prevention of disease. During pregnancy, blood studies are done routinely and iron prescribed as necessary, not only for the immediate value, but also because anemia predisposes to puerperal infection. A great deal of emphasis is placed on health teaching at this time, particularly in regard to general hygiene. The patient is advised to avoid all possible sources of infection. Some physicians advise against tub baths in the last weeks of pregancy, because the bath water may introduce surface bacteria from the body into the vagina, particularly in multiparas. It is well for the nurse to recognize that this idea is still prevalent in many circles, although it is now believed to have little validity. The greatest hazard of tub baths in these last weeks of pregnancy arises because climbing in and out of the tub is awkward and sudden changes in balance might result in a fall and, thus, the likelihood of physical trauma. Coitus should be avoided during the last two months of pregnancy, and vaginal douches after the fifth month. Contacts with upper respiratory infections should always be avoided.

During labor, care should be exercised to limit bacteria from extraneous sources. In the hospital, cleanliness and good housekeeping are imperative, but, nevertheless, individual care technic reduces the chance of contamination from other patients. Each patient should have all of "her own" equipment, which includes her own bedpan. This bedpan should be cleansed after each use and sterilized once a day. Scrupulous hand washing on the part of all personnel after contacts with each patient will do much to prevent the transfer of infection from one patient to another. Strictest rules should be enforced for surgical cleanliness during labor and delivery. No one with an infection of the skin or the respiratory tract should work in the maternity department. The nasopharynx of attendants is the most common source of contamination of the birth canal. Masks should be worn any time that the external genitalia are exposed for inspection or examination or treatments, in the labor room as well as in the delivery room. To be effective, masks must cover the nose and the mouth and be clean and dry; thus they must be changed frequently and should not hang around the neck when not in use.

During the puerperium the same careful precautions should be carried out. For many days following the delivery, the surface of the birth canal is a vulnerable area for pathogenic bacteria. The birth canal is well protected against the invasion of extraneous bacteria by the closed vulva, unless this barrier is invaded. Patients should be taught the principles of perineal hygiene and how to give themselves self-care. The nurse should remember never to use her fingers to separate the labia in giving perineal care, because this permits the cleansing solution to enter the vagina.

Types of Puerperal Infection

Generally speaking, puerperal infection can be divided into two main types: (1) *local processes* and (2) *extensions of the original process*. When a lesion of the vulva, the perineum, the vagina, the cervix or the endometrium becomes infected, the infection may remain localized in these wounds. However, the original inflammatory process may extend along the veins (the most common way) and cause thrombophlebitis and pyemia, or through the lymph vessels to cause peritonitis and pelvic cellulitis.

Lesions of the Perineum, the

Vulva and the Vagina. These lesions are highly vulnerable areas for bacterial invasion in the early puerperium and so may become infected. The most common of these is a localized infection of a repaired perineal laceration or episiotomy wound. The usual symptoms are elevation of temperature, pain and sensation of heat in the affected area and burning on urination. The area involved becomes red and edematous, and there is profuse seropurulent discharge. If a wound of the vulva becomes infected, the entire vulva may become edematous and ulcerated. Infections involving the perineum, the vulva and the vagina cause the patient considerable discomfort and alarm. These local inflammatory processes seldom cause severe physical reactions, provided that good drainage is established and the patient's temperature remains below 38.4° C. (101° F.). To promote good drainage, all stitches must be removed so that the surface is laid open. Because the drainage itself is a source of irritation and contamination, the wound must be kept clean and the perineal pads changed frequently. Care must be exercised in cleansing the wound to see that none of the solution runs into the vagina. It is understood, of course, that vaginal douches would never be given at this time. Treatments such as sitz baths or the perineal heat lamp are generally used for the relief of pain. Penicillin or one of the sulfonamides is prescribed to combat the infection. If drainage is impaired the patient will not only have more pain but she also may have a chill, followed by a sudden elevation of temperature.

Endometritis. This is a localized infection of the lining membrane of the uterus. Bacteria invade the lesion, usually the placental site, and may spread to involve the entire endometrium. When endometritis develops it usually manifests itself about the third or fourth day after delivery. In the milder forms the patient may have no complaints or symptoms other than a rise in temperature to about 38.4° C. (101° F.) which persists for several days and then sub'-sides. On the other hand, the more virulent infections are often ushered in by chills and high fever, with a comparable rise in pulse rate. In the majority of cases the patient experiences a chilly sensation, or actual chills, at the onset and often complains of malaise, loss of appetite, headache, backache and general discomfort. It is not unusual for the patient to have severe and prolonged after-pains. The uterus is invariably large and is extremely tender when palpated abdominally. The lochial discharge is increased in amount and distinguished from normal lochia by its dark brown appearance and foul odor. To promote drainage of this discharge the patient should be placed in Fowler's position. If the infection remains localized in the endometrium, it is usually over in about a week or 10 days. But when extension of the infection occurs to cause peritonitis, pelvic thrombophlebitis or cellulitis, the disease may persist for many weeks, often with dramatic temperature curves and repeated chills.

Thrombophlebitis. This is an infection of the vascular endothelium with clot formation attached to the vessel wall. It may be of two types: pelvic thrombophlebitis, an inflammatory process involving the ovarian and the uterine veins, or femoral thrombophlebitis, in which the femoral, the popliteal or the saphenous vein is involved. The latter type of thrombophlebitis is often spoken of as "phlegmasia alba dolens" (painful white inflammation) and also very frequently as "milk leg"—a term once given to the condition by physicians in the belief that it was due to the collection of milk in the affected leg. Early ambulation may be a factor in preventing this complication.

FEMORAL THROMBOPHLEBITIS. This condition presents a special group of signs and symptoms. It is a disease of the puerperium characterized by pain, fever and swelling in the affected leg.

These symptoms are due to the formation of a clot in the veins of the leg itself, which interferes with the return circulation of the blood. When "milk leg" develops it usually appears about 10 days after labor, although it may manifest itself as late as the 20th day. As in all acute febrile diseases occurring after labor, the secretion of milk may cease when phlegmasia alba dolens develops.

The disease is ushered in with malaise, chilliness and fever, which are soon followed by stiffness and pain in the affected part. If it is in the leg, the pain may begin in the groin or the hip and extend downward, or it may commence in the calf of the leg and extend upward. In about 24 hours, the leg begins to swell, and although the pain then lessens slightly, it is always present and may be severe enough to prevent sleep. The skin over the swollen area is shiny white in color.

The acute symptoms last from a few days to a week, after which the pain gradually subsides and the patient slowly improves.

The course of the disease covers a period of from 4 to 6 weeks. The affected leg is slow to return to its normal size and may remain permanently enlarged and troublesome.

The prognosis is usually favorable. In some of the very severe cases, however, abscesses form, and the disease may become very critical or even be fatal. In very rare instances the clot may be dislodged and carried to the heart, causing instant death.

The treatment of femoral thrombophlebitis consists in rest, elevation of the affected leg, the use of icebags along the course of the affected vessels, sedatives, as indicated, for the pain, and penicillin. Anticoagulants, such as heparin and Dicumarol, may be prescribed to prevent further formation of thrombi. A "cradle" should be used to keep the pressure of the bedclothes off the affected part. Under no circumstances should a nurse rub or massage the affected part; and it should be handled with the utmost care when changing dressings, applying a bandage, making the bed or giving a bath. As the acute stage subsides, nourishing food and the most carefully regulated hygienic conditions are needed to build up the patient's strength. As recovery is usually tedious, skillful nursing care is required to preserve the tissues of the body.

PELVIC THROMBOPHLEBITIS. This is a severe complication in the puerperium. The onset usually occurs about the second week following delivery with severe, repeated chills and dramatic swings in temperature. The infection is usually caused by anaerobic streptococci, and although it is difficult to obtain a positive blood culture, bacteria are present in the blood stream during chills. Penicillin therapy is used because it is effective in treating most strains of this organism, and as long as the chills and the fever persist, blood transfusions may be given. Heparin and Dicumarol may be prescribed to prevent the formation of more thrombi. A further problem is likely to arise with metastatic pulmonary complications, such as lung abscesses or pneumonia.

These patients are usually mentally depressed and discouraged. If the nurse is conscious of this complication, she will make every effort to keep the patient contented and have her realize the value of immobilization, even though the convalescent period is prolonged. The nurse may also make suggestions to the family as to ways in which they may be helpful.

Peritonitis. Peritonitis is an infection, either generalized or local, of the peritoneum. Here, as a rule, the infection reaches the peritoneum from the endometrium by traveling via the lymphatic vessels; but peritonitis may also result from the extension of thrombophlebitis or parametritis. The clinical course of pelvic peritonitis resembles that of surgical peritonitis. The patient has a high fever, rapid pulse and, in general, has

the appearance of being profoundly ill. She is usually restless and sleepless and has constant and severe abdominal pain. Hiccups, nausea and vomiting, which is sometimes fecal and projectile, may be present. Antibiotic therapy is given to combat the infection, analgesic drugs for discomfort and mild sedative drugs to relieve the restlessness and apprehension. If there is intestinal involvement, oral feedings are withheld until normal intestinal function is restored; meanwhile, fluids are administered intravenously. Blood transfusions and oxygen therapy may be indicated for supportive treatment. The record of intake and output must be kept, and, in order to be of value to the physician, the elimination of fluids from the skin by sweating should be noted accurately.

Pelvic Cellulitis, or Parametritis. This is an infection which extends along the lymphatics to reach the loose connective tissue surrounding the uterus. It may follow an infected cervical laceration, endometritis or pelvic thrombophlebitis. The patient will have a persistent fever and marked pain and tenderness over the affected area. The problem is usually unilateral but may involve both sides of the abdomen. As the process develops, the swelling becomes very hard and finally either undergoes resolution or results in the formation of a pelvic abscess. If the latter occurs, as the abscess comes to a point, the skin above becomes red, edematous and tender. Recovery is usually prompt after the abscess is opened.

Signs and Symptoms

It is highly important that the nurse recognize and report early signs and symptoms of puerperal infection in order that proper treatment may be instituted without delay. When puerperal infection develops, one of the first symptoms usually seen is a rise in temperature. Although temperature elevations in the puerperium may be caused by upper respiratory infections, urinary tract infections and the like, the majority are due to puerperal infection. Puerperal morbidity is the term used to include all puerperal fevers. The Joint Committee on Maternal Welfare in this country has defined puerperal morbidity as a "temperature of 100.4° F. (38° C.), the temperature to occur on any two of the first ten days postpartum, exclusive of the first 24 hours, and to be taken by a standard technic at least four times daily." The symptoms may vary, depending on the location and the extent of the infectious process, the type and the virulence of the invading organisms and the general resistance of the patient. The affected area is usually painful, reddened and edematous and the source of profuse discharge. The patient may complain of malaise, headache and general discomfort. As mentioned above, the temperature is elevated, and in the more severe infections, chills and fever may occur. In its typical form, each of the clinical types of puerperal infection presents a very characteristic set of signs and symptoms, although occasionally one form of the disease is combined with another. The distinctions between these different types of infections are of importance, because the clinical course, the treatment and the prognosis depend on the particular form of infection. For this reason these aspects of the various puerperal infections have been discussed in the preceding pages.

Treatment

The use of the sulfonamides and penicillin therapy has brought about radical changes in the treatment and the prognosis of puerperal infection. These drugs are effective in combating most of these infections, but, nevertheless, the management and the care of patients with puerperal infections are highly important and demand the utmost in skill. Penicillin is effective against the hemolytic streptococcus, the Welch bacillus and the staphylococcus. Since penicillin is not effective against the colon bacillus

and certain strains of staphylococci, sulfadiazine or Gantrisin are usually prescribed for infections caused by these organisms. Resistant staphylococcal infections are often vulnerable to erythromycin used in conjunction with Gantrisin. The dosage of these drugs depends on the severity of the disease and the type of the offending organism. Wound cultures are frequently taken to gain information about the organism; and in severe cases blood cultures may be taken, but if they are to be of real diagnostic value they must be taken at the time of the chill. The infected lesions are treated the same as those of any surgical wound. Drainage must be established, and since this discharge is of a highly infectious nature, care must be taken to see that it is not spread and that all contaminated pads and dressings are wrapped and burned.

The curative treatment, of course, will be directed by the physician, but good nursing care is essential. The patient should be kept as comfortable and quiet as possible, for sleep and rest are important. Conserving the patient's strength in every way, giving her nourishing food, increased amounts of fluids, fresh air and sunshine will help to increase her powers of resistance. To promote drainage the head of the bed should be kept elevated, a measure which also contributes to the patient's comfort. In cases of endometritis it is usually customary to apply icebags to the head and the abdomen at intervals.

Care must be exercised to prevent the spread of the infection from one patient to another. Isolation of infected patients from others is desirable in order to protect the healthy maternity patients; ideally, the patient with puerperal infection should be away from the maternity divisions. If it is impossible to arrange for such complete segregation, the nurse must consider every patient with puerperal infection as "in isolation" and follow scrupulous technic accordingly. Regardless of the situation, the nurse who is caring for a patient with puerperal infection (or any infection, for that matter) should not attend other maternity patients. The hands of all attendants need special attention and should be scrubbed thoroughly after caring for a mother who has an infection. In certain cases strict isolation technic, with special gowns, masks and rubber gloves, is essential. Clean isolation gowns, masks and gloves should be available for all persons who attend the isolated patient and after being used should be left in the room and disposed of in special hampers or containers. Under no circumstances should this apparel be worn outside the patient's room. Since it is assumed that the nurses who care for these patients are fully acquainted with principles of good isolation technic, this aspect of care will not be pursued further here.

SUBINVOLUTION OF THE UTERUS

Subinvolution is the term used to describe the condition which exists when normal involution of the puerperal uterus is retarded. The causes contributing to this condition may be (1) lack of tone in the uterine musculature, (2) imperfect exfoliation of the decidua, (3) retained placental tissue and membranes, (4) endometritis and (5) presence of uterine fibroids. Subinvolution is characterized by a large and flabby uterus; lochial discharge prolonged beyond the usual period, sometimes with profuse bleeding; backache and dragging sensation in the pelvis; and disturbance of health until corrected. Since this abnormality is the result of local conditions, an important phase of the treatment rests in correcting the causative factor. Oxytocic medication, such as ergonovine, may be administered to maintain the uterine tone and prevent the accumulation of clots in the uterine cavity, and hot vaginal douches may be prescribed for several days. When the condition is due to disturbances of the endometrium or retained secundines,

dilatation and curettage may be necessary. If the uterus is displaced, it may delay normal involution and should be corrected by a suitably fitting pessary.

Early ambulation is believed to have decreased the incidence of subinvolution. And, since it is recognized that breast feeding stimulates uterine contractions, the fact that a mother is not breast feeding may be an influencing factor when subinvolution occurs.

HEMORRHAGE

These complications are discussed in Chapter 19.

DISORDERS OF THE BREASTS
Engorgement of the Breasts

Any time after the third postpartal day, after lacteal secretion is established, engorgement of the breasts may occur. The onset is usually rapid, and, as the breasts become distended, dilated veins may be visible under the skin, and on palpation the breasts feel hard and nodular. This condition, commonly called "caked breasts" by the laity, is likely to occur in mothers who are breast feeding as well as in those who are not. At one time it was believed that this was brought about because the lobules of the breast gland became overdistended with milk, but engorgement is really an exaggeration of the normal venous and lymph stasis of the breasts which occurs in relation to lactation (see "The Breasts" in Chap. 13). The breasts become tense and swollen for a day or so, with the result that the mother experiences throbbing breast pains which may extend into the axilla. The breasts are sometimes so immensely distended and painful that some analgesic medication, such as codeine, may be required. The condition may be relieved by supporting the breasts properly with a tight breast binder or brassière, worn day and night, and by applying icecaps, at intervals, over the affected areas. When the breasts are well supported, they are not only more comfortable but also, if pendulous, the support aids in preventing congestion caused by the interference with the circulation (see Fig. 181). Immediate treatment of engorged breasts is important, because if the condition is allowed to persist it may threaten the mother's future milk supply. With prompt attention, the engorgement usually subsides after 24 to 48 hours. If the mother is breast feeding, the regular emptying of the breasts by suckling and adequate breast care will then be all that is necessary.

The mother who is desirous of breast feeding may have additional problems when she is trying to nurse her infant. Because of the fullness of the breasts and the simultaneous flattening of the nipple, the infant may be unable to get a proper grasp on the areola and nipple. Sometimes the use of the breast pump at very low pressure, and for only a few minutes, prior to the feeding will bring the nipple out sufficiently to permit the infant to grasp it. It must be remembered that too vigorous use of the breast pump or frequent and prolonged nursing periods are irritating to the breast, as well as highly discomforting to the mother. When the engorgement is pronounced, it may be helpful to apply hot compresses to the breasts before the nursing period.

Drying Up the Breasts

When the mother is not breast feeding, for one reason or another, measures must be taken to inhibit lacteal secretion. This is discussed in Chapter 14.

Abnormalities in Mammary Secretion

It is obvious to the nurse who has had experience taking care of new mothers and their infants that there are marked individual variations in the amount of milk secreted by the breast in almost every case. In most instances it depends on the degree of development of the glandular portions of the breast rather than on the individual's general health

or the physical appearance of these organs. A mother with large, well-formed breasts may be eager to breast feed her infant but produces such a meager quantity of breast milk that she is unable to do so. On the other hand, another mother with small, flat breasts may have a remarkably good milk supply and be able to suckle her infant successfully. Obese women with exceedingly large breasts, the bulk of which is fatty tissue, usually do not have a good supply of breast milk for their infants.

When there is an absolute lack of mammary secretion, the condition is called *agalactia*. This condition rarely occurs and is seldom seen; in fact, one of the authors has seen it only once in 13 years. As a rule, there is at least a small amount of mammary secretion, but it is so scant that, despite all efforts to stimulate lactation, the quantity would be inadequate to supply the nourishment required for the infant. Since in the latter instance it is a case of hyposecretion rather than an absolute lack of it, perhaps in time it will be more properly called hypogalactia. One point should be made clear here. When one speaks of abnormalities in mammary secretions, this does not refer to temporary episodes which may momentarily affect lactation but in no way affect the mother's ability to continue on with breast feeding. For example, many new mothers, especially primiparas, who have been breast feeding their infants quite successfully in the hospital find that when they are discharged home there is a sudden diminution in their milk supply. More than likely this is due to the anxiety and fatigue involved with the experience, because once they are settled and rested at home, the milk supply usually resumes normally. This happens so frequently that new mothers are warned that it might occur.

Occasionally the other extreme in lactation is observed, in that the mammary secretion is excessive, so-called *polygalactia*. When this secretion is so copious that it constantly leaks from the nipples it is called *galactorrhea*. The latter condition is not common, but when it does occur it may be hazardous to the mother's health if it continues over a prolonged period. The condition is best treated by measures which are similar to those used to "dry up the breasts," i.e., limit the fluid intake, use a tight breast binder and apply icecaps to the breasts, in this instance immediately after breast feeding. In addition, the failure to empty the breasts completely at each feeding may help to check the excessive secretion.

Abnormalities of the Nipples

Variations in what is considered to be normal in the nipple, which is cylindrical in shape and projects well beyond the center of the areolar surface, are not unusual and present no difficulty until the mother wants to breast feed her infant. The *flat nipple*, i.e., a slightly rounded projection above the breast surface, or the *depressed nipple*, i.e., one which is slightly depressed below the breast surface, are difficult for the infant to grasp with its mouth. The *inverted nipple* is the most pronounced variation, because this nipple is actually inverted, and in this state it is impossible for the infant to grasp it. When these abnormalities exist, the mother should begin corrective measures during pregnancy, such as described by Hoffman (p. 159). Afterward, the use of an electric breast pump or a rubber nipple shield at the beginning of each nursing period may be of value to help draw the nipple out. This may require considerable patience and persistence on the part of the mother, but, with encouragement and help from the nurse, she may be successful. However, a real danger may arise if persistent efforts at breast feeding are attempted and are unsuccessful, because the breasts become engorged and/or the nipples become sore, with resultant fissures or erosions on the surface. These raw, cracked surface areas make breast feeding a very painful experience for the mother and, moreover, provide a portal of entry for pathogenic bacteria which may give rise to mastitis.

Mastitis

Mastitis, or inflammation of the breast, may vary from a "simple" inflammation of the tissues to a suppurative process which results in abscess formation in the glandular tissue. Mastitis is always the result of an infection, usually caused by *Staphylococcus aureus* or hemolytic streptococcus organisms. The disease in most instances is preceded by fissures or erosions of the nipple or the areola, which provide a portal of entry to the subcutaneous lymphatics, although, under conducive conditions, organisms present in the lactiferous ducts can invade the tissues and cause mastitis.

Symptoms. Puerperal mastitis may occur any time during lactation but usually occurs about the third or fourth week of the puerperium. There is usually marked engorgement of the breast preceding mastitis, although engorgement per se does not cause the infection. When the infection occurs, the patient complains of acute pain and tenderness in the breast and often experiences general malaise, a chilly sensation or, in fact, may have a chill followed by a marked rise of temperature and an increased pulse rate. On inspection, the breast appears hard and reddened. The obstetrician should be notified at once and treatment instituted promptly in the hope that resolution may take place before the infection becomes localized as an abscess.

Treatment. Puerperal mastitis is preventable, for the most part, by prophylactic measures. An important measure is initiated when the expectant mother learns about breast hygiene and begins to take special care of her breasts during the latter months of pregnancy (see Chap. 8). After delivery, appropriate breast care will further help to prevent the development of lesions, but if they do occur, proper treatment must be given promptly. Any time the mother complains of sore, tender nipples, they should be inspected immediately. At this time there may be no break in the surface, but if the condition is neglected, the nipple may become raw and cracked. The alert nurse can often detect even a very small crack in the surface of the nipple if she inspects it carefully. Once a break in the skin occurs, the chances of infection mount, because pathogenic organisms are frequently brought to the breast by the hands or may reach the breast from the patient's nightgown or bedclothes.

With early treatment by antibiotics or chemotherapeutic agents, the inflammatory process may be brought under control before suppuration occurs. Penicillin is effective in treating acute puerperal mastitis if the therapy is started promptly, and often symptoms subside within 24 to 48 hours. The breasts should be well supported with a tight breast binder rather than a brassière. While the breasts are so painful, small side pillows used for support may give the mother some measure of comfort. Icecaps may be applied over the affected part, but if in time it becomes apparent that suppuration is inevitable, heat applications may be ordered to hasten the localization of the abscess. Most obstetricians advise that breast feeding be discontinued immediately in cases of mastitis.

If the treatment outlined above is unsuccessful, measures will have to be taken to remove the pus when abscess formation occurs. The obstetrician may prefer to aspirate the pus rather than resort to incision and drainage in some cases. When incision and drainage is done, the abscess should be well walled off. The operation is performed under general anesthesia, so the nurse must prepare the patient for surgery accordingly. In operating, the incision is made radially, extending from near the areolar margin toward the periphery of the gland, in order to avoid injury to the lactiferous ducts. After the pus is evacuated, a gauze drain is inserted. Following the operation, the care of the patient is essentially the same as that for a surgical patient. Complete recovery is usually prompt.

Epidemic Puerperal Breast Abscess

During the last decade a type of puerperal breast abscess has been seen, both in this country and abroad, which is unlike the type described above. In this new manifestation, the offending organism is also *Staphylococcus aureus,* but an antibiotic-resistant strain which has been identified by bacteriophage typing as 52/42B/80/81 and called the "epidemic" strain. Another difference is related to the portal of entry of these micro-organisms. In these cases there is no history of nipple lesions, and the infection is introduced through apparently normal lactiferous ducts in the breast, not through the connective tissue. An infant who has been exposed to the epidemic strain of the staphylococcus, and has the organisms present in his nose and throat, can introduce the infection to the mother's breast in the process of nursing. Once these organisms are introduced into the mother's breast, milk provides a superb culture medium for them. Efforts to prevent puerperal mastitis cannot be limited to the care of the mother's breasts but must extend to the hospital nursery where the infant may acquire the virulent organism. In the nursery such equipment as soap-solution containers, cribs, mattresses, blankets, linens and floors can harbor the organisms. Some methods to help control the spread of infection at its source include rigid nursery aseptic technic on the part of all personnel, measures to prevent the spread of organisms from infant to infant, such as proper spacing of cribs, and the exclusion of carriers from the maternity divisions as soon as they are identified. It should be remembered that in maternity hospitals the nasopharynx of new-born infants tends to become readily infected with *Staphylococcus aureus,* and, moreover, the infection may persist for some weeks after the infant leaves the hospital. Where intensive studies have been carried out and puerperal mastitis or breast abscess appeared after discharge from the hospital, the cultures of the mothers' nares on admission to the hospital did not show evidence of the epidemic strain of the organism. In these cases the infant was the source of infection, because the offending organism was cultured from the nose, the throat and the skin of the infants.

Symptoms. The symptoms of epidemic puerperal breast abscess develop slowly and subtly and usually appear about the third or fourth week after delivery. The condition is characterized by high fever; the breast becomes very tender, swollen and indurated and suppurates rapidly. The surface of the breast may not be consistently reddened because the abscess is often deep. In some cases the infection may involve more than one portion of the breast, or both breasts.

Treatment and Care. The underlying principles for the care of this form of breast abscess are essentially the same as those described in puerperal mastitis. Breast feeding should be discontinued immediately, for obvious reasons. Since the offending organism here is antibiotic-resistant, the effects of antibiotic therapy are of questionable value. Nearly all of these infections are susceptible to chloramphenicol, erythromycin and bacitracin but have identical antibiotic sensitivity with resistance to tetracycline, streptomycin and penicillin. The staphylococcus develops antibiotic resistance easily. In the beginning, the treatment of these infections with erythromycin usually resulted in prompt improvement in the condition, but now erythromycin-resistant strains of coagulase-positive staphylococci have been isolated from infections of mothers

and their infants. When suppuration occurs in the breast, incision and drainage is usually done as soon as localization of the abscess becomes evident, in order to limit the extent of tissue destruction. When this has been done, special measures must be employed for the control of infection. To protect the surrounding area of the breast, it should be washed with a soap containing hexachlorophene, because such cleansing reduces the occurrence of staphylococci to some degree. This soap is also advocated for hand washing and baths. When warm moist applications to the wound are prescribed, vigilance and care must be exercised so that the underlying skin does not become macerated. Aside from the unnecessary discomfort that this would cause the mother, such maceration would provide another portal of entry for micro-organisms. When such infections occur, either in the mother or her infant, the nurse should emphasize health teaching in her care of the mother, not only concerning hygienic measures for the prevention of skin infections, but also the urgency for prompt treatment of any member of the family if carbuncles, boils, burns or other skin lesions develop.

The *epidemiologic aspects* of antibiotic-resistant infections of infants and their mothers are far reaching and a major problem, because when these infections occur, nearly all the hospitals in the community may be affected for varying periods of time. A few years ago this was considered a "hospital" infection, but now it may be found throughout a general community. Once the organism is introduced into a family, this organism can be the cause of disease in the family over a long period of time. For example, the infant may acquire the infection in the maternity nursery, 4 weeks later the mother may develop a breast abscess, and 5 months later the father may develop a boil—all caused by this epidemic strain of staphylococcus. Flaws in nursery "clean technic" in hospital nurseries have long been cited as the cause of spreading skin infections in the newborn, but when these epidemic infections have occurred in hospital nurseries, and the staff has scrutinized their technic and improved it wherever possible, the results have not been as gratifying as one would hope for, because the epidemics have disappeared and appeared again after a period of time. In fact, large numbers of infections have occurred despite meticulous nursery technic. It must be remembered that these infections are not confined to the maternity service but may be spread by carriers to or from other clinical services in the hospital as well as to other members of the family and the community. The infection is thought to be airborne and is easily spread by droplet contamination from the nasopharynx of carriers of these micro-organisms. Scrupulous technic in giving patient care in the hospital is undoubtedly an important factor in prevention and control, both in the nurseries or on postpartal divisions, but this alone will not solve the problem. Washing with hexachlorophene has already been mentioned as a means to reduce the occurrence of staphylococcal infections, but this has not reduced the colonization of the organisms in the nasopharynx of individuals. The housekeeping functions which are routine in every institution are of vast importance, both from the standpoint of procedure and personnel, and should be investigated and improved as much as possible. The nurse will find it advantageous to pursue the current literature regarding antibiotic-resistant staphylococcal infections, because there is a wealth of information in the professional journals and space here does not permit an adequate discussion of the subject. Some references have been listed among the suggested readings at the end of this chapter.

BLADDER COMPLICATIONS

The two most common bladder complications in the puerperium are retention of urine and residual urine. In the former, the patient is unable to void at all; in the latter, she is able to void certain amounts of urine but is unable to empty the bladder.

Retention of urine, or the inability to void, is more frequently seen after operative delivery. It often lasts 5 or 6 days but may persist for 2 weeks or longer. The main cause is probably due to edema of the trigone, which may be so pronounced that it obstructs the urethra. Very temporary urinary retention may be due to the effects of analgesia and anesthesia received in labor. As already stressed, the nurse should make every effort to have the patient void within 6 hours after delivery (see Chap. 14). If the patient has not done so within 8 hours, the physician usually will order catheterization. In some hospitals this is routine if voiding has not occurred within 8 hours postpartum. The nurse should remember that it may not be prudent for her to wait for a designated lapse of time to indicate when the bladder should be emptied; rather she must be observant for evidence indicating the degree of bladder distention, because the bladder may fill in a shorter span of time than has been specified and this should be reported to the physician. At this particular period the bladder has increased capacity, and, because it is usually not as sensitive to distention as prior to pregnancy, overdistention and incomplete emptying may occur, thus the problem of residual urine frequently results. Repeated catheterization may be necessary for several days; or the physician may request the insertion of an indwelling catheter which will provide constant drainage.

When the mother continues to void small amounts of urine at frequent intervals, the nurse may suspect that these voidings are merely an overflow of a distended bladder and that there is residual urine there. The physician will order catheterization for residual urine, and, to be completely accurate, this must be done within 5 minutes after the patient voids. If 60 cc. or more of urine still remains in the bladder after the patient has voided, it is usually considered that the voiding has been incomplete. It is not uncommon for the catheterization to yield 800 cc. or more of residual urine. Large amounts of urine (from 60 to 1,500 cc., as shown by catheterization) may remain in the bladder, even though the patient may think she has completely emptied her bladder when she voided. The condition is due primarily to lack of tone in the bladder wall and is more likely to occur when the mother's bladder has been allowed to become overdistended during labor. A distended bladder requires prompt attention because of the resultant trauma; moreover, it may be a predisposing cause of postpartal hemorrhage.

In many cases of residual urine the patient is without symptoms other than scanty urination, but in others there may also be suprapubic or perineal discomfort. The treatment of this condition is usually confined to catheterization after each voiding until the residual urine becomes less than 30 cc. In severe cases constant drainage by means of an indwelling catheter may be employed.

The normal bladder is very resistant to infection, but when stagnant urine remains in a traumatized bladder and infectious organisms are present there is danger of cystitis. When cystitis occurs the patient often has a low-grade fever, frequent and painful urination and marked tenderness and discomfort over the area of the bladder. The physician will order a catheterized specimen of urine for microscopic examination, and if pus cells are present in association with residual urine, the diagnosis of cystitis is confirmed. Since it is important in the presence of bladder infection to avoid accumulations of stagnant urine in the bladder, an indwelling bladder catheter may be inserted. In addition, chemotherapeutic agents are prescribed and fluids should be forced.

PUERPERAL PSYCHOSES

These are discussed in Chapter 9, The Mental Hygiene of Pregnancy.

PULMONARY EMBOLISM

Pulmonary embolism is usually due to the detachment of a small part of a thrombus which is washed along in the blood current until it becomes lodged in the right side of the heart. In many cases the thrombus originates in a uterine or a pelvic vein, although its origin may be in some other vessel. When the embolus occludes the pulmonary artery, it obstructs the passage of blood into the lungs, either wholly or in part, and the patient may die of asphyxia within a few minutes. If the clot is small the initial episode may not be fatal, although repeated attacks may prove so. The condition may follow infection, thrombosis, severe hemorrhage or shock, and it may occur any time during the puerperium, especially after sudden exertion.

Symptoms. The symptoms of pulmonary embolism are sudden intense pain over the heart; severe dyspnea; unusual apprehension; syncope; feeble, irregular or imperceptible pulse; pallor in some cases, cyanosis in others; and eventually air hunger. Death may occur at any time from within a few minutes to a few hours, according to the amount or degree of obstruction to the pulmonary circulation. If the patient survives for a few hours, it is likely that she may recover.

Treatment. The treatment consists, first of all, in preventing the accident by careful attention to all details of surgical asepsis and to the proper management of labor and delivery. Following delivery, early ambulation may be an additional prophylactic measure, since circulatory stasis is undoubtedly a causative factor. In some instances it is almost impossible to prevent a fatal attack, because the patient may be recovering without elevation of temperature and without complications and yet, on the seventh or tenth day, suddenly cries out, passes into a coma and succumbs.

When embolism occurs, rapid emergency measures to combat anoxia and shock must be carried out promptly. Oxygen is administered without delay and anticoagulants are given. Morphine may be helpful to relieve the patient's apprehension and is usually given. It is essential that the patient be kept absolutely quiet and on her back, for the slightest movement may cause fatal results. If the patient survives the attack, absolute rest is mandatory, in the hope that meanwhile the clot may be absorbed. Dicumarol therapy will be continued to prevent recurrent emboli. During this time the patient must be kept warm, quiet, comfortable and as free from worry as possible. She may be given a light, nourishing diet during early convalescence.

SUGGESTED READING

Adams, Ralph, et al.: Control of infections within hospitals, J.A.M.A. 169: 1557, 1959.

Bookmiller, Mae, and Bowen, George: Textbook of Obstetrics and Obstetric Nursing, ed. 3, Philadelphia, Saunders, 1958.

Carrington, Elsie R., and Sivak, Alice M.: Epidemic puerperal breast abscess: I. Preventive and therapeutic aspects; II. Nursing care, Am. J. Nursing 58:1683, 1958.

Davis, M. E., and Scheckler, C. E.: DeLee's Obstetrics for Nurses, ed. 16, Philadelphia, Saunders, 1957.

Duckman, Simon, and Hubbard, John F.: The role of fluids in relieving breast engorgement without the use of hormones, Am. J. Obst. & Gynec. 60:200, 1950.

Eastman, Nicholson J.: Williams Obstetrics, ed. 11, New York, Appleton, 1956.

Greenhill, J. P.: Obstetrics, ed. 11, Philadelphia, Saunders, 1955.

Guibeau, Joseph A., et al.: Aureomycin in obstetrics, J.A.M.A. 143:520, 1950.

McElin, T. W., et al.: Puerperal hematomas, Am. J. Obst. & Gynec. 67:356, 1954.

Navori, C. A.: Severe hemorrhage and maternal death associated with amniotic fluid embolism, Am. J. Obst. & Gynec. 67:432, 1954.

Newton, Michael, and Newton, Niles R.: Postpartum engorgement of the breast, Am. J. Obst. & Gynec. 61:664, 1951.

Ravenholt, Reimert T., et al.: Staphylococcal infections in the hospital and community (Symposium), Am. J. Pub. Health 48:277, 1958.

Redfield, R. L., and Bodini, K. R.: Air embolism following knee-chest position, J.A.M.A. 113:671, 1939.

Rienzo, John S.: The use of hormones for prevention of breast engorgement and lactation, Am. J. Obst. & Gynec. 66:1248, 1953.

Shaffer, T. E., et al.: Staphylococcal infections in newborn infants: I. Study of an epidemic among infants and nursing mothers, Pediatrics 18:750, 1956.

Van Blarcom, Carolyn C., and Ziegel, Erna: Obstetrical Nursing, ed. 4, New York, Macmillan, 1957.

Wolfe, S. A., and Pedowitz, P.: Late postpartum hemorrhage, Am. J. Obst. & Gynec. 53:84, 1947.

Wysham, D. N., et al.: Staphylococcal infections in an obstetric unit: I. Epidemiologic studies of pyoderma neonatorum; II. Epidemiologic studies of puerperal mastitis, New England J. Med. 257:304, 1957.

Zilboorg, Gregory: Clinical issues of postpartum psychopathologic reactions, Am. J. Obst. & Gynec. 73:305, 1957.

CONFERENCE MATERIAL

1. What provisions are made in regard to the care of the infant when the mother develops a puerperal infection in the hospital? At home? What are the implications for the nurse making a home visit?

2. As you consider the situation in which you are working, what measures could be instituted by the hospital or public health agency to further the prevention and the control of infection? What is the role of the nurse in this endeavor?

3. If the mother develops a rash 3

days after delivery and a diagnosis of scarlet fever has been made, what would you consider to be the method of managing this problem?

4. An infant has been exposed to infection caused by staphylococci of the epidemic strain while in the hospital nursery. What instructions should be given the mother concerning the prevention and the control of infection following their discharge from the hospital?

5. How do you account for the maternal mortality rate due to postpartal complications? What contribution can the nurse make toward improving these conditions?

6. If you have a patient whose preg-nancy was complicated by cardiac disease (or tuberculosis, or syphilis or diabetes), and who is discharged from the hospital in satisfactory condition following delivery, what would be the responsibility of the hospital and the public health agency in the community for this patient's health supervision? Who has the responsibility for initiating referrals to related health agencies?

7. What routine procedures are employed in maternity care for the detection and the control of venereal disease? How would you go about finding out which states in the U. S. have legislation governing premarital and antepartal health examinations? What is the existing legislation in your state?

Study Questions

UNIT SEVEN: ABNORMALITIES OF OBSTETRICS

Read through the entire question and place your answers in the parentheses.

1. Which of the following signs and symptoms should the nurse anticipate when a pregnant patient has a history of heart disease?
A. Dyspnea
B. Slow pulse rate
C. Decrease in blood pressure
D. Hemorrhage
Select the number corresponding to the correct letter or letters.
    1. A only
    2. B only
    3. A, C and D
    4. All of them

                                                  (——1——)

2. Which of the following factors influence the answer which you have given in Question No. 1?
A. Increased need for oxygen intake
B. Increased blood volume
C. Toxic damage to the heart
D. Failure of kidneys to excrete
Select the number corresponding to the correct letters.
    1. A and B
    2. A and C
    3. B, C and D
    4. All of them

                                                  (——1——)

3. Which of the following signs and symptoms would the patient with a ruptured fallopian tube manifest?
A. Hegar's sign
B. Intense pain
C. Profound shock
D. Irregular fetal heart tones
E. Vaginal bleeding
Select the number corresponding to the correct letters.
    1. A and B
    2. A, C and D
    3. B, C and E
    4. B, D and E

                                                  (——3——)

4. Which of the following factors must exist before an erythroblastotic infant can be produced?

Note: The key to the correct answers to these questions is given on page 533.

A. Rh-negative mother
B. Rh-positive father
C. Rh-positive fetus
D. Rh-positive substance from the fetus must find its way into the mother's blood stream to build up antibodies.
E. Mother must have had a previous Rh-positive pregnancy or transfusion.
Select the number corresponding to the correct letters.
    1. A and D
    2. A, C and D
    3. B, C and E
    4. All of them

(———4———)

5. What is the best known method to prevent erythroblastosis fetalis?
A. Early determination of Rh factor of parents
B. Transfusing the mother during pregnancy
C. Transfusing all Rh-negative fathers
D. Transfusing all Rh-negative babies
E. Repeated small transfusions of Rh-positive blood to the mother
Select the number corresponding to the correct letter or letters.
    1. A only
    2. A and B
    3. B, C and D
    4. C, D and E

(———1———)

6. Which of the following statements concerning diabetes complicated by pregnancy are correct?
A. The size of the placenta tends to be in direct relationship to the size of the infant.
B. Toxemia occurs more frequently than in nondiabetic pregnancies.
C. Deliveries are always performed by cesarean section, usually 2 weeks prior to term.
D. The fetus tends to be large.
E. Hypoglycemia occurs in the infant following delivery.
Select the number corresponding to the correct letters.
    1. A and B
    2. B, D and E
    3. B, C, D and E
    4. All of them

(———2———)

7. Which of the following are causes of bleeding in the first and second trimesters of pregnancy?
A. Menstruation
B. Abortion
C. Abruptio placentae
D. Placenta previa
E. Ectopic pregnancy
Select the number corresponding to the correct letters.
    1. A and B
    2. A, B and D
    3. A, B and E
    4. B, C, D and E

(———3———)

8. How is inevitable abortion distinguished from threatened abortion?
A. Dilatation of the cervical canal
B. Rupture of the membranes
C. Pain
D. Bleeding
Select the number corresponding to the correct letter or letters.
   1. A only
   2. B only
   3. A, B and D
   4. All of them

(——————)

9. What is the effect of tetanic contractions on the pregnant uterus?
A. Descent and rotation are hastened
B. Ruptured uterus is imminent
C. Fetal distress may occur
D. Uterine inertia may follow
E. Perineal lacerations may occur
Select the number corresponding to the correct letter or letters.
   1. A only
   2. B only
   3. A, C and D
   4. B, C and E

(·——————)

10. Insofar as the toxemias are concerned, which of the following symptoms during labor should be reported to the physician promptly?
A. Hard, painful uterine contractions
B. Epigastric pain
C. Dimness of vision
D. Headache
E. Decrease in urinary excretion
Select the number corresponding to the correct letters.
   1. A, C and D
   2. A, C and E
   3. B, C and D
   4. B, C, D and E

(——————)

11. Which of the following conditions contribute to postpartal hemorrhage?
A. Toxemias of pregnancy
B. Overdistention of the uterus due to twins or hydramnios
C. Unwise management of the third stage of labor
D. Involution
E. Retained placental fragments
Select the number corresponding to the correct letters.
   1. A and C
   2. A, B and D
   3. B, C and E
   4. All of them

(———₃———)

12. A patient in the first stage of labor develops secondary uterine inertia. Which of the following are important in the treatment of this condition?
A. Pitocin
B. Sedation
C. Fluids
D. Bed rest
E. Ambulation
Select the number corresponding to the correct letters.
   1. A, B and D
   2. A, C and E
   3. B, C and D
   4. B, C and E

(——3——)

13. To which of the following causes may urinary tract infections during the puerperium be attributed?
A. Poor hygiene
B. Urinary retention
C. Uterine inertia
D. Subinvolution
E. Trauma sustained during delivery
Select the number corresponding to the correct letters.
   1. A and B
   2. A, B and E
   3. B, D and E
   4. All of them

(——2——)

14. Which of the following are the chief dangers from sore, cracked nipples?
A. Infection of the infant from nursing
B. Invasion of bacteria resulting in abscess of the nipple
C. Invasion of bacteria through the nipple into the breast tissue, resulting in abscessed breast
D. Formation of scar tissue which will prevent normal nursing thereafter
E. Formation of a permanent fissure in the nipple
Select the number corresponding to the correct letters.
   1. A and C
   2. B and C
   3. B, D and E
   4. B, C, D and E

(——2——)

15. Which of the following veins is likely to be involved in puerperal thrombophlebitis?
A. Splenic vein
B. Popliteal vein
C. Renal vein
D. Ovarian vein
E. Saphenous vein
Select the number corresponding to the correct letters.
   1. A, B and D
   2. B, C and E
   3. B, D and E
   4. All of them

(——3——)

16. In the spaces provided in Column 2, write the term or the phrase which best fits each statement in Column 1.

Column 1	Column 2
A. A suppurative process in the glandular structure of the breast	A. _mastitis_
B. A localized infection of the lining membrane of the uterus	B. _endometritis_
C. An infection of the loose connective tissue which surrounds the uterus	C. _parametritis_
D. Failure of the puerperal uterus to be restored to its normal proportions as rapidly as expected	D. _subinvolution_
E. Exaggeration of the normal venous and lymphatic stasis of the breasts following the development of lacteal secretion	E. _engorgement_

Note: The key to the correct answers to these questions is given on page 533.

UNIT EIGHT

Abnormalities of the Fetus and the Newborn

Asphyxia Neonatorum
Injuries
Infections
Malformations
Hemolytic Disease of the Newborn
Miscellaneous Disorders

CHAPTER TWENTY-ONE

Disorders of the Newborn

ASPHYXIA NEONATORUM

Normally, the infant cries immediately after delivery—often when the shoulders are being born. If respiration has not begun within 30 seconds or so after birth, the condition usually is referred to as *asphyxia neonatorum*. This complication may show various gradations from brief, transitory apnea (absence of respiration) to fatal respiratory failure. In the milder cases the infant's face and often the entire body are of a livid hue, and the vessels of the umbilical cord are distended with blood; the tone of the muscles is good, so that any attempt to move the extremities or open the mouth will meet with some resistance. This stage of the process is known as *asphyxia livida*. In severe cases the infant's face and body are of a deathlike pallor, the vessels of the cord empty and the muscles relaxed so that the infant is entirely limp. This stage is known as *asphyxia pallida*.

Failure of the infant to breathe at birth usually is due to one of three main causes, or to a combination of them:

1. Anoxia (deprivation of oxygen)
2. Cerebral injury
3. Narcosis

Anoxia. Since the infant in utero is entirely dependent on the placenta for its oxygen supply, any interference with the function of that organ or with that of the umbilical cord will put the infant in grave danger because of anoxia. If the oxygen supply is entirely cut off for more than a very few minutes, fetal

death in utero results; if only partially curtailed, the infant is born in an asphyxiated state and (like all asphyxiated persons) does not breathe.

Intra-uterine asphyxia may be produced in a number of ways. The umbilical cord may prolapse and become pinched between the pelvic brim and the fetal head, with the result that the umbilical vein becomes compressed and unable to carry oxygen to the infant. Premature separation of the placenta often disrupts placental function entirely so that the baby suffers complete deprivation of oxygen. Extremely severe uterine contractions may so squeeze the placental site as to jeopardize the infant's oxygen supply.

Cerebral Injury. This is a very common cause of apnea at birth, particularly after difficult deliveries. Not only may the associated brain hemorrhage damage the respiratory center itself, but other vital centers may be injured. Cerebral injury at birth may be caused by difficult operative delivery, such as midforceps operations, version and extraction and breech extraction. Likewise, disproportion between the size of the head and that of the pelvis may bring about such compression of the fetal skull as to damage the brain. Cerebral injury may also result from long, difficult labor when no instruments are used.

Narcosis. The narcosis produced in the fetus by analgesic and anesthetic drugs given to the mother is a frequent cause of sluggish respiration at birth. As a rule, however, this is quite tran-

473

sitory, and statistics indicate that these infants do as well subsequently as infants whose mothers received no such drugs. This explains why nurses with adequate experience should supervise these patients closely.

Prevention of Asphyxia Neonatorum

Preventive treatment is very important but is largely the responsibility of the obstetrician. It begins with the first antepartal visit when he measures the pelvis and makes sure that it is large enough to allow passage of the infant's head without compression. Good diet and hygiene contribute greatly to the health of the infant at birth. During labor, the physician can do much to prevent asphyxia of the infant by care in the use of analgesic and anesthetic drugs and by avoiding as much as possible the more difficult types of operative delivery. Moreover, by listening regularly to the fetal heart tones, the attendant may detect early signs of impending fetal distress (slow and/or irregular rate), and, with this warning, it may be possible for the physician to deliver the infant before serious trouble develops. The passage of meconium-stained amniotic fluid is another sign of fetal distress but is of no value in breech presentations, since the passage of meconium—ordinarily pure meconium—is the rule in breech cases.

Many physicians believe that the administration of vitamin K to the mother late in pregnancy and during labor tends to prevent cerebral hemorrhage in the newborn by improving the clotting power of the fetus' blood. This antihemorrhagic vitamin passes readily through the placenta and raises the prothrombin concentration of the fetal plasma which is ordinarily low. Since prothrombin is known to be essential to proper blood coagulation, this measure is theoretically a sound one, and the practical experience of a number of obstetricians suggests that it may prove to be a valuable procedure.

Treatment of Asphyxia Neonatorum

In treating an infant which does not breathe at birth, there are 5 main principles to be kept in mind.

1. Gentleness. These infants are often in a state of shock, and rough attempts to resuscitate them—as by vigorous spanking or other overvigorous methods of external stimulation—may do more harm than good. Methods of physical stimulation should be limited to gentle rubbing of the back and, at the most, to light patting of the buttocks. When anoxia is present, oxygen is necessary to overcome it, and the use of measures which act as external irritants will not oxygenate the tissues.

2. Warmth. Heated cribs and other means of maintaining body warmth, such as hot-water bottles and warm blankets, must be in readiness. This is particularly important to remember because the measures employed to resuscitate infants, unless care be taken, tend to expose their completely naked bodies (accustomed to the temperature in

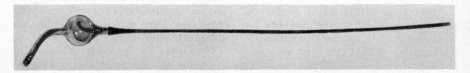

Fig. 261. Catheter and glass bulb with a trap, for aspirating mucus in the treatment of asphyxia. (Chicago Lying-in Hospital)

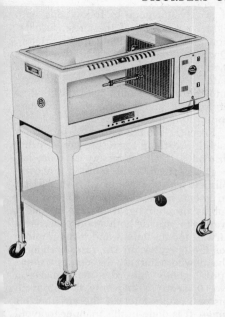

Fig. 262. An explosion-proof baby incubator, constructed especially for use in the delivery room, provides an environment in which desirable levels of heat, humidity and oxygen can be maintained. (The Gordon Armstrong Company, Inc., Cleveland, Ohio)

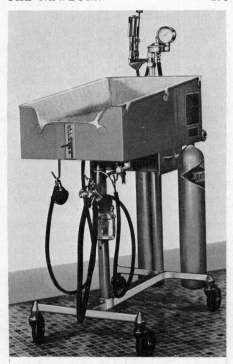

Fig. 263. Kreiselman infant resuscitator (Ohio Chemical and Surgical Equipment Co., Madison, Wis.)

utero) to room temperature; and this may aggravate the state of shock. The body of the infant should be kept covered as much as possible.

3. Posture. Most obstetricians hold the infant up by the feet momentarily after birth in order to expedite drainage of mucus from the trachea, the larynx and the posterior pharynx. The baby is then placed on its back in a slight Trendelenburg position (head turned aside, lower than buttocks), also to favor gravity drainage of mucus.

4. Removal of Mucus. Cleansing the air passages of mucus and fluid is essential, since effective respiration cannot be accomplished through obstructed air passages. The head-down position will promote drainage of mucus and fluid from the respiratory passages, but postural drainage alone is often not adequate for this purpose, and suction of one type or another is frequently necessary. An ordinary catheter is used, size 12 to 14 French; in premature infants a smaller size (8 to 10) is advisable. A glass trap (Fry) is inserted into the catheter to arrest mucus which otherwise might be drawn into the operator's mouth (Fig. 261). Milking the trachea upward will help bring mucus and fluid into the posterior pharynx, where it may be aspirated by the catheter. Gentleness is essential, since the mucous membrane of the infant's mouth is delicate. Although the physician occasionally does so, the nurse should not introduce the catheter farther than the posterior pharynx. Mechanical suction devices are provided with most of the modern machines for infant resuscitation and are very convenient (Fig. 263).

5. Artificial Respiration. If the newborn infant fails to cry or the infant's muscle tone fails to improve within 2 minutes following delivery, the infant *must* receive oxygen promptly. The infant's head should be lowered and positioned to extend the neck; consequently the infant's natural air passage is straightened. As oxygen is administered by mask, the infant's chin should be supported by pressing upward with the fourth and fifth fingers under the angles of the infant's jaw. Mechanical devices for the controlled administration of oxygen are the most efficient, but resuscitation may be carried out in a number of ways when such equipment is not available. Gentle compression of the chest with the hand followed by sudden release may be tried a few times if the person in attendance fully understands this method of manipulation, but unless this produces spontaneous breathing immediately, more efficient methods should be employed.

Probably the oldest method of resuscitation is mouth-to-mouth insufflation, but this is disapproved by some physicians because the method may be dangerous, both from the possibility of rupturing pulmonary alveoli and the risk of infection. Although this procedure is ordinarily performed by the doctor, the nurse may be asked to carry it out if the available physicians are busy attending the mother. The operator stands or sits back of the infant's head. After placing 3 or 4 layers of gauze on the infant's nose and mouth, the operator bends over the infant and puts his opened mouth over the infant's mouth and nose, the gauze intervening. He now exhales gently into the infant's respiratory tract.

It is advantageous to follow this with light compression of the chest, insufflation and compression being alternated. One does not "blow" into the baby's mouth but simply exhales more or less naturally. As mentioned above, blowing into the baby's mouth with any degree of force is highly dangerous and may rupture pulmonary alveoli.

Recently a modification of mouth-to-mouth breathing for resuscitation, using instead a mouth-to-airway technic, has been described.* This method is accomplished with the use of an S-shaped instrument assembled from 2 standard rubber oropharyngeal airways in such a way as to provide both an oropharyngeal airway for the infant and a mouthpiece for the operator. In the resuscitation of the newborn infant, the operator must "puff" gently into the mouthpiece, a No. 0 airway, using only the air from his oral cavity and not the air from his lungs. It is done in this manner to avoid damage to the infant's lungs. As soon as the chest rises, the operator takes his mouth off the mouthpiece and allows the infant to exhale passively before proceeding with the next "puff" of breath into the airway.

Many hospitals are now using mechanical devices for the resuscitation of the newborn. Such apparatus permits the administration of pure oxygen to the baby's lungs at pressures which are controlled mechanically within safe limits.

Atelectasis

Prior to birth, the lungs contain no air and are in a state of collapse. With the first breath, expansion of the lung tissue begins and continues progressively for several days until all parts of the lung are expanded. Feeble respiratory action after birth may expand the lungs only partially, leaving large areas in a collapsed state. This condition is known as "atelectasis." It is particularly

* Safar, P., and McMahon, M.: Mouth-to-airway artificial respiration, J.A.M.A. **166**:1459, 1958.

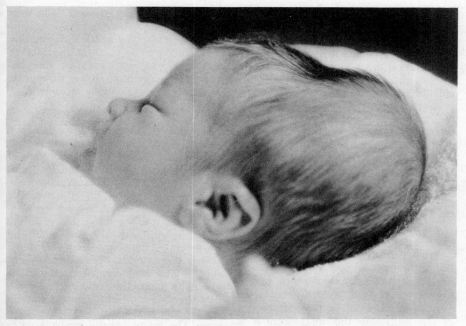

Fig. 264. Caput succedaneum. (MacDonald House, University Hospitals of Cleveland)

common in premature infants. Cyanosis is usually present because the small areas of expanded lung are inadequate to oxygenate the blood properly. Atelectasis is treated best by continuous administration of oxygen, frequent changes of position and occasional attempts to stimulate deeper respiration. However, the outlook in most of these cases is poor.

Hyaline Membrane Disease

Hyaline membrane disease is a syndrome of neonatal respiratory distress in which the alveoli and the alveolar ducts are filled with a sticky exudate, a hyaline material, which prevents aeration. Although it is known that the hyaline material is a protein, the cause of hyaline membrane formation is not definitely known. The condition is observed most frequently in premature infants and infants delivered by cesarean section. A small percentage of infants born at full term are observed to develop this condition, but it is never found in stillborn infants.

The infant may breathe normally at birth and show no signs of respiratory difficulty, but within periods varying from minutes to several hours after birth he develops respiratory distress. This occurs because the hyaline material is deposited and obstructs the flow of air and the exchange of oxygen and carbon dioxide. The cardinal symptoms are cyanosis and dyspnea. If the clinical picture reverses itself promptly, recovery is likely. The infant's color will return to normal, and his respirations will become rhythmic and easy. But if he develops progressive respiratory difficulty and cyanosis and marked sternal retractions increase, death may occur within 48 hours.

Treatment primarily consists of placing the infant in an incubator to facilitate the administration of oxygen and the maintenance of high humidity as soon as the first signs and symptoms are observed. Since infants delivered by cesarean section are prone to develop this disease, they should be placed in an incubator with oxygen and high humidity immediately upon delivery as a prophylactic measure. Moreover, the immediate care for these infants should include the aspiration of stomach contents, as well as oropharyngeal suctioning to remove mucus and fluid from the nose and the mouth.

INJURIES

Caput Succedaneum

Prolonged pressure on the head during a protracted first stage of labor, where the membranes rupture before the cervix is fully dilated, causes an edematous swelling of the soft tissues of the scalp over the area where it is encircled by the cervix (Fig. 264). This is called "caput succedaneum," and in its milder forms is very common—so common that it may be regarded as normal.

It is due to an extravasation of serum into the tissues of the scalp at the portion surrounded by the cervix during labor and free from pressure. The term is not confined to vertex cases; the corresponding swelling which forms on any presenting part is also, for the sake of uniformity, known as caput succedaneum. The condition always disappears within a few days without treatment.

Cephalhematoma

Another swelling of the scalp which resembles caput succedaneum in certain respects is caused by an effusion of blood between the bone and the periosteum (Fig. 265). This explains why the swelling appears directly over the bone. It is most common over the parietal bones. It is seldom visible when the infant is born and may not be noticed for several hours or more after delivery, since subperiosteal bleeding occurs slowly. The cephalhematoma increases gradually in size until about the seventh day after labor, when it remains stationary for a time and then begins to disappear. The infant usually recovers without treatment. It may be due to pressure in normal labor, or by forceps; but also it is seen occasionally in breech cases in which no instruments were used or prolonged pressure exerted on the aftercoming head. Such cases, however, are not common.

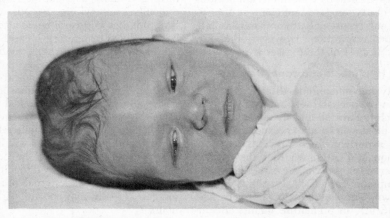

Fig. 265. Cephalhematoma. (MacDonald House, University Hospitals of Cleveland)

Intracranial Hemorrhage

Synonyms for this condition are cerebral hemorrhage and brain hemorrhage. In contradistinction to the two conditions just described, intracranial hemorrhage is one of the gravest complications encountered in the newborn. It may occur any place in the cranial vault but is particularly likely to take place as the result of tears in the tentorium cerebelli with bleeding into the cerebellum, the pons and the medulla oblongata. Since these structures contain many important centers (respiratory center, etc.), hemorrhage in these areas is very often fatal.

Intracranial hemorrhage occurs most often after prolonged labor, especially in primiparae, and is particularly likely to take place in difficult forceps deliveries and in version and extractions. It is also seen more commonly in precipitate deliveries as the result of the rapid propulsion of the infant's head through the birth canal. It is due primarily to excessive or unduly prolonged pressure on the fetal skull. This causes excessive molding of the head and such overriding of the cranial bones that the delicate supporting structures of the brain (tentorium cerebelli, falx cerebri, etc.) are torn, with consequent rupture of blood vessels.

The development of symptoms in cerebral hemorrhage may be sudden or gradual. If the hemorrhage is severe, the infant is usually stillborn; if less marked, apnea neonatorum may result, often with fatal outcome. Many infants which are resuscitated with difficulty at birth succumb later from brain hemorrhage. On the other hand, the infant may appear normal after delivery and develop the first signs of intracranial hemorrhage several hours or several days later.

The nurse should be familiar with the common signs of cerebral hemorrhage, which are described as follows.

1. **Convulsions.** These may vary from mild, localized twitchings to severe spasms of the whole body. Twitching of the lower jaw is characteristic, particularly when associated with salivation.

2. **Cyanosis.** This may be persistent but is more likely to occur in repeated attacks.

3. **Abnormal Respiration.** Grunting respiration is characteristic; or it may be irregular, of Cheyne-Stokes type, or very rapid and shallow, or very slow. Very slow breathing usually is associated with cyanosis, suggests respiratory paralysis due to pressure on the medulla oblongata and is a grave sign.

4. **A Sharp, Shrill, Weak Cry.** This is similar to that seen in meningitis.

5. **Flaccidity.** If persistent, this usually portends a fatal outcome.

Treatment. Prevention is most important but is largely the responsibility of the physician. It consists in protecting the infant from trauma, particularly in difficult operative delivery. As stated previously, many obstetricians believe that the administration of vitamin K to the mother before delivery decreases the likelihood of cerebral bleeding. Moreover, following operative delivery, often it is given to the infant hypodermically as a prophylactic measure.

Curative treatment is rarely effective, since considerable damage, as a rule, already has been done to the brain tissue when the signs of the condition first develop. Complete rest, with the very minimum amount of handling, is imperative. Infants suspected of having a cerebral hemorrhage should not nurse the breast and should not be weighed or bathed. Since shock is often present, external heat is frequently indicated. Feeding should be carried out in such a manner as to impose on the infant the least possible effort; some of these infants have to be gavaged. Usually the physician will order some form of sedative for convulsions and will prescribe the administration of oxygen for cyanosis. The head of the infant should be kept a few inches above the level of the hips, because this position is believed to lower intracranial pressure. Moreover, the infant should *not* be placed in Trendelenburg position after delivery.

Facial Paralysis

Pressure by forceps on the facial nerve may cause temporary paralysis of the muscles of one side of the face so that the mouth is drawn to the other side. This will be particularly noticeable when the infant cries. The condition is usually transitory and disappears in a few days, often in a few hours.

Arm Paralysis

Injury to the brachial plexus, inflicted in the course of breech extraction, may cause paralysis of one arm. In the majority of cases, this disappears within a few weeks but may be permanent. It is called "Erb's paralysis" (or "Erb-Duchenne's paralysis"). In order to reduce tension on the brachial plexus, the physician usually will place the arm in a splint or cast in an elevated, neutral position.

Fractures and Dislocations

Fracture of a long bone or dislocation of an extremity may be the result of a version; or it may occur following a breech delivery in which the arms were extended above the head and are brought down into the vagina. Fractures of the clavicle ("collar bone") or of the jaw, or dislocation of either of these bones, may follow forcible efforts to extract the aftercoming head in cases of breech presentation.

Fractures in the newborn baby usually heal rapidly, but it is often difficult to keep the parts in good position during repair. Dislocation should be reduced at once, or there will be great danger of permanent deformity in the joint. Follow-up supervision is necessary in order to prevent permanent deformity. Physiotherapy under orthopedic direction is important.

INFECTIONS
Ophthalmia Neonatorum

This is a serious condition which may result in total blindness, but if suitable treatment is adopted at the very outset of the disease and intelligently carried out, usually the sight can be saved. The entire treatment is, of course, under the direct supervision of the physician.

Ophthalmia neonatorum is usually of gonorrheal origin and is characterized by a profuse, purulent discharge due to infection, generally from the genital canal at the time of birth. This is not always the case, however, and the lack of proper hygiene by the physician or the nurse or the mother may carry the infection to the eyes of the baby. Until the use of silver nitrate prophylaxis was established, from 25 to 30 per cent of all children in schools for the blind suffered impaired sight as the result of a gonorrheal infection.

If the infection occurs at the time of birth, the disease appears within 2 or 3 days; but as the septic discharge may be introduced into the eye at a later period by neglect of the proper care of the infant, the onset may be later. Both eyes are usually affected; and at first they are suffused with a watery discharge and considerable inflammation of the eyelids. Within 24 hours the lids become very much swollen, and a thick, creamy, greenish pus is discharged. Later, unless treatment has been instituted early, the swelling becomes so marked that the eyes cannot be opened, opacities of the cornea occur, the conjunctiva is ulcerated and then perforated, and the eye collapses and finally atrophies.

The preventive treatment consists in the use of 1 per cent silver nitrate, which is instilled into the eyes immediately after birth, or penicillin is administered in the form of aqueous drops (5,000 units per cc.) or ophthalmic ointment (100,000 units per Gm.), as already discussed in Chapter 12. Penicillin is widely reported as being as effective as silver nitrate for use at birth. Penicillin may also be given as intramuscular injections. If the infection persists, intensive penicillin administration should be carried out. Thanks to this drug, gonorrheal ophthalmia, which used to be one of the most stubborn and grave of afflictions and demanded the utmost in elaborate and prolonged nursing and medical care, is now cured within from 12 to 24 hours. The swelling and the pus usually disappear in even less time than this.

Ophthalmia neonatorum is a distinctly infectious disease, and there is extreme danger of conveying it to others. This applies not only to other infants' eyes but to the genital tract of other mothers. Even the eyes of the nurse herself may become infected, unless she is most conscientious in her methods. The infant should be isolated, and all articles used should be sterilized. Gloves, cap and gown should be worn by the nurse, and she should handle all dressings with forceps. Staphylococcus of resistant types occasionally cause purulent discharge; all such cases should be under the care of a physician until recovery.

Impetigo

Impetigo is a skin disease of infectious origin and not infrequently occurs in epidemic form in the nursery. For this reason, it is often called "impetigo contagiosa." The condition manifests itself by the eruption of small, semiglobular vesicles or pustules. While these may appear on any part of the body, they are most frequently encountered on moist opposing surfaces, such as the folds of the neck, the axilla and the groin. Thence they may spread rapidly by auto-inoculation to any part of the body. The lesion is small and varies from the size of a pinhead to a diameter of half an inch. It contains yellow pus. The bacterium involved is usually the staphylococcus or the streptococcus.

The treatment is essentially preventive, and cases rarely occur if the nursery technic has been meticulous. The nurse and the physician must wash their hands carefully before handling any infant, and every possible source of skin infection must be eliminated. Constant vigilance is necessary if these cases are to be pre-vented. Treatment consists of prompt isolation of the infant and local treatment of the lesions. Since these lesions tend to appear on moist or opposing skin surfaces, the infant must be kept clean and dry. Daily baths using hexachlorophene (pHisoHex) are given. Usually the blebs are broken and the areas painted with alcohol, gentian violet, Zephiran or some antiseptic solution.

As soon as a lesion develops which resembles impetigo even slightly, strict isolation of the infant is imperative. The physician should be notified at once. If properly treated, the superficial lesions heal quickly and with little scarring. Parenteral antibiotic therapy may be given prophylactically. A high nutritional level must be maintained, and scratching should be controlled. It is important for the nurse to remember that it is the fluid within the bleb which spreads the infection. When impetigo develops in a nursery it may be stubborn to eradicate, and occasionally it may even become necessary to close the nursery for a few weeks.

Thrush

Thrush is an infection of the mouth caused by the organism *Candida albicans*, the organism which causes monilial vaginitis in the mother (see Chap. 8). The infant may acquire the infection as it passes through the birth canal of a mother so infected. However, the infection may be transferred from infant to infant on the hands of attendants and is favored by lack of cleanliness in feeding, in the care of the mother's nipples, or in the care of the bottles and the nipples. It is most likely to occur in weak, undernourished babies. The condition appears as small white patches (due to the fungus growth) on the tongue and in the mouth. These white plaques may be mistaken at first for small curds of milk. The infant's mouth must be kept clean, but great gentleness is required to avoid further injury to the delicate epithelium, and any attempt to wipe away the plaques will usually cause bleeding.

Some physicians advise painting the spots with an aqueous solution of 1 per cent gentian violet, in which case the spots are touched gently with a sterile, soft cotton swab saturated with the medication. Another method of treatment is with nystatin, an antibiotic specific for infections caused by the monilial organism, *Candida albicans*. Mycostatin, an oral suspension of nystatin (100,000 units per cc.), is dropped into the infant's mouth and thus comes in contact with the affected areas. The usual dosage of Mycostatin is from 1 to 4 cc. 3 or 4 times daily, as prescribed by the physician. The nurse will recall that nystatin is poorly absorbed from the gastro-intestinal tract and is excreted almost entirely in the feces after oral administration.

Special care must be taken with the bottles and nipples used for infants who have thrush. These bottles and nipples must be kept separated from the others in the nursery until they are soaked in antiseptic solution, washed thoroughly and boiled before they are cared for in the routine way with bottles and nipples of other infants.

Epidemic Diarrhea of the Newborn

During recent years, a number of highly fatal epidemics of diarrhea have occurred in nurseries for the newborn throughout the country. Among infants so affected, almost half have died. The mortality rate in premature infants is twice the rate in full-term infants. The onset is sudden, with profuse, watery yellow stools which increase in frequency. Associated with the diarrhea, a precipitous weight loss occurs—often a pound within 24 hours. The appearance of the infant changes rapidly from that of a healthy baby to one of a markedly dehydrated and emaciated infant. In a severe case, death may occur in a day, but more often the baby lingers on in a semicomatose condition for 4 or 5 days. The spread of the disease is very rapid, and half the infants in a nursery may

succumb within a fortnight. Many of the epidemics accordingly are described as "explosive" in character.

The disease seems to be a special type of diarrhea which affects newborn infants and is quite different from the diarrhea from which older infants sometimes suffer. The symptoms and the mortality rate differ from bacterial types of dysentery or diarrhea. One of the most important predisposing factors is overcrowding in the nurseries. Faulty nursery technic is another—that is, failure to wash the hands before touching a baby, failure to sterilize rubber nipples properly, etc. The guiding principle involved is that everything coming in contact with the baby's mouth and nose should be in a surgically aseptic condition. All obstetric and nursing technics must be planned accordingly. Various health departments have set up rigid regulations along these lines in the hope of preventing epidemics. No visitors should be allowed while newborn infants are being fed or nursed by their mothers, and no visitors under 14 years should be allowed at any time. Small units for infant and maternity patients are desirable. Aseptic technic should be rigid.

When a case is discovered, immediate and absolute isolation is necessary; therefore, the infant should be transferred from the newborn nursery. A culture of the stools is done to find out the causative organism. This is done so that specific therapy can be instituted as soon as possible.

In many cases chemotherapy is used, along with supportive fluid therapy by the intravenous or subcutaneous route. Oral fluids—water, 5 per cent glucose in water, or Lytren (a commercially prepared electrolyte fluid replacement for oral use)—are given in small amounts. Whole blood is given by transfusion if indicated. Recently, Neomycin has been used in an effort to rid the intestinal tract of bacteria that might be irritating. Penicillin and streptomycin are sometimes administered to prevent or control the secondary infection that might occur in these debilitated infants.

If necessary, the nursery should be closed to new admissions until the epidemic clears up. These nurseries are washed and sometimes even painted before being opened again for new admissions. In the prevention of this disease, there seems to be nothing more effective than strict aseptic nursery technic. Hand washing with soap or pHisoHex and water after changing diapers, before feeding the infant and after handling the infant or any of its equipment is a rigid rule that should be stressed.

If an outbreak occurs, there should be a follow-up of all infants discharged in the preceding 2 weeks, and any infants needing treatment should be readmitted to the pediatric service of the hospital. All infants exposed at the time of an outbreak should be given prophylactic therapy. Complete control of this disease, which formally led to closing of the nursery, can be gained by prompt reporting, rigid technics and immediate treatment.

Syphilis

Syphilis of newly born infants shows lesions only if the child has early prenatal syphilis. They may be present at birth or may appear from a few days up to 4 months of age, predominantly on the face, the buttocks, the palms and the soles. Mucous patches occur in the mouth, and condylomata about the anus. These lesions are highly infectious. The eruption is usually maculopapular and not quite so generalized as in acquired syphilis. Bullae may appear on the palms and the soles, a type of lesion never found in acquired syphilis. The palms and the soles may desquamate as a result of the lesions. Less frequently seen are papular lesions or purely macular or, very rarely, vesicular or somewhat pustular ones. The nails may be deformed, and alopecia may be present. In such cases the blood test for syphilis is usually strongly positive. In addition to the cutaneous manifestations of syphilis, other signs and symptoms may arouse suspicion of the presence of the disease. The infant becomes restless, develops rhinitis (snuffles) and a hoarse voice. The baby does not gain weight as it should. The lymph nodes are enlarged, especially the epitrochlear nodes. The liver and the spleen are enlarged, as are also the ends of the long bones.

In the treatment of syphilis of the newborn, the physicians will rely chiefly on penicillin, which has largely replaced the arsenic and bismuth formerly used.

Babies born to mothers who have been treated early in the antepartal period for syphilis are seldom born with the disease.

Staphylococcal Infection

At the present time there is growing concern about the spread of staphylococcal infection in hospitals and its increasing resistance to antibiotic therapy. The newborn nursery is one of the most vulnerable areas because of the infants' low tolerance to infections.

In recent studies of staphylococcal infection of the newborn, the epidemic strain of the organism has been found not only in skin lesions of the infected infants but also in the nasopharynx of a high percentage of apparently well infants. Nurseries at this time must be considered potential epidemic centers. Many factors contribute to the large numbers of infants found to harbor these organisms. *Crowding* of infants in a nursery has always been a serious problem and a contributing factor in any epidemic disease outbreak. The usually recommended minimum of 24 to 30 square feet of space per infant may actually not be adequate to prevent spread of infection. *Hospital personnel* have been found to be carriers of staphylococcus coagulase-positive organisms. These organisms are highly resistant to most antibiotics in current use, and when they are transmitted to patients may result in such manifestations as skin lesions, pneumonia, septicemia and other forms of infections from mild to those of extremely serious nature. In many studies there appears to be a direct transmission of the offending organisms from hospital personnel to infant, from infant to infant, from infant to mother and to the family at home, and even into the community (see Chap. 20). Hospital sanitation must be critically appraised, since these organisms may be air-borne and can exist in many contaminated or unclean surfaces of the nurseries, wards and other hospital areas. The type of walls, floors and equipment used must be of materials which can be easily and satisfactorily cleaned. Housekeeping per-

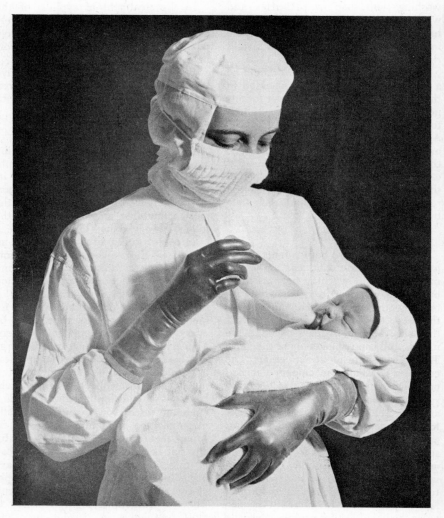

Fig. 266. An infant with any infectious disease should be cared for with isolation technic.

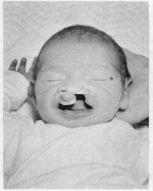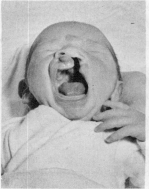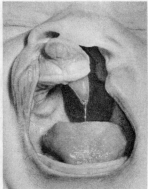

Fig. 267. Harelip and complete cleft palate. In this case surgical closure of the harelip was performed less than 18 hours following birth, with excellent results. (MacDonald House, University Hospitals of Cleveland)

sonnel, their equipment and methods must be constantly evaluated and supervised. There is no substitute for cleanliness, aseptic technic and isolation of infected patients and staff in controlling the spread of infection.

Manifestations of staphylococcal infection of the newborn frequently appear as pyoderma, stuffy noses, pneumonia and conjunctivitis. Few infants develop serious staphylococcal disease without preceding or accompanying pyoderma.

Infants with obvious infection should be isolated immediately and strict aseptic technic used in their care (Fig. 266). Therefore, the principles of communicable disease nursing must be understood and carried out by all personnel coming in contact with the newborn infants in hospital nurseries.

MALFORMATIONS

In one case in 200, approximately, an infant is born with some kind of malformation. Congenital deformities may range from minor abnormalities such as supernumerary digits to grave malformations, incompatible with life, such as anencephalus (absence of brain), hydrocephalus (excessive amount of fluid in the cerebral ventricles with tremendous enlargement of head) and various heart abnormalities. In 1957, 15,801 infants (14.1%) died because of congenital malformations. In the case of hydrocephalus, grave dystocia may occur because of the inability of the huge head to pass the pelvic inlet. Congenital malformations of the heart are a common cause of cyanosis in the newborn. Clubfoot, imperforate anus and meatus, harelip and cleft palate are other fairly frequent congenital deformities.

The graver congenital malformations are always a cause of keen disappointment to the family and sometimes produce serious psychological disturbances in the mother. Such cases demand the utmost in sympathy and understanding on the part of the nurse, who will do well, as a rule, to endeavor tactfully to direct the mother's thoughts to other interests.

Harelip and Cleft Palate

Before the baby with harelip or cleft palate, or both, is referred for surgical treatment, he will need special care during feeding. Nursing (sucking) is difficult and may be impossible, depending on the degree of malformation (Fig. 267). For some infants soft rubber nipples with large holes may be used. Others may need to be fed with a medicine dropper or even by gavage feeding. Because of difficulty in swallowing, great care must be exercised to prevent choking and nasal vomiting, but food is especially important in preparation for surgery. Therefore, definite time must be allowed to give adequate care to these infants. It is generally accepted that these deformities are due to some arrest in the development of the fetus as early as the eighth to the twelfth week of gestation. The cause is not known, although studies have indicated that there is a genetic influence in many cases.

Frenum Linguae

The frenum linguae is a vertical fold of mucous membrane under the tongue which is normally short and tight in the newborn infant. If this membrane is *too* short, the activity of the tongue is limited, so-called "tonguetie," and this interferes with sucking and later with the child's speech. This condition should be observed at the time of the initial physical examination or during the inspection bath. The physician will "snip" the margin of the membrane with sterile blunt scissors if necessary.

Spina Bifida

Spina bifida is a rather common malformation and is due to the congenital absence of one or more vertebral arches, usually at the lower part of the spine. This allows the membranes covering the spinal cord to bulge, forming a soft, fluctuating tumor filled with cerebrospinal fluid. The tumor is diminished by pressure and enlarges when the baby cries. The condition is usually fatal, although a few recoveries have been recorded. When the tumor is very small and shows no signs of increasing in size, it may merely be protected from injury and infection by carefully applied dress-ings; but the more severe cases must be treated surgically.

Umbilical Hernia

Umbilical hernia, or rupture at the umbilicus, may appear during the first few weeks of life. The associated protrusion of intestinal contents may be made to disappear entirely on pressure, but it reappears when the pressure is removed or when the baby cries. This is due to a weakness or an imperfect closure of the umbilical ring and is often associated with non-union of the recti muscles. The condition usually disappears spontaneously, but should the protrusion of omentum persist, the abdomen may be strapped, using a 2-inch strip of adhesive plaster or a suitable cord bandage. Some mothers may need to be discouraged from placing a coin or a button beneath the umbilical dressing, a practice used many years ago as a "home remedy." This has no value and prohibits adequate approximation of the margins of the hernia.

Obstructions of the Alimentary Tract

Imperforate Anus. This abnormality consists of atresia of the anus, with the rectum ending in a blind pouch. Careful examination of the infant in the delivery room usually reveals the condition, but it may be discovered by the nurse when attempting to take the first rectal temperature. Surgical treatment is, of course, imperative.

Pyloric Stenosis. This is a congenital anomaly and usually manifests its symptoms from the first few days to the second or the third week by the onset of vomiting which becomes projectile in character and occurs within 30 minutes after every feeding. The infant loses weight, the bowel elimination lessens, highly colored urine becomes scanty, and the symptoms of dehydration appear. Upon examination, gastric peristalsis is present and the pyloric "acorn-like" tumor can be palpated. Usually, thick cereal feedings are prescribed. If no improvement is noted it is necessary to resort to surgery. Since it is not usually an emergency operation,. there is sufficient time for supportive treatment to prepare the infant for surgery by vein and hypoclysis. The preoperative preparation includes intravenous blood and plasma. If the hemoglobin is below 70 per cent, transfusion is indicated. Gastric lavage, from 1 to 2 hours before operation, should be done until returns are clear. Maintaining body heat before and after the operation is essential. Transfusion should be given if indicated. The physician usually orders from 5 to 10 cc. of water to be given within a few hours, then alternated with 10 cc. of milk. As soon as the baby is gaining and consuming from 3 to 4 ounces at each feeding, he is ready for discharge.

Obstruction of the Duodenum and the Small Intestine. These conditions are relatively easy to diagnose. Vomiting occurs with the first feeding, and no meconium is eliminated. The vomitus may or may not be bile-stained, depending on whether the obstruction is high or low in the intestinal tract. If the obstruction is low, usually there is marked distention. A roentgenogram is used to confirm the diagnosis, and immediate surgery is indicated. However, the newborn infant should be allowed at least 12 hours for the respiration and kidney function to become established. The operation is usually accompanied by continuous venous drip and plasma, and blood should be available if needed. Postoperative care includes maintaining body temperature, intravenous fluids until peristalsis is established (about a week), followed by feedings as given in pyloric stenosis. If distention occurs, nasoduodenal suction may be necessary. If the distention is severe, the infant should be in an oxygen tent.

Intussusception. Acute intussusception is the most frequent type of intestinal obstruction and often may be unrecognized. There is usually intermittent abdominal pain, mild or severe, accompanied by blood and mucous intestinal elimination; and the baby may vomit. Upon abdominal examination a mass can be palpated. Immediate surgery is usually indicated. In preparation for surgery a gastric lavage is done, and an indwelling gastric catheter is inserted. Shock, if present, should be treated. Fluids are replaced by the intravenous route. Hypoclysis may be given for 24 hours, followed by water by mouth. Feedings may be started on the third day if retained. Antibiotics may be ordered for the first 3 to 5 days and vitamin C to stimulate healing.

German Measles as a Cause of Malformations

As the result of observations made in an Australian epidemic of German measles in 1941, it seems clear that when German measles occurs during the first 3 months of pregnancy, a substantial proportion of the fetuses will show malformation, principally cataracts, heart disease, deaf-mutism and microcephaly. It should be noted that the disease which produces these harmful effects is German measles, or rubella, and not rubeola measles, which has no such action. It should also be observed that German measles exerts these effects mainly when it occurs very early, usually before the twelfth week of pregnancy; and even then not all infants are affected. Just what proportion of babies are injured cannot be stated in the present stage of our knowledge. All that can be said is that when an expectant mother suffers from German measles during the first 12 weeks of pregnancy, there is a good —but by no means certain—chance that the infant will suffer from one of the malformations mentioned.

HEMOLYTIC DISEASE OF THE NEWBORN

Erythroblastosis Fetalis

Erythroblastosis fetalis is a severe hemolytic disease of the newborn most often due to Rh incompatibility. The name is derived from *erythros*, "red," and *blastos*, "a formative cell." It occurs approximately once in every 200 deliveries. The disease may manifest itself in different degrees of severity. About one fifth of the Rh-positive infants born of sensitized Rh-negative mothers may have no clinical manifestations. Others may be mildly or severely affected. If the mother's antibody titer is low, the infant will likely have a mild form of the disease. In mild cases of erythroblastosis fetalis, slight jaundice and anemia may be present at birth or may become evident within a few hours thereafter. These symptoms may be the only clinical manifestations. In more severe cases, the jaundice and the anemia are more exaggerated, and the liver and the spleen may be enlarged. Marked anemia with consequent pallor is a characteristic feature. In making observations the nurse should bear in mind that if the jaundice is pronounced it may mask the developing pallor.

When severe jaundice is present, there is risk of serious damage to the brain, known as *kernicterus*. This condition is associated with the high level of bilirubin. The infant who has symptoms of kernicterus will take its feedings poorly and show increasing signs of lethargy and loss of normal Moro reflex. It may have convulsions and opisthotonos, often accompanied by a shrill high-pitched cry. Kernicterus due to Rh incompatibility is often fatal, and if the infant survives it almost always suffers from severe forms of mental retardation and spastic paralysis, and its hearing may be impaired.

The most severe manifestation of erythroblastosis affecting the newborn is *hydrops fetalis*. With this condition the infant is tremendously edematous, has marked anemia, jaundice and enlargement of the liver and the spleen. Such infants may be stillborn, otherwise they invariably succumb shortly after birth.

Erythroblastosis fetalis is very likely to repeat itself in subsequent pregnancies, and some unfortunate mothers give birth to a series of such infants. Its cause is immunologic in character and is based on the fact that the mother in these cases develops in her blood certain antibodies which attack a substance in the baby's red blood corpuscles known as the "Rh factor" (see Fig. 249).

The Rh Factor. To understand the phenomenon which causes erythroblastosis fetalis, the nurse must have a knowledge and understanding of the Rh factor. This has already been discussed in some detail in Chapter 18.

Once in every several hundred pregnancies, as the result of an extraordinary combination of chance factors, the Rh substance may be responsible for a chain of events which exerts a harmful effect on the fetus. A number of circumstances must be present before this singular action on the fetus can be exerted. In the first place, the mother must be Rh negative. As indicated in Chapter 18, there is only 1 chance in 7 that any member of the white race belongs to this minority group. In the second place, her husband must be Rh positive; the chances are good—6 out of 7—that he does belong to the positive group, but he may not. In the third place, the fetus must be Rh positive; because the husband is Rh positive it does not necessarily follow that the baby is positive, because if any large group of Rh-positive men are studied it will be found that the spermatozoa of about one half are partly Rh negative and will produce an Rh-negative infant. In the fourth place—and this is the crux of the matter —the Rh substance from the Rh-positive fetus must find its way through the placenta and into the blood stream of the mother and build up antibodies therein, as occurs with an Rh-positive blood transfusion. Once these antibodies are developed in the mother they pass through the placenta into the fetal blood stream where they cause varying degrees of damage to the infant's red blood cells. Finally, the woman must have had a previous pregnancy or a previous blood transfusion because, as we have seen, it takes some time for the antibodies to develop.

From the above facts the following rather comforting conclusions can be drawn. Six out of 7 women are Rh positive, and for them there is no possibility whatsoever of complications occurring from this source. Likewise in first pregnancies, even if the expectant mother is Rh negative, the possibility of trouble developing is quite remote unless she has had a previous blood transfusion with Rh-positive blood. But if a woman is Rh negative and has had previous pregnancies or previous transfusions, what is her outlook in subsequent pregnancies? So many factors enter into this question that it is impossible to answer it with great precision, but all authorities agree that the vast majority even of this group—from 90 to 95 per cent—go through pregnancy after pregnancy without any suggestion of a complication.

Treatment in Erythroblastosis. In live births, that is, except in *hydrops fetalis*, the life of the infant may be saved by exchange transfusion with Rh-negative blood. This provides new red cells and removes the harmful maternal antibodies and products of hemolysis which produce jaundice. Transfusions should be given promptly. The exchange transfusion is accomplished through a polyethylene catheter inserted into the umbilical vein, or other large vein such as the saphenous. Small amounts of the infant's blood are withdrawn (approximately 10 to 15 cc. at a time) and equal amounts of the Rh-negative donor's blood injected. This procedure is continued until most of the circulating blood of the infant is replaced.

When there is any possibility that exchange transfusion may be required for the infant, the obstetrician invariably will leave the umbilical cord stump longer than usual. Moist saline dressings should be applied to the cord stump immediately and should be kept on constantly until the report of the Coombs Test is obtained and it is negative or until exchange transfusion is completed in cases where it is indicated.

Those infants with hemolytic disease who do not require exchange transfusion should be observed carefully for development of anemia for at least 3 weeks following birth, even when they appear to be doing satisfactorily. The physician will continue to have scheduled determinations of hemoglobin levels done during this period.

The infant with erythroblastosis is usually lethargic, due to the anemia and generalized weakness, and should have his position changed frequently to prevent atelectasis. Furthermore, special precautions must be exercised to protect this infant from intercurrent infection. There is some disagreement as to whether or not mothers giving birth to erythroblastotic infants should breast feed their babies. However, in Nelson's 7th edition of the *Textbook of Pediatrics** it is stated: "Erythroblastosis fetalis is not a contraindication to breast feeding, if the infant's general condition warrants it, since antibodies in the mother's milk are inactivated in the intestinal tract and do not contribute to further hemolysis of the infant's red blood cells."

The prognosis is favorable for the infant with erythroblastosis fetalis if he survives the first week without developing signs of kernicterus, provided that the severe anemia is given watchful attention and treatment. One may anticipate that hemoglobin and erythrocyte levels will be normal by the time the infant reaches the age of 5 months.

ABO Incompatibility

A relatively mild type of hemolytic disease of the newborn is associated with ABO incompatibility. In this disease the

* Page 115.

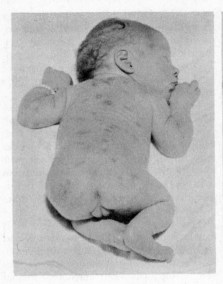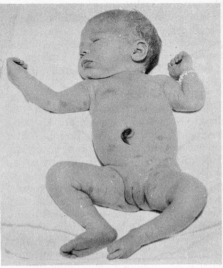

Fig. 268. Erythema toxicum. This "newborn rash" develops more frequently on the back, the shoulders and the buttocks. (MacDonald House, University Hospitals of Cleveland)

father's blood group is A or B and the mother's is Type O. At the time of conception the fertilized ovum receives the genes from both parents, and because the A and B genes are dominant over O, the infant will develop Type A or B blood. During the placental exchange of intra-uterine life, the anti-A or anti-B agglutinins of the mother's blood cross the placental barrier and attack the red blood cells of the infant. Hemolysis of these cells occurs, resulting in severe jaundice and anemia.

This disease occurs in first as well as in subsequent pregnancies, but rarely is it as severe as the hemolytic disease caused by Rh incompatibility. The Coombs' test is invariably negative.

Exchange transfusions are done, as necessary, to keep the serum bilirubin level below 20 mg. per 100 cc. The blood for transfusion should be of appropriate Rh type and Type O, the mother's blood group and not the infant's.

MISCELLANEOUS DISORDERS

Icterus Neonatorum

Icterus neonatorum is an exceedingly common condition during the first week of life and, as the name implies, is characterized by jaundice. Physiologic jaundice is dependent on the normal neonatal rise in the serum bilirubin level. It makes its appearance, as a rule, on the second or the third day of life and disappears without treatment about the sixth or seventh day. Almost 1 baby in 3 shows icterus, which is often called "physiologic jaundice." Most authorities attribute it to inadequate liver function and the destruction of red cells which takes place during the first week of life. The mother may be assured that the condition is due to a normal process and will clear up within a few days.

Erythema Toxicum

Erythema toxicum, sometimes referred to as the newborn rash, is a blotchy

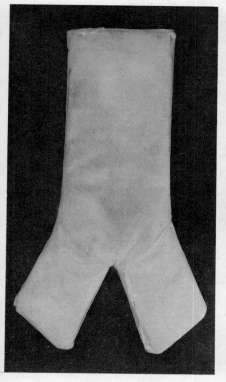 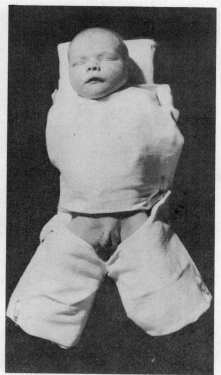

Fig. 269. Preparation of the infant, restrained for circumcision. (*Left*) Board, padded and covered with oilcloth, as used in many hospitals for circumcision. (*Right*) The infant, restrained on the board with towels, ready for circumcision.

erythematous rash which may appear in the first few days of life (Fig. 268). The erythematous areas, which develop more frequently on the back, the shoulders and the buttocks, have a small blanched wheal in the center. The cause of this skin disturbance is obscure and no treatment is necessary. The rash is transient and likely to change appreciably within a few hours and may disappear entirely within a day or so.

Milia

Milia are pinpoint-sized pearly white spots which occur commonly on the nose and the forehead of the newborn infant. When touched gently with the tip of the finger, these spots feel like tiny, firm seeds. They are due to retention of sebaceous material within the sebaceous glands, and if they are left alone will usually disappear spontaneously during the neonatal period. Mothers often mistake milia for "whiteheads" and may attempt to squeeze them if the nurse or the physician has not warned them against such practice.

Phimosis

In many male infants the orifice in the foreskin of the penis is so small that the foreskin cannot be pushed back over the glans. This condition is known as "phimosis." While it is rarely of suffi-

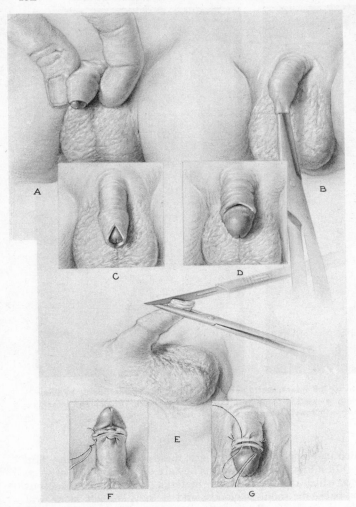

Fig. 270. Technic of circumcision, using hemostat, scalpel and sutures. After cleansing penis and surrounding area, the prepuce is stripped back with the help of a partial dorsal slit (A to D). The prepuce is now clamped and excessive prepuce cut off (E). The suture material used is plain 00 or 000 catgut in a very small needle (F and G), but some physicians prefer silk.

cient degree to obstruct the outflow of urine or cause any immediate symptoms, it is undesirable because it prevents proper cleanliness. Phimosis may be corrected either by stretching the orifice of the foreskin with a hemostat, or by circumcision. Both of these procedures are carried out by the physician, but sometimes the nurse is asked to stretch the foreskin gently every day after having first received detailed instructions from the physician. Preparation of an infant

for circumcision as well as two common methods of performing the operation are depicted in Figures 269-271.

Hemorrhage from Cord

Hemorrhage from the cord may be of two types: (1) primary, due to the slipping or loosening of the ligature or umbilical clamp, and (2) secondary, coming from the base of the cord when it separates from the body of the baby. In

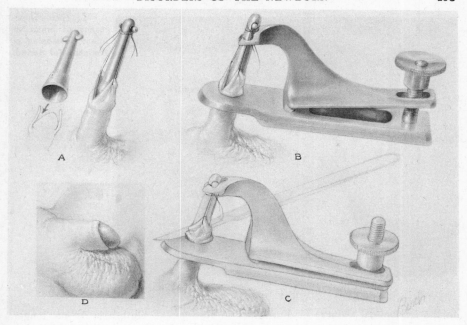

Fig. 271. Technic of circumcision with Yellen clamp. After cleansing area and stripping back prepuce as shown in Figure 270, the cone of the Yellen clamp is placed over the glans and the prepuce put on a stretch with sutures (A). The prepuce is now drawn through the beveled hole of platform (B). Screwing down clamp crushes prepuce, producing hemostasis. Three to 5 minutes of such pressure is necessary to prevent subsequent bleeding. The excess of the prepuce is then cut away (C) and the clamp removed (D). (Yellen, H. S.: Am. J. Obst. & Gynec. 30:146)

the first instance, the bleeding is from the end of the cord and not from its base and can be controlled by the proper application of a fresh ligature. The secondary hemorrhage, from the base of the cord, occurs at about the fifth to the eighth day when separation takes place. It is often preceded by a slight jaundice; it is not an actual flow of blood but a persistent oozing which frequently resists treatment. This variety of hemorrhage, which is of rare occurrence, is usually due to one of two causes: (1) the baby may be syphilitic, or (2) the peculiar condition known as the "hemorrhagic diathesis" may be present. In this condition, the baby's blood shows

no disposition to coagulate, and bleeding from any denuded surface is persistent and often profuse.

The nurse's responsibility in the treatment of secondary hemorrhage from the cord consists in applying a sterile dressing to the bleeding surface. The physician should be notified promptly; and if, by the time he arrives, the use of the dressing has not effectually controlled the oozing, he will doubtless ligate the base of the umbilicus. When this form of bleeding is at all severe and persistent, recovery is doubtful; and even if the umbilical hemorrhage is controlled, bleeding may appear in the nose, the mouth, the stomach, the intestines

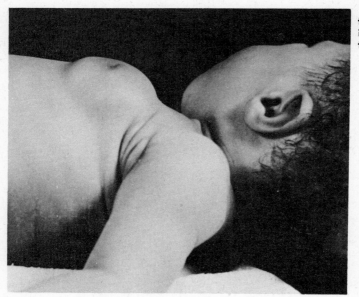

Fig. 272. Hypertrophy of breast in infant developing in the neonatal period.

or the abdominal cavity; or purpuric spots may develop on various parts of the body. The prompt administration of vitamin K has greatly improved the prognosis in these cases.

Retrolental Fibroplasia

Retrolental fibroplasia is an acquired disease, associated with prematurity, in which retinal pathology occurs in those infants receiving continuous oxygen therapy in high concentration. This disease is characterized by proliferation of endothelial cells in the layer of nerve fibers in the periphery of the retina. This leads to the formation of new vessels, and the retina becomes edematous and elevated and finally retinal detachment may follow. Because most of the damage is mechanical, one cannot determine the extent of detachment that will occur. When the condition is detected early and proper measures are instituted promptly, i.e., reduction in concentration of oxygen administered, the condition in the infant may regress at any stage of the disease, or, on the other hand, partial or complete blindness may result.

Retrolental fibroplasia is no longer considered to be a major problem because it rarely occurs today. Extensive research carried on within the past two decades, since retrolental fibroplasia was first described, has established the cause and the means of prevention of the disease. It is now a fact that almost all cases of retrolental fibroplasia in the premature infant are the result of intensive oxygen therapy. Today oxygen is administered to an infant in the lowest concentration compatible with life and is discontinued as soon as feasible. The maximum oxygen concentration of the incubator housing the premature infant is kept at less than 40 per cent, with rare exceptions, and this is done only for as long as it is *absolutely* necessary (see Oxygen Therapy, p. 358).

Breast Engorgement

Engorgement of the breasts is common during the neonatal period, in both male and female infants (Fig. 272). It is due to the same causes which bring about mammary engorgement in the mother—that is, endocrine influence. In the case of the infant, its breasts have been acted upon throughout pregnancy by the estrogenic hormone which passes to it through the placenta from the mother. This is the same hormone which prepares the mother's breasts for lactation. When it is withdrawn after birth, changes in the infant's breasts take place similar to those in the mother.

Mammary engorgement in the newborn subsides without treatment, but sometimes persists for 2 or 3 weeks.

Menstruation

Menstruation occasionally occurs in newborn girls and is due to estrogenic hormone, as described above. It usually amounts only to slight spotting and need cause no special concern.

SUGGESTED READING

Allen, Fred H., et al.: Erythroblastosis Fetalis, Boston, Little, 1958.

Biggs, Alfred D.: Emergencies of the newborn, Bull. Maternal Welfare 5: 18, 1958.

Book, J. A., and Reed, S. C.: Empiric risk figures in mongolism, J.A.M.A. 143:730, 1950.

Callon, Helen: How the nurse can combat staphylococcal infections, Nursing World 132:8, 1958.

Dale, Mary B.: Antibiotic-resistant staphylococcus: a health department survey, California's Health 16:201, 1958.

Davidson, H. H., Hill, Justina H., and Eastman, N. J.: Penicillin in the prophylaxis of ophthalmia neonatorum, J.A.M.A. 145:1052, 1951.

Dill, David B.: Symposium on mouth to mouth resuscitation, J.A.M.A. 167: 317, 1958.

Drorbaugh, James, and Fogg, Marguerite: Respiratory distress in the newborn infant, Am. J. Nursing 56:1559, 1956.

Eastman, N. J.: Obstetrical factors in the etiology of cerebral palsy, Connecticut Med. 23:316, 1959.

Hamra, M. L.: Congenital dysplasia and dislocation of the hips; nursing care in the hospital, Am. J. Nursing 56:1276, 1956.

Hospital Acquired Staphylococcal Disease, Proceedings of the National Conference—September 1958, U. S. Dept. of Health, Education and Welfare, Public Health Service, Washington, D. C.

Illness and Mortality Among Infants During the First Year of Life (Pub. Health Monograph No. 81), U. S. Dept. of Health, Education and Welfare, Public Health Service, Washington, D. C., 1955.

Jeans, P. C., Wright, F. H., and Blake, F. G.: Essentials of Pediatrics, ed. 6, Philadelphia, Lippincott, 1958.

Long, John C., Jr.: Are birthmarks malignant?," Am. J. Nursing 55:955, 1955.

Lynch, Matthew, et al.: Hyaline membrane disease, J. Pediat. 48:602, 1956.

McCall, M. L.: Diagnosis of Rh and ABO incompatibility, Clin. Obst. & Gynec. 1:709, 1958.

MacCollum, Donald W., et al.: Care of the child with cleft lip and cleft palate, Am. J. Nursing 58:211, 1958.

Miller, Herbert C., et al.: Respiratory activity and function in newborn infants dying with pulmonary hyaline membranes, Pediatrics 22:665, 1958.

Nelson, Waldo E.: Textbook of Pediatrics, ed. 7, Philadelphia, Saunders, 1959.

Ravenholt, Riemert T., and Ravenholt, Alto H.: Staphylococcal infection in the hospital and community, Am. J. Pub. Health 48:277, 1958.

Ryan, Elizabeth K.: Nursing care of the patient with spina bifida, Am. J. Nursing 51:28, 1951.

Safar, Peter, et al.: A comparison of the mouth-to-mouth and mouth-to-airway methods of artificial respiration with the chest-pressure arm-lift methods, New England J. Med. 258:671, 1958.

Shaffer, Thomas: The cyanotic infant, Ohio State M. J. 51:444, 1955.

Shannon, Victoria: When children are born with defects, Children 2:27, 1955.

Shapiro, J. M., et al.: Incidence of retrolental fibroplasia: past and present, J. Pediat. 48:640, 1956.

Taschdjian, B. S., and Kozinn, P. J.: Laboratory and clinical studies on candidiasis in the newborn infant, J. Pediat. 50:426, 1957.

Vaughan, Victor C.: Current status of

hemolytic disease of the newborn, Postgrad. Med. 18:115, 1955.

West, Jessie Stevenson: Congenital Malformation and Birth Injuries, Assoc. for Aid of Crippled Children, 345 E. 46th St., New York, 1954.

Wiener, A. S., *et al.*: Treatment of erythroblastosis fetalis with special reference to Rh-Hr factors other than Rho, J. Pediat. 49:381, 1956.

CONFERENCE MATERIAL

1. In your own hospital setting, scrutinize and evaluate the facilities for and the care of the newborn infants in relation to the prevention of infection.

2. A mother's first-born infant has a cleft lip and cleft palate. The infant is apparently normal otherwise. The distraught mother can only see "my poor deformed baby girl" and blames herself for this "tragedy" because she did not follow her physician's instructions during pregnancy, particularly in relation to good nutrition. How might the nurse handle the nursing problems in this situation?

3. How do you account for the high infant mortality during the neonatal period?

4. What community agencies in your city render services for handicapped children? What is the procedure for making the referral to such agencies? How can the public health nurse function most effectively in such cases?

5. What legislation in your city or state has contributed to reducing the incidence of congenital syphilis?

Study Questions

Read through the entire question and place your answer in the parentheses.

1. When the newborn infant does not breathe at birth, and modern equipment for infant resuscitation is not available, which of the following procedures are sometimes resorted to?
   A. Hold the infant in the palm of one hand, with head, legs and arms hanging forward, thus compressing the chest wall. Then turn the infant over on its back, in the other hand, in which position the head, legs and arms hang backward, thus expanding the chest.
   B. With one hand grasp the infant by the ankles and hold him suspended head downward, while the other hand is used to "milk the trachea" or gently rub the infant's back.
   C. Mouth-to-mouth insufflation, exhaling through clean dry gauze directly into the infant's mouth at intervals corresponding to those of normal respiration.
   D. Alternately, plunge the infant into tubs of hot and cold water.
   E. Immerse the infant's body in a tub of hot water (110° F.) to prevent chilling and simultaneously dash a little cold water upon the infant's face and chest.
   Select the number corresponding to the correct letters.
   1. A and C
   2. B and C
   3. B and D
   4. C and E

   (————)

2. The nurse sometimes observes swelling of the newborn infant's scalp which may be due to caput succedaneum or cephalhematoma. Which of the following statements are true concerning cephalhematoma?
   A. It is due to an extravasation of serum into the tissues of the scalp.
   B. It is seldom visible when the infant is born and may not be noticed for several hours or more after delivery.
   C. The infant usually recovers without treatment.
   D. It always disappears within a few days.
   E. It gradually increases the size until about a week after the infant's birth, when it remains stationary for a time and then begins to disappear.
   Select the number corresponding to the correct letters.
   1. A and B
   2. A, C and D
   3. B, C and D
   4. B, C and E

   (————)

3. What are some of the signs of cerebral hemorrhage which may be observed by the nurse caring for infants in the newborn nursery?
   A. Convulsions.

497

B. Slow, deep, rhythmic respiration.
C. Twitching of extremities.
D. Flushed face with circumoral pallor.
E. Weak, whining cry.
Select the number corresponding to the correct letter or letters.
1. A only
2. A and C
3. B, C and E
4. All of them

(————)

4. A newborn infant develops respiratory distress several hours after birth, and the diagnosis of hyaline membrane disease is made. Which of the following statements have bearing on this condition?
A. The infant was born prematurely.
B. The infant is cyanotic and dyspneic.
C. Progressive respiratory difficulty is evidenced by increased cyanosis and marked sternal retractions.
D. Treatment primarily consists of the administration of oxygen and maintenance of high humidity.
E. A protein material is obstructing the flow of air and the exchange of oxygen and carbon dioxide in the lungs.
Select the number corresponding to the correct letters.
1. A, B and C
2. B, D and E
3. C, D and E
4. All of them

(————)

5. Which of the following manifestations of staphylococcal infection may appear in the newborn infant?
A. Impetigo.
B. Milia.
C. Conjunctivitis.
D. Erythema toxicum.
E. Breast engorgement.
Select the number corresponding to the correct letters.
1. A and C
2. A and D
3. B, C and E
4. All of them

(————)

6. Which of the following conditions are congenital disorders?
A. Phimosis.
B. Chloasma.
C. Frenum linguae.
D. Retrolental fibroplasia.
E. Seborrhea capitis.
Select the number corresponding to the correct letters.
1. A and C
2. B, C and D
3. B, D and E
4. All of them

(————)

7. The most effective treatment of erythroblastosis is accomplished by blood transfusion. Which one of the following is the best method to use?
   A. Exchange transfusion with Rh-negative blood.
   B. Exchange transfusion with Rh-positive blood.
   C. Exchange transfusion with blood plasma.
   D. Repeated small transfusions with Rh-negative blood.
   E. Repeated small transfusions with Rh-positive blood.
   F. Repeated small transfusions with blood plasma.

(————)

8. Hemolytic disease of the newborn may be produced by the union of parents with which of the following blood types?
   A. Rh-positive mother with Rh-negative father.
   B. Rh-negative mother with Rh-negative father.
   C. Rh-negative mother with Rh-positive father.
   D. Type O mother with Type A father.
   E. Type A mother with Type B father.
   Select the number corresponding to the correct letters.
      1. A and C
      2. B and D
      3. C and D
      4. All of them

(————)

9. Which one of the following infectious diseases, when contracted by the mother during the first trimester of pregnancy, will most often produce congenital anomalies in the infant?
   A. Scarlet fever.
   B. Rubella (German measles).
   C. Diphtheria.
   D. Rubeola (Measles).
   E. Typhoid fever.

(————)

10. Some disorders which affect the infant in the neonatal period are manifestations of endocrine influence. Which of the following conditions would this include?
   A. Menstruation in female infants.
   B. Icterus neonatorum.
   C. Engorgement of the breasts in male and female infants.
   D. Hyaline membrane disease.
   E. Erythroblastosis fetalis.
   Select the number corresponding to the correct letter or letters.
      1. A only
      2. A and C
      3. B, C and D
      4. B, D and E

(————)

Note: The key to the correct answers to these questions is given on page 533.

UNIT NINE

Related Information

CHAPTER TWENTY-TWO

Home Delivery

Even though, at the present time, the vast majority of mothers in this country are delivered in hospitals, there is still a small percentage of deliveries attended by physicians and qualified midwives at home, the majority of which take place in rural areas. Therefore, the nurse should know how a home delivery is conducted. In an emergency, too, the nurse may need this knowledge and experience. For the nurse who is interested in special preparation for maternity care, the schools of nurse-midwifery, such as the Maternity Center Association School of Nurse-Midwifery in New York, the Frontier Graduate School of Midwifery in Kentucky, the Catholic Maternity Institute in New Mexico and the Puerto Rico Department of Health, offer education and training for the conduct of home deliveries. More recently, graduate nursing programs leading to Master of Science degrees and certification in nurse-midwifery have been developed by Catholic University of America School of Nursing, Columbia University Faculty of Medicine Department of Nursing and Yale University School of Nursing.

When a home delivery is preferred, such factors as the normalcy of the patient, accessibility of the obstetrician, facilities at home and available care are important considerations.

PREPARATIONS FOR HOME DELIVERY

Preparations for home delivery should be begun early in pregnancy to enable the family to make adequate preparations. Today, in many areas the public health nurse visits the patient in her home routinely during the antepartal period and assists the physician in the management and care of the mother. When there is a home delivery service, these nurses may attend the delivery with the physician. The nurse can be most helpful with preparations for delivery because of her special knowledge.

Many obstetricians give their patients a list of supplies that they will need for delivery at home, but where the matter is left to the parents and the nurse, the following suggestions may be helpful. Even when the mother has been able to avail herself of the opportunity of attending a Mothers' Club or expectant parents' classes and of obtaining suggestions, she may desire to discuss some of them, along with personal problems, with the obstetrician and the nurse.

Supplies for the Mother

The supplies provided by the mother will necessarily vary in the individual situation. The following list contains supplies which will be needed:

Sheets and pillowcases (4)

Bath towels and washcloths (4)

Waterproof material—large enough to protect the mattress (about 1½ yards square). Rubber sheeting, plastic or white table oilcloth are preferable, although heavy brown paper can be used.

Receiving blanket for the infant

Delivery pads (4 to 6). These bed pads are made from 12 thicknesses of newspaper opened to full size (sewed together at the edges) and covered with freshly laundered old or new muslin. The corners of the cover may be mitered, so that it can be removed and laundered when necessary and fresh newspaper inserted (Fig. 273). Quilted pads or large-size paper diapers may also be purchased for this purpose.

Newspapers. A supply of clean newspapers should be saved for the many uses to which they can be put at this time.

Newspaper bags. The large newspaper bags are especially useful at the time of delivery (Fig. 274).

Small enamel wash basins (2 or 3) for solutions and sponges used in cleansing the patient's genitals, to receive the placenta, and a hand basin.

Large pail with cover

Covered kettles or stew pans (2), one for cooled boiled water and one for boiling water

Ladle or dipper

Enema can with tubing and rectal tip

Board for placing under mattress of delivery bed (table leaf or ironing board without legs may be used)

Hot-water bottle and cover

Bedpan

Pair of white stockings (may be inexpensive variety)

Nightgowns or pajama tops (3 or 4)

Brassières (3 or 4) (may be improvised from straight binders, 10 in. wide, or large smooth cotton towels)

Sanitary pads (2 to 3 doz.). If they cannot be purchased, they may be made from freshly laundered, soft, absorbent material, folded and ironed ready for use.

Sanitary belts or T-binders (3 or 4)

Safety pins: 1 doz. small and 1 doz. large

Pitcher or Mason jar with cover

Sterile absorbent cotton (1 lb.) in original package, unopened

Sterile gauze squares 4″ x 4″ (1 doz.)

Mineral oil

Plain white petroleum jelly (tube)

Soap

New nail brush and orangewood stick

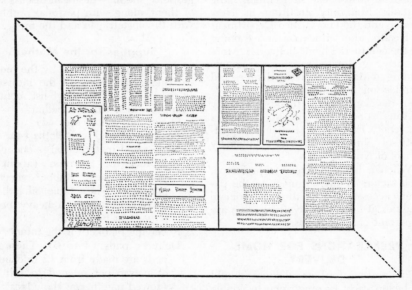

Fig. 273. Newspaper pad made of 12 thicknesses of newspaper sewed together at the outer edges and covered with unbleached muslin (viewed from underside). The muslin covers are mitered at the corners so that they may be removed, laundered and used again.

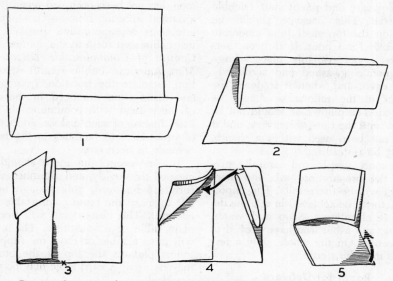

Fig. 274. Steps in making a newspaper bag. These are useful receptacles for waste material. They may be made in small and large sizes.

Umbilical tape or bobbin tape (narrow cotton) for tying cord (1 yd.)
Scissors
Roll of toilet tissue, unopened

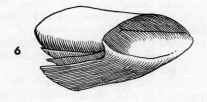

Home Preparations

In preparing for a home delivery, the nurse should explain and demonstrate to the mother how to prepare the articles that are to be used during delivery, viz., sheets to be used for the bed and draping, towels and bedpads of the homemade variety. These articles should be washed with soap and water, dried in the sun if possible, ironed and folded so that the ironed surfaces are folded upon each other. The ironed surface should be used for the field of delivery. These articles should be put away in a pillowcase or wrapped in a piece of ironed paper. The other articles needed at the time of delivery should be laid aside ready for use. Packages of absorbent cotton, gauze squares, sanitary pads and toilet tissue should be put away unopened.

Packages of sterile delivery supplies may be available from a local health agency, or it may be possible to have a package, assembled at home, autoclaved at a local hospital. Although autoclaving is most desirable, it is possible to sterilize dressings, etc., in the oven at home. The simplest method is to place the materials in small muslin bags, or bags of some other heavy white cotton material, and then place these bags in an old pillowcase and pin it shut (double wrapped). This package should be baked on the top shelf in a moderate oven, 325° for 1 hour. If an oven thermometer is not available, place a large white potato (washed and scrubbed) in the oven, and when it is done, the supplies in the pillowcase should be sterilized. The pillowcase should not be opened until the time of delivery, and if it has not been used within a month, it must be resterilized.

The more simple and carefully prepared the preparations are, the more efficient will be the results. The important factor to be achieved in a home delivery is cleanliness. Soap and water, sunshine and a hot iron have proved to be effective. On the whole, only a few articles must be sterile.

Room for Delivery

Deciding on the room in which the patient is to be delivered is one of the "preparations." It should be the room in which the patient will be most comfortable. Many mothers during this period have to assume certain responsibilities for the management of the household, so it means much to be where the household affairs can be directed with the least exertion.

Ideally, it should be a room that is light, airy, quiet, cheerful and comfortable, conveniently near a bathroom. The room furnishings should be simple, so that they are easy to keep clean, as cleanliness is one of the first essentials of good obstetric care. The bed should be so placed that it can be approached from either side, and so that the light is convenient either day or night. Ample light is a necessity.

The nurse may help select the room, but the choice is limited or even fixed by the possibilities of the house. Naturally, the nurse will avoid putting the family to any unnecessary inconvenience, but always her first thought must be in the interest of her patient.

The nurse should make sure that the room has not been occupied recently by a patient suffering from any contagious, infectious or suppurative disease. The instructions set forth in the manual *The Control of Communicable Disease in Man,* American Public Health Association, regulate the isolation, quarantine and disinfection practiced in the care of the patient with communicable disease. In case of such disease, adaptation of procedures to facilities in the home is made as necessary.

In any event, the room should be cleaned thoroughly, and all unnecessary furniture removed, only enough being left to make the room comfortable and cheerful. The obstetrician will need a plain table or a substitute. The nurse will need a table or chair for supplies, unless perhaps the top of the bureau may be used. A card table may be very practical.

Preparation of the Delivery Bed

The mother's bed should be comfortable. The springs should be in good condition, and the mattress firm and level. A single bed is preferable to the wider or double bed, because it is easier for the obstetrician and the nurse to care for the mother. If the bed is low, it may be raised to a more convenient height by using blocks. The bed should be so arranged that after the labor the mother may be made clean and comfortable without too much disturbance. The best way to accomplish this is first to prepare the bed as it is to be used after delivery and then to add the necessary preparations on top for the labor and the delivery.

The mattress should be supported by means of boards placed between it and the springs, so that it will be perfectly firm and level and not sag. Table leaves, a flat ironing board or plain board may be used for this purpose. Such supports should lie crosswise under the mattress at a point directly under the mother's buttocks and should be removed at the conclusion of the delivery. A firm, flat mattress helps to prevent the patient's hips from sinking into the bed.

The mattress should be covered with a piece of waterproof material, if available; if not, heavy brown paper, newspaper or water-repellent paper may be used. Over this covering, a white cotton sheet should be placed and tucked in securely along the edges. The top sheet, the blanket and the spread should be fan-folded to the foot of the bed, where they will be convenient to cover the mother immediately after the delivery. Covered newspaper or moisture-proof pads afford excellent protection and are so arranged that they protect the bed at the time of delivery, and a fresh one is left under the mother after delivery.

If these preparations are first demonstrated and their uses explained to the patient and her husband, they may be better able to make adequate preparations and have them ready at the time of labor.

Special Equipment

The physician and the nurse probably will have all the supplies needed for the delivery other than those provided by the mother. As stated previously, sometimes these supplies are approved by a local health agency. The Maryland State Department of Health, Division of Public Health Nursing, provides its staff with a nurse's bag and, since it provides a home delivery service, also makes available a nurse-midwife's delivery bag which contains the following:

1. Newspaper pads
   Safety pins
2. Sterno outfit
3. Box of medicines:
   A. Syntocin (2 amp.)
   B. Methergine (2 amp.)
   C. Ergotrate tablets (50)
   D. Silver nitrate 1% (2 wax amp.)
   E. Vitamin K (2 amp.)
   F. File
   G. Chromic catgut #2 (2 tubes)
4. Sterile gloves:
   Size 7 (2 pairs)
   Size 7½ (2 pairs)
5. Sterile pack containing:
   A. Hand towel (1)
   B. Doctor's gown (1)
   C. Leggings (2) with towel clips (2)
   D. Towels (6)
   E. Gauze squares 3" × 3" (12)
   F. Cord dressings (2) with cord ties (4)
   G. Perineal pads (package)
   H. Towels for pelvic examination (package of 5)
6. Case of instruments:
   A. 1-2 cc. syringe with No. 25 needles (2)
   B. Mayo scissors (1)
   C. Metal box with needles

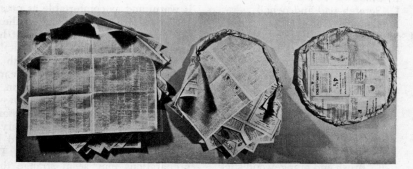

Fig. 275. The evolution of a newspaper Kelly pad. When used under a patient, it is lined with a piece of waterproof material and a towel.

    D. Sponge holder (1)
    E. Kelly clamps (2)
7. Muslin case with scales, tape measure, bottle of cord tape, 3 × 3 gauze squares (2 pkgs.)
8. Large basins (2)
    Liter cup (1)
    Bag of cotton (to be placed in cup)
9. Enamel covered container
10. Muslin case containing:
    A. Applicators, tongue depressors, razor and box of blades, and finger cots
    B. No. 14 catheters (2):
        1 for bladder catheterization
        1 for suctioning the infant
    C. No. 28 rectal tube with glass connecting tip (1)
    D. Rubber bulb syringe (1)
11. Muslin case containing enema equipment
12. Muslin case containing:
    A. Aprons (2)
    B. Caps (2)
    C. Masks (4)
13. Brown folder containing:
    A. Delivery bag list
    B. Labor and delivery procedure
    C. Standing orders
    D. Procedure for care of premature infants
    E. Birth certificate book
    F. Labor and delivery records (12)
    G. Infant records (6)
    H. Baby's Care (6)
    I. Small envelopes (12)
    J. Scratch pad and pencil
    K. Laundry lists (12)
14. Side pockets of bag:
    No. 1 Thermometers
        A. Mouth thermometer
        B. Rectal thermometer
    No. 2. K. Y. jelly
    No. 3.
        A. Alcohol 70%
        B. Green soap
        C. Bottle of antiseptic No. 3
        D. Mercury cyanide
        E. Brush and orangewood stick
        F. Paper napkins (12)
        G. Paper towels (12)
        H. Aromatic spirits of ammonia

If an anesthetic other than Trilene is to be given, the nurse may need to cover the wire mask (Fig. 140). A cone may be improvised with a wire sieve, but should not be made from newspaper because of the danger involved (see Chap. 11, Analgesia and Anesthesia in Labor).

DELIVERY IN THE HOME

During the antepartal period, the patient and her husband will have prepared the needed supplies and made preparations so that labor should be conducted with comparatively little inconvenience and confusion. They have been instructed concerning the symptoms of labor and when to call the physician and the nurse. Many physicians wish to be with the mother from the onset of labor; however, this will have been arranged beforehand, and if the nurse's arrival precedes that of the physician, she will make her observations of the mother's condition and proceed accordingly.

A few preparations cannot be made until labor begins, such as boiling the 2 kettles of water (for 20 minutes) in covered vessels and setting 1 aside to cool. It is a good idea also to boil a ladle or dipper in the kettle that is set aside to cool. The bed and the crib should be prepared and the delivery supplies arranged (Fig. 276). The nurse should also see that the provisions for lighting the room are ample, and that the room is warm and as comfortable as possible.

The underlying principles for the care of the mother being delivered at home are the same as those for hospital delivery (see Chap. 12), although procedures will necessarily have to be modified because of the home situation. The patient will probably have taken a warm sponge bath, but it may be necessary to assist her with it if this is necessary and time permits. The patient should have special preparation for delivery. These preparations may seem strange to the patient, so the nurse should explain procedures and any developments carefully, so the mother will have less cause to

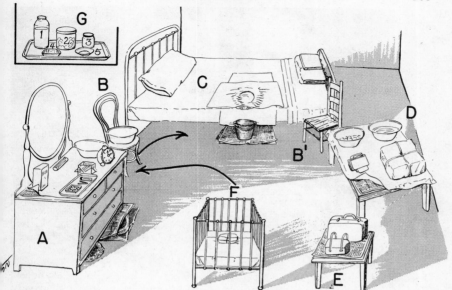

Fig. 276. Delivery room in the home, in readiness for the mother in labor.

A. Bureau (newspaper protecting the surface, cloth on top):
   1. Flashlight
   2. Perineal pads
   3. Paper waste bag
   4. Clock
   5. Basin
   6. Enamel tray containing: (a) Thermometer in solution in glass tube, (b) Thumb forceps, (c) Cotton balls in tray

B. Chair at head of bed for enema equipment. *Note.* This chair will be moved down toward the center of the bed later to support the mother's legs for the actual delivery.

B' Second chair to be moved toward the center of the bed to support the mother's legs for the delivery.

C. Bed protected with paper pad, Kelly newspaper pad and cloth cover for the delivery. Sheet fanned-folded to foot of bed, extra blanket and sheet. (Bed is made for delivery with the mother lying crosswise.)

D. Table (protected with newspaper covered by cloth):
   1. Basin of antiseptic solution
   2. Basin with sterile cotton balls in water
   3. Sterile gloves and towels
   4. Sterile pack (for contents see "Special Equipment" in this chapter)

E. Small table (protected with newspaper) for nurse's bag and delivery bag (see "Special Equipment" for contents)

F. Crib containing small bundle of infant's clothes and blankets. *Note.* The crib is moved in place of chair B when that space is available.

G. Improvised toilet tray for the infant:
   1. Jars (3) for boiled water, cotton balls and small cotton swabs
   2. Soap dish
   3. Dish for mineral oil

Note. This tray should be readily available for use when needed for the infant's initial care. Before this time there may be no place for it because the bureau and small table surfaces are occupied by the essentials for the delivery.

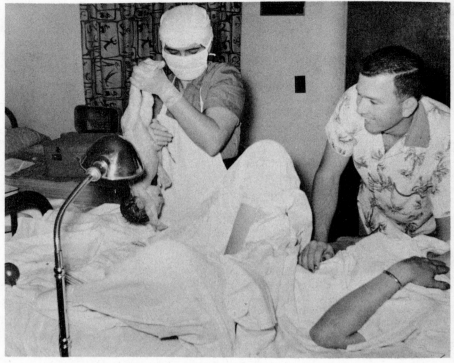

Fig. 277. The certified nurse-midwife conducting a home delivery. The father at the bedside encourages his wife and simultaneously derives considerable satisfaction from his participation in the birth of their baby. (Catholic Maternity Institute, Santa Fe, N. Mex.)

become anxious. According to the physician's specific orders, a low soapsuds enema may be given to empty the lower intestine in order to make more room for the descending head and to prevent fecal discharge during the delivery. The vulva should be shaved and the external genitalia cleansed with aseptic technic. The mother may need to have it explained that the former practice of keeping a perineal pad on while in labor has been largely discarded because of the danger of carrying infection, notably the colon bacillus, to the parturient canal from the anal region.

During the first stage of labor the mother is usually allowed to be up and about until labor becomes very active or the membranes rupture. The physician may suggest liquids to be given freely and that light nourishment be offered, such as tea and toast or crackers, if delivery is not imminent. As labor progresses, careful explanation will provide comfort and reassurance.

The nursing care of the mother in labor at home is essentially the same as in the hospital. Observations of the mother's temperature, pulse, respirations, blood pressure, intake and output and the progress of labor are made consistently. The fetal heart tones should be checked routinely, and the mother should be watched closely for any complication which might develop. If membranes rupture in the first stage of labor, the danger of prolapse of the cord must be kept in mind. In addition, if the physician is not present, he should be notified immediately, as would be the case if anything unusual developed. If the physician needs to be called for this reason, it should be done without alarming the mother, especially if this is her first labor. From the beginning of true labor, the mother should use a commode or bedpan and should be encouraged to empty her bladder at fairly frequent intervals to avoid bladder distention, as well as to keep her more comfortable.

As soon as it is apparent that the mother is nearing the second stage of labor, she should be put to bed, if she has not been already. The nurse should now have everything in readiness for delivery, if possible. On the arrival of the physician, he will, in all probability, want to make a rectal or a vaginal examination at once in order to determine the amount of dilation of the cervix and the progress the mother has made. For the examination, the patient should be in lithotomy position, lying on the side of the bed convenient for the physician. The nurse should drape the mother so that she is well protected, but with the perineal region well exposed. Some physicians prefer to make the examination with the patient lying on her back, but across the bed, with the buttocks resting on the edge of the mattress and the patient's feet supported by two chairs. A pillow may be placed under the patient's head for comfort. When a vaginal examination is to be made, the preparation of the perineal area will be according to the wishes of the physician. Although the technic for local preparation of the patient for vaginal examination varies, if the nurse always regards the perineal region as a site for operation and cleanses the immediate area accordingly, she has followed an important principle for safe care.

All instruments required for the delivery are usually provided by the physician and are brought to the home in sterile packages. However, if such equipment as catheters, hypodermic syringes and needles and the various instruments are not sterile, these are boiled in a tightly covered container for 20 minutes. Sterile packages should not be laid open, or sterile equipment laid out, until just before they are to be used for the delivery.

The Delivery. The activities of the nurse in assisting the physician at delivery will be directed by the physician. Because of the vast differences in home situations, the details in each case are so variable that it would be impossible to describe them here. In general, the conduct of normal labor, as described in Chapter 12, should serve as a guide for the care of the mother and her infant.

Delivery by the Nurse

In certain cases the nurse will find it necessary to manage the entire labor herself, either because of precipitate delivery or through delay in securing the services of a physician.

It is needless to say that labor in such cases progresses rapidly, and that almost before anything else can be done, the contractions are recurring with such frequency and severity that the mother must be put to bed and be given the undivided attention of the nurse. If time permits, much can be done for the comfort of the mother while preparations are made for delivery. Undoubtedly, the calmness of the nurse at the bedside will be transferred to the mother.

It seldom happens that the nurse and her patient are entirely alone; usually the husband, some relative or friend in the home can be called upon to assist and bring the necessary things to the bedside. In an emergency, when there has been no previous preparation, an ordinary pair of scissors and pieces of clean, soft, white cord or tape may be boiled and used for tying and cutting the cord. As there is usually never any special hurry about tying and cutting the umbilical cord, there is time for scissors and tape to be boiled. Time may be saved by using only enough water to cover the instruments, but it must be sufficient to allow for evaporation. Also, anything which will float, such as the tape, should be weighted down with the scissors. The pan may be covered with a second pan, thus sterilizing both.

If the patient is fully dressed, as may be the case in precipitate delivery, the nurse should do what she can to protect the patient's clothing and the bedding and maintain cleanliness to the best of her ability. The procedure is, of course, the same as when the physician is present; but since the nursing care is wholly different, it may help her to have the steps described as they are in the section on "Emergency Delivery by the Nurse" in Chapter 12, in order to aid her until help arrives.

SUGGESTED READING

Bookmiller, Mae, and Bowen, George: Textbook of Obstetrics and Obstetric Nursing, ed. 3, Philadelphia, Saunders, 1958.

Davis, M. E., and Scheckler, C. E.: DeLee's Obstetrics for Nurses, ed. 16, Philadelphia, Saunders, 1957.

Frontier Nursing Service, Wendover, Ky.: Thirty Years Onward (1925-1955), 1955.

Maryland State Dept. of Health, 301 West Preston St., Baltimore, Md.: Division of Public Health Nursing, Manual of Nursing and Special Procedures, 1955.

Maryland State Dept. of Health, Bureau of Preventive Medicine: Midwifery in the Counties of Maryland, The Maryland Law, Senate Bill No. 115, Enacted 1924, and Regulations of the State Board of Health Governing the Licensing of Midwives, Adopted Feb. 1, 1957.

Newman, Margaret: The "mountain granny" bows out, Nursing Outlook 6:680, 1958.

U. S. Children's Bureau: Prenatal Care (Pub. No. 4), Washington, D. C., U. S. Government Print. Off., 1949.

Van Blarcom, Carolyn C.: Obstetrical Nursing (rev. by E. Ziegel), ed. 4, New York, Macmillan, 1957.

CHAPTER TWENTY-THREE

Obstetrics During Emergency

When any large-scale emergency arises, it is usually sudden and calls for immediate action, whether it is caused by hurricane, flood, fire or war. In the event of such catastrophe, babies are likely to be born rapidly, and many women may abort. When organized rescue work is hampered, it may fall to those who are in the immediate area to manage as best they can. The nurses in the area should be able to assist with measures for the safety and the welfare of maternity patients and their newborn infants.

All nurses who have completed the basic course in maternity nursing are familiar with antepartal care, the con-duct of labor and the immediate care of the newborn infant, but their preparation has been carried out, for the most part, in an organized environment (such as a hospital) where supplies, equipment and medical direction are available. It requires considerable imagination on the part of a nurse to conceive of an emergency situation in which she might be required to work. Communities may be isolated and temporarily left to their own resources if telephone and radio communications are wrecked; roads may be impassable if they are inundated by water and blocked by débris, and an area may be without safe water, means of power and medical supplies.

Disaster Insurance for Mothers and Babies*

by Sara E. Fetter, John Whitridge, Jr., and Col. John Welch

Insuring the lives and health of pregnant women and newborn infants during national or extensive local disasters requires planning for this purpose predicated on the belief that plans and preparations *prior* to disasters are essential and imperative.

With the advent of the H-bomb and the rapid advance in the development of ballistics and intercontinental missiles, the earlier concept of planning for the care of pregnant women and newborn infants, based on the Hiroshima experience, has changed in some ways, because the degree and the extent of man-made hazard have increased. Pro-

* Reprinted from The Bulletin of Maternal Welfare 4:9, 1957.

tection from radioactive fallout must be provided; evacuation from expected target areas will be 20 to 50 miles distant, instead of the 8 to 10 miles originally considered necessary, and, in all probability, the care of women in labor must be provided en route. Large-scale plans are under way for evacuees to be cared for in reception areas—including pregnant women and newborn infants. As the national defenses are strengthened and increased, there is logical expectation that there may be prior warning of an attack and time to put into effect large-scale evacuation of priority groups, such as pregnant women, to pre-designated reception areas. However, evacuation is cumbersome, time-consuming and requires several hours advance warning. Provision must also be made for protection in shelters, pits, etc., to care for those who cannot be evacuated.

Although early planning for the protection of the civilian population recognized the need for pacts of mutual assistance mostly with State co-ordination, disaster planning now includes nationwide and continental participation. The concept is still valid that official state and community agencies, in co-operation with civil defense planners, medical and welfare, assume the major responsibility, not only for planning prior to disasters, but for the administration and operation of emergency services for expectant mothers and infants through local and regional health units.

In planning for the safeguarding of mothers and newborn infants prior to a disaster, certain assumptions can be made and specific factors considered:

Pregnant women will be subject to all of the risks and injuries to which men and nonpregnant women will be exposed. Their general care should be in accordance with provisions made for the population at large. However, their obstetric care does require additional planning and facilities for it should be separate from hospital and emergency facilities for casualties. Two lives are at stake, lives of particular import to the future of the country. The need for care of the pregnant woman is predictable, since sooner or later she must inevitably be delivered, and in the process will need medical attention to a greater or lesser extent. In the vast majority of instances, probably in 90 per cent of all cases, the birth process, whether it results in a viable infant or abortion, will be essentially uncomplicated. The most formidable complications to be encountered with any frequency will be hemorrhage, obstructed or prolonged labor, infection, mild and severe toxemias of pregnancy with convulsions and miscellaneous medical and surgical conditions accompanying pregnancy.

It is estimated that at any given time, approximately 2 per cent of the total population will consist of women in various stages of pregnancy. In applying this prevalence rate to a given geographic area, allowance must be made for the character of the area, since the rate will, of course, be affected by the presence of large industrial plants and offices employing large numbers of males.

On the basis of the Hiroshima experience with the A-bomb, it can be anticipated that approximately one quarter of all surviving pregnant women on the periphery of the atomic explosion will abort or deliver shortly thereafter. Furthermore, approximately 10 per cent of pregnant women within range of the effects of a nuclear explosion will have abortions or premature deliveries.

It is possible, therefore, that in the affected blast area there may be as many as 500 to 700 deliveries or abortions per 100,000 population shortly after an explosion. In areas more remote from the explosion, the number of deliveries or abortions will more nearly approximate that occurring during normal times.

If the foregoing concepts are accepted and remain valid in disaster planning, what then should be the planning for minimal essential care for mothers and newborn infants in disaster situations? To the extent that it is possible, the facilities which are normally available for pregnant women during the antepartal delivery and postpartal periods should be available.

Preparation for the care of mothers and babies during a disaster requires that thought be given and plans made for the training of families for their own protection and survival and for the training of a large percentage of the population to carry out minimal essentials of care to save the lives of other people.

It can be assumed that in any major disaster, physicians, nurses and other specially trained professional personnel will be almost completely absorbed in the task of caring for casualties; normal women in labor at such times will have to rely largely on nonprofessional personnel for their needs. Just who will these nonprofessional people be? They will have to be other women who have received instruction in the procedures described. In other words, each community must contain a corps of lay women who understand the basic concepts contained in this brief review and have been given at least minimal training in providing this type of care. Preparation for civil defense is a family affair. Every citizen and every family needs to have the information necessary to protect himself, his family and his community well in advance of a disaster or an enemy attack. Those responsible for planning and implementing disaster plans have the unique responsibility for making this information available to individuals in communities in a way which they can understand and accept.

The only hope we have for the saving of lives of mothers and newborn infants depends on the family's ability to carry out the plans made with and for them.

Every expectant mother needs to know her physician's expectation of the kind of delivery she will have, so that if she needs any special facilities she will be able to go where these are available. She needs to understand the care she and her baby will need during delivery and immediately afterward.

There are differences of opinion about how much information pregnant women should have about their own condition and the conduct and the outcome of the delivery. It is assumed that in the event of large-scale disasters, women will have to carry much of the responsibility for their own safety. Therefore, adequate information about what to do, where to go and what constitutes essential equipment will be comforting to them rather than alarming.

Essential equipment is quite minimal and is available to almost every woman in her own home. A package should be made up and kept accessible with other emergency supplies. Contents include a clean sheet, towels, washcloth and soap; blankets, clothing, a nipple and a bottle for the baby; a pair of blunt scissors; 2 pieces of clean linen tape, 6 inches long and ¼ inch wide, wrapped separately from the other articles, and a package of powdered milk for the mother.

Those who are giving care to pregnant women need to understand that the pregnant woman's normal dependent needs may be greatly enhanced by separation from and concern for her husband and family and by increased fear for herself and her baby. Understanding in meeting this exaggerated need for mothering and providing a warm accepting environment will increase the confidence of the pregnant woman in her ability to have her baby and will comfort her and relieve some of her fear and apprehension. Every effort should be made to have someone with the patient throughout labor. The emotional support which patients in labor (who have had some preparation) derive from each other should be utilized.

Essentials of care during the first stage of labor include the maintenance of physical and emotional reserves, the interpretation of the progress of labor to the patient and the family, the provision of rest and fluids, the maintenance of asepsis and preparation for the second stage of labor, including frequent emptying of the bladder.

There should be constant review of progress and observation of signs of complications. As the patient approaches the completion of the first stage of labor, she will need special care and encouragement and should not be left alone. If care is delegated, it should be assigned to a nursing auxiliary or to a relative or a friend who is kindly, understanding and responsible.

During the second stage of labor, constant observation, encouragement and interpretation are all important. A clean delivery area should be maintained, and there should be continual observation of the patient's general condition for signs of exhaustion and other complications. The maternal pulse rate and the quality should be observed.

A progress report to the supervising physician should be made by the person giving the care. In the absence of the physician during the delivery, the nurse, the nurse-midwife or the attendant who is helping the patient can teach her that when the baby's head is in sight to take a deep breath at the beginning of each contraction, to hold her breath and exert downward pressure, while the infant's head is controlled. As soon as the contraction is over, the patient should be encouraged to relax completely and wait for the next contraction.

Supportive care is especially important. The back can be rubbed for low back pain and the legs stretched for muscle cramps. The explanation of the progress of labor often provides the encouragement which the patient needs to complete the second stage of labor with minimal emotional stress.

When the head crowns, the perineum should be supported and protected with a clean towel if a sterile towel is not available. Gentle pressure is applied against the head as it emerges to prevent too rapid delivery of the head, which is supported as it is born. Immediate removal of the membranes from around the baby's head is important. If the umbilical cord is around the neck, it is slipped over the head whenever it can be done easily. The mucus should be wiped from the baby's mouth and nose. Occasionally, spontaneous rotation of the head to one side or the other will not take place within a reasonable period of time. Under such circumstances, gentle rotation of the head in the direction toward which it tends to go more easily will suffice to bring one shoulder anteriorly behind the symphysis.

To deliver the anterior shoulder of the baby, the head is grasped with both hands, and gentle but steady pressure toward the floor is applied until the anterior shoulder slips under the symphysis pubis and the upper portion of the arm can be seen. Then the direction of traction is reversed upward in order to deliver the posterior shoulder over the perineum. The above maneuvers should be carried out slowly and carefully; there is no pressing need to hurry.

The baby's body is supported as it is born and is wrapped in a warm sterile towel or clean cloth and placed on the mother's abdomen with the head lower so that the mucus will drain out. Pulling on the cord should be avoided. The mother will want to know about the baby and see it as soon as it is born. If the baby does not cry immediately, or if there is mucus, the nose and the mouth should be cleared and postural drainage instituted. Gentle rubbing of the back helps to stimulate the baby's breathing. When the cord stops pulsating it is tied in two places and cut between the two ties. After the cord is cut, the baby is warmly wrapped and placed in the mother's arms.

During the delivery of the baby and the beginning of the third stage of labor there should be constant observation of the mother's general condition and of signs indicating the separation of the placenta. If the attendant assisting with the delivery places her hand on the mother's fundus, she can report the changes to the person conducting the delivery. When the uterus rises upward in the abdomen and becomes globular and firm, and the umbilical cord extends 3 or 4 inches out of the vagina and there is a gush of blood, the patient can be asked to bear down with the next contraction. This pressure is usually sufficient to expel the placenta, which is received in a clean receptacle. In order to express the placenta it may be necessary occasionally to apply gentle pressure on the fundus of the uterus when it is well contracted. The direction of pressure should be toward the vaginal outlet. Following the expulsion of the placenta, if the uterus tends to become soft and bleeding occurs, the uterus should be massaged vigorously with the finger tips to promote uterine contraction, and the baby put to the breast.

The placenta and membranes should be examined to determine whether there are any missing portions.

If the uterus remains small and firm, nothing should be done, other than to keep the hand on the fundus for 1 hour following the delivery of the baby. The patient should be made comfortable, given nourishment, encouraged to void and allowed to rest.

As soon as the mother can be left, the baby should be identified, according to the method established by the particular health department, and carefully examined for injuries and congenital malformations.

Essentials of nursing care of the baby include gentle handling, observation of breathing, color, appearance, activity, skin and body temperature, stools, weight (if possible) and umbilical cord for bleeding and healing; provision should be made for warmth, proper food and protection from infection.

Mother and newborn baby should be considered an inseparable unit. If a mother cannot take care of her baby, full-time mothering care must be provided to enhance the baby's chances of survival and promote his well-being. Irregularities in breathing, mucus in air passages, weak sucking reflex, skin irritation and unstable temperature-regulating mechanism point to the importance of constant observation and an environment adapted to meet the needs of the individual infant.

The infant should be put to breast 24 hours after birth and at 4-hour intervals for periods of 5 minutes until the milk supply is established. Once the supply of milk is sufficient to satisfy the infant, feedings should be given as often as necessary to meet his need. Artificial feedings may be necessary until the mother's milk supply is adequate or in instances where the mother is unable to nurse the infant.

The newborn is particularly susceptible to infection. Anyone with any evidence of infection, such as rash, diarrhea or upper respiratory infection, should not give infant care.

When the infant is found to be premature and in need of special care, or to have congenital malformations, the emergency facilities which have been developed for such conditions should be utilized.

When the mother and infant are to be discharged from the place where care has been given during labor and delivery, it is essential for arrangements to be made with the family and others for the mother to be relieved of responsibilities except the care of her baby and herself. The mother, the family and the attendant should know where and whom to call if she or the baby have any conditions or symptoms needing medical care.

To increase the number of people with some training in the care of pregnant women and newborn infants, the existing educational programs need to be expanded. These include mother and baby care classes, such as those given by the Red Cross and other health agencies, parent education groups, home nursing classes, first-aid training, classes for baby sitters and junior and senior high school students and the midwifery training programs. Planning for training and the achievement of the training of persons who carry this responsibility in a disaster are not easy.

During a disaster, it is assumed that it will be the responsibility of nurses, certified nurse-midwives and licensed nonprofessional midwives to carry on an intensive program of on-the-job training of whomever is available to help and to supervise the care of mothers and babies.

SUGGESTED READING

Green, Josephine M.: Emergency care of the obstetric patient, Nursing Outlook 6:694, 1958.

Hogan, Aileen: Bomb-born babies, Pub. Health Nursing 43:383, 1951.

——: If disaster strikes—are we ready?, Briefs 21:8, 1957.

Maryland State Dept. of Health, Div. Pub. Health Nursing: Suggested Content for the Training Program in Civil Defense Nursing, Parts III and IV, Maryland State Dept. of Health, Jan., 1952.

New York State Dept. of Health, Bureau of Maternal and Child Health: Assisting at the Birth of a Baby If No Doctor Is Available, New York State Dept. of Health, 1954.

Rayner, Jeanette F.: How do nurses behave in disaster?, Nursing Outlook 6:572, 1958.

Work Conference on Disaster Nursing: Text of addresses, Norfolk, Va., Nov. 12-16, 1956.

CHAPTER TWENTY-FOUR

History of Obstetrics*

In the course of one chapter it is impossible to give a detailed history of obstetrics. This does not purport to be a complete account of the progress of obstetrics through the ages but merely a skeletal outline upon which the interested may place significant facts by additional reading. Sufficient references will be given as to where more complete information can be obtained.

For greater simplicity and more ready understanding, the ages of obstetrics have been divided arbitrarily as set forth at the beginning of this chapter.

OBSTETRICS AMONG PRIMITIVE PEOPLES

We know little about obstetrics among the primitive races, but from careful study of the customs of the aboriginal American Indians and the African Negroes are able to learn some of the customs which were part of the obstetric practice of the ancients. Childbirth in primitive times was a relatively simple process. The mother retired to a place apart from the tribe and there gave birth to her child without great difficulty. It is known that intertribal marriages were relatively rare; therefore, there was not the conglomeration of mingled races which exists today. A realization of this fact alone makes possible an understanding of the relative simplicity of childbirth under these circumstances. The fetal head and body were accommodated

satisfactorily within the anatomic range of the maternal pelvis. The lack of mixed marriages prevented the resultant disproportion between passenger and pelvic passages. It became customary for women who had attended other women in labor to be asked to assist or accompany more of them, and they became the primitive counterpart of our latter-day midwife. The only real danger a primitive mother faced was that of abnormal presentation, which usually terminated fatally for both mother and child. Toxemias and other complications are largely the products of more advanced civilization and were rarely if ever met among primitive peoples.

EGYPTIAN OBSTETRICS

In Egypt, a highly organized state of society existed, and with it there arose a more complicated, if not more advanced, type of obstetrics. The priesthood in Egypt was interested in all the activities of society, and obstetrics was not neglected. They had a supervisory interest in it and took an active part in the care of abnormal or operative cases. They are known to have had obstetric forceps, performed cesarean sections on dead mothers, and podalic version was a part of their art.

ORIENTAL OBSTETRICS

Hindu medicine was probably the first authentic system of medicine to be given to the world. One of their most prolific writers and earliest men of whom

* By Douglas E. Cannell, M.B., B.Sc. (Med.), F.R.C.S. (C), Toronto, Canada.

we have written record is Susrata. The
exact date of his existence is still a matter of dispute, but he is variously stated
to have worked and written between
600 B.C and A.D. 500, more probably
about the latter date. His knowledge of
menstruation and gestation was quite
modern. He knew and described intelligently the management of normal and
abnormal labor. He described the use of
forceps and cesarean section upon dead
mothers to remove living children, and
gave excellent prenatal and postpartal
advice. He advised cleanliness on the
part of the obstetrician; cutting the
beard, the hair and the nails closely; the
wearing of clean gowns; and thorough
disinfection of the operating rooms prior
to operation or delivery. His surgical
antiseptic technic seems remarkable to
modern students.

Chinese obstetrics was largely of a
legendary nature until the publication
of a Chinese household manual of obstetrics, Ta Sheng P'Ien, which, according to the author's own statement, "is
correct and needs no change or addition
of prescription." There were mono-
graphs on obstetrics prior to this, but
none so complete. Many of his statements are unfounded; in fact, the knowledge is scanty or incorrect, but the
author had the saving grace of objecting
to unnecessary interference and coun-
seled patience in the treatment of labor.
He had a poor opinion of midwives in
general, stating that "the majority of
them are fools." The reviews of Chinese
obstetrics and obstetric drugs by Max-
well are excellent and give a detailed
account of an interesting phase of obstetrics, which for lack of space we are
forced to dispense with in this account.

GRECIAN OBSTETRICS

Prior to Hippocrates, the Asclepie-
ads, or followers of Aesculapius, the
Father of Medicine, had a slight and
largely supervisory interest in obstetrics.
Abortions were not illegal. There is little
definite knowledge concerning this period, but it seems probable that obstetric
treatment was of a primitive nature.

The Hippocratic Period. During
this age, normal obstetric cases were
handled by midwives under the supervision of the physicians. Abnormal labor
was entirely in the hands of the medical
profession. To Hippocrates is accredited
the Hippocratic oath which is still a
part of the exercises for all students
graduating from medical school. Treat-
ises upon obstetrics attributed to Hippocrates are the oldest records available
of the Western World's obstetric methods.

Greco-Roman Obstetrics. This period was one of progress which was due
largely to the work of Celsus, Aëtius
and Soranus (second century). The last
reintroduced podalic version and is responsible for the first authentic records
of its use in the delivery of living children. He gave an excellent technical
description of the procedure and the
indications for its use.

BYZANTINE, MOHAMMEDAN, JEWISH AND MEDIEVAL PERIODS

These may be said to have been characterized by a complete absence of
progress, and as a corollary, a retrogression and loss of previously known practice resulted. This was due in large part
to the general failure of science in the
medieval period, but the interference of
the Roman Church in secular matters,
particularly those of a scientific nature,
must be held responsible for a large
share of it. The paucity of operative
treatment in difficult labor may be
judged from the recommendations contained in the only textbook of the day
on obstetrics and gynecology, which
read as follows: "Place the patient in a
sheet held at the corners by four strong
men, with her head somewhat elevated.
Have them shake the sheet vigorously
by pulling on the opposite corners, and

with God's aid she will give birth." However, hospitals and nursing services were organized in this age.

While the ancient Jews gave very little assistance to the woman during labor and delivery, they were interested in the hygiene of pregnancy and cleanliness at the time of childbirth. Hygiene and sanitation were apparently a part of their religion. At the time of difficult deliveries, the women "were comforted until they died." The stool or obstetric chair was used at this time and continued to be used until about the nineteenth century A.D. Reference is made to this chair in the Bible, in the first chapter of Exodus, "when you do the office of the midwife to the Hebrew women, and see them upon the stools . . ."

THE RENAISSANCE PERIOD

The Renaissance was characterized by advances in medicine and obstetrics commensurate with those in other fields. During this time we have the first English text on obstetrics, the *Byrthe of Mankynde,* published by Raynalde. Both it and its German counterpart by Roesslin are copies of Soranus, and with their publication podalic version was reintroduced to obstetric practice. Many famous men were responsible for the progress in obstetrics—among them Leonardo da Vinci (who made the first accurate sketches of the fetus in utero) and Vesalius (who accurately described the pelvis for the first time).

To Ambrose Paré, the dean of French surgeons and obstetricians, must go the chief credit for making podalic version a useful and practicable procedure. Due to his skill, he preferred its use to cesarean section in difficult labor. By his careful studies of its indications and technic, he made possible the removal of obstetrics from the hands of the midwives, where it had rested since the fall of the Roman Empire, and its establishment as an independent branch of medicine.

Regulations were enacted for the practice of midwives, and schools were established during this period for their training. Paré's work on version and his discouragement of cesarean section were opportune.

Sections had been practiced since antiquity upon dead mothers, but the first authentic section performed upon a living mother is credited to Trautman, of Wittenberg, in 1610. This was done upon a woman with a large ventral hernia which contained the uterus. Prior to this, Nufer, a sow gelder, is reputed to have performed the operation on his wife, after obstetricians and midwives had failed to deliver her. It has been stated that Jane Seymour was delivered by a section done by Frère, a noted surgeon of the time, at the request of Henry VIII. That she died a few days after the birth of Edward VI adds credence to the story, but no absolute confirmation is available. Due to the frightful mortality from hemorrhage, sepsis, etc., it did not become popular in spite of the advocacy of the Church. Through the following centuries it was done occasionally, but not until the advent of uterine sutures and aseptic technic did it become a practical procedure.

The origin of its name has been ascribed to Julius Caesar, but, as his mother lived many years after his birth, this seems improbable—considering the high mortality of all abdominal operations before the time of Lister. A more accurate explanation is that Numa Pompilius, one of the earlier Roman kings, passed a law making it compulsory to perform the operation upon all mothers who died while pregnant in order that the mother and the child might be buried separately. This was known as the "Lex Regis" and with the advent of the Caesars as the "Lex Caesaris"—and subsequently "cesarean section." The name has been attributed to "cedere," the Latin verb meaning "to cut," but the former explanation seems to be more reasonable.

THE SEVENTEENTH CENTURY

This century was notable for many famous obstetricians. Mauriceau, of Paris, was the first to correct the view that the pelvic bones separated in normal labor. He was also the first man to refer to epidemic puerperal fever. His description of an obstetrician, or rather of the qualities an obstetrician should possess, is both interesting and amusing. He stated:

He must be healthful, strong and robust; because this is the most laborious of all the Operations of Chirurgery; for it will make one sometimes sweat, so he shall not have a dry Thread, tho' it were the coldest Day in Winter. . . . He ought to be well shaped, at least to outward appearance, but above all, to have small hands for the easier Introduction of them into the Womb when necessary; yet strong, with the Fingers long, especially the Fore-finger, the better to reach and touch the inner orifice. He must have no Rings on his Fingers, and his Nails well pared, when he goeth about the Work, for fear of hurting the Womb. He ought to have a pleasant Countenance, and to be as neat in his Clothes as in his person, that the poor women who have need of him be not affrighted at him. Some are of the opinion, that a Practitioner of this Art ought on the contrary to be slovenly, at least very careless, wearing a great Beard, to prevent the Occasion of the Husband's Jealousy that sends for him. Truly some believe this Policy augments their Practice but 'tis fit they should be disabused; for such a Posture and Dress resembles more a Butcher than a Chirurgeon, whom the woman apprehends already too much, that he needs not such a Disguise. Above all he must be sober, no Tipler, that he may at all times have his Wits about him. . . ."

Van Deventer, of Holland, has been called the Father of Modern Obstetrics and is credited with the first accurate description of the pelvis, its deformities and their effect on parturition. He also shares with Ould, of Dublin, the first description of the mechanism of labor. As time passed, customs changed, and the term "accoucheur" replaced the objectionable "midman" and "man-midwife." Obstetric forceps were invented, probably about 1580, by Peter Chamberlen but were kept as a family secret until 1813 in an effort of the Chamberlens to monopolize the field. In 1699, Hugh Chamberlen sold one half of the instrument to Amsterdam but added fraud to infamy by selling the vector or worthless half. Prior to that, in 1670, he had demanded the equivalent of $7,500 for the secret and, in an attempt to show their worth, had killed a woman and baby before Mauriceau, who craftily chose for the demonstration a woman with a distorted pelvis, upon whom he previously had planned to do a cesarean section. After some hours of fruitless effort, Chamberlen failed in his attempts at delivery, with the resultant double fatality. When the Chamberlen forceps were finally revealed to the profession in 1813, their need had been met by other men, and the Chamberlens were thus justly punished for the discredit they had brought upon their calling.

THE EIGHTEENTH CENTURY

The eighteenth century was marked by a succession of famous men such as Palfyne, the Hunters, Smellie, White and others. The first named is credited with the invention of obstetric forceps, as he presented a copy in 1770 to the Academy of Medicine of Paris.

Smellie taught obstetrics with a manikin and made improvements on the obstetric forceps in use at that time, adding a steel lock and curved blades. He also laid down the first principles for their use and differentiated by measurement between contracted and normal pelves.

William Hunter, though a pupil of Smellie, was opposed to the use of forceps, and frequently exhibited his rusted blades as evidence of their uselessness.

In conjunction with his brother, he laid the foundation of our modern knowledge of placental anatomy.

Charles White published an obstetric thesis advocating the scrubbing of the hands and general cleanliness on the part of the accoucheur; he was the pioneer in aseptic midwifery. John Harvie, 90 years before Credé, advocated external manual expression of the placenta, and it is known that a similar procedure was in use in Dublin at that time. One of the most active and famous English obstetricians of the time, John Clarke, had has fame commemorated in this epitaph:

Beneath this stone, shut up in the dark
Lies a learned man-midwife y'clep'd Dr.
    Clarke.
On earth while he lived by attending
    men's wives,
He increased population some thousands
    of lives;
Thus a gain to the nation was gain to
    himself
An enlarged population, enlargement of
    pelf.
So he toiled late and early, from morn-
    ing to night,
The squalling of children his greatest
    delight;
Then worn out with labours, he died
    skin and bone
And his ladies he left all to Mansfield
    and Stone.

There were many famous obstetricians on the Continent in this period, chief among them being Baudelocque, who invented the pelvimeter and named and described positions and presentations. In America, prejudices against men in midwifery were carried over from Europe; as late as 1857 a demonstration before the graduating class at Buffalo roused such a storm of criticism that the American Medical Association had to intervene. Their judgment was that any physician who could not conduct labor by touch alone should not undertake midwifery.

This eighteenth century produced such men as Moultrie, Lloyd and Shippen. The last was a pupil of Smellie and Hunter; in 1762, he opened a school for midwifery in Philadelphia, and, since he provided convenient lodgings for the accommodation of poor women during confinement, he may be said to have established the first lying-in hospital in America. With Morgan, he founded the School of Medicine of the University of Pennsylvania, becoming its first Professor of Anatomy, Surgery and Midwifery.

THE NINETEENTH AND THE TWENTIETH CENTURIES

The increased knowledge, interest and ability which physicians brought to obstetrics were largely offset by the increased mortality due to puerperal fever. During the seventeenth, the eighteenth and the nineteenth centuries it became a pestilence, at times wiping out whole communities of puerperal women. The mortality rates varied in the best European clinics at Paris and Vienna from 10 to 20 per cent. The origin and the spread of the disease were little understood or studied. Obstetricians wasted futile hours on a study of minor alterations in instruments or technic and ignored the vast loss of life from puerperal fever. Oliver Wendell Holmes, of Harvard, first presented his views on the contagiousness of puerperal fever in 1843, and in 1855 he reiterated them in a monograph on *Puerperal Fever as a Private Pestilence*. This was, and still remains, a medical classic on the subject. His statements aroused great controversy in America, and he received a great deal of abuse and criticism from Meigs and Hodge, two of the foremost American obstetricians of the day. One of them stated that it was ridiculous to conceive of any gentleman carrying contamination on his hands from patient to patient.

The following is Holmes' summary of his observations on the prevention of puerperal sepsis. Written in 1843, before the discovery of any human pathologic organism, and before the adoption of disinfection in surgical procedures, it is a truly remarkable summary.*

1. A physician holding himself in readiness to attend cases of midwifery, should never take any active part in the postmortem examination of cases of puerperal fever.

2. If a physician is present at such autopsies, he should use thorough ablution, change every article of dress, and allow twenty-four hours or more to elapse before attending to any case of midwifery. It may be well to extend the same caution to cases of simple peritonitis.

3. Similar precautions should be taken after the autopsy or surgical treatment of cases of erysipelas, if the physician is obliged to unite such offices with his obstetrical duties, which is in the highest degree inexpedient.

4. On the occurrence of a single case of puerperal fever in his practice, the physician is bound to consider the next female he attends in labor, unless some weeks, at least, have elapsed, as in danger of being infected by him, and it is his duty to take every precaution to diminish her risk of disease and death.

5. If within a short period two cases of puerperal fever happen close to each other, in the practice of the same physician, the disease not existing or prevailing in the neighborhood, he would do wisely to relinquish his obstetrical practice for at least one month, and endeavor to free himself by every available means from any noxious influence he may carry about with him.

6. The occurrence of three or more closely connected cases, in the practice of one individual, no others existing in the neighborhood, and no other sufficient causes being alleged for the coincidence, is prima facie evidence that he is the vehicle of contagion.

7. It is the duty of the physician to take every precaution that the disease shall not be introduced by nurses or other assistants, by making proper inquiries concerning them, and giving timely warning of every suspected source of danger.

* From Abraham Levinson, Pioneers of Pediatrics.

8. Whatever indulgence may be granted to those who have heretofore been the ignorant causes of so much misery, the time has come when the existence of a *private pestilence* in the sphere of a single physician should be looked upon not as a misfortune but as a crime; and in the knowledge of such occurrences, the duties of the practitioner to his profession should give way to his paramount obligations to society.

While Holmes first conceived the correct idea of the nature of the disease, it is to Ignaz Philipp Semmelweiss that the glory must go of finally proving without question the nature of its source and transmission. He was an assistant in the Viennese clinic for women, and while his associates fussed with unimportant details of technic, he was studying and mourning the tremendous death rate among puerperal women in the clinic. He observed that the death rate in Clinic I where women were delivered by medical students or physicians was always higher than that of Clinic II where midwives officiated or received instruction. After fruitless study and manifold changes in technic in order to follow more closely that of Clinic II, the cause of the disease was brought home to him in a desperate and startling fashion. His friend, Kalletschka, an assistant in pathology, died after performing an autopsy upon a victim of puerperal fever, during which Kalletschka had sustained a slight cut on his finger.

At postmortem the findings were identical with those of puerperal sepsis, and Semmelweiss concluded that the disease was transmitted from the dead, by contact from the physicians and the students, who often went directly from the postmortem room to deliveries. Accordingly, he immediately instituted and enforced a ruling which made it obligatory that all physicians and students wash their hands in a solution of chloride of lime after attending autopsies and before examining or delivering mothers. In seven months he had reduced the mortality in Clinic I from 12 to 3 per cent, and in the subsequent year had a mortality lower than Clinic II, a hitherto unheard-of feat. Subsequently, he observed that puerperal sepsis could be transmitted from patient to patient by contact of contaminated material, or attendants, as well as from the postmortem room, and in 1861 he published his immortal work on *The Cause, Concept and Prophylaxis of Puerperal Fever.*

Medicine provides pitiful figures in profusion, but none, it seems, met such a cruel reception and ultimate fate as Semmelweiss. His colleagues (for the most part, but with a few notable and loyal exceptions) distorted and criticized his teachings. Had they stopped there it might have been bad enough, but they carried their distaste for his views to the stage of persecution. He was forced to leave Vienna and go to Budapest, where a similar attitude—if possible a more malignant one—awaited him. A disappointed man, he died in 1865 from a brain abscess which may have originated in an infection similar to that of his friend Kalletschka. To the tragedy of his life, his death added satire. His work, however, has lived on; Pasteur and Lister added to it; and with a more modern and tolerant age his worth has been recognized.

The organisms causing puerperal fever probably were seen by several early workers beginning with Mayrhofer, who, in 1863, described "cylindrical vibrios" or "strings of pearls" in the lochia of puerperal sepsis. In 1864, 310 deaths occurred in the 1,350 confinement cases in the Maternité hospital in Paris, and that "Vestibule of Death" had to be closed in 1865.

Pasteur, in 1879, saw "cocci in chain" in cases of puerperal sepsis and contributed definitely to our knowledge of the causal streptococci, demonstrating to doctors the "presence of the invisible foe" in a drop of blood obtained by a "simple pin-prick on the finger tip of the unhappy woman doomed to die the next day" and recommending methods of aseptic technic for their control.

The nineteenth and the twentieth centuries were largely notable for their utilization of drugs to alleviate the pains of childbirth. The use of ether as an anesthetic was first discovered in America, but it was first utilized for childbirth by Simpson in Great Britain. He brought back the lost art of version by making it a safer procedure and eventually substituted chloroform for ether. As with almost every advance in medicine, it was opposed bitterly. The opposition was loudest and most vehement from the clergy, but, in 1853, Queen Victoria accepted it for delivery and by her action silenced most of the criticism. Nitrous oxide had been used in 1880 and has continued to be popular ever since that time.

Obstetric analgesia and anesthesia have made great strides during the twentieth century (see Chap. 11, Analgesia and Anesthesia in Labor).

The present century will be remembered largely for the development of antepartal clinics and the more concentrated care of the expectant mothers that came with them. The application of advances in general medicine, metabolism and public health to obstetrics has led to a marked decrease in mortality and morbidity from cardiac, pulmonic, metabolic, venereal and associated medical conditions complicating pregnancy. The consideration of adequate vitamin, mineral and caloric contents in connection with the diet of pregnant and puerperal women has not only decreased the morbidity but also has enhanced the health of all mothers and children who receive adequate obstetric care.

Many other contributions have been made and are being added constantly to the science of obstetrics, not the least of which is more intensive training and study in this specialty demanded by the public as well as the medical profession. The advent of routine external expression of the placenta, silver nitrate prophylaxis in the eyes of the newborn, purified ergot and pituitary preparations in hemorrhage control and prevention are but a few of the methods and medications which have marked the early twentieth century.

The morphologic and anthropologic studies of Naegele, Roberts, Williams, Goodwin, Caldwell, Moloy and others have done much to improve our understanding of the various types of pelves and some of their importance in labor. Roentgenologic pelvimetry and cephalometry have greatly advanced our knowledge of the probable course of labor and delivery; Thoms, Caldwell and Moloy, Hanson, Jarcho and countless others have contributed to our advances in this field (see Chap. 2).

In a necessarily brief and incomplete fashion, an endeavor has been made to touch upon some of the more interesting phases of the history of obstetrics—a delightful and fascinating subject.

Background and Development of Antepartal Care in the U.S.

As we know it today, antepartal care developed into its present status through devious avenues of investigation and many by-paths of interrelated activity and work. Individuals, both from the profession and the laity, as well as private and municipal organizations, contributed time, money and interest until, at last, Government action was obtained.

The background of our present maternity situation is of interest both as a history and a story. Antepartal care in the United States had its beginnings in the days of slavery. The intelligent slave-owners paid special attention to the diet and the care of pregnant slaves. Healthy slaves were more valuable, were worth more money and produced stronger offspring. From this beginning, the chronologic efforts which led to our present-day antepartal care follow.

1866. A story was written which concerned cruelty to a child. Some thoughtful person referred the case to *The Society for the Prevention of Cruelty to Animals*. Henry Bergh, a former diplomat to Russia, was the founder and director of this association and was influential in having the judgment pronounced on the ground that a child was a human animal. This incident stimulated interest in the general treatment of children.

1873. *The New York Diet Kitchen Association,* the oldest public health organization in America, was opened at the request of doctors from "de Milt Dispensary" on the lower East Side of New York City. It was first organized as a soup kitchen, and milk, gruel, beef tea and cooked rice were taken to the sick in their homes, with the idea of restoring health. In 1892, they began to make formulas for sick babies and still later dispensed free milk or sold it at 3 cents a quart. Maria L. Daniels was the first nurse director and contributed much for many years to public health progress. In 1926, this group was organized as *The Children's Health Service of New York*. The organization grew with the times, changing its program from curing the sick to preventive work—keeping well babies well. While the organization devoted its major effort to work with babies and preschool children, it also included antepartal care in its program.

1876. The beginning of child-welfare legislation in the United States was the Act passed by the New York State Legislature, granting to *The Society for the Prevention of Cruelty to Children* a charter giving it wide power with regard to the protection of child life. The inception of this legislation was based on the incident of the "child as a human animal" (1866).

1893. The first *Infant Milk Station* in the United States was established in New York City by Nathan Strauss. Through his persistence, milk was finally made "safe" through pasteurization; and many such stations were set up.

1900. *The United States Census Bureau* was made a permanent organization. Up to this time, *vital statistics* were considered to be of so little importance in the United States that, as soon as the population was tabulated and classified, the bureau was disbanded, to be reestablished and reorganized every 10 years.

1906. *The United States Census Bureau* published mortality statistics which drew attention to the appalling loss of life among babies and children. Up to this time, very little thought had been given to maternity and infant protection.

1907. Due to the growing interest, Mr. George H. F. Schrader was stimulated to give money to *The Association for Improving Conditions of the Poor* (now the *Community Service Society*) for the salaries of two nurses to do antepartal work. This was the first consistent effort to prevent deaths of babies by caring for the mothers *before* the babies were born. Two reasons were given as to why antepartal care would be of value: (1) nurses in convalescent homes for postpartal mothers thought that if patients had better care during pregnancy, the health of mothers would be improved; (2) social workers going into the homes felt that they were not adequately prepared to advise pregnant mothers.

1907. *The New York Milk Committee* was organized. Its object was the reduction of infant mortality through the improvement of the city's milk supply. It established milk depots which proved

beyond question their great value in the reduction of infant mortality by dispensing clean pasteurized milk and by educating mothers.

1908. In this year the *Division of Child Hygiene* was established in New York City, the first in the United States, and it was important enough to be recognized nationally. Josephine Baker, M.D., was appointed chief. This was a pioneer achievement, and the methods that were evolved had no precedent.

1909 to 1914. At approximately this time, Mrs. William Lowell Putnam, of Boston, promoted a demonstration of organized antepartal care. It was called *The Prenatal Care Committee* of the Women's Municipal League. They worked in co-operation with the Boston Lying-In Hospital through Robert L. DeNormandie, M.D., of Harvard Medical School, Dr. Ruggles, of the then Homeopathic Hospital, and the Instructive District Nurses Association. The committee functioned long enough to establish the fact that good obstetric care was not possible without antepartal care.

1909. In this year *The American Association for the Study and Prevention of Infant Mortality* was organized and held its first meeting in New Haven, Connecticut. This committee was composed of both professional and lay members and devoted itself entirely to problems connected with child life, particularly to studying and trying to correct the high mortality rate. At this time there were no records of birth or deaths, and the causes of deaths were unknown. The education of physicians and nurses was shamefully unsatisfactory; there was no public health in the schools, and practically no activity on the part of municipal, state or the Federal Government to prevent infant mortality. The first president of this association was J. H. Mason Knox, M.D., and Gertrude B. Kipp was the first secretary. The committee consisted of the Honorable Herbert Hoover, Livingston Ferrand, M.D.,

L. Emmet Holt, M.D., Richard Bolt, M.D., and Philip Van Ingen, M.D. The work of this organization was of profound significance. In 1918, its expanding activities caused it to change its name to *The American Child Hygiene Association,* and in 1923 the name was changed to the *American Child Health Association.* In 1935, after having contributed to every angle of this pioneer work, the association was disbanded.

1909. *The First White House Conference,* on "The Dependent Child," was called by President Theodore Roosevelt. These investigations resulted in the establishment of the U. S. Children's Bureau in 1912. According to some authorities, this conference was called through the influence of a public health nurse.

1910. *The Census Bureau* published another report, this time on the mortality of infants under one year of age and at "special ages." As a result of this report maternity hospitals made an effort to improve the care given to infants.

1911. In New York City *the first strictly municipal baby-health stations* were organized under the jurisdiction of the Department of Health, and the full cost of the work was borne by the municipality. Soon the dispensing of milk was of minor importance, and emphasis was placed on prevention—keeping well babies well. They are now called *Child-Health Stations.*

1911. *The New York Milk Committee* (1907) made an investigation at the baby-health stations and found that 40 percent of all infant deaths (112 per 1,000) occurred within the first month of life before the mothers registered their babies at the health stations. This indicated the necessity for care *before* birth. The committee then decided to carry on an experiment in antepartal work. (See 1917.) They were convinced that much could be hoped for as a result of organized antepartal care.

1912. *The Babies' Welfare Association* (formerly *The Association of Infant Milk*

Stations [1893]) represents the first comprehensive and successful attempt to co-ordinate the various child-welfare agencies in any community. All of the organizations of this type agreed to co-ordinate their activities by preventing duplication and overlapping without interfering with the organizations. In 1922, the name was changed to the *Children's Welfare Federation* of New York City. It continues to act as a clearing house and, among its other activities, manages the *Mother's Milk Bureau.*

1912. The *U. S. Children's Bureau* was established. It began in the Department of Commerce and Labor; in 1913 it was made a part of the Department of Labor and, in 1946, was transferred to the Federal Security Agency. This was created by Congress through a Federal Act (Government sanction). This bureau was to set up special machinery to study and protect the child and to study all matters pertaining to the welfare of children and child life among all classes of our people, to assemble and accumulate factual information and to disseminate this information throughout the country. Miss Julia Lathrop was chosen as chief. Much of the success of this bureau is credited to Miss Lathrop's vision. Fortunately, her successor, Miss Grace Abbott, continued the work with equal zeal.

1915. *The Birth Registration Area* was established as a Federal Act. The information is compiled in a uniform manner, giving the birth and the death statistics on which are based our information on mortality rates. The New England States, New York, Pennsylvania, Michigan, Minnesota and the District of Columbia, were the first states to comply. At the present time all 50 states and the District of Columbia require registration of every birth. (See pp. 4-5 and Tables 1 and 2.)

1915. Dr. Haven Emerson, Health Commissioner of New York City, appointed a special committee (Ralph W. Lobenstine, M.D., Clifton Edgar, M.D., and Philip Van Ingen, M.D.), in co-operation with the New York Milk Committee, to make an analysis of the facilities for maternity care in the city. The result of the survey showed that there was little antepartal work and no uniformity and that only a very small number of pregnant mothers were receiving care. It showed also that hospitals took care of 30 per cent of the deliveries, midwives delivered 30 per cent, general practitioners delivered 30 per cent, and private doctors, who might be classified as obstetricians, delivered 10 per cent. Previous to this time little or nothing had been done to regulate or control the midwives.

1916. *The National Society for the Prevention of Blindness* was created after much pioneer work and investigation, locally and throughout the states, by Carolyn Van Blarcom, R.N. She was chosen to be the executive secretary. Through these investigations it was learned that by far the greatest cause of blindness was ophthalmia neonatorum. These findings led to the passing of a law compelling all physicians and midwives to use prophylaxis in newborn babies' eyes. Also, as a direct result of Miss Van Blarcom's surveys, a school for lay midwives was started (Belleview School for Midwives, now out of existence). Miss Van Blarcom took out a midwife's license and was the first nurse in the United States so to register. The first obstetrical nursing textbook to be written by a nurse is to Miss Van Blarcom's credit. Her latest contribution to the better care of mothers and babies was to secure for Johns Hopkins Hospital the E. Bayard Halsted Fund for medical research.

1917. The Women's City Club of New York City and the New York Milk Committee opened three antepartal centers. The one sponsored by the Women's City Club was organized as the *Maternity Service Association* and, with Frances Perkins as the first executive secretary and Miss Mabel Choate as president, provided stimulating leadership. Dr. Ralph W. Lobenstine, a famous obstetrician, gave much time, labor, authority and direction as chairman of the medical board. In 1918, this organization was incorporated as the Maternity Center Association and carried out the first extensive piece of organized antepartal work in the United States. Miss Anne Stevens was director. Miss Annie W. Goodrich's wise counsel, as a member of the nursing committee, gave impetus to the organization's accomplishments. Louis I. Dublin, Ph.D., associated with this movement from the beginning, made an analysis of the first 4,000 records collected by the association. This revealed the startling fact that, through antepartal care, 50 per cent of the lives of mothers might be saved and 60 per cent of the lives of babies. Antepartal training and experience was extended to nurses throughout the world. This piece of intensive antepartal work fired increased interest in the care of mothers and babies. In 1929, the Maternity Center Association opened a school for the training of nurse midwives.

1919. *The Second White House Conference* was called by President Woodrow Wilson, as a result of the activities of the U. S. Children's Bureau. It was organized in five sections. Each section was interested in a different phase of maternity and child care.

1919. *The American Committee on Maternal Welfare* was founded. The object of the committee was:

To awaken and stimulate the interest of members of the medical profession in cooperating with public and private agencies for the protection of the health of mothers and their offspring before and during pregnancy and labor and after confinement to the end that the conditions which menace and interfere with the health or life of the mother or infant may be improved or prevented, disease and disorder corrected, health promoted and life saved; to teach the principles and practices of general and personal hygiene and health to parents and to improve and generalize the standards and methods of training physicians, nurses and others dealing with the problems of maternity.

The Committee was incorporated as a nonprofit organization in 1934 for the purpose of studying the maternal mortality rate in the U. S. and the management of obstetric problems generally. For more recent progress, see 1957.

This organization publishes the magazine *The Bulletin of Maternal and Infant Health*. It also promotes the American Congress of Obstetrics and Gynecology, which is held every three years. Seven such Congresses have been held, in 1939, 1942, 1947, 1950 (the first International Congress to be held in the U. S.), 1952, 1954 and 1957.

1921. *The Sheppard-Towner Bill* was passed by Congress, an Act for the Promotion of the Welfare and Hygiene of Maternity and Infancy, to be administered by the Children's Bureau. This bill was introduced in the 65th Congress by Congresswoman Jeanette Rankin of New Jersey. It was reported out of committee favorably but failed to pass. A second bill was introduced in the 66th Congress. It passed in the Senate but, through delays, was not considered by the House. In the first session of the 67th Congress the bill was again introduced by Senator Sheppard and Congressman Towner and, after much agitation, finally passed—an epoch in child-welfare legislation. An appropriation of $1,240,000 per year was granted for five years. The Cooper Bill, passed in 1927, extended it for two more years. This law was accepted by all of the states except three. This legislation gave a tremendous impetus to the education not only of the laity but also of the physicians. Because of this legislation there was created at once, in the states which did not already have them, departments, now quite uniformly labeled Divisions or Bureaus of Maternity and Child Health. In 1935, the Social Security Act

was passed, following the plan of the Sheppard-Towner Bill. This Act appropriated $3,800,000. In 1939, the Social Security Act was amended, increasing the appropriation to $5,820,000. The amount has been increased gradually, and by 1952 (82nd Congress), $30,000,000 was appropriated for Maternal and Child Health, Crippled Children and other Child Health Services.

1923. *The National Committee for Maternal Health* was formed with Robert L. Dickinson, M.D., as secretary and later as president. This was a clearing house and a center of information on certain medical aspects of human fertility. The object was to gather and analyze material, to stimulate research, and to issue reports to the medical profession and persuade it to take a leading part in the scientific investigations of these problems in preventive medicine. No other group existed for this purpose. It was dissolved in 1950.

1923. *The Margaret Sanger Research Bureau* came into being, an affiliation of the Planned Parenthood Federation of America, Inc., for research in the field of infertility, contraception and marriage counseling.

1923. Mary Breckinridge began her investigations in Kentucky, which led to the organization of the *Frontier Nursing Service*. With this concentrated effort of all phases of maternity and infant care, the striking results proved the value of prenatal care. Through her vision, determination and unfaltering energy, Mary Breckinridge has made this organization one of world-wide renown. In 1936, the Frontier Nursing Service opened a school for the training of nurse midwives.

1925. *The Joint Committee on Maternal Welfare* was formed. This consisted of the American Gynecological Society, the American Association of Obstetrics and Gynecology and Abdominal Surgeons and the American Child Health Association (1909). Later the section of Obstetrics, Gynecology and

Abdominal Surgeons of the American Medical Association was represented. They issued a pamphlet entitled *An Outline of Delivery Care*. This stimulated the Children's Bureau to publish a concise pamphlet, *Standards of Prenatal Care* (1925), an outline for the use of physicians, which did much to standardize routine procedures.

1930. *The Third White House Conference* was called by President Herbert Hoover. Mr. Hoover's interest in child welfare was very evident. The conference was very comprehensive and far-reaching and was devoted to all aspects of maternity and child care. The Children's Charter was adopted and became a Federal Act. The 45,000,000 children were analyzed in chart form to show the paramount importance of care during pregnancy and the early years.

1938. *The Conference on Better Care for Mothers and Babies* was called by the Children's Bureau. This was the first time that representatives from the states, private and public organizations, both lay and professional people, met to pool ideas.

1939. The *Maternity Consultation Service* in New York City was organized to further prenatal education and care.

1940. The *Fourth White House Conference* on Children in a Democracy was called by President Franklin D. Roosevelt. It considered the aims of our American civilization for the children in whose hands its future lies; how children can best be helped to grow into the kind of citizens who will know best how to preserve and protect our democracy. By 1940, the 48 states, the District of Columbia, Puerto Rico, Alaska and Hawaii (then Territories) were co-operating with the Children's Bureau in its administration of child-welfare services.

1940. *The Cleveland Health Museum* was opened to the public—the first health museum in the Western Hemisphere. It is significant in the maternity field because, in its workshops, it is reproducing the *Dickinson-Belskie models*,

acquired in 1945. Dr. Bruno Gebhard, Director, says that, in his belief, the use of this sculptural series in professional and lay education will advance knowledge on this all-important subject more quickly and more accurately than any other visual means thus far available.

1943. *The Emergency Maternity and Infancy Care Program* was launched to care for the wives and the babies of enlisted men in the armed forces. From $17,000,000 to $45,000,000 per year was appropriated. This Act also furthered interest in prenatal and child care.

1946. The *World Health Organization* —an agency of the United Nations—became a reality. At the first meeting in Paris, 64 nations signed the constitution. The membership now (1958) totals 85 countries and 3 associated members. The object of the organization is "the attainment of the highest possible level of health of all the peoples." So far, much has been accomplished toward that end.

1950. *The Fifth White House Conference,* with emphasis on children and youth, was called by President Harry S. Truman.

1950. *The Fred Lyman Adair Foundation* of the American Committee on Maternal Welfare was established. Its purpose is to collect funds from charitable sources to underwrite research and educational projects in this field.

1955. The *American College of Nurse-Midwifery* was established as an organization of nurse-midwives to study and evaluate the activities of nurse-midwives, to plan and develop educational programs meeting the requirements of the profession and to perform other related functions. In 1957, the College became a member of the International Confederation of Midwives, a midwifery organization with members from some 30 countries throughout the world.

1957. The *American Association for Maternal and Infant Health* (formerly the American Committee on Maternal Welfare) was activated at the Seventh American Congress held in July. Prompted by the spectacular improvements and advances in maternity care which have taken place since its founding, the Board of Directors of the Committee voted unanimously to change the name, the role and the character of the organization. The new American Association for Maternal and Infant Health provides close integration of the various disciplines which participate in providing modern maternity care, and will serve as a forum for their mutual problems related to maternal and infant health.

1960. The *Sixth White House Conference,* concerned with the nation's children and youth, has been called by President Dwight D. Eisenhower to be held in March, 1960. The theme and focus of this "Golden Anniversary" Conference will be "Opportunities for Children and Youth to Realize Their Full Potential for Creative Life in Freedom and Dignity."

Although there is yet much to be done, encouraging advances have been made over the years. During this seemingly disconnected sequence of activities, from cruelty to a child, care of the sick, keeping the well babies well, mortality studies and then to antepartal care, the aim for well mothers and healthy babies has finally been reached.

Today, in contrast with the past, the general public, including mothers and fathers, through education and publicity, realizes the need for antepartal care. Hospitals have established antepartal clinics with their many clinical facilities. Physicians encourage early antepartal supervision in order to keep the mother well and to prevent complications during the maternity cycle.

The credit for the advancement of antepartal care and child care in the United States cannot be assigned to any individual or any one organization. Our present improved conditions are the results of extended public health educa-

tion, organized efforts through private and public agencies (national, state and local), the intelligent interest and cooperation of public-spirited citizens who gave time and real sums of money, public officials, physicians, nurses, social workers, teachers, dentists and many others who made possible the putting into action of these ideas.

The outgrowth has led to continuous new researches, technics and current statistical studies of mortality and morbidity and means of prevention.

SUGGESTED READING

Bookmiller, Mae, and Bowen, George: Textbook of Obstetrics and Obstetric Nursing, ed. 3, Philadelphia, Saunders, 1958.

Corbin, Hazel: Maternity care today and tomorrow, Am. J. Nursing 53:201, 1953.

Cowan, M. Cordelia: Yearbook of Modern Nursing 1956, New York, Putnam, 1956.

——: Yearbook of Modern Nursing 1957-1958, New York, Putnam, 1958.

Findley, Palmer: Priests of Lucina, Boston, Little, 1939.

Graham, Harvey: Eternal Eve, Garden City, Doubleday, 1951.

Heaton, C. E.: Obstetrics and gynecology in America, North Carolina M. J. 8:35, 1947.

Heaton, Claude: Fifty years of progress in obstetrics and gynecology, New York State J. Med. 51:83, 1951.

Hingson, Robert L., and Hellman, Louis M.: Anesthesia for Obstetrics, Philadelphia, Lippincott, 1956.

Kirkwood, Samuel B.: Twenty years of maternity care, Children 2:133, 1955.

Mack, Harold C.: Back to Sacajawea, Am. J. Obst. & Gynec. 69:933, 1955.

Speert, Harold: Obstetric and Gynecologic Milestones, New York, Macmillan, 1958.

Van Blarcom, Carolyn C.: Obstetrical Nursing (rev. by E. Ziegel), ed. 4, New York, Macmillan, 1957.

Williams, Whitridge: Sketch of the History of Obstetrics in America, New York, 1903. (Reprinted from American Gynecology 5:1903.)

Answer Key for Study Questions

UNIT ONE

1: 3
2: A
3: B
4: A. External conjugate
   B. Diagonal conjugate
   C. Intercristal
   D. Conjugata vera
   E. Intertuberous diameter
5: A. D
   B. D
   C. C
6: C
7: A. 4
   B. 3
   C. 1
   D. 2
8: C
9: B
10: A. 2
    B. 2
    C. 3
11: B
12: C
13: C
14: D
15: 2
16: A
17: A. L.O.T.
    B. L.O.A.
    C. R.O.P.
    D. L.S.P.
    E. R.M.A.
    F. R.A.D.P.

UNIT TWO

1: 2
2: A. 3
   B. 3
3: B
4: B
5: F
6: C

7: C
8: A. 2
   B. 3
9: A. 1
   B. 3
   C. 3
10: A. 3
    B. 1
11: B
12: D
13: A
14: D
15: 1
16: 2
17: D

UNIT THREE

1: A. Full dilatation
   B. Effacement
   C. Amnesic
   D. Uterine atony
   E. Episiotomy
   F. Lightening
2: Situation No. 1: 3
   Situation No. 2: 2
   Situation No. 3: 2
3: A. 2
   B. 3
   C. 2
4: 1
5: 3
6: C
7: B
8: 4
9: 2
10: 1
11: 3
12: A. 3
    B. 2
13: A. 3
    B. 1
    C. 4
    D. 4

UNIT FOUR

1: 3
2: 2
3: 1: G
   2: D
   3: B
   4: C
   5: G
   6: G
   7: D
   8: G
4: 4
5: 2
6: 1
7: 3
8: 1

UNIT FIVE

1: 1
2: 2
3: D
4: E
5: B
6: C
7: C
8: D
9: 2
10: 3
11: 3
12: 2
13: 1
14: 1
15: 2

UNIT SIX

1: 3
2: 2

3: 2
4: 1
5: 3
6: 1

UNIT SEVEN

1: 1
2: 1
3: 3
4: 4
5: 1
6: 2
7: 3
8: 1
9: 2
10: 4
11: 3
12: 3
13: 2
14: 2
15: 3
16: A. Mastitis
    B. Endometritis
    C. Pelvic cellulitis or parametritis
    D. Subinvolution
    E. Engorgement

UNIT EIGHT

1: 2
2: 4
3: 2
4: 4
5: 1
6: 1
7: A
8: 3
9: B
10: 2

Glossary

Note: The pronunciations as indicated in the following paragraph in this Glossary follow Webster's International Dictionary.

āle, châotic, câre, ădd, ăccount, ärm, ȧsk, sofȧ; ēve, hẽre, êvent, ĕnd, silĕnt, makẽr; īce, ĭll, charĭty; ōld, ȯbey, ôrb, ŏdd, sȯft, cŏnnect; fōōd, fŏŏt; out; oil, cūbe, ûnite, ûrn, ŭp, circŭs, menü; chair; go; sing; then, thin; naṭure; verdŭre; k = ch in German ich or ach; bon; yet; zh = z in azure

abdominal (ăb-dŏm′ĭ-năl). Belonging to or relating to the abdomen.

  a. delivery, delivery of the child by abdominal section. See *cesarean section.*

  a. gestation, ectopic pregnancy occurring in the cavity of the abdomen.

  a. pregnancy. See *gestation* above.

ablatio placentae. See *abruptio placentae.*

abortion. The termination of pregnancy at any time before the fetus has attained a stage of viability, i.e., before it is capable of extra-uterine existence.

abruptio placentae (ăb-rŭp′shĭ-ō plȧ-sen′tē). Premature separation of normally implanted placenta.

acromion (ȧ-krō′mĭ-ŏn). An outward extension of the spine of the scapula, used to explain presentation of the fetus.

adnexa (ăd-nĕk′sȧ). Appendages.

  a., uterine (ū′tẽr-ĭn), the fallopian tubes and ovaries.

afibrinogenemia (ȧ-fī″brin-ō-jen-ē′mē-ȧ). Lack of fibrinogen in the blood.

after-birth (ȧf′tẽr-bûrth″). The structures cast off after the expulsion of the fetus, including the membranes and the placenta with the attached umbilical cord; the secundines.

after-pains (ȧf′tẽr-pāns″). Those pains, more or less severe, after expulsion of the after-birth, which result from the contractile efforts of the uterus to return to its normal condition.

agalactia (ăg′ȧ-lăk′shĭ-ȧ). Absence or failure of the secretion of milk.

allantois (ȧ-lăn′tō-ĭs). A tubular diverticulum of the posterior part of the yolk sac of the embryo; it passes into the body stalk through which it is accompanied by the allantoic (umbilical) blood vessels, thus taking part in the formation of the umbilical cord; and later, fusing with the chorion, it helps to form the placenta.

amenorrhea (ȧ-mĕn″ō-rē′ȧ). Absence or suppression of the menstrual discharge.

amnesia (ăm-nē′zhĭ-ȧ). Loss of memory.

amnion (ăm′nĭ-ŏn). The most internal of the fetal membranes, containing the waters which surround the fetus in utero.

amniotic (ăm″nĭ-ŏt′ĭk). Pertaining to the amnion.

  a. sac, the "bag of membranes" containing the fetus before delivery.

analgesia (ăn″ăl-jē′zĭ-ă). Drug which relieves pain, used during labor.

androgen (ăn′drô-jĕn). Any substance which possesses masculinizing activities, such as the testis hormone.

android (ăn′droid). The term adopted for the male type of pelvis.

anencephalus (ăn″ĕn-sĕf′ȧ-lŭs). Form of monstrosity with absence of a brain.

anovular (ăn-ōv′ŭ-lẽr). Not accompanied with the discharge of an ovum; said of cyclic uterine bleeding.

anoxia (an-ox′e-ah). Oxygen deficiency; any condition of absence of tissue oxidation.

antenatal (ăn-tê-nā′tăl). Occurring or formed before birth.

antepartal (ăn″tê-pär′tal). Before labor and delivery or childbirth; prenatal.

areola (ȧ-rē′ō-lȧ). The ring of pigment surrounding the nipple.

  secondary a., a circle of faint color sometimes seen just outside the original areola about the fifth month of pregnancy.

articulation (är-tĭk″ū-lā′shŭn). The fastening together of the various bones of the skeleton in their natural situation; a joint. The articulations of the bones of the body are divided into two principal groups—*synarthroses,* immovable articulations, and *diarthroses,* movable articulations.

Aschheim-Zondek test (ăsh″hĭm-tsŏn′dĕk). A test for the diagnosis of pregnancy. Repeated injections of small quantities of urine voided during the first weeks of pregnancy produce in infantile mice, within 100 hours, (1) minute intrafollicular ovarian hemorrhage and (2) the development of lutein cells.

asphyxia (ăs-fĭk'sĭ-á). Suspended animation; anoxia and carbon dioxide retention resulting from failure of respiration.

   a. neonatorum (nē"ô-ná-tō'rŭm), "asphyxia of the newborn," deficient respiration in newborn babies.

attitude (ăt'ĭ-tūd). A posture or position of the body. In obstetrics, the relation of the fetal members to each other in the uterus; the position of the fetus in the uterus.

axis (ăk'sĭs). 1. A line about which any revolving body turns. 2. **Pelvic a.**, the curved line which passes through the centers of all the anteroposterior diameters of the pelvis.

bag of waters. The membranes which enclose the liquor amnii of the fetus.

ballottement (bă-lŏt'mĕnt). Literally means tossing. A term used in an examination when the fetus can be pushed about in the pregnant uterus.

Bandl's ring (Bän'dls). A groove on the uterus at the upper level of the fully developed lower uterine segment; visible on the abdomen after hard labor as a transverse or slightly slanting depression between the umbilicus and the pubis. Shows overstretching of lower uterine segment. Resembles a full bladder.

Bartholin's glands (Bär'tô-lĭn). Glands situated one on each side of the vaginal canal opening into the groove between the hymen and the labia minora.

bicornate uterus (bī-kôr'năt). Having two horns which, in the embryo, failed to attain complete fusion.

bimanual (bī-măn'ŭ-ăl). Performed with or relating to both hands.

   b. palpation, examination of the pelvic organs of a woman by placing one hand on the abdomen and the fingers of the other in the vagina.

blastoderm (blăs'tô-dûrm). Delicate germinal membrane of the ovum.

   b. vesicle, hollow space within the morula formed by the rearrangement of cells, and by proliferation.

Braxton-Hicks sign. Painless uterine contractions occurring periodically throughout pregnancy, thereby enlarging the uterus to accommodate the growing fetus.

B.-H. version, one of the types of operation designed to turn the baby from an undesirable position to a desirable one.

breech (brēch). Nates or buttocks.

   b. delivery, labor and delivery marked by breech presentations.

bregma (brĕg'má). The point on the surface of the skull at the junction of the coronal and sagittal sutures.

brim (brĭm). The edge of the superior strait or inlet of the pelvis.

caked breast. See *engorgement*.

caput (kă'pŭt). 1. The head, consisting of the cranium, or skull, and the face. 2. Any prominent object, such as the head.

   c. succedaneum (sŭk"sê-dā'nê-ŭm), a dropsical swelling which sometimes appears on the presenting head of the fetus during labor.

catamenia (kăt-á-mē'nĭ-á). See *menses*.

caudal (kô'dăl). The term applied to analgesia or anesthesia resulting from the introduction of the suitable analgesic or anesthetic solution into the caudal canal (nonclosure of the laminae of the last sacral vertebra).

caul (kôl). A portion of the amniotic sac which occasionally envelops the child's face at birth.

cephalhematoma (sĕf"ăl-hē"má-tō'-má). A tumor or swelling between the bone and the periosteum caused by an effusion of blood.

cephalic (sê-făl'ĭk). Belonging to the head.

   c. presentation, presentation of any part of the fetal head in labor.

cervix (sûr'vĭks). Necklike part; the lower and narrow end of the uterus, between the os and the body of the organ.

cesarean section (sê-zâ'rê-ăn). Delivery of the fetus by an incision through the abdominal wall and the wall of the uterus.

Chadwick's sign (tshăd'wĭks). The violet color on the mucous membrane of the vagina just below the urethral orifice, seen after the fourth week of pregnancy.

change of life. See *climacteric*.

chloasma (klô-ăz'mă). Pl. *chloasmata*. A cutaneous affection exhibiting spots and patches of a yellowish-brown color. The term chloasma is a vague one and is applied to various kinds of pigmentary discoloration of the skin.

c. gravidarum, c. uterinum, chloasma occurring during pregnancy.

chorio-epithelioma (kō'rĭ-ō-ĕp-ĭ-thē-lĭ-ō'-mȧ). Chorionic carcinoma; a tumor formed by malignant proliferation of the epithelium of the chorionic villi.

chorion (kō'rĭ-ŏn). The outermost membrane of the growing zygote, or fertilized ovum, which serves as a protective and nutritive covering.

chromosome (kro'mo-sōm). One of several small, dark-staining and more or less rod-shaped bodies which appear in the nucleus of the cell at the time of cell division and particularly in mitosis.

circumcision (sûr"kŭm-sĭzh'ŭn). The removal of all or part of the prepuce, or foreskin of the penis.

cleft palate (klĕft păl'ĭt). Congenital fissure of the palate and the roof of the mouth.

climacteric (klĭ-măk'tĕr-ĭk). A particular epoch of the ordinary term of life at which the body undergoes a considerable change; especially, the menopause or "change of life."

clitoris (klĭ'tȯ-rĭs). A small, elongated, erectile body, situated at the anterior part of the vulva. An organ of the female homologous with the penis of the male.

coitus (kō'ĭt-ŭs). Sexual intercourse; copulation.

colostrum (kȯ-lŏs'trŭm). A substance in the first milk after delivery, giving to it a greenish or yellowish color.

c. corpuscles, large, granular cells found in colostrum.

colporrhaphy (kŏl-pōr'ȧ-fĭ). 1. The operation of suturing the vagina. 2. The operation of denuding and suturing the vaginal wall for the purpose of narrowing the vagina.

colpotomy (kŏl-pŏt'o-mĭ). Any surgical cutting operation upon the vagina.

conception (kŏn-sĕp'shŭn). The impregnation of the female ovum by the spermatozoon of the male, whence results a new being.

condyloma (con-dil-o'mah). Pl. *condylomata.* A wartlike excrescence near the anus or the vulva; the flat, moist papule of secondary syphilis.

confinement (kŏn-fĭn'mĕnt). Term applied to childbirth and the lying-in period.

congenital (kŏn-jĕn'ĭ-tĕl). Born with a person; existing from or from before birth, as, for example, congenital disease, a disease originating in the fetus before birth.

conjugate (kŏn'jŏŏ-gȧt). The anteroposterior diameter of the pelvic inlet.

contraception (kŏn"trȧ-sĕp'shŭn). The prevention of conception or impregnation.

coronal (kŏr'ȯ-nȧl). Belonging to, or relating to, the crown of the head.

c. suture, the suture formed by the union of the frontal bone with the two parietal bones.

corpus luteum (kôr'pŭs lū'tĕ-ŭm). The yellow mass found in the graafian follicle after the ovum has been expelled.

cotyledon (kŏt"ĭ-lē'dŭn). Any one of the subdivisions of the uterine surface of the placenta.

cul-de-sac (kōōl'dē-săk') **of Douglas.** A pouch between the anterior wall of the rectum and the uterus.

cyesis (sī-ē'sĭs). Pregnancy.

decrement (dĕk'rē-mĕnt). Decrease; also the stage of decline.

delivery (dē-lĭv'ēr-ĭ). [French, *délivrer,* to free, to deliver.] 1. The expulsion of a child by the mother, or its extraction by the obstetric practitioner. 2. The removal of a part from the body; as *delivery* of the placenta.

dizygotic (dĭ"zī-gŏt'ĭk). Pertaining to or proceeding from two zygotes (ova).

Döderlein's bacillus (ded'er-līnz). The large gram-positive bacterium occurring in the normal vaginal secretion.

Douglas' cul-de-sac (kōōl'dē-săk'). A sac or recess formed by a fold of the peritoneum dipping down between the rectum and the uterus. Also called *pouch of Douglas* and *recto-uterine pouch.*

ductus (dŭk'tŭs). A duct.

d. arteriosus (är-tē"rĭ-ō'sŭs), "arterial duct," a blood vessel peculiar to the fetus, communicating directly between the pulmonary artery and the aorta.

d. venosus (vē-nō'sŭs), "venous duct," a blood vessel peculiar to the fetus, establishing a direct communication between the umbilical vein and the descending vena cava.

Duncan (dŭng'kȧn) **mechanism.** The position of the placenta, with the maternal surface outermost; to be born edgewise.

dystocia (dĭs-tō'shĭ-ȧ). Difficult, slow or painful birth or delivery. It is distinguished as *maternal* or *fetal* according as the difficulty is due to some deformity on the part of the mother or on the part of the child.

d., placental, difficulty in delivering the placenta.

eclampsia (ĕk-lămp'sĭ-*à*). Acute "toxemia of pregnancy" characterized by convulsions and coma which may occur during pregnancy, labor or the puerperium.

ectoderm (ĕk'tŏ-dûrm). The outer layer of cells of the primitive embryo.

ectopic (ĕk-tŏp'ĭk). Out of place.

e. gestation, gestation in which the fetus is out of its normal place in the cavity of the uterus. It includes gestations in the interstitial portion of the tube, in a rudimentary horn of the uterus (cornual pregnancy) and cervical pregnancy as well as tubal, abdominal and ovarian pregnancies. See also *extra-uterine pregnancy.*

e. pregnancy, same as *ectopic gestation.*

effacement (ĕ-fās'mĕnt). Obliteration. In obstetrics, refers to thinning and shortening of the cervix.

ejaculation (ê-jăk"ŭ-lā'shŭn). A sudden act of expulsion, as of semen.

embryo (ĕm'brĭ-ō). The product of conception in utero from the 3rd through the 5th week of gestation; after that length of time it is called the fetus.

empathy (ĕm'pà-thĭ). The projection of one's own consciousness into that of another. Empathy may be distinguished from sympathy in that the former state includes relative freedom from emotional involvement.

endocervical (ĕn'dŏ-sûr'vĭ-kàl). Pertaining to the interior of the cervix of the uterus.

endometrium (ĕn"dŏ-mē'trĭ-ŭm). The mucous membrane which lines the uterus.

engagement (ĕn-gāj'mĕnt). In obstetrics, applies to the entrance of the presenting part into the superior pelvic strait and the beginning of the descent through the pelvic canal.

engorgement (ĕn-gôrj'mĕnt). Hyperemia; local congestion; excessive fullness of any organ or passage. In obstetrics, refers to an exaggeration of normal venous and lymph stasis of the breasts which occurs in relation to lactation.

entoderm (ĕn'tŏ-dûrm). The innermost layer of cells of the primitive embryo.

enzygotic (ĕn-zĭ-gŏt'ĭk). Developed from the same fertilized ovum.

episiotomy (ĕp"ĭs-ĭ-ot'ŏ-mĭ). Surgical incision of the vulvar orifice for obstetric purposes.

Erb's paralysis. Partial paralysis of the brachial plexus, affecting various muscles of the arm and the chest wall.

ergot (ûr'gŏt). A drug having the remarkable property of exciting powerfully the contractile force of the uterus, and chiefly used for this purpose, but its long-continued use is highly dangerous. Usually given in the fluid extract.

erythroblastosis fetalis (ê-rĭth"rŏ-blăs-tō'sĭs). A severe hemolytic disease of the newborn usually due to Rh incompatibility.

estrogen (ĕs'trŏ-jĕn). A hormone secreted by the ovary and the placenta.

extraperitoneal (ĕks"tră-pĕr-ĭ-tŏ-nē'ăl). Situated or occurring outside the peritoneal cavity.

extra-uterine (ĕks"tră-ū'tĕr-ĭn). Outside of the uterus.

e. pregnancy, pregnancy in which the fetus is contained in some organ outside of the uterus, i.e., tubal, abdominal and ovarian pregnancies.

fallopian (fă-lō'pĭ-ăn). [Relating to G. *Fallopius,* a celebrated Italian anatomist of the sixteenth century.]

f. tubes, the oviducts—two canals extending from the side of the fundus uteri.

fecundation (fē"kŭn-dā'shŭn). The act of impregnating or the state of being impregnated; the fertilization of the ovum by means of the male seminal element.

fertility (fĕr-tĭl'ĭ-tĭ). The ability to produce offspring; power of reproduction.

fertilization (fûr-tĭ-lĭ-zā'shŭn). The fusion of the spermatozoon with the ovum; it marks the beginning of pregnancy.

fetus (fē'tŭs). The baby in utero from the end of the fifth week of gestation until birth.

fimbria (fĭm'brĭ-à). A fringe; especially the fringelike end of the fallopian tube.

fontanel (fŏn"tà-nĕl'). The quadrangular space between the frontal and two parietal bones in very young infants. This is called the *anterior f.* and is the familiar "soft spot" just above a baby's forehead. A small, triangular one (*posterior f.*) is between the occipital and parietal bones.

foramen (fŏ-rā'mĕn). A hole, opening, aperture or orifice—especially one through a bone.

which menstruation ceases; the "change of life."

menorrhagia (mĕn″ŏ-rā'jĭ-á). An abnormally profuse menstrual flow.

menses (mĕn'sēz). [Pl. of Latin *mensis*, month.] The periodic monthly discharge of blood from the uterus; the catamenia.

menstruation (mĕn″strōō-ā'shŭn). The monthly period of the discharge of a red fluid from the uterus; the function of menstruating. It occurs from puberty to the menopause.

mentum (mĕn'tŭm). The chin.

mesoderm (mĕs'ŏ-dûrm). The middle layer of cells derived from the primitive embryo.

metrorrhagia (mē-trŏ-rā'jĭ-á). Abnormal uterine bleeding.

migration (mī-grā'shŭn). In obstetrics refers to the passage of the ovum from the ovary to the uterus.

milia (mĭl'ē-á). Plural of *milium*.

milium (mĭl'ē-ŭm). A small white nodule of the skin, usually caused by clogged sebaceous glands or hair follicles.

milk-leg. See *phlegmasia alba dolens*.

miscarriage (mĭs-kăr'ĭj). Abortion.

molding (mōld'ĭng). The shaping of the baby's head so as to adjust itself to the size and shape of the birth canal.

monozygotic (mŏn″ŏ-zī-gŏ'tĭk). Pertaining to or derived from one zygote.

    m. twins (mŏn″ŏ-zī-gŏ'tĭk). Pertaining to or derived from one zygote.

mons veneris (mŏnz vĕn'ĕ-rĭs). The eminence in the upper and anterior part of the pubes of women.

Montgomery's tubercles (mŭnt-gŭm'ĕr-ĭz). Small, nodular follicles or glands on the areolae around the nipples.

multigravida (mŭl″tĭ-grăv'ĭ-dá). A woman who has been pregnant several times, or many times.

multipara (mŭl-tĭp'á-rá). A woman who has borne several, or many, children.

navel (nāv'ĕl). The umbilicus.

neonatal (nē″ŏ-nā'tăl). Pertaining to the newborn, usually considered the first four weeks of life.

nevus (nē'vŭs). A natural mark or blemish; a mole, a circumscribed deposit of pigmentary matter in the skin present at birth (birthmark).

nidation (nĭ-dā'shŭn). The implantation of the fertilized ovum in the endometrium of the pregnant uterus.

nullipara (nŭ-lĭp'á-rá). A woman who has not borne children.

occipitobregmatic (ŏk-sĭp″ĭt-ŏ-brĕg-măt'-ĭk). Pertaining to the occiput (the back part of the head) and the bregma (junction of the coronal and sagittal sutures).

oligohydramnios (ŏl″ĭ-gŏ-hī-drăm'nĭ-ŏs). Deficiency of amniotic fluid.

omphalic (ŏm-făl'ĭk). Pertaining to the umbilicus.

oocyesis (ō'ŏ-sī-ē'sĭs). Ovarian pregnancy.

ophthalmia neonatorum (ŏf-thăl'mĭ-á). Acute purulent conjunctivitis of the newborn usually due to gonorrheal infection.

os (ŏs). Pl. *ora* (ō'rá). Mouth.

    o. externum (*external os*), the external opening of the canal of the cervix.

    o. internum (*internal os*), internal opening of canal of cervix.

    o. uteri, "mouth of the uterus."

ova. Plural of ovum.

ovary (ō'vá-rĭ). The sexual gland of the female in which the ova are developed. There are two ovaries, one at each side of the pelvis.

ovulation (ō-vŭ-lā'shŭn). The growth and discharge of an unimpregnated ovum, usually coincident with the menstrual period.

ovum (ō'vŭm). 1. An egg, particularly a hen's egg. 2. The female reproductive cell. The human ovum is a round cell about $\frac{1}{120}$ of an inch in diameter, developed in the ovary.

oxytocic (ŏk″sĭ-tō'sĭk). 1. Accelerating parturition. 2. A medicine which accelerates parturition.

oxytocin (ŏk-sĭ-tō-sĭn). One of the two hormones secreted by the posterior pituitary.

palsy (pôl'zĭ). A synonym for paralysis, used in connection with certain special forms.

    Bell's p., peripheral facial paralysis due to lesion of the facial nerve, resulting in characteristic distortion of the face.

    Erb's p., the upper-arm type of brachial birth palsy.

para (pär'ä). The term used to refer to past pregnancies which have produced an infant which has been viable, whether or not the infant is dead or alive at birth.

parametrium (păr-á-mē'trĭ-ŭm). The fibrous subserous coat of the supravaginal portion of the uterus, extending laterally be-

GLOSSARY

tween the layers of the broad ligaments.

parity (păr'ĭ-tĭ). The condition of a woman with respect to her having borne children.

parovarian (pär-ô-vâr'ĭ-ăn). Pertaining to the residual structure in the broad ligament between the ovary and the fallopían tube.

parturient (pär-tū'rĭ-ĕnt). Bringing forth; pertaining to child-bearing. A woman in childbirth.

parturition (pär"tŭ-rĭsh'ŭn). The act or process of giving birth to a child.

patulous (păt'ŭ-lŭs). Spreading somewhat widely apart; open.

pelvimeter (pĕl-vĭm'ĕ-tĕr). An instrument for measuring the diameters and capacity of the pelvis.

pelvimetry (pĕl-vĭm'ê-trĭ). The measurement of the dimensions and capacity of the pelvis.

penis (pē'nĭs). The male organ of copulation.

perineorrhaphy (pĕr"ĭ-nē-ŏr'ȧ-fĭ). Suture of the perineum; the operation for the repair of lacerations of the perineum.

perineotomy (pĕr'ĭ-nē-ŏt'ō-mĭ). A surgical incision through the perineum.

perineum (pĕr"ĭ-nē'ŭm). The area between the vagina and the rectum.

peritoneum (pĕr"ĭ-tô-nē'ŭm). A strong serous membrane investing the inner surface of the abdominal walls and the viscera of the abdomen.

phimosis (fĭ-mō'sĭs). Tightness of the foreskin.

phlegmasia alba dolens (flĕg-mā'zhĭ-ȧ ăl'bȧ (dō'lĕnz). Phlebitis of the femoral vein, occasionally following delivery.

Pitocin (pĭ-tŏ'sĭn). A proprietary solution, the oxytocic principle of the posterior lobe of the pituitary gland.

placenta (plȧ-sĕn'tȧ). The circular, flat, vascular structure in the impregnated uterus forming the principal medium of communication between the mother and the fetus.

    ablatio p. See *abruptio placentae.*

    abruptio p., premature separation of the normally implanted placenta.

    previa p., a placenta which is implanted in the lower uterine segment so that it adjoins or covers the internal os of the cervix.

polygalactia (pŏl"ē-gȧ-lăk'shē-ȧ). Excessive secretion of milk.

polyhydramnios (pŏl"ĭ-hĭ-drăm'nĭ-ŏs). Hy-

dramnios; excess in the amount of the amniotic fluid.

position (pô-zĭsh'ŭn). The situation of the fetus in the pelvis; determined by the relation of some arbitrarily chosen portion of the fetus to the right or the left side of the mother's pelvis.

postnatal (pōst-nā'tȧl). Occurring after birth.

postpartal (pōst-pär'tal). After delivery or childbirth.

preeclampsia (prē-ĕk-lămp'sĭ-ȧ). A disorder encountered during pregnancy or early in the puerperium, characterized by hypertension, edema and albuminuria.

pregnancy (prĕg'năn-sĭ). [Latin, *praegnans,* literally "previous to bringing forth."] The state of being with young or with child. The normal duration of pregnancy in the human female is 280 days, or 10 lunar months, or 9 calendar months.

premature infant. An infant which weighs 2,500 Gm. or less at birth.

prepuce (prē'pūs). The fold of skin which covers the glans penis in the male.

    p. of the clitoris, the fold of mucous membrane which covers the glans clitoridis.

presentation (prē"zĕn-tā'shŭn). Term used to designate that part of the fetus nearest the internal os; or that part which is felt by the physician's examining finger when introduced into the cervix.

primigravida (prĭ"mĭ-grăv'ĭ-dȧ). Pl. *primigravidae* (prĭ"mĭ-grăv'ĭ-dē). A woman who is pregnant for the first time.

primipara (prĭ-mĭp'ȧ-rȧ). Pl. *primiparae* (prĭ-mĭp'ȧ-rē). A woman who has given birth to her first child.

primordial (prĭ-môr'dĭ-ăl). Original or primitive; of the simplest and most undeveloped character.

prodromal (prŏ-drŏ'măl). Premonitory; indicating the approach of a disease.

progesterone (prŏ-jĕs'tĕr-ōn). The pure hormone contained in the corpora lutea whose function is to prepare the endometrium for the reception and development of the fertilized ovum.

prolactin (prŏ-lăk'tĭn). A proteohormone from the anterior pituitary which stimulates lactation in the mammary glands.

prolan (prŏ'lăn). Zondek's term for the gonadotropic principle of human-pregnancy urine, responsible for the biologic pregnancy tests.

promontory (prŏm'ŭn-tō"rĭ). A small projection; a prominence.

p. of the sacrum, the superior or projecting portion of the sacrum when in situ in the pelvis, at the junction of the sacrum and the last lumbar vertebra.

pseudocyesis (sū"dō-sī-ē'sĭs). An apparent condition of pregnancy; the woman really believes she is pregnant when, as a matter of fact, she is not.

puberty (pū'bĕr-tĭ). The age at which the generative organs become functionally active.

pubic (pū'bĭk). Belonging to the pubis.

pubiotomy (pū'bĭ-ŏt'ō-mĭ). The operation of cutting through the pubic bone lateral to the median line.

pubis (pū'bĭs). The os pubis or pubic bone forming the front of the pelvis.

pudendal (pū-dĕn'dăl). Relating to the pudenda.

pudendum (pū-dĕn'dŭm). [Latin, *pude're,* to have shame or modesty.] The external genital parts of either sex, but especially of the female.

puerperium (pū"ĕr-pē'rĭ-ŭm). The period elapsing between the termination of labor and the return of the uterus to its normal condition, about six weeks.

quickening (kwĭk'ĕn-ĭng). The mother's first perception of the movements of the fetus.

rabbit test. See *Friedman test.*

Rh. Abbreviation for *Rhesus,* a type of monkey. This term is used for a property of human blood cells, because of its relationship to a similar property in the blood cells of *Rhesus* monkeys.

Rh factor. A term applied to an inherited antigen in the human blood.

Ritgen maneuver (rĭt'gĕn). Delivery of the infant's head by lifting the head upward and forward through the vulva, between contractions, by pressing with the tips of the fingers upon the perineum behind the anus.

Schultze's mechanism (shōōlt'sĕz). The expulsion of the placenta with the fetal surfaces presenting.

secundines (sĕk'ŭn-dīn). The afterbirth; the placenta and membranes expelled after the birth of a child.

segmentation (sĕg"mĕn-tā'shŭn). The process of division by which the fertilized ovum multiplies before differentiation into layers occurs.

semen (sē'mĕn). 1. A seed. 2. The fluid secreted by the male reproductive organs.

show (shō). 1. Popularly, the blood-tinged mucus discharged from the vagina before or during labor.

Skene's gland. Two glands just within the meatus of the female urethra; regarded as homologues of the prostate gland in the male.

smegma. A thick cheesy secretion found under the prepuce and in the region of the clitoris and the labia minora.

souffle (sōōf'f'l). A soft, blowing, auscultatory sound

funic s., a hissing souffle synchronous with the fetal heart sounds and supposed to be produced in the umbilical cord.

placental s., a souffle supposed to be produced by the blood current in the placenta.

spermatozoon (spûr"mă-tō-zō'ŏn). Pl. *spermatozoa* (spûr"mă-tō-zō'ă). The motile, microscopic sexual element of the male, resembling in shape an elongated tadpole. The male reproductive cell.

stillborn (stĭl'bôrn"). Born without life; born dead.

stria (strī'ă). Pl. *striae* (strī'ē). A Latin word signifying a "groove," "furrow" or "crease."

s. gravidarum (grăv-ĭ-där'ŭm), shining, reddish lines upon the abdomen, thighs and breasts during pregnancy.

subinvolution (sŭb'ĭn-vŏ-lū'shŭn). Failure of a part to return to its normal size and condition after enlargement from functional activity, as subinvolution of the uterus which exists when normal involution of the puerperal uterus is retarded.

succedaneum (sŭk'sĕ-dā'nĕ-ŭm). See *caput.*

superfecundation (sū'pĕr-fĕ-kŭn-dā'shŭn). The fertilization at about the same time of two different ova by sperm from different males.

superfetation (sū'pĕr-fĕ-tā'shŭn). The fecundation of a woman already pregnant.

symphysis (sĭm'fĭ-sĭs). The union of bones by means of an intervening substance; a variety of synarthrosis.

s. pubis (pū'bĭs), "symphysis of the pubis," the pubic articulation or union of the pubic bones which are connected with each other by interarticular cartilage.

synchondrosis (sĭng″kŏn-drō′sĭs). A union of bones by means of a fibrous or elastic cartilage.

testicle (tĕs′tĭ-k′l). One of the two glands contained in the male scrotum.

thrush. An infection caused by the fungus *Candida albicans* characterized by whitish plaques in the mouth.

tonguetie. See *lingua frenum*.

toxemia (tŏks-ē′mĭ-á). The toxemias of pregnancy are disorders encountered during gestation, or early in the puerperium, which are characterized by one or more of the following signs: hypertension, edema, albuminuria, and in severe cases, convulsions and coma.

trichomonas (trĭk-ŏm′ŏ-năs). A genus of parasitic flagellate protozoa.

   t. vaginalis, a species sometimes found in the vagina, especially when the secretion is acid.

trophectoderm (trŏf-ĕk′tŏ-dûrm). The outer layer of cells of the early blastodermic vesicle; it develops the trophoderm—the feeding layer.

umbilical (ŭm-bĭl′ĭ-kăl). Pertaining to the umbilicus.

   u. arteries, the arteries which accompany and form part of the umbilical cord.

   u. cord [Latin, *funis umbilicalis*], the cord connecting the placenta with the umbilicus of the fetus, and at the close of gestation principally made up of the two umbilical arteries and the umbilical vein, encased in a mass of gelatinous tissue called "Wharton's jelly."

   u. hernia, hernia at or near the umbilicus.

   u. vein, forms a part of the umbilical cord.

uterus (ū′tēr-ŭs). The hollow muscular organ in the female designed for the lodgement and nourishment of the fetus during its development until birth.

vagina (vá-jī′ná). [Latin, a sheath.] The canal in the female, extending from the vulva to the cervix of the uterus.

vernix caseosa (vûr′nĭks kā″sĕ-ō′sá). "Cheesy varnish." The layer of fatty matter which covers the skin of the fetus.

version (vûr′shŭn). The act of turning; specifically, a turning of the fetus in the uterus so as to change the presenting part and bring it into more favorable position for delivery.

vertex (vûr′tĕks). The summit or top of anything. In anatomy, the top or crown of the head.

   v. presentation, presentation of the vertex of the fetus in labor.

vestibule (vĕs′tĭ-būl). A triangular space between the labia minora; the urinary meatus and the vagina open into it.

viable (vī′á-b′l). A term in medical jurisprudence signifying "able or likely to live"; applied to the condition of the child at birth.

villus (vĭl′ŭs). A small vascular process or protrusion growing on a mucous surface, such as the chorionic villi seen in tufts on the chorion of the early embryo.

vulva (vŭl′vá). The external genitals of the female.

Wharton's jelly (hwôr′tŭnz). [Thomas *Wharton*, English anatomist, died 1673.] The jellylike mucous tissue composing the bulk of the umbilical cord.

witches' milk (wĭch′ĕz). A milky fluid secreted from the breast of the newly born.

womb (wōōm). See *uterus*.

zona pellucida (zō′ná pĕll-ū′sĭd-ä). A transparent belt; translucent or shining through.

zygote (zī′gŏt). A cell resulting from the fusion of two gametes.

CONVERSION TABLE FOR WEIGHTS OF NEWBORN

(Gram equivalents for pounds and ounces)

For example, to find weight in pounds and ounces of baby weighing 3315 grams, glance down columns to figure nearest 3315 = 3317. Refer to number at top of column for pounds and number to far left for ounces = 7 pounds, 5 ounces.

Pounds→ Ounces↓	3	4	5	6	7	8	9	10
0	1361	1814	2268	2722	3175	3629	4082	4536
1	1389	1843	2296	2750	3203	3657	4111	4564
2	1417	1871	2325	2778	3232	3685	4139	4593
3	1446	1899	2353	2807	3260	3714	4167	4621
4	1474	1928	2381	2835	3289	3742	4196	4649
5	1503	1956	2410	2863	3317	3770	4224	4678
6	1531	1984	2438	2892	3345	3799	4252	4706
7	1559	2013	2466	2920	3374	3827	4281	4734
8	1588	2041	2495	2948	3402	3856	4309	4763
9	1616	2070	2523	2977	3430	3884	4338	4791
10	1644	2098	2551	3005	3459	3912	4366	4819
11	1673	2126	2580	3033	3487	3941	4394	4848
12	1701	2155	2608	3062	3515	3969	4423	4876
13	1729	2183	2637	3090	3544	3997	4451	4904
14	1758	2211	2665	3118	3572	4026	4479	4933
15	1786	2240	2693	3147	3600	4054	4508	4961

OR, to convert grams into pounds and *decimals* of a pound, multiply weight in grams by .0022. Thus, 3317 × .0022 = 7.2974, i.e., 7.3 pounds, or 7 pounds, 5 ounces.

To convert pounds and ounces into grams, multiply the pounds by 453.6 and the ounces by 28.4 and add the two products. Thus, to convert 7 pounds, 5 ounces, 7 × 453.6 = 3175; 5 × 28.4 = 142; 3175 + 142 = 3317 grams.

Index

547

AID FOR VISUALIZATION

1 cm.

2 cm.

3 cm.

6 cm.

8 cm.